Handbook of Research on Advanced Techniques in Diagnostic Imaging and Biomedical Applications

Themis P. Exarchos
University of Ioannina, Greece

Athanasios Papadopoulos
University of Ioannina, Greece

Dimitrios I. Fotiadis
University of Ioannina, Greece

Medical Information Science
REFERENCE

MEDICAL INFORMATION SCIENCE REFERENCE

Hershey · New York

Director of Editorial Content:	Kristin Klinger
Senior Managing Editor:	Jamie Snavely
Managing Editor:	Jeff Ash
Assistant Managing Editor:	Carole Coulson
Typesetter:	Kim Barger
Cover Design:	Lisa Tosheff
Printed at:	Yurchak Printing Inc.

Published in the United States of America by
Information Science Reference (an imprint of IGI Global)
701 E. Chocolate Avenue, Suite 200
Hershey PA 17033
Tel: 717-533-8845
Fax: 717-533-8661
E-mail: cust@igi-global.com
Web site: http://www.igi-global.com/reference

and in the United Kingdom by
Information Science Reference (an imprint of IGI Global)
3 Henrietta Street
Covent Garden
London WC2E 8LU
Tel: 44 20 7240 0856
Fax: 44 20 7379 0609
Web site: http://www.eurospanbookstore.com

Library of Congress Cataloging-in-Publication Data

Handbook of research on advanced techniques in diagnostic imaging and biomedical applications / Themis P. Exarchos, Athanasios Papadopoulos, and Dimitrios I. Fotiadis, editors.

p. ; cm.

Includes bibliographical references and index.

Summary: "This book includes state-of-the-art methodologies that introduce biomedical imaging in decision support systems and their applications in clinical practice"--Provided by publisher.

ISBN 978-1-60566-314-2 (hardcover)

1. Imaging systems in medicine--Data processing--Handbooks, manuals, etc. 2. Diagnostic imaging--Digital techniques--Handbooks, manuals, etc. I. Exarchos, Themis P., 1980- II. Papadopoulos, Athanasios, 1971- III. Fotiadis, Dimitrios Ioannou.

[DNLM: 1. Diagnostic Imaging--methods--Handbooks, manuals, etc. 2. Diagnostic Imaging--trends. 3. Image Processing, Computer-Assisted--methods. WN 180 H2365 2009]
R857.O6H367 2009
616.07'54--dc22

2008050005

British Cataloguing in Publication Data
A Cataloguing in Publication record for this book is available from the British Library.

Editorial Advisory Board

List of Contributors

Table of Contents

Detailed Table of Contents

Recent advances in computer science provide the intelligent computation tools needed to design and develop Diagnosis Support Systems (DSSs) that promise to increase the efficiency of physicians during their clinical practice. This chapter provides a brief overview of the use of computational intelligence methods in the design and development of DSSs aimed at the differential diagnosis of hepatic lesions from Computed Tomography (CT) images. Furthermore, examples of DSSs developed by our research team for supporting the diagnosis of focal liver lesions from non-enhanced CT images are presented.

Indicative features of an fMRI data set can be evaluated by methods provided by theory of random matrices (RMT). RMT considers ensembles of matrices and yields statements on the properties of the typical Eigen systems in these ensembles. The authors have studied the particular ensemble of random correlation matrices that can be used as a noise model for the empirical data and that allows us thus to select data features that significantly differ from the noisy background. In this sense RMT can be understood as offering a systematic approach to surrogate data. Interestingly, also the noise characteristics change between different experimental conditions. This is revealed by higher-order statistics available from RMT. The authors illustrate the RMT-based approach by an exemplary data set for the distinction between a visuomotor task and a resting condition. In addition it is shown for these data that the degree of sparseness and of localization can be evaluated in a strict way, provided that the data are sufficiently well described by the pairwise cross-correlations.

Diffusion Magnetic Resonance Imaging (diffusion MRI) can provide important information about tissue microstructure by probing the diffusion of water molecules in a biological tissue. Although originally proposed for the characterization of cerebral white matter connectivity and pathologies, its implementation has extended to many other areas of the human body. In a parallel development, a number of diffusion

The objective of this chapter is to propose a quantitative hysteroscopy imaging analysis system in gynaecological cancer and to provide the current situation about endoscopy imaging. Recently works, involves endoscopy, gastroendoscopy, and colonoscopy imaging with encouraging results. All the methods are using image processing using texture and classification algorithms supporting the physician diagnosis. But none of the studies were involved with the pre-processing module. Also, the above studies are trying to identify tumours in the organs and no of the are investigates the tissue texture. The system supports a standardized image acquisition protocol that eliminates significant statistical feature differences due to viewing variations. In particular, the authors provide a standardized protocol that provides texture features that are statistically invariant to variations to sensor differences (color correction), angle and distance to the tissue. Also, a Computer Aided Diagnostic (CAD) module that supports the classification of normal vs abnormal tissue of early diagnosis in gynaecological cancer of the endometrium is discussed. The authors investigate texture feature variability for the aforementioned targets encountered in clinical endoscopy before and after color correction. For texture feature analysis, three different features sets were considered: (i) Statistical Features, (ii) Spatial Gray Level Dependence Matrices, and (iii) Gray Level Difference Statistics. Two classification algorithms, the Probabilistic Neural Network and the Support Vector Machine, were applied for the early diagnosis of gynaecological cancer of the endometrium based on the above texture features. Results indicate that there is no significant difference in texture features between the panoramic and close up views and between different camera angles. The gamma correction provided an acquired image that was a significantly better approximation to the original tissue image color. Based on the texture features, the classification algorithms results show that the correct classification score, %CC=79 was achieved using the SVM algorithm in the YCrCb color system with the combination of the SF and GLDS texture feature sets. This study provides a standardized quantitative image analysis protocol for endoscopy imaging. Also the proposed CAD system gave very satisfactory and promising results. Concluding, the proposed system can assist the physician in the diagnosis of difficult cases of gynaecological cancer, before the histopathological examination.

Patient anatomy, biochemical response, as well functional evaluation at organ level, are all key fields that produce a significant amount of multi modal information during medical diagnosis. Visualization, processing and storage of the acquired data sets are essential tasks in everyday medical practice. In order to perform complex processing that involves or relies on image data a robust as well versatile data structure was used as extension of the Visualization Toolkit (VTK). The proposed structure serves as a universal registration container for acquired information and post processed resulted data. The structure is a dynamic multidimensional data holder to host several modalities and/or Meta data like fused image sets, extracted features (volumetric, surfaces, edges) providing a universal coordinate system used for calculations and geometric processes. A case study of Treatment Planning System (TPS) in the stereotactic radiotherapy (RT) based on the proposed structure is discussed as an efficient medical application.]

The aim of this chapter is to analyze the recent advances in image processing and machine learning techniques with respect to facial expression recognition. A comprehensive review of recently proposed methods is provided along with an analysis of the advantages and the shortcomings of existing systems. Moreover, an example for the automatic identification of basic emotions is presented: Active Shape Models are used to identify prominent features of the face; Gabor filters are used to represent facial geometry at selected locations of fiducial points and Artificial Neural Networks are used for the classification into the basic emotions (anger, surprise, fear, happiness, sadness, disgust, neutral); and finally, the future trends towards automatic facial expression recognition are described.

The authors of this chapter present an overview on recent developments in the field of clinical applications of the functional infrared imaging. The functional infrared imaging is a relatively recent imaging methodology introduced for the study for biomedical purposes of the functional properties and alterations of the human thermoregulatory system. The methodology is based on the modeling of the bio-heat exchange processes and the recording of thermal infrared data by means of advanced technology. Some innovative applications of functional infrared imaging to diagnostics, psychometrics, stress measurements and psycho-neurophysiology will be presented, with special emphasis to the potentialities and the capabilities that such technique may bring to biomedical investigations.

The completion of the Human Genome Project and the emergence of high-throughput technologies at the dawn of the new millennium, are rapidly changing the way we approach biological problems. DNA microarrays represent a promising new technological development, widely used for the investigation and identification of genes associated with important biological processes. The chapter is divided in two parts: the first discusses current methods for the acquisition and quantitation of the microarray image while the second focuses in the analysis and interpretation of the microarray signals (standardization, normalization, statistical analysis etc.)

Microarray technology allows the comprehensive measurement of the expression level of many genes simultaneously on a common substrate. Typical applications of microarrays include the quantification

Wavelet-, Fourier-, and spatial domain-based texture classification methods have been used successfully for classifying zoom-endoscopic colon images according to the pit pattern classification scheme. Regarding the wavelet-based methods, statistical features based on the wavelet coefficients as well as structural features based on the wavelet packet decomposition structures of the images have been used. In the case of the Fourier-based method, statistical features based on the Fourier-coefficients in ring filter domains are computed. In the spatial domain, histogram-based techniques are used. After reviewing the various methods employed we start by extracting the feature vectors for the methods from one color channel only. To enhance the classification results the methods are then extended to utilize multichannel features obtained from all three color channels of the respective color model used. Finally, these methods are combined into one multiclassifier to stabilize classification results across the image classes.

In this chapter the state of the art is presented in the domain of automatic identification and classification of bodies on the basis of their deformed images obtained via microscope. The approach is illustrated by means of the case of automatic recognition of third-stage larvae from microscopic images of them in high deformation instances. The introduced methodology incorporates elements of elasticity theory, image processing, curve fitting and clustering methods; a concise presentation of the state of the art in these fields is given. Combining proper elements of these disciplines, the authors first evaluate the undeformed shape of a parasite given a digital image of a random parasite deformation instance. It is demonstrated that different orientations and deformations of the same parasite give rise to practically the same undeformed shape when the methodology is applied to the corresponding images, thus confirming the consistency of the approach. Next, a pattern recognition method is introduced to classify the unwrapped parasites into four families, with a high success rate. In addition, the methodology presented here is a powerful tool for the exact evaluation of the mechano-elastic properties of bodies from images of their deformation instances.

Elastography or elasticity imaging can be defined as the science and methodology of estimating the mechanical properties of a medium (including soft tissue). In this chapter, an overview of elastography and its relation to tissue pathology will be presented. The basic principles of the static and dynamic methods will be described with special emphasis on the dynamic methods that rely on the acoustic radiation force of ultrasound. Of interest are the low-frequency narrowband shear waves that can be generated by a modulated radiation force produced by the interference of two continuous-wave (CW) ultrasound beams of slightly different frequencies. The advantages of using narrowband shear waves to estimate the viscoelastic properties of tissue will be discussed. Furthermore, an implementation of the inverse-problem approach will be presented and it will be shown how harmonic maps of the local shear modulus and viscosity can be reconstructed based on both the fundamental and higher-harmonic components of the propagated narrowband shear waves.

The aim of this chapter is to provide an overview about models and methodologies used for the Dynamic Contrast Enhancement (DCE) analysis. DCE is a non-invasive methodology aimed to diagnostic the nature of a lesion on the base of the perfusion's dynamic of specific contrast agents. The idea at the base of DCE is that, in several pathological tissues, including tumors and inflammatory diseases, the angiogenic process is abnormal, hence the characterization of vascularisation structure may be used to support the diagnosis. In this chapter, the authors will describe the basic DCE procedures and introduce some of its most innovative evolution based on the pharmacokinetic analysis technique (PK), and the empirical model (EM). Even if DCE is still a medical research topic, there is large interest for this type of approach in biomedical applications as witnessed by the availability of specific tools in the last generation top-class US, CT, and MR machines.

The accurate estimation of point correspondences is often required in a wide variety of medical image processing applications including image registration. Numerous point correspondence methods have been proposed, each exhibiting its own characteristics, strengths, and weaknesses. This chapter presents a comparative study of four automatic point correspondence methods. The four featured methods are the Automatic Extraction of Corresponding Points approach, the Trimmed Iterated Closest Points scheme, the Correspondence by Sensitivity to Movement technique and the Self-Organizing Maps network.

All methods are presented, mainly focusing on their distinct characteristics. An extensive set of dental images, subject to unknown transformations, was employed for the qualitative and quantitative evaluation of the four methods, which was performed in terms of registration accuracy. After assessing all methods, it was deduced that the Self-Organizing Maps approach outperformed in most cases the other three methods in comparison.

Various approaches have been taken to detect anomalies, with certain particularities in the medical image scenario, linked to other terms: content-based image retrieval, pattern recognition, classification, segmentation, outlier detection, image mining, as well as computer-assisted diagnosis, and computer-aided surgery. This chapter presents, a review of anomaly detection (AD) techniques and assessment methodologies, which have been applied to medical images, emphasizing their peculiarities, limitations and future perspectives. Moreover, a contribution to the field of AD in brain computed tomography images is also given, illustrated and assessed.

The authors present in this chapter an overview on evaluation of medical image compression. The different methodologies used in the literature are presented. Subjective evaluation uses some a priori knowledge such as the judgment of experts or the ability to realize a correct diagnosis. Objective evaluation generally takes into account the value of metrics: the PSNR is an example of such a criterion. The goal of hybrid evaluation is to realize a reliable judgment while having a simple computation. The authors discuss on the benefits and drawbacks of these approaches. The European Project called OTELO in which they were involved, gives feedback on ultrasound image compression.

Medical images are often characterized by high complexity and consist of high resolution image files, introducing thus several issues regarding their handling. Current compression schemes produce high compression rates, sacrificing however the image quality and leading this way to unenviable examination. Region of Interest (ROI) coding has been introduced as an efficient technique for addressing such

Preface

Diagnostic imaging in biomedicine is based on several techniques and processes aiming at the enhancement of experts' capability to evaluate imaging data. Diagnostic imaging combines image processing and decision support methods to improve and accelerate case-specific advice in clinical environments.

Decision support today focuses on diagnosis, prognosis, therapy and follow-up recommendations and is usually based on simple and easily acquired features met in biomedical data. The latest breakthroughs in imaging technologies in medicine lead to an explosion of the imaging data available. New techniques and methods addressing mainly acquisition and processing of information from medical and biological images appeared and the integration of biomedical image data into decision support systems is a challenging task. This mainly supports the decision on the patient's health status and the quality of the extracted diagnosis and prognosis.

Despite the wide application of decision support systems in medicine, only a few such systems have been developed for biomedical imaging. One of the reasons is the difficulty in representing anatomical or functional units of the images in formal features. Dealing with this uncertain and imprecise information increases the complexity of decision support systems. Furthermore, each imaging modality and each type of pathology requires the development of dedicated low-level feature extractors. Although, standard computer-vision techniques may be used (template matching, region growing, etc.), specific methodologies and algorithmic approaches need to be developed. These difficulties, combined with the computational cost associated with biomedical imaging applications, have prevented, so far, the development of fully automated image guided decision support systems. By producing a formal and structured representation of the images, imaging decision support systems enable new applications such as the automated generation of anatomical and functional atlases or the content-driven image retrieval. The abundance of information derived from cross-sectional imaging modalities, such as computed tomography (CT), magnetic resonance imaging (MRI), single photon emission computerized tomography (SPECT), positron emission tomography (PET), or conventional planar imaging technologies such as digital X-ray, and ultrasound highlights the need for the design and the development of decision support systems based mainly on multiple imaging data. Such tools improve diagnostic accuracy and overall reproducibility by providing a second opinion and objective measurements of normal and abnormal patterns.

This handbook features the most current research findings in all aspects of biomedical imaging, diagnostic and decision support methodologies, from theoretical and algorithmic problems to successfully designed and developed biomedical image guided decision support systems. The handbook is intended for all those working in the field of medical image analysis and information technologies in biomedicine. It provides different approaches and levels of knowledge for experienced researchers, graduate students, computer engineers, and medical practitioners interested in emerging intelligent diagnostic tools and systems. The handbook serves as the basis for understanding the future of decision support technologies and services based on biomedical imaging, exemplifying the impact of knowledge extraction on clinical environments.

The objective of this Handbook is to present state of the art in the field and present advances which:

- Bridge the gap between medical and biological imaging with clinical decision support systems.
- Integrate biomedical images in the most efficient way in existing decision support systems.
- Present a unified framework for image analysis in medical and biological applications.
- Enhance the readers' capability in designing decision support systems which employ biomedical images.

This book is divided into three sections. The first introduces the readers to some advanced image-based decision support applications. This part addresses the utilization of existing methodologies and techniques to several clinical areas with increased needs for computer-aided assistance. An overview of computational methods and tools applied in decision support systems is presented. Integration of imaging data as well as new approaches on cardiac, intracoronary and cardiac MRI data are analyzed extensively. In addition, clinical decision support systems for the interpretation of hepatic lesions, oncology samples and breast imaging are presented, along with a quantitative analysis of hysteroscopy imaging in gynecological cancer. The second section of the book presents novel methodologies in the field of biomedical imaging. 3D quantitative radionuclide dosimetry and combination of geometry and image data appear to have great interest in the area of radiation therapy. Diffusion tensor imaging, infrared imaging as well as DNA microarray analysis are new issues. Research studies based on the mechano-elastic properties of matter and elastographic applications are also presented. In the third section, methodological approaches of image processing and their medical applications are presented.

Themis P. Exarchos
Athanasios Papadopoulos
Dimitrios I. Fotiadis
University of Ioannina, Greece
August 2008

About the Editors

Dr. **Themis P. Exarchos** was born in Ioannina, Greece in 1980. He received the diploma degree in computer engineering and informatics from the Engineering School of the University of Patras in 2003. He received a PhD degree from the University of Ioannina in 2009; his PhD thesis is entitled *Data Mining and Healthcare Decision Support System*. He is a member of the Unit of Medical Technology and Intelligent Information Systems at the University of Ioannina, working in research and technology development projects. His research interests include data mining, decision support systems in healthcare, biomedical applications including biomedical imaging and bioinformatics. Dr. Exarchos is the author of more than fifty papers in scientific journals and conference proceedings.

Dr. **Athanassios Papadopoulos** received his degree in physics from the department of physics of the University of Patras, Greece in 1994. He completed his MSc in medical physics at University of Surrey, U.K. He received his Ph.D from the Department of Medical Physics from University of Ioannina, Greece in 2006. He is serving as a radiation physicist in the Department of Nuclear medicine of University Hospital of Ioannina, Greece. He is a member of the research group of the "Foundation for Research and Technology-Hellas / Biomedical Research Institute" and the Unit of Medical Technology and Intelligent Information Systems. His major research interests include medical image processing, medical decision support, computer-aided detection and diagnosis, machine learning and data mining. Lately his work is related to the use of vital signs of the human body, their analysis and use of intelligent methods for diagnosis or prognosis. Dr. Papadopoulos is the author of two book chapters and more than twenty papers in scientific journals and international conference proceedings.

Dimitrios I. Fotiadis is the director of the Unit of Medical Technology and Intelligent Information Systems, department of materials science and engineering and an associated member of Biomedical Research Institute. He holds diploma in chemical engineering from the National Technical University of Athens (1985) and a PhD in chemical engineering and materials science from the University of Minnesota, Minneapolis, USA (1990). He served as visiting researcher at the RWTH, Aachen, Germany and the Massachusetts Institute of Technology, Boston, USA. He has published more than 120 papers in scientific journals, 250 papers in peer-reviewed conference proceedings, more than 20 chapters in books and he is the editor of 14 books. His work has received more than 800 citations. His research interests include modelling of human tissues and organs, intelligent wearable devices for automated diagnosis and bioinformatics. He is the chairman of the board and CEO of the Science and Technology Park of Epirus, National Representative of Greece in FP7 and he coordinates several R&D projects funded by the EC and other bodies.

Chapter I
Computational Methods and Tools for Decision Support in Biomedicine:
An Overview of Algorithmic Challenges

Ioannis N. Dimou
Technical University of Crete, Greece

Michalis E. Zervakis
Technical University of Crete, Greece

David Lowe
University of Aston, UK

Manolis Tsiknakis
Foundation of Research and Technology Hellas, Heraklion Crete, Greece

ABSTRACT

The automation of diagnostic tools and the increasing availability of extensive medical datasets in the last decade have triggered the development of new analytical methodologies in the context of biomedical informatics. The aim is always to explore a problem's feature space, extract useful information and support clinicians in their time, volume, and accuracy demanding decision making tasks. From simple summarizing statistics to state-of-the-art pattern analysis algorithms, the underlying principles that drive most medical problems show trends that can be identified and taken into account to improve the usefulness of computerized medicine to the field-clinicians and ultimately to the patient. This chapter presents a thorough review of this field and highlights the achievements and shortcomings of each family of methods. The authors' effort has been focused on methodological issues as to generalize useful conclusions based on the large number of notable, yet case-specific developments presented in the field.

INTRODUCTION

Contemporary and future methods of healthcare delivery will be exploiting new technology, novel sensing devices and a plethora of modes of information generated by distributed data sources. This raw data is inevitably increasing in volume and complexity at a rate faster than the ability of primary healthcare providers to access and understand it. Several countries are currently considering issues of integrated personalised healthcare and the application of 'intelligent' data mining methodologies in providing medical decision support to the clinician (and the individual), using principled pattern recognition methodologies.

Within such an environment, the domain of medical imaging, with its various structural (CT, MRI, U/S) and functional (PET, fMRI) modalities, is probably on the top of the list with respect to the amount of raw data generated. Most of these modalities are explored in other chapters of this volume. Even though image inspection by human experts enables the accurate localization of anatomic structures and/or temporal events, their systematic evaluation requires the algorithmic extraction of certain characteristic features that encode the anatomic or functional properties under scrutiny. Such imaging features, treated as markers of a disease, can subsequently be integrated with other clinical, biological and genomic markers, thus enabling more effective diagnostic, prognostic and therapeutic actions. It is the purpose of this chapter to address issues related to the decision making process, to trace developments in infrastructure and techniques, as well as to explore new frontiers in this area.

The Medical Informatics Revolution

During the last decades we are witnessing a gradual shift in the medical field. Medical professionals are increasingly being supported by advanced sensing equipment. These instruments provide objective information and assist in reducing the margin of error in diagnosis and prognosis of diseases. Detailed imaging techniques provide accurate anatomic and/or functional maps of the human body, and advanced signal processing methods performing biosignal and biochemical analyses are now largely automated, faster and increasingly accurate. In the broader medical research field, larger datasets of patients including multiple covariates are becoming available for analysis.

Figure 1 outlines the information flow in a medical decision support system. At an initial stage, a large amount of data is collected from various sensors and pre-processed. This data is accessibly stored in a structured format and fused with other information, such as expert knowledge. At a higher level, patterns are sought in the full dataset and translated in an intelligent way to produce meaningful and helpful reasoning. This output supports healthcare professionals during their prognostic, diagnostic and other decision making tasks. At the end of this process, feedback to the system in the form of expert evaluation or validity of analysis can be incorporated to improve performance.

This relative data abundance has resulted in a corresponding explosion of scientific papers referring to thorough statistical analysis with data mining and pattern classification techniques. New findings are more easily made available to the scientific community through the internet and cheap processing power aids the development of complex models of diseases, drugs, and effects.

In this context the field of medical informatics emerges as the intersection of information technology with the different disciplines of medicine and health care. It deals with the resources, devices, and methods required to optimize the acquisition, storage, retrieval, analysis and use of information in health and biomedicine (VanBemmel & Musen, 1997). Medical informatics tools include not only computers but also clinical guidelines, formal medical terminologies, and information, communication and decision support systems. It

Figure 1. Medical informatics decision support system dataflow

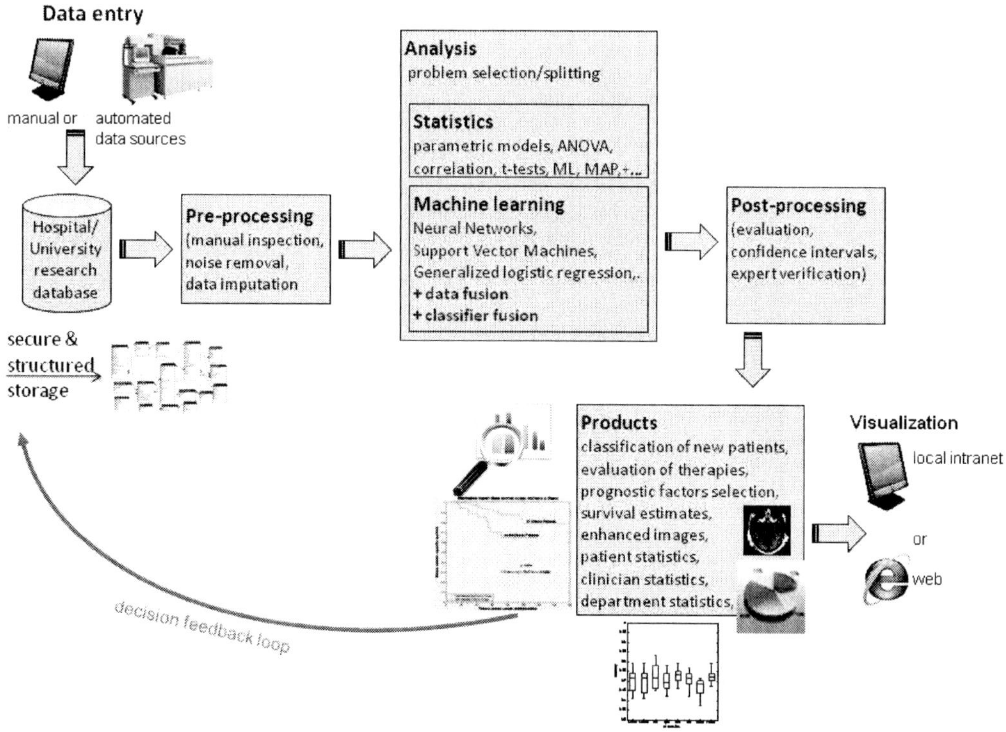

is by now evident that medical informatics do not just provide information but also summarize it in an intelligent and comprehensive form.

Current State in Medical Informatics

According to the latest statistics, an increasing number of health care institutions are initiating the shift to informatics both for internal use and for patient accessibility. Funding for Healthcare Information Technologies (HIT) is at an all time high reaching in some countries 3.5% of their healthcare budget (Steele, 2002). In most cases, such efforts are not standardized within countries and the expectations are much lower at a global scale. Although initially driven by requirements to support logistics, billing, and patient administration, today's healthcare information systems face a growing interest for higher level applications such as diagnostic decision support and treatment evaluation.

Serious efforts have been made in the last five years in creating standards for a patient's Electronic Health Record (EHR) (Katehakis, Tsiknakis, & Orphanoudakis, 2002) to facilitate data exchange not only between hospitals, labs and clinicians, but also between institutions and countries. The task of structuring an individual's medical status and history in a common format has been undertaken by a number of vendors. There are three main organizations creating standards related to EHR: HL7, CEN TC 215 and ASTM E31. HL7 operating in the United States, develops the most widely used health care-related electronic data exchange standards in North America (HL7 RIM, Clinical Document Architecture, CDA), while CEN TC 215 operating in 19 European member states, is the pre-eminent healthcare information technology standards developing organization in Europe. Both HL7 and CEN collaborate with the ASTM that operates in the United States and is mainly used by commercial laboratory vendors. ASTM's Continuity of Care Record (CCR) standard has recently been criticised for being too focused on patient file transfer in contrast to CDA's adaptability to emerging future needs and applications (Ferranti, Musser, Kawamoto, & Hammond, 2006). In the medical imaging field DICOM is the most widely used standard (Bidgood, & Horii, 19970). A broader framework termed *integrating healthcare enterprises* (IHE, www.ihe.com) is an initiative by healthcare professionals and industry to improve the way computer systems in healthcare share information. IHE promotes the coordinated use of established standards such as DICOM and HL7 to address specific clinical need in support of optimal patient care. Systems developed in accordance with IHE communicate with one another better, are easier to implement, and enable care providers to use information more effectively.

The combination of EHR standards with the upward trend in funding for HIT creates good prospects in the field. However a decisive factor in the expansion of such technologies in the applied domain is their acceptance by the healthcare personnel. There is some scepticism regarding the extensive use of computerized tools for decision support. Starting from individual data safety to reliability of automated systems, to proper training and acceptance, the attitude of clinicians is often positive only in institutions focused on research.

A Diversity of Applications

Within such a context and mentality, a number of key application areas can be identified in which automated data processing is already or can be effectively applied. Disease diagnosis is probably the most important application of informatics in medical decision making. It involves the evaluation of criteria that can discriminate between different pathologies. Prognosis of the onset of pathology is also among the leading applications of pattern recognition tools in medicine (Bates, 2002). Its utility ranges from preemptive advice to statistical analysis of risk for insurance companies. At subsequent stages, following a patient's initial diagnosis, treatment evaluation is a key issue, which involves monitoring of disease progress and correlation of observed results with the treatment plan; the objective being to quantify the effect of the chosen treatment on the pathology.

From a similar perspective, modelling of patient survival utilizes ideas from statistical risk and survival analysis and censoring models to estimate the probability of a health event (i.e. relapse, death) –due to a specific disease– of a patient at a specific time (Taktak, Fisher, & Damato, 2004). It is also used for patient grouping and allocation to specialized reference centres. Moreover the statistical results from the survivability analysis are used to optimize follow-up monitoring of patients in a personalized manner.

At a lower level, electronic health records (EHR) are gradually becoming a reality providing near real-time data access, and thus dramatically expanding the clinician's opportunities for timely response. Although not an application in itself, these clinical information systems and the related standards elevate the functionality of upper layers of decision support systems by providing a unified structured and meaningful representation of multimodal and diverse data.

From a broader epidemiological standpoint, automated data processing has made possible the large scale analysis of populations with the objective of identifying disease traits and epidemiological patterns that were previously beyond the reach of a single researcher.

All the above applications share common analytic aspects but at the same time pose a number of difficulties for the biomedical engineers, as they indicate a transition from disease management to personalized treatment (Cimino,

& Shortliffe, 2006). Can we put together rational structures for the way clinical evidence is pooled, communicated, and applied to routine care? What tools and methods need to be developed to help achieve these aims in a manner that is practicable, testable, and in keeping with the fundamental goal of healthcare - the relief from disease? In the following sections we present a perspective on the current state-of-the-art in automated data analysis and decision support.

BACKGROUND

Need for Intelligent Knowledge Extraction Tools

Advanced biosensing methods and technologies have resulted in an explosion of information and knowledge about diseases and their treatment. As a result, our ability to characterize, understand and cope with the various forms of diseases is growing. At the same time, errors in U.S. hospitals cause from 44,000 to 98,000 deaths per year, putting medical errors, even at the more conservative estimate, above the eighth leading causes of death (Steele, 2002).

It seems that difficulties and failures of medical decision-making in everyday practice are largely failures in *knowledge coupling*, due to the over-reliance on the unaided human mind to recall and organize all the relevant details (Hsinchun, Fuller, Friedman, & Hersh, 2005). They are not, specifically and essentially, failures to reason logically with the medical knowledge once it is presented completely and in a highly organized form within the framework of the patient's total and unique situation. If we are to reduce errors and provide quality of care, we must transform the current healthcare enterprise to one in which caregivers exercise their unique human capacities within supportive information systems that compensate for their inevitable human limitations.

Therefore, tools to extend the capacity of the unaided mind are required to couple the details of knowledge about a problem with the relevant knowledge from combined, evidenced and validated clinical and genomic data repositories.

Underlying Technologies

In this direction there are a number of technologies that serve as foundations upon which the upper layer services can be built. At the data collection level, most researchers and clinicians face the need for common protocols to standardise and assist data collection, allow online incorporation of new cases and comparison of results over diverse population sets. Much like the EHR eases the transfer of health records, common data collection standards (Potamias, & Moustakis, 2001) are needed to facilitate interoperability of not only patient data but also analysis and presentation tools at levels ranging from institutional to international level.

The emerging GRID (Huang, Lanza, Rajasekaran, & Dubitzky, 2005) technologies are of great utility in the wide application field of collecting, storing, processing, and presenting the medical data in a way transparent to the end user. Utilizing bandwidth, computational power and other resources optimally, the GRID promises a cost effective solution to the unification of the medical informatics landscape. Although presently limited to research purposes, its use is undoubtedly going to extend the limits of artificial intelligence in medicine.

Moving to a more abstract (re)presentation layer, the development of medical and genomic ontologies and their alignment is a requirement for storing and handling huge datasets in a structured and logically founded way. A lot of research effort has been devoted recently towards this direction primarily in connection to DNA analysis (Alonso-Calvo, & Maojo, 2007), as explained in the last section.

Specific Challenges

The breadth and depth of information already available in both medical and genomic research communities, present an enormous opportunity for improving our ability to study disease-mechanisms, reduce mortality, improve therapies and meet the demanding individualization of care needs. The inability to *share* both data and technologies developed by MI and BI research communities and by different vendors and scientific groups, is therefore severely hampering the discovery process (Martin-Sanchez et al., 2004).

Among the challenges that characterize medical data pattern analysis one can identify data missingness as a key concept (Perez, Dennis, Gil, Rondon, & Lopez, 2002). *Missing data* occur due to a number of reasons: inconsistent data entry, poor protocol design, death censoring, inadequate personnel familiarization with the system and inconsistent sensing equipment between collection centres. The patterns of missing data depend on the specific causes of this effect. The optimal way to handle this is in turn based upon the pattern and the covariance of the effect with other model factors. As discussed in a related review paper (Burton, & Altman, 2004), most often in published clinical research this phenomenon is handled inadequately. Cases or covariates with missing data are discarded or imputed in naïve ways resulting in added bias to the statistical findings. Safe imputation of medical datasets is realistically achievable up to certain missingness ratios. Above these thresholds the affected covariates have to be discarded. In particular, Expectation Maximization (EM) imputation, data augmentation and multiple imputation are considered effective and statistically sound methods to compensate for this problem.

Apart from incomplete data, *noise* is also a crucial factor in medical informatics data. The human body has itself largely varying characteristics. Sensing equipment also introduce an additional noise component (Bruce, 2001). On top of that, examiners assess the raw information in a subjective way depending on the context, their experience and other factors. The final quantifiable and electronically storable result is far from an ideal measurement. Taking this into account, any biomedical pattern recognition system has to be robust with respect to noise. Common practice dictates that the noise component should be removed as early as possible in the processing sequence. As an additional measure, cross validation of research results can be used in the post-processing phase to minimize output variance.

Closely related to the reliability of the input information is the concept of *uncertainty quantification*. Researchers observe very strong uncertainties in data, models, and expert opinions relating to clinical information (Ghosh, 2004). Being able to quantify this factor in every step of the computational process makes it possible to infer bounds on the final decision support outcome. This is far from theoretical. The real world decisions that a healthcare professional has to make require that the information used is as concise as possible. Confidence intervals are already used in commercial imaging diagnostic support software packages. More advanced techniques as Bayesian Belief networks and Dempster-Schafer theory of evidence are still under research.

Finally, a usually overlooked part of any medical problem is that the outcome usually affects human lives. In practice this makes the *misclassification cost largely asymmetric* (Freitas, Costa-Pereira, & Brazdil, 2007). A false negative patient diagnosis costs far more than a false positive one (usually not even measurable in medical expenses). Yet, in most clinical classification research papers, cost functions are assumed symmetric as a default for simplicity reasons. Another important problem is that the *models' assumptions* are not always analysed in detail. It is common practice to assume Gaussian distributions or equal class priors due to their mathematical tractability, although they are not applicable to all contexts.

Biomedical datasets usually consist of features of *different modalities*. Data types can range from CT images, to EEGs, to blood tests, to microarray data or experts' opinions (Acharya, Wasserman, Stevens, & Hinojosa, 1995). All have different dimensionalities and dynamic ranges and require different pre-processing, data mapping and feature extraction and representation methods.

The data is often collected through large scale multicenter studies. The participating centres are usually *distributed* geographically and have to submit new samples online. This creates the need for on-site data reduction in order to be able to transmit and store high volumes of patient data. A pattern classifier should be scalable or modular or be able to run in an automated way before the data has to be transmitted to a core facility.

In such a distributed setting a number of security topics become very important. In our case the term security is considered to be information systems security, which covers all aspects of data or information protection. The measures applied to protect information systems include:

- **Authentication & Authorisation:** Ensuring that the distributed data or other resources are accessible only to those people who are authorised to do so.
- **Confidentiality:** The data produced or handled is not exposed to unauthorised persons.
- **Accountability:** The ability to create an Audit Trail, to observe and chronologically log all actions undertaken by users (patient history data entry, treatment logging, etc).
- **Non-repudiation:** Strongly related to accountability is non-repudiation, which involves preventing an individual or entity from denying having performed a particular action related to data (records tampering, lowering security level, releasing).
- **Privacy:** Since much work to be carried out deals with clinical data concerning patients' private information, it should be assured that privacy is well protected. For example: In many cases researchers are able to complete their work without knowing the identity of the patients concerned in their study. This can be accomplished through de-identification and pseudonymisation (Taira, Bui, H. Kangarloo, Taira, Bui, & E. Kangarloo, 2002).

The latter topic, patients' privacy, has a great impact on current research efforts due to the nature of post-genomic data and the existing legislation concerning this type of information. Data protection measures need to comply with laws and ethical guidelines, while reassuring patients about the proper protection of their sensitive information. Conversely, data protection measures must not be so restrictive that they inhibit the work of researchers.

Answering the above needs will evidently enhance the scope and results of medical informatics as a practical healthcare tool.

METHODS FOR PROCESSING MEDICAL DATA

Having established some of the main challenges to be addressed by the biomedical informatics research community, we will in the following section present the available methods for processing multilevel medical data.

Functional Taxonomies

Medical data dimensionalities can be high, 1-D time series, 2-D images, 3-D body scans, 4-D spatio-temporal sequences. How this data is processed depends on the eventual functionality required to be reached by the technological tools. The first high level division of techniques depends upon whether or not one is aware of the type or class of ailment, or whether one is more concerned with a generic investigation of health state.

If the problem cannot be posed in a way that one can ascribe an explicit target value of a prognostic or medical indicator, then we are dealing with an *unsupervised* problem. For instance, in dealing with the visualization of a population of thousands of people based on features extracted from ECG waveforms, specific ailments might be irrelevant and we are more interested in how the population is dispersed as a distribution. This would be the visualization problem of unsupervised density estimation. Using such an unconditional distribution would be useful at the individualized level for detecting whether an individual should be considered somehow anomalous, or an outlier of the population. Such information could then be used as a warning signal for further investigation of that individual. Figure 2 depicts a functional hierarchy of unsupervised processing tasks, along with exemplar algorithms that implement these functional tasks.

In feature extraction, most techniques are focused either in decomposing the biomedical data into components (ICA, PCA) so that the noise and the signal may be more easily discriminated, or in transforming data into another more appropriate representation (Projection Pursuit, PCA), or simply in data reduction without reducing the relevant signal content. *Clustering* relies on the existence of similarity or dissimilarity measures for separating cases that exhibit a pathology from the general population, taking into account prior knowledge (Bathula, Papademetris, & Duncan, 2007) and cause-effect relationships. Some fuzzy classification techniques can additionally account for multiple concurrent pathological causes.

A common such application is the use of ICA for feature extraction from modalities such as electroencephalograms (EEGs) and functional magnetic resonance imaging (fMRI) signals. As an example, (Moosmann, Eichele, Nordby, Hugdahl, & Calhoun, 2008) present such an application with extensions to synchronous visualization and data fusion. The two signal sources first undergo preprocessing to including correction of head motion related image offsets, temporal filtering and appropriate masking to deal with eye, pulse and magnetic susceptibility artifacts. Independent components are then estimated, back-reconstructed, averaged across data-sets and compared to the original sources

Figure 2. Functional separation of unsupervised tasks.

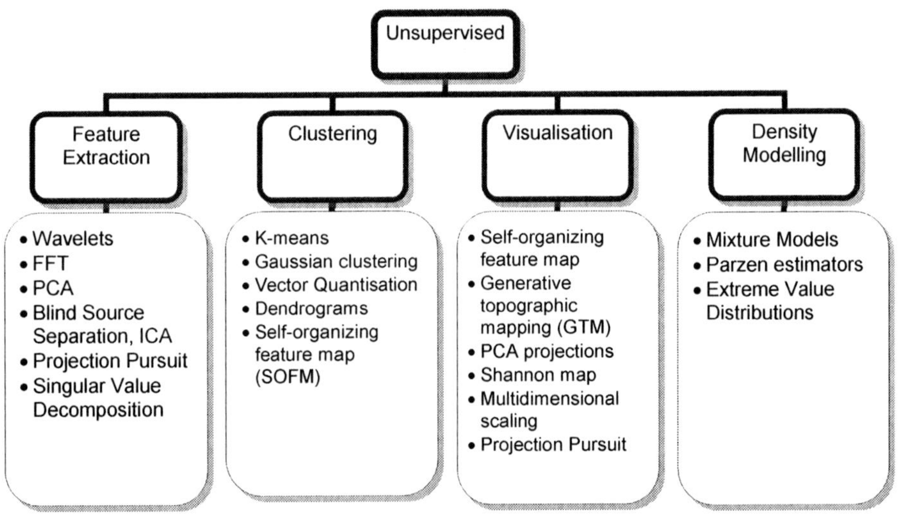

with linear regression. This 2-stage process creates both robust feature representations and classification outcomes.

Visualization of high dimensional biomedical data is an important and under-researched area. It is a difficult task since the projection of high-dimensional data onto low dimensional spaces in which data can be visualized requires compromises that necessarily distort the data. Amongst the more common visualization methods are projections onto dominant principal component spaces, the self-organising feature map (SOFM), the Generative Topographic Map, and a group of methods which explicitly exploit *relative dissimilarity* between feature vectors rather than their absolute distances (Serocka, 2007). Another important application of unsupervised methods is related to *density modelling*. This is an explicit attempt to describe the probabilistic structure of medical data in situations that we do not have gold standard target data vectors. In this domain, one is usually interested in describing the unconditional probability distribution of patient's characteristics without knowledge of explicit disease characteristics or states.

If on the other hand one focuses on a specific class of ailment (e.g. benign or malignant cancer), then we are concerned with a *supervised* problem. Supervised problems are exemplified by classification and prediction problems where one is able to collect data involving *ground truth target vectors* for patients with known established outcomes. In supervised approaches labelled data is used as a source for constructing generic models which can then be applied to individuals from a population in which these target labels are not yet known. Many approaches in supervised biomedical tasks come under the categories of *prediction and classification*. Because we have access to a dataset of labelled patient data, parametric or nonparametric models can be constructed in attempting to reproduce the generator of the labelled data without reproducing the noise itself. The basic difference between classification and prediction tasks is in the nature of the target variable; in classification tasks one is concerned with the estimation of a binary vector, whereas in generic prediction the target is typically a continuously varying quantity, such as life expectancy. In this view, supervised classification extends to *function approximation*. Data modelling aims to provide some form of regularization or smoothing to allow noise and outliers to be eliminated. Figure 3 depicts this functional taxonomy of supervised tasks along

Figure 3. Functional separation of supervised tasks, with algorithm examples.

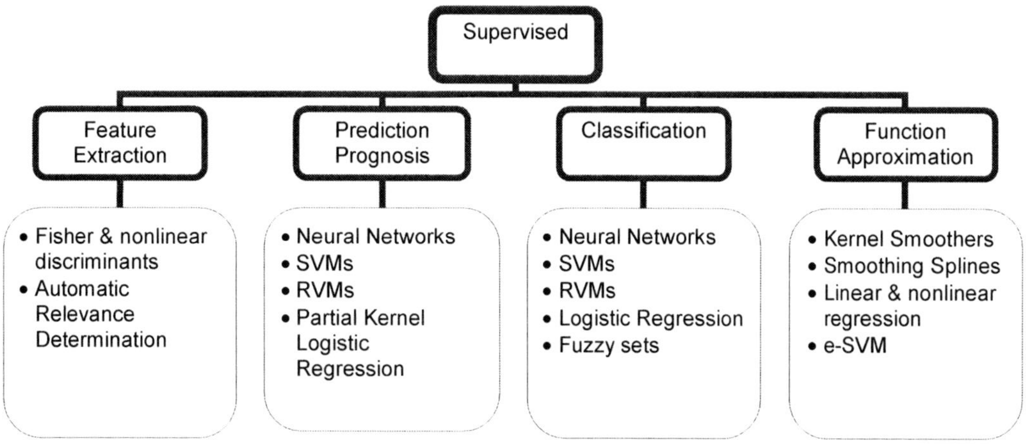

with examples of common algorithms used in each area.

As an illustrative example we can briefly describe the case of classification of SPECT images of Alzheimer's disease patients (Fung, & Stoeckel, 2007). In this medical imaging classification problem certain preprocessing has to be applied in order to remove noise, amplify edges, centre the region of interest and perform spatial and space normalization before the actual classification mechanism is applied. A support vector machine was trained to identify regions using spatial information. The SVM was primarily used for feature selection by choosing subregions in which cerebral activity deviates highly from a set of baseline images (pre-labeled dataset). Figure 4 shows the extracted rectangular regions of voxels overlaid on the respective SPECT image.

Model Selection and Evaluation Techniques

Model selection and assessment are crucial common aspects that cut across the supervised/unsupervised boundary and relate to evaluation strategies of algorithmic approaches. In biomedical data processing it is essential to construct low bias models that are robust to fluctuations (in data and model parameters) for stability. Overtraining of adaptive models, or over-parameterization of parameterized models are two examples of situations to be avoided, in particular in biomedical data processing. Methods for model assessment involve issues linked to the bias-variance dilemma and regularization, either explicitly through the cost functions being used or implicitly through restricting the model class. However, more and more in the intermediate levels of biomedical data processing, the use of single models is being replaced by methods of averaging. This is motivated from the Bayesian perspective of marginalization rather than selection. By averaging over model predictions or over models trained on different data samples drawn from the same distribution, it is possible to compensate for weak or overtrained models. Common methods of averaging include Bootstrap, Boosting, Bagging, Stacking, Bayesian averaging and approximate methods based on sampling, such as Markov chain Monte Carlo methods.

Many novel and promising models are presented and evaluated in the published literature in a way that leaves doubt regarding the variance, reproducibility and reliability of the results (Mur-

Figure 4. Rectangular regions picked by the algorithm overlaid on a SPECT image of an Alzheimer's disease patient.

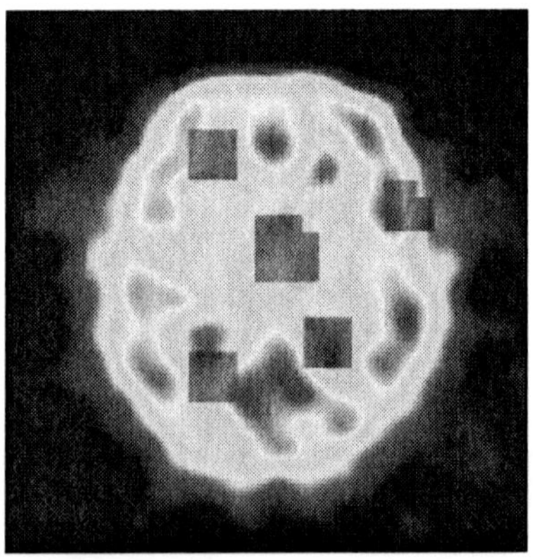

phy, 2004). Showing high accuracies on a specific dataset instance is not important unless supported by analysis that verifies statistical robustness. A large amount of research work and debate has been devoted to the choice of performance metrics (Eberhart, & Dobbins, 1990). Optimistically, diagnostic or prognostic models should aim to produce the class-conditional probabilities for combinations of disease occurrence and feature or test presence. Assessment and evaluation needs to also reflect the full tradeoffs between selecting prognostic classes depending upon a threshold, such as the Receiver Operating Characteristic (ROC) curve (Lasko, Bhagwat, Zou, & Ohno-Machado, 2005). Alternatives to the misclassification probabilities are the *predictive values*, which quantify the clinical relevance of the test and involve the reverse conditioning of probabilities. Another description of the prognostic value of a test (or model) is in terms of positive and negative *Likelihood ratios* (McGee, 2002). These are specifically relevant since they quantify the increase in knowledge about a disease gained through the output of a diagnostic model.

Apart from the above performance metrics, the medical informatics community faces the need to standardize measures for clustering, visualization, model comparisons and optimization. Such common metrics that should be considered involve scoring metrics (Wilcoxon and Kruskal-Wallis statistics), prediction error variance, entropy measures, mutual information, Kullback-Leibler divergence and dissimilarity metrics, such as Standardised Residual Sum of Squares (STRESS).

Data and Decision Fusion

In pattern analysis it is known that there is no single best algorithm for a specific dataset. Classifier ensembles have in recent years produced promising results, improving accuracy, confidence and most importantly improved feature space coverage in many practical applications. In biomedical problems the combination of multiple classifiers has been effectively applied for diagnosis, gene selection and patient grouping (Dimou, Manikis, & Zervakis, 2006). The driving principle behind this type of approach is that a combination of elementary classifiers can map a feature space effectively, provided that the outcomes are interpreted and combined in a statistically appropriate way. Classifier fusion methods are described and reviewed in (Ruta & Gabrys, 2000). A common pitfall in using ensembles is that the base classifiers' outcomes are in many cases not interpretable as probabilities. This limits the choice of the available combiners if the objective is to provide statistical bounds on the fused output. Therefore, researchers should pay attention to the assumptions of each fusion method. The low ratio of positive to negative cases in clinical datasets poses an additional problem for both individual classifiers and combiners. Adjusting for prior class distributions is an efficient way to handle this asymmetry.

Data fusion will also play an important part of clinical decision support, mainly in imaging related applications. Combining the various types of available information into a single decision boundary is important if all available information is to be utilized (Barillot, Lemoine, Le Briquer, Lachmann, & Gibaud. 2003). In achieving this goal the relative weight of each datasource and contextual information need to be accounted for.

FUTURE TRENDS

Medical Data Integration

The nature and amount of information now available opens directions of research that were once in the realm of science fiction. Pharmacogenomics (Roses, 2002), diagnostics (Sotiriou, & Piccart, 2007) and drug target identification are just a few of the many areas that have the potential to use this information to dramatically change the scientific landscape in the life sciences.

During this information revolution, the data gathering capabilities have greatly surpassed the data analysis techniques. If we were to imagine the Holy Grail of life sciences, we might envisage a technology that would allow us to fully understand the data at the speed at which it is collected. Sequencing, localization of new genes, functional assignment, pathway elucidation, and understanding the regulatory mechanisms of the cell and organism should be seamless. In a sense, knowledge manipulation is now reaching its pre-industrial age. The explosive growth in the number of new and powerful technologies within proteomics and functional genomics (Celis, 2003) can now produce massive amounts of data. However, data interpretation and subsequent knowledge discovery require explicit and time consuming involvement of human experts. The ultimate goal is to automate this knowledge discovery process.

The process of heterogeneous database integration may be defined as "*the creation of a single, uniform query interface to data that are collected and stored in multiple, heterogeneous databases.*" Several varieties of heterogeneous database integration are useful in biomedicine. The most important ones are:

- *Vertical integration.* The aggregation of semantically similar data from multiple heterogeneous sources. For example, a virtual repository that provides homogeneous access to clinical data that are stored and managed in databases across a regional health information network (Martín, Bonsma, Anguita, Vrijnsen, García-Remesal, Crespo et al., 2007).
- *Horizontal integration.* The composition of semantically complementary data from multiple heterogeneous sources. For example, a system that supports complex queries across genomic, proteomic, and clinical information sources for molecular biologists.

From the theoretical point of view, there exist three types of database integration methods (Sujansky, 2001), namely 1) Information Linkage (IL), 2) Data Transformation (DT) and 3) Query Translation (QT). While IL uses cross references to establish proper links among the data sources, DT creates a centralized repository with a unified schema representing the integration (e.g. Data Warehouses). Conversely, QT focuses the transformation effort in the query and the retrieved results—i.e. a query formulated for the integration is divided into a set of sub-queries, appropriate for the underlying databases. After these queries are launched, retrieved results are integrated and presented to the user in a unified manner. IL is used by a variety of online sources, such as MEDLINE, GENBANK, OMIM, Prosite, etc. DT has been widely used in industrial solutions. However, given the disparate and evolving nature of data in the biomedical domain, the existing privacy issues and the significant size of the databases, QT approaches are more appropriate for mediation solutions in the field.

Approaches to Solve Syntactic and Semantic Heterogeneities among Biomedical Databases

Ironically, huge gains in efficiency in the "front end" of the discovery pipeline have created huge "down stream" inefficiencies because the data cannot be accessed, integrated, and analyzed quickly enough to meet the demands of drug R&D. The industry has outgrown traditional proprietary data capture and integration methods solve only part of the problem. First generation integration solutions that centred on the concept of local repositories have not scaled well, are costly to maintain, and ultimately are limited in long-term usefulness.

To achieve the aforementioned objectives and goals a new breed of techniques, systems and software tools are required for two main reasons:(a) to convert the enormous amount of data collected by geneticists and molecular biologists into information that physicians and other health-care providers can use for the delivery of care and the converse, and (b) to codify and anonymize clinical phenotypic data for analysis by researchers.

Towards the goal of seamless information and data integration (for sharing, exchanging and processing of the relevant information and data items) the need for uniform information and data representation models is raised. The Resource Description Framework (RDF) and XML technology offers the most suitable infrastructure framework towards seamless information/data integration. Based on an appropriate RDF Query Language the generated XML documents can be parsed in order to: (i) homogenize their content (according to the adopted data-models and ontologies); and (ii) apply dynamic querying operations in order to generate sets of data on which intelligent data processing operation could be uniformly applied.

Syntactically homogeneous access to distributed data sources is typically provided by way of wrappers (Thiran, Hainaut, & Houben, 2005; Hernandez, & Kambhampati, 2004). One of the main challenges in building wrappers is the variation in the query functionality of the underlying data sources. Data sources may not only use different data models and support syntactically different query mechanisms, but the query capabilities can differ as well. This makes it difficult to support a common query language, an essential step towards syntactic homogeneity. There are two extreme approaches. A highly expressive common query language can be chosen. This, however, makes it difficult to implement wrappers for sources with primitive query capabilities. On the other hand, if a very basic common query language is chosen, significant and unnecessary performance penalties are introduced as the capabilities of the underlying data sources are not effectively used.

As neither approach is ideal, an intermediate solution is proposed in (Martín, Bonsma, Anguita, Vrijnsen, García-Remesal, Crespo et al., 2007). A powerful common query language is chosen, but wrappers may choose to only support a subset of the queries, based on the capabilities of the underlying data source. Each wrapper describes the queries it supports using the Relational Query Description Language (RQDL) developed for this purpose. An RQDL specification consists of a set of query templates that represent parameterized queries that are supported. Benefits of this approach are that wrappers can provide and expose exactly the query functionality that corresponds to that of the underlying data source. A drawback is the increased complexity associated with interpreting and reasoning about the query capabilities of each source. It is generally recognized that writing wrappers requires significant programming effort, and as a result research efforts have been devoted to automating parts of this (Thiran, Hainaut, & Houben, 2005).

The largest barrier to heterogeneous database integration is the variety with which similar data are represented in different databases, i.e., semantic or representational heterogeneity. It is appropriate to consider several types of representational heterogeneity that schema integration techniques must resolve. The most general type of heterogeneity is related to the data models themselves. Aggregating data from relational, hierarchical, object-oriented, and flat file databases into a single representation is the first step in schema integration. However, even if all database systems were to use the relational model, significant semantic heterogeneity would remain. Semantic differences occur when the meanings of table names, field names and data values across local databases are similar but not precisely equivalent.

Semantic interoperability, as an important practical problem, has been tackled from many different angles (Martín, Bonsma, Anguita, Vrijnsen, García-Remesal, Crespo et al., 2007). Methods to achieve semantic interoperability largely fall into the following three categories: model alignment, using semantic tags or metadata, and developing shared conceptual references or ontologies. The first approach, model alignment, creates mappings among models to support their semantic interoperability (Klein, 2001). The second method is to use semantic tags or metadata, such as the Dublin Core Metadata Initiative. The third approach, which is also the ideal solution to semantic interoperability, is to develop core ontology or a shared conceptual reference model to serve as the common ground for all systems.

CONCLUSION

In this chapter we have identified common algorithmic aspects in biomedical data processing by reference to a more generic taxonomy of approaches to pattern recognition. In biomedical data analysis, whether the task is time series or image analysis, microarray processing or histology analysis, there are common themes that emerge, such as the desire to reduce noise, reduce dimension, transform to more suitable representations for subsequent interpretation, extract similarities, and exploit dissimilarities.

In many areas there have been significant advances in international research, notably in the areas of neural networks, optimisation and image analysis, and Bayesian approaches to inference. However, several bottlenecks can be identified. Among them is the development of methods that have been genuinely devised to support medical decision making. To this end, tools and techniques that engage clinicians to all stages from data acquisition, to processing, validation and interpretation of results should be largely encouraged.

Biomedical data is notoriously unreliable, noisy, distributed and incomplete. Many tools and methods, however, assume data integrity. There are a proportionally insufficient number of methods which explicitly deal with uncertainty, both in the inputs and the outputs. Only a few methods exist that present predictions along with uncertainties in those predictions.

Developments in other areas, such as complexity, communications and information theory probably have a great deal to offer to biomedical data processing, as algorithmic requirements cross the discipline boundaries. What we have presented in this report is merely a summary of current common aspects reflecting future promise along with an indication that much more research is required in effectively dealing with the pattern processing waterfall. Advances are required in areas such as (a) biomedical ontologies, (b) ontology based integration of heterogeneous biomedical data, and (c) service oriented computational frameworks capitalizing on modern technologies (i.e. Grid) enabling the fast and efficient processing of biomedical data.

ACKNOWLEDGMENT

Research supported by EU: BIOPATTERN (FP6-2002-IST 508803), INFOBIOMED (IST-507585).

REFERENCES

Acharya, R., Wasserman, R., Stevens, J., & Hinojosa, C. (1995). Biomedical imaging modalities: a tutorial. *Computerized Medical Imaging and Graphics, 19*(1), 3-25.

Alonso-Calvo, R., & Maojo, V. (2007). An Agent and Ontology-based System for integrating Public Genomic Databases. *J Biomed Inform., 40*(1), 17-29.

Barillot, C., Lemoine, D., Le Briquer, L., Lachmann, F., & Gibaud B. (1993). Data fusion in medical imaging: merging multimodal and multipatient images, identification of structures and 3D display aspects. *European Journal of Radiology, 17*(1), June, 22-27.

Bates, D. W. (2002). The quality case for information technology in healthcare. *Medical Informatics and Decision Making*, 2(7).

Bathula, D. R., Papademetris, X., & Duncan, J. S. (2007). Level set based clustering for analysis of functional MRI data. *4th IEEE International Symposium on Biomedical Imaging: From Nano to Macro*, (pp. 416-419).

Bidgood W. D., & Horii, S. C. (1997). Understanding and Using DICOM, the Data Interchange Standard for Biomedical Imaging. *Journal of the American Medical Informatics Association, 4*, 199-212.

Bruce, E. N. (2001). *Biomedical Signal Processing and Signal Modelling*, Wiley-Interscience, New York, NY, (pp. 13-18).

Burton A., & Altman D.G. (2004). Missing covariate data within cancer prognostic studies: a review of current reporting and proposed guidelines. *British Journal of Cancer*, *91*, 4–8.

Celis, J. E. (2003). Integrating Proteomic and Functional Genomic Technologies in Discovery-driven Translational Breast Cancer Research. *Molecular & Cellular Proteomics*; *2*, 369-77.

Cimino, J. J., & Shortliffe E. H. (2006). Biomedical Informatics: Computer Applications in Health Care and Biomedicine. *Health Informatics*, *3*, 120-134

Dimou, I., Manikis, G., & Zervakis, M. (2006). Classifier Fusion approaches for diagnostic cancer models, *Proceedings of the 28th IEEE, EMBS Annual International Conference*, New York City, USA, Aug 30-Sept 3, (pp. 5334-5337).

Eberhart, R. C., & Dobbins, R. W. (1990). Neural network performance metrics for biomedical applications, *Proceedings of Third Annual IEEE Symposium on Computer-Based Medical Systems*, (pp. 282-289).

Ferranti, J. M., Musser, R. C., Kawamoto, K., & Hammond, W. E. (2006). The clinical document architecture and the continuity of care record: a critical analysis. *J Am Med Inform Assoc.*, *13*(3), 245-52.

Freitas, A., Costa-Pereira, A., & Brazdil, P. (2007). Cost-sensitive decision trees applied to medical data. *In Lecture Notes in Computer Science (including subseries Lecture Notes in Artificial Intelligence and Lecture Notes in Bioinformatics). 4654 LNCS,* 303-312.

Fung, G., & Stoeckel, J. (2007). SVM feature selection for classification of SPECT images of Alzheimer's disease using spatial information. *Knowledge and Information Systems*, *11*(2), 243–258.

Ghosh, A. K. (2004). On the challenges of using evidence-based information: The role of clinical uncertainty. *Journal of Laboratory and Clinical Medicine*, *144*(2):60-64.

Hernandez, T., & Kambhampati, S. (2004). Integration of biological sources: Current systems and challenges. *ACM SIGMOD*, *33*(3), 51-60.

Hsinchun, C., Fuller, S. S., Friedman, C., & Hersh, W. (Ed.). (2005). *Medical Informatics: Knowledge Management and Data Mining in Biomedicine.* (Integrated Series in Information Systems), Springer.

Huang, C. H., Lanza, V., Rajasekaran, S., & Dubitzky, W. (2005). HealthGrid - Bridging life science and information technology. *Journal of Clinical Monitoring and Computing*, *19*(4-5), 259-262.

Katehakis, D. G., Tsiknakis, M., & Orphanoudakis, S. (2002). *Towards an Integrated Electronic Health Record - Current Status and Challenges, Business Briefing: Global Healthcare 2002*, The Official Publication of the World Medical Association, January 2002.

Klein, M., (2001). Combining and relating ontologies: an analyis of problems and solutions. In: Gomez-Perez A et al., editors. *Workshop on ontologies and information sharing, IJCAI'01*, Seattle.

Lasko, T. A., Bhagwat, J. G., Zou, K. H., & Ohno-Machado, L. (2005). The use of receiver operating characteristic curves in biomedical informatics. *Journal of Biomedical Informatics 38*(5), 404-415.

Martín, L., Bonsma, E., Anguita, A., Vrijnsen, J., García-Remesal, M., Crespo, J., Tsiknakis, M., & Maojo, V. (2007). Data Access and Management in ACGT: Tools to Solve Syntactic and Semantic Heterogeneities Between Clinical and Image Databases. In: *Advances in Conceptual Modeling – Foundations and Applications*, (pp. 24-33).

Martin-Sanchez, F., et al (2004). Synergy between medical informatics and bioinformatics: facilitating genomic medicine for future health care. *Journal of Biomedical Informatics, 37*(1), 30-42.

McGee, S. (2002). Simplifying likelihood ratios. *Journal of General Internal Medicine: Official Journal of the Society for Research and Education in Primary Care Internal Medicine, 17*(8), 646-9.

Moosmann, M., Eichele, T., Nordby, H., Hugdahl, K., & Calhoun, V. D. (2008). Joint independent component analysis for simultaneous EEG-fMRI: Principle and simulation. *International Journal of Psychophysiology, 67*(3), 212-221.

Murphy, J. R. (2004). Statistical errors in immunologic research. *Journal of Allergy and Clinical Immunology, 114*(6), 1259-1263.

Perez, A., Dennis, R. J., Gil, J. F. A., Rondon, M. A., & Lopez, A. (2002). Use of the mean, hot deck and multiple imputation techniques to predict outcome in intensive care unit patients in Colombia. *Statistics in Medicine, 21*, 3885-3896.

Potamias, G., & Moustakis, V. (2001). Knowledge Discovery from Distributed Clinical Data Sources: The Era for Internet-Based Epidemiology. In *Procs 23rd Annual International Conference of the IEEE Engineering in Medicine and Biology Society*, Istanbul, Turkey, (pp. 25-28).

Roses, A. D. (2000). Pharmacogenomics and the practice of medicine. *Nature*; *405*, 857-65.

Ruta D., & Gabrys B. (2000). An overview of classifier fusion methods. *Computing and Information Systems*, 7, 1-10.

Serocka, P. (2007). Visualization of High-Dimensional Biomedical Image Data In: *Advances in Multimedia Information Processing.* Springer.

Sotiriou, C., & Piccart, M. J. (2007). Taking gene-expression profiling to the clinic: when will molecular signatures become relevant to patient care. *Nature Reviews*; *7*, 545-53.

Steele, A. (2002). *Medical Informatics Around the World: An International Perspective Focusing on Training Issues.*, Universal Publishers, ISBN: 1581126344.

Sujansky W. (2001). Heterogeneous database integration in biomedicine. *J Biomed Inform, 34*(4), 285–98.

Taira, R. K., Bui, A. A. T., Kangarloo, H. K. R., Taira, A., Bui, H., & Kangarloo, E. (2002). Identification of Patient Name References within Medical Documents Using Semantic Selectional Restrictions. *Proc AMIA Fall Symposium*, (pp. 757-761).

Taktak, A. G., Fisher, A. C., & Damato, B. (2004). Modelling survival after treatment of intraocular melanoma using artificial neural networks and Bayes theorem. *Physics in Medicine and Biology, 49*, 87–98.

Thiran, P., Hainaut, J. L., & Houben, G. J. (2005). Database Wrappers Development: Towards Automatic Generation. In: *Proc of the Ninth Euro-*

pean Conference on Software Maintenance and Reengineering (CSMR'05), 207-216.

VanBemmel, J. H., & Musen, M. A. (Ed.) (1997). *Handbook of Medical Informatics*. Stanford University, Stanford, Springer.

KEY TERMS

Information Fusion: The utilization of all available information at multiple abstraction levels (measurements, features, decisions) to maximize an expert system's performance.

GRID Computing: A service scheme that facilitates the utilization of the processing and storage resources of many computers as a common infrastructure for specific application domains (scientific etc.).

Medical Informatics: Study, invention, and implementation of structures and algorithms to improve communication, understanding and management of medical information.

Principal Components Analysis (PCA): Transformation often used to reduce multidimensional data sets to lower dimensions for analysis (also known as Karhunen-Loève or Hotelling transform).

Prognostic/Diagnostic Models: Mathematical/ algorithmic models designed to provide early detection of disease.

Electroencephalogram (EEG): Measurement of postsynaptic electrical activity produced by the brain's neurons.

Functional Magnetic Resonance Imaging (fMRI): Method to measure the haemodynamic response related to neural activity in the brain or spinal cord.

Receiver Operating Characteristic: Curve that connects all points defined of corresponding sensitivity-specificity values for varying threshold levels. It is used to visualize a trained classifier's overall performance irrespective of specific decision thresholds.

Single Photon Emission Computed Tomography (SPECT) Imaging: A nuclear medicine tomographic imaging technique using gamma rays.

Chapter II
Integrating Imaging and Clinical Data for Decision Support

William Hsu
University of California, Los Angeles, USA

Alex A. T. Bui
University of California, Los Angeles, USA

Ricky K. Taira
University of California, Los Angeles, USA

Hooshang Kangarloo
University of California, Los Angeles, USA

ABSTRACT

Though an unparalleled amount and diversity of imaging and clinical data are now collected as part of routine care, this information is not sufficiently integrated and organized in a way that effectively supports a clinician's ability to diagnose and treat a patient. The goal of this chapter is to present a framework for organizing, representing, and manipulating patient data to assist in medical decision-making. We first demonstrate how probabilistic graphical models (specifically, Bayesian belief networks) are capable of representing medical knowledge. We then propose a data model that facilitates temporal and investigative organization by structuring and modeling clinical observations at the patient level. Using information aggregated into the data model, we describe the creation of multi-scale, temporal disease models to represent a disease across a population. Finally, we describe visual tools for interacting with these disease models to facilitate the querying and understanding of results. The chapter concludes with a discussion about open problems and future directions.

INTRODUCTION

More patient data is being gathered, given the adoption of the electronic medical record (EMR), the availability of clinical tests, and the growing rates of chronic diseases (Wyatt & Wright, 1998). Modern medical records are not only comprised of traditional data (*e.g.*, clinical notes, labs), but also digital images (*e.g.*, computed tomography, magnetic resonance imaging) and other graphical representations (*e.g.*, pulmonary function graphs). Notably, medical imaging is becoming the predominant *in vivo* tool for objectively documenting patient presentation and clinical findings. Patient care is largely dependent upon imaging to understand disease processes and to establish tangible evidence of treatment response. However, even within imaging, the scope of data collected can range from the cellular level (*e.g.*, molecular imaging) to tissue level (*e.g.*, histopathology), up to the level of the organism itself (*e.g.*, conventional radiology). As the quantity and diversity of collected data continues to grow, the task of consolidating this information in a way that improves patient care becomes a challenge: clinicians need effective tools to organize, access, and review the data. For instance, current methods for querying image data are limited to a set of keywords (*e.g.*, stored as part of the image header), but much of the clinically useful information about a disease is contained within the image itself (*e.g.*, mass volume, border, shape). Advances in image processing have resulted in sophisticated algorithms for automated content extraction (Pham, Xu, & Prince, 2000), enabling the characterization, segmentation, and classification of pixel data to extract meaningful features from an image (*e.g.*, regions of edema). However, the extraction of meaningful features from patient data alone is insufficient. While imaging data provides a phenotypic description of disease progression, the combination of imaging and other clinical observations has the potential to better model and predict disease behavior. A collective understanding of how features from different levels are needed: a finding observed at the phenotype level can be explained as an emergent manifestation of multiple findings at the genotype level. For instance, the cellular level serves as the basis for describing genetic/proteomic irregularities that lead to larger scale effects that are seen at the tissue, organ, and organism levels. While research in the area of intelligent data analysis (IDA) has explored content extraction and representation, current approaches have significant limitations: 1) they do not capture the context in which the data was collected; 2) the data is not represented in a way that facilitates a computer's ability to reason with the information; and 3) a lack of tools exists for facilitating the querying and understanding of the stored data.

This chapter describes efforts, particularly those undertaken by the Medical Imaging Informatics Group at the University of California, Los Angeles (UCLA), to address these issues by transforming clinical observations into a representation enabling a computer to "understand" and reason with the data. Computer understanding, in this context, is defined as being able to determine the relative importance of a given data element (*e.g.*, necrosis size) in the patient record in relation to a phenomenon of interest (*e.g.*, brain tumor). The chapter is organized as follows: Section 2 provides an overview of IDA and recent work in the area towards creating expert systems. While various techniques for representing medical knowledge exist, this chapter focuses on probabilistic graphical models. Section 3 introduces a phenomenon-centric data model (PCDM) that structures clinical observations at the patient level by organizing findings (*i.e.*, collected data) around a given phenomenon (*i.e.*, medical problem). Section 4 describes the process of generating multi-scale, temporal disease models using dynamic Bayesian belief networks to represent a disease across a population: these steps are illustrated in the context of our efforts to develop tools that help assess and manage patients with brain tumors. Subsequently, Section 5 discusses a novel interface for querying these models using a visual paradigm to facilitate the composition of queries related to image features. The chapter concludes by describing open problems in the area and identifying potential directions for future work.

BACKGROUND

The field of intelligent data analysis (also commonly referred to as *knowledge discovery*) has matured over the past as a product of several disciplines, including statistics, computer science, pattern recognition, and artificial intelligence (Hand, 1998). Unlike data mining, which focuses on specific algorithms and techniques for solving a particular problem, IDA encompasses a wide range of tasks from content extraction and organization of data, through to reasoning with the data and visualizing the results (R. Bellazzi & Zupan, 2001; Holmes & Peek, 2007). The specific goals of IDA within medicine are: 1) to extract useful information from collected patient data; 2) to organize this data in a meaningful representation that facilitates retrieval and medical decision making tasks; and 3) to assist in the interpretation of patient data by presenting the information in a context-sensitive manner (Lavrac et al., 1998). IDA accomplishes these goals using a number of techniques such as decision trees, neural networks, support vector machines, and Bayesian networks. Comprehensive reviews on the topic of data mining for diagnosis and prediction may be found in (Bath, 2003; Chen et al., 2005; Riccardo Bellazzi & Zupan, 2008).

Representing medical knowledge in a computer-understandable form (*i.e.*, a model) poses several key challenges: 1) the uncertainties inherent to medical knowledge must be captured; 2) the models must be sufficiently intuitive so that domain experts understand the explanations proposed by the system; and 3) the models must be practically analyzable using algorithms that are computationally tractable. Although various data mining techniques address these challenges with varying degrees of success, we argue that probabilistic graphical models are best capable to meet these requirements. A probabilistic graphical model provides a normative method for modeling uncertain phenomena, with the corresponding computational techniques for comprehensive, detailed model analysis. A graphical model is comprised of a set of nodes, which are connected by arcs. Each node represents a random variable, and each arc represents a probabilistic relationship between nodes. Having roots in both probability theory and graph theory, probabilistic models are solvable either using purely algebraic manipulation or by using diagrammatic representations of probability distributions. Importantly, graphical models also provide a readily understood visual representation of the relationships among variables; assumptions made in the model (*e.g.*, conditional independence relationships between variables) are explicitly encoded into the graph structure. For the remainder of this chapter, we focus on probabilistic graphical models, specifically Bayesian belief networks, as the method for modeling clinical observations.

Bayesian Belief Network

A Bayesian belief network (BBN) is an instance of a graphical model, which offers a complete and intuitive representation of uncertain domain knowledge (Pearl, 1988). Formally, a BBN is a directed acyclic graph (DAG) whose nodes represent evidence variables and arcs represent associations (or in some cases, causal links) between nodes. When the model is instantiated, each node is set to a specific value. The arcs in the DAG represent the probabilistic influences between the variables. A variable X_i is dependent on its parents and children in the DAG but is conditionally independent of any of its non-descendents given its parents, a property known as the Markov condition.

Formally, the structure of the DAG is a representation of a factorization of the joint probability distribution. Each variable X_i in the DAG is specified by a set of conditional probability distributions: P(***X*** | parents(***X***)). Each of these distributions describes the joint effect of a specific combination of values for the parents of X_i on the probability distribution over the values of X_i. These sets of conditional probability distributions define a joint probability distribution that is factorized over the graph's topology using the following equation:

$$P(U) = \prod_{X} P(X \mid parents(X))$$

Using this equation, knowledge bases that have been formerly computationally intractable because of their large joint probability space are now realizable as the space can be more compactly represented using the Markov property. Indeed, because of its ability to capture uncertainty in medical data and to answer a wide range of clinical queries, BBNs are an increasingly popular formalism for representing models of disease (Shwe et al., 1991; Heckerman, Horvitz, & Nathwani, 1992). Work in utilizing BBNs in biomedicine (Lucas, van der Gaag, & Abu-Hanna, 2004) can be roughly classified into three categories:

- **Diagnostic and prognostic reasoning:** Applications of BBNs encompass a range of broad fields such as internal medicine, to more specific areas such as tumor classification, pulmonology, neuroimaging, and mammography (Kahn et al., 1997; Friston et al., 2002; Kline et al., 2005). Several projects, such as MUNIN and Pathfinder, have used BBNs to provide classification of presenting symptoms and/or objective clinical findings (Andreassen et al., 1999). Another class of applications attempt to predict values based on a patient's presentation and/or a potential intervention. Many of these applications support limited prognostic queries, which are addressed more thoroughly in (Nikiforidis & Sakellaropoulos, 1998; Sebastiani et al., 2005).
- **Treatment selection (decision support):** Closely related to the prognostic usage of BBNs is decision support, allowing a user to view different scenarios to optimize some criteria and select a plan of action (Herskovits & Gerring, 2003; Leibovici et al., 2000). This set of applications utilizes a broader class of BBNs called influence diagrams and can be seen as a global optimization problem across the network (Meyer et al., 2004).
- **Functional linkage:** BBNs are being pursued in bioinformatics and to model biological phenomenon (Friedman et al., 2000), such as modeling and analyzing cellular networks and computing genetic linkages.

While popular in medicine, traditional Bayesian belief networks are limited because they require clinical data and disease processes – which are intrinsically temporal in nature – to be condensed and represented using a single node. Addressing this shortcoming, dynamic Bayesian networks (DBN) (Murphy, 2002) are an extension of BBNs that model time-variant states, which are common in functional magnetic resonance imaging (fMRI) (Battle, Chechik, & Koller, 2007), gene expression networks, and other bioinformatics-related problems (Yu et al., 2004). DBNs are a generalized version of hidden Markov Models (HMMs): they are similar to HMMs but have the advantage of separating out hidden state variables and thus reducing the number of probabilities required to express state transitions. Formally, let X_t be a vector representing the set of unobservable state variables at some time, t, and Et denote the set of observable evidence at time t. A DBN, depicted in Figure 1, is defined in three parts: the initial prior distribution, $P(X_0)$;

Figure 1. A general example of a dynamic Bayesian belief network with two time slices.

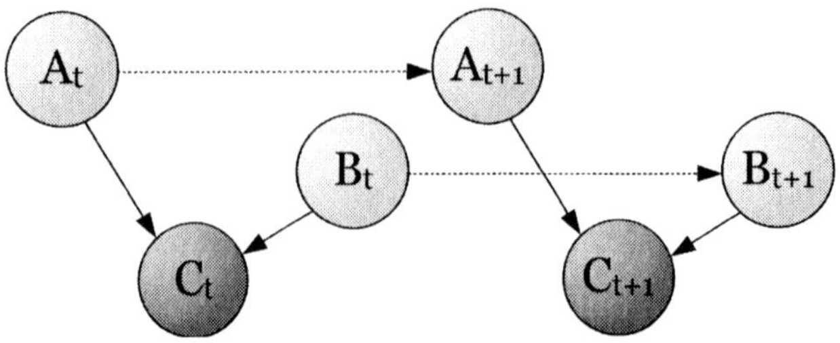

the sensor model, $P(E_t \mid X_t)$, which gives the conditional distribution of the evidence variables for a given time point, t; and the transition model, $P(X_{t+1} \mid X_t)$, which details how the current state affects a future state.

The remainder of this chapter presents a framework for organizing clinical observations into a representation that enable computers (*i.e.*, expert systems) to assist in clinical decision making that builds upon these past works and formalisms. The framework is described in the context of assessing and managing patients with primary malignant brain tumors. Patient data is used to populate a *phenomenon-centric data model* (PCDM), which in turn is used to generate a disease model from a neuro-oncology research database maintained at the UCLA Medical Center. In addition to radiology, pathology, surgical, lab, demographic, imaging, and medical information, the database contains outcome information such as Karnofsky score, time to progression (TTP), and time to survival (TTS) for each patient. We demonstrate how the database is reorganized following the PCDM to facilitate temporal and investigative exploration of the data.

ORGANIZING PATIENT DATA

The first step towards organizing clinical data is the creation of a clinical repository. To be useful, the repository must make possible quick retrieval of patient data, while accommodating the changing needs of the hospital environment (Johnson, 1996). Though various schemas (*e.g.*, entity-value-attribute with classes and relationships (EAV/CR) (Nadkarni et al., 1999)) have been proposed that address these conditions, their approaches, while highly generalizable, do not explicitly contain the contextual details about collected data (*e.g.*, degree of certainty, reason for collection) and their relationships, nor natively support temporal manipulation of the data (Adlassnig et al., 2006). To address these shortfalls, (Bui, Taira, El-Saden, Dordoni, and Aberle 2004) has introduced an extended entity-relationship (ER) data model called a *phenomenon-centric data model* (PCDM) based on the principle that knowledge discovery is an exploratory process, going from an unknown, described phenomenon to documented conclusions through iterative refinement of theories. The core PCDM consists of three classes of entities:

1. Phenomena & findings. Central to the data model, a phenomenon is defined as the center of an investigation, such as a medical problem of interest (*e.g.*, patient complains of a migraine). A set of findings is associated with a phenomenon and is anything that is observable (*e.g.*, slurred speech).
2. Theories & evidence. A theory attempts to account for a phenomenon, and is often a working conjecture (*i.e.*, a hypothesis).

The theory is a logical explanation based on all available evidence and observations. Theories explain the facts, but are not the facts themselves, instead representing how facts are related. Findings are thus a type of evidence used to support these hypotheses, linking causes and effects. Evidence can also be derived from different sources (*e.g.*, an x-ray image showing a bone fracture, a population-based study).

3. States, properties, & behaviors. A finding is simply an object: its description is given by a state entity, which acts as a vector of specific properties. This abstraction defines a finding at a single point in time in terms of objective features (*e.g.*, the size of an observed tumor). The degree of certainty associated with an observation, error bounds, and noise models are captured as part of the property entity. Changes between states are defined as a behavior – that is, a change in a given property (*e.g.*, decrease in tumor size) over time.

Figure 2 depicts the core entities of the PCDM and how entities are linked together. These entities serve as high-level templates, from which subclassed objects are created for specific medical problems. The PCDM also utilizes streams (Bui, 2000; Dionisio et al., 1996) as a way of capturing temporal data sequences in the patient record. A stream comprises a set of (valid and logical) time-based data elements occurring at a single point in time (*e.g.*, a lab value's timestamp) or duration (*e.g.*, a drug regimen over weeks). The evolution of findings associated with a phenomenon is represented using a stream, enabling representation of the behavior of a finding's properties as they change over time. Streams can also be used to capture a clinician's differential diagnosis and the progression of evidence towards a final diagnosis.

PCDM for Neuro-Oncology

Data elements from the existing neuro-oncology database can be reorganized into a PCDM. Image features (tumor, edema, necrosis, cystic

Figure 2. A portion of the PCDM that illustrate core entities of the PCDM.

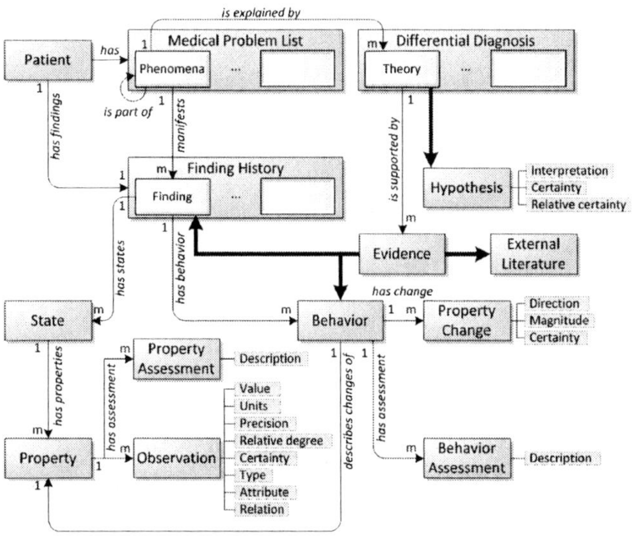

components) and pathology results (histology, tumor genetic markers) are modeled as findings. Because of the temporal nature of these findings, they are represented in streams; for instance, the stream construct is used to model individual image studies acquired at different time points. In addition, each finding is associated with one or more states that provide information on a finding's properties and the context in which properties are observed. For example, image studies include attributes such as acquisition protocol parameters and scanner/site information. Theories and evidence entities associate problems and findings to provide an explanation of why certain findings occur: a theory entity is used to relate (increased) edema, signs of necrosis, and other image findings to an underlying cause (*e.g.,* chemotherapy, steroids). These entities define the structure of the data model using a combination of expert opinion and scientific literature. Behavior entities capture changes in properties for a given finding; an example would be capturing the quantitative differences in tumor burden of the patient as treatment progresses. Figure 3 illustrates a portion of the PCDM for neuro-oncology. The structure of the PCDM captures information from different data sources and across multiple levels of detail. In particular, relationships among image features in the neuro-oncology database and other clinical variables are explicitly defined, providing contextual information on what factors contribute to the observed image features. This integrative and comprehensive representation of patient data is then used to guide the creation of a disease model.

CREATING DISEASE MODELS

The purpose of creating a disease model is to formalize the representation of knowledge about the disorder such that computers are able to reason with the information and provide meaningful answers to queries from clinicians. In this section, we describe a methodology for developing temporal, multi-scale disease models that integrate heterogeneous data collected during routine patient care. We advocate a gradated approach for

Figure 3. An instance of the PCDM for neuro-oncology.

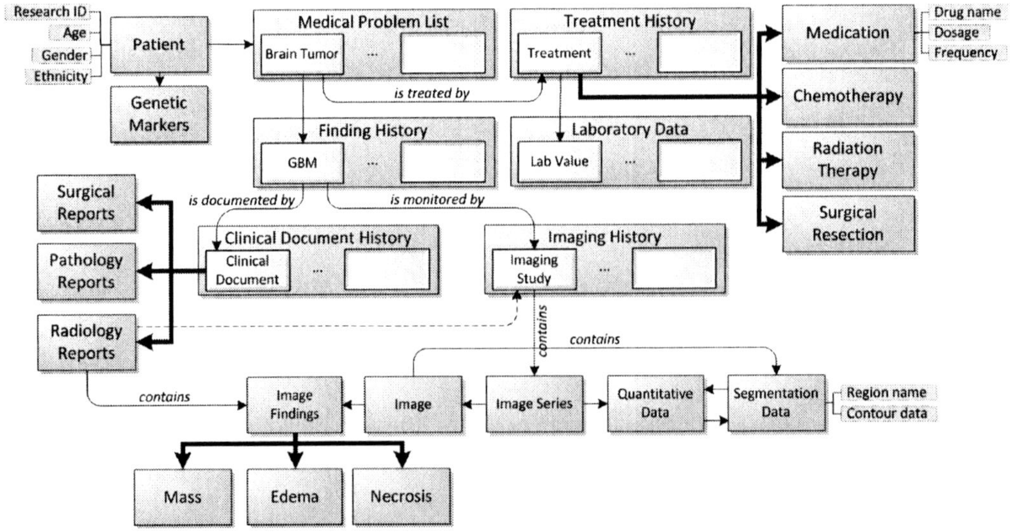

model construction, which: 1) allows the model to be built progressively as new variables are made available (*e.g.*, the discovery of new genomic tests, new quantitative imaging parameters); and 2) permits an evaluation to be done at each step to assess improvements in answering queries. Generation of a disease model proceeds iteratively using information stored in the PCDM through the following four steps:

1. **Variable selection:** Variables are commonly identified using sources such as clinical data repositories, expert opinion, public data sources, and published literature. Entities in the PCDM (*e.g.*, findings) can be translated into variables in the model. Once a variable is identified, it is codified using standardized representations (*e.g.*, Unified Medical Language System (UMLS), RadLex, Common Data Model, etc.) (Zou et al., 2003). The use of common terminology enables the model to be linked with external knowledge sources (*e.g.*, Gene Ontology, Fundamental Model of Anatomy) (Rubin, Shah, & Noy, 2008).
2. **Network structure:** After model variables have been specified, the next step is to define the associations between variables. Such links correspond closely to a scientific hypothesis relating a cause (*e.g.*, an intervention) to an effect. The network topology may be defined using the structure of the PCDM, expert opinion, scientific literature, or inferred computationally given sufficient data. While the PCDM is a wide range of semantic relationships, only a subset of these relationships is delineated in a BBN: the concepts representing theories and hypotheses within the PCDM are bound to a directed path within the BBN, establishing the rationale for the observations and findings.
3. **Discretization:** To address complexity issues in large static models, continuous variables need to be divided into a finite number of states using either univariate methods (*e.g.*, equal-width binning, quantiles) or class-based methods (*e.g.*, minimum description length processing), both of which are reviewed in (Monti, 1999). When dealing with temporal data, an additional discretization step is taken to represent variables at different time points. Variables are divided into temporal clusters based on the time point associated with each value. These clusters are then used to define the transition states in the DBN.
4. **Parameter estimation:** Given the qualitative description of the BBN topology, the last construction step, parameter estimation, involves computing the conditional probability tables (CPTs) for each variable (or prior probabilities for root nodes). Computation of CPTs typically occurs in two ways: calculated from clinical data using an expectation maximization (EM) algorithm; or elicited from scientific literature and experts. While data stored in the PCDM may be used to compute the probabilities, two potential issues arise: 1) not all patients may have information for a given variable (*e.g.*, if a patient does not have genetic information); and 2) the database may not contain sufficient data to represent the probability distribution. While obtaining opinions from domain experts may be used to overcome these issues, such an approach can introduce a bias into the values (Monti & Carenini, 2000). Parameter fitting algorithms such as EM, Gibbs sampling, and gradient ascent may be used to learn CPTs with missing data. In the situation where few outcomes are available relative to the number of covariates, the use of propensity scores (Glynn, Schneeweiss, & Stürmer, 2006), which are the conditional probability of assignment to a specific state given a vector of observed covariates, may improve estimates of their values.

Imaging-Centric Temporal Disease Model for Brain Tumors

Drawing upon the PCDM for neuro-oncology, we created a disease model that predicts how changes in image features and treatment selection over time affect a patient's time to progression (TTP) and time to survival (TTS). During the variable selection process, we identified findings in the PCDM that were related to demographics (*e.g.*, age, gender), image features (*e.g.*, edema, contrast enhancement, mass effect), and treatments (*e.g.*, resection extent, dosage of chemotherapy) and represented them as variables in the model. Using the temporal clusters defined in the PCDM, we divided the DBN into two logical time slices based on the patient's TTP: the first cluster representing status and treatment before initial progression, and the second temporal cluster representing progression and subsequent changes in treatment protocol. The structure of the model is based on the associations between findings defined in the PCDM. To parameterize the model, we used a subset of 200 patients from the database that had glioblastoma multiforme (GBM) and an initial treatment of a chemotherapy drug called temozolomide. The resulting DBN is depicted in Figure 4. The transition model included all nodes except the non-temporal data (age, gender, race, tumor location), which were held static, and TTS was influenced by the values of the TTP over both time slices. Using a 10-fold cross validation where we trained the model on 90% of the data and tested the model on the remaining 10% and averaged the results over ten trials, the accuracy for predicting the initial TTP, second TTP, and TTS was 83%, 85%, and 87% respectively. To determine whether modeling time improved model performance, we evaluated a static BBN's ability to predict TTS. Using the same variables as the DBN, we generated a model that aggregated all of the temporal clusters and found that the model achieved 79% accuracy. To provide a baseline comparison for our results, we used logistic regression to model the same variables as the previous two models and determined that the logistic regression predicted the initial TTP, second TTP, and TTS with an accuracy of 72%, 84%, and 86%, respectively.

Figure 4. DBN for neuro-oncology. Only the first time slice (t_0) is shown. All nodes in the network were duplicated in two time states (i.e., t_0, t_1) except demographic variables, tumor location, and time to survival. Time to survival was influenced by both time to progression at t_0 and t_1.

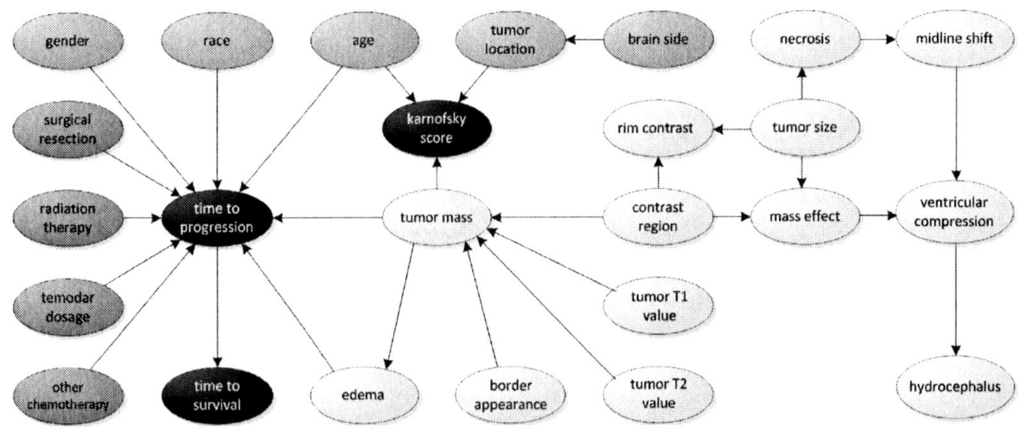

APPLICATIONS

Up to this point, we have presented a framework for establishing a clinical repository that organizes patient data, using this data to create a disease model across a population. However, this process is only useful when users (*i.e.,* clinicians) can easily interact with these models to obtain relevant information that helps them make informed decisions about a patient's case. While much literature has been published on building BBNs to answer clinical queries, little has been written about the interface that clinicians use to pose queries to the model. Such an interface must effectively support the full spectrum of user activities (*e.g.,* reviewing a patient for the first time, diagnosis and treatment planning, a follow-up visit, etc.). BBN visualizations typically employ the DAG as the pictorial representation upon which queries are composed and results presented (*e.g.,* using node monitors). The problem with current types of visualizations being explored is: 1) that as the complexity of the BBN grows, understanding variable interaction is difficult at best; and 2) that the variables are visually abstracted and thus lose contextual meaning. We suggest the development of *surrogate interfaces*; these interfaces provide users with a familiar environment to intuitively pose queries and automatically translate the user's queries into parameters that can be used to instantiate the model. One such system is TraumaSCAN (Ogunyemi, 2006), in which the user interacts with a three-dimensional model of the body to place entry and exit wounds for injuries from gunshots; then, in combination with inputted patient findings, the system performs reasoning on a Bayesian model to predict the most probable symptoms and conditions arising from the specified injuries.

Visual Query Interface

Given the visual and spatial nature of medical images (*e.g.,* size, shape, location), a visual query-by-example interface seems well-suited to the task, allowing for composition of a query image (such as in content-based image retrieval systems, (Shyu et al., 1999)). Past studies show that visual querying has a shallower learning curve, allows more expressive queries (*vs.* text keywords), and generates more accurate results (Catarci, Costabile, & Matera, 1995). We introduce the *visual query interface*, which improves interaction with the BBN in two ways: 1) it provides visual tools for users to pose graphical queries to represent image features; and 2) it uses the network structure of the model to guide users through the query formulation process. The fundamental elements in a visual query are *graphical metaphors* (Marcus, 1998), which correspond to visual representations of variables specified in the disease model. Graphical metaphors range from capturing nominal inputs (*e.g.,* male/female) to representing visual features (*e.g.,* edema shape and size). For non-spatial constructs (*e.g.,* gender), the graphical metaphor may simply be an icon: selecting this icon enables the user to add this variable to the query and indicate a value. For entities involving visual features, invoking the graphical metaphor from the toolbar will allow the user to draw the corresponding entity in a sketch editor. The system then automatically translates the arrangement of graphical metaphors into parameters that are used to instantiate the BBN.

The process of posing a visual query is as follows: from a normal or patient imaging study, the user selects a representative slice or location to pose the query; the user iteratively constructs a query by drawing upon the available set of metaphors to capture various visual features of the disease; and the final visual query is translated into an object representation that is used to set the states of variables in the model as the basis of a maximum a posteriori query.

A disadvantage of existing visual query interfaces is that users are presented with a potentially large set of graphical metaphors but receive little or no guidance on how to effectively utilize these metaphors to construct a query. This problem is commonly faced in programs that contain a multitude of commands; for instance, Microsoft addresses this issue in Office through Ribbon (McCormack et al., 2007), a method for dynamically displaying available functionality based on task. Similarly, we introduce the *adaptive toolbar* (Hsu & Bui, 2006), which uses the inherent structure and CPTs of the underlying BBN to selectively present metaphors. This approach reduces the potential visual clutter associated with presenting the entire set of metaphors simultaneously and assists users in selecting which metaphor is best suited for a particular query. The determination of whether a metaphor is (un)related is influenced by the relationships among the variables in the BBN. Each metaphor is mapped to a corresponding variable in the model. Selection of a metaphor, and thus the variable, computes the Markov blanket for the BBN node; variables in the Markov blanket are then selected for presentation in the toolbar. Figure 5 illustrates the main query editor interface and the adaptive toolbar concept. The figure depicts the system being used in a neuro-oncology context: users are presented with a normal brain atlas (ICBM452), from which axial/coronal/sagittal slices can be selected (Figure 5b). Above the editor, the adaptive toolbar presents available metaphors based on context: as the user selects structures (*e.g.*, white matter) or metaphors (*e.g.*, edema metaphor) in the editor, related metaphors are presented in the toolbar while unrelated metaphors are removed (Figure 5a). For example, when the rim contrast metaphor is selected, the user is prompted to define whether the border is thick or thin. This adaptive presentation of relevant metaphors not only simplifies the process of creating a query by reducing visual selection clutter but also enforces logical rules regarding the order that metaphors are selected to formulate a query.

Figure 5: Left side depicts the visual query interface. The adaptive toolbar (a) is dynamically updated to guide the user, allowing for composition using the query-by-example paradigm in the visual editor (b). The toolbar uses the underlying BBN to select the appropriate graphical metaphors at any given time. The right side illustrates how the adaptive toolbar guides the query formulation process.

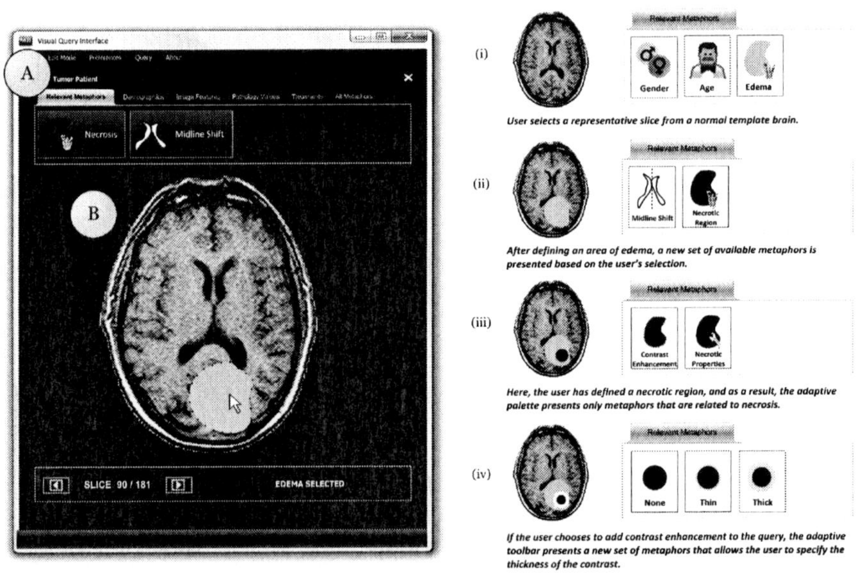

FUTURE TRENDS

The latest breakthroughs made by imaging technologies have not only provided a wealth of new information about a disease but also underscored the need for novel approaches that are scalable, extensible, and capable of helping users with understanding this information:

- **Improved methods for analyzing clinical data.** The development of advanced medical imaging techniques has resulted in the discovery of new variables that characterize disease behavior. Models should be modular and extensible so that new variables may be easily incorporated into existing models. In addition, techniques need to be scalable: as more data is generated about a patient, algorithms must be capable of handling the increased quantities of data. Fully automated methods are needed to identify and extract features; manual or semi-automated algorithms are too costly and time consuming to generate meaningful amounts of data for population-level modeling. Finally, models should be adaptable: they should have the ability to accommodate data from a single clinical site to a large quantity of data from a clinical trial that involves multiple sites.
- **Development of novel visualizations.** The utility of building comprehensive, integrated models are realized when tools and visualizations that assist users with knowledge exploration and discovery are available. These tools should draw upon imaging and clinical observations to provide insight into a user's clinical questions. In the book *Visual Thinking*, (Arnheim, 2004) contends that perception is highly intertwined with the process of reasoning. If the user is unable to quickly perceive the meaning of an image or display, the information is useless. New visualizations need to not only facilitate the user's ability to understand the data but also direct the user towards new avenues of research with the goal of discovering new knowledge.

Building upon these themes, our goal is to leverage DBNs as a way to represent temporal information, allowing users to understand changes that occur in a patient through the course of a disease. As part of future work, we will address limitations of our modeling paradigm: 1) the model is highly sensitive to the method of discretization and sample size; 2) it assumes that data is missing at random; and 3) the results may be confounded by hidden variables. We also intend to expand the development of new visualizations that improve the interaction between the user and underlying model.

CONCLUSION

Medical imaging is an objective method for characterizing and tracking disease progression. As new techniques are developed for imaging the human body at various levels of detail (*e.g.*, cellular to organ), large amounts of data are collected about a patient. However, the full utility of this information to assist in diagnosis, prognosis, and treatment is unrealized without a means to understand this information in the context of all the other clinical observations. Clinical reports, laboratory values, and pathology results provide contextual information that shed additional light into the high-level features captured in radiological images. Recent developments in intelligent data analysis have made it possible to automate the accurate characterization and extraction of unique features from images and clinical reports. Unfortunately, current efforts to organize this information have not addressed the need for handling the integration of data acquired at multiple sources and at different levels of detail. A unified framework that encompasses the entire process from organizing, representing, and interacting with patient data is needed.

In this chapter, we introduced a *phenomenon-centric data model* as a way to organize all of the data collected about individual patients into a comprehensive model that defines how observations are related to one another. Drawing upon this unified model, we described the generation of multi-scale, temporal disease models that represent a disease at the population-level and support a variety of clinical queries related to the diagnosis and treatment of a patient given his/her unique findings. Finally, we presented a *visual query interface* as an intuitive novel method for posing clinical queries visually by manipulating graphical metaphors. While we have presented the framework in the context of neuro-oncology, the framework is generalizable to other medical domains. Ultimately, a comprehensive framework such as the one presented provides clinicians with a powerful tool for effectively integrating and understanding the information that is mined from the large quantities of medical data and has the potential for improving patient care.

ACKNOWLEDGMENT

The authors would like to thank Dr. Timothy Cloughesy for providing access to the UCLA Neuro-Oncology Database. This work is supported in part by funding from the National Institutes of Health P01-EB000216 and T15-LM007356.

REFERENCES

Adlassnig, K.-P., Combi, C., Das, A. K., Keravnou, E. T., & Pozzi, G. (2006). Temporal representation and reasoning in medicine: Research directions and challenges. *Artif Intell Med, 38*(2), 101-113.

Andreassen, S., Riekehr, C., Kristensen, B., Schonheyder, H. C., & Leibovici, L. (1999). Using probabilistic and decision-theoretic methods in treatment and prognosis modeling. *Artif Intell Med, 15*(2), 121-134.

Arnheim, R. (2004). *Visual Thinking*. Berkeley, CA: University of California Press.

Bath, P. (2003). Data mining in health and medical information. *Annual Review of Information Science and Technology, 38*, 331-369.

Battle, A., Chechik, G., & Koller, D. (2007). Temporal and Cross-Subject Probabilistic Models for fMRI Prediction Tasks. In B. Scholkopf (Ed.), *Advances in Neural Information Processing Systems 19: Proceedings of the 2006 Conference* (pp.121-128). Cambridge: MIT Press.

Bellazzi, R., & Zupan, B. (2001). Intelligent data analysis--special issue. *Methods Inf Med, 40*(5), 362-364.

Bellazzi, R., & Zupan, B. (2008). Predictive data mining in clinical medicine: Current issues and guidelines. *Int J Medical Informatics, 77*(2), 81-97.

Bui, A. A. (2000). *A multimedia data model with generalized stream constructs.* (Ph.D. Dissertation, University of California, Los Angeles, 2000).

Bui, A. A., Taira, R. K., El-Saden, S., Dordoni, A., & Aberle, D. R. (2004). Automated medical problem list generation: Towards a patient timeline. *Medinfo, 11*(Pt 1), 587-591.

Catarci, T., Costabile, M. F., & Matera, M. (1995). Visual metaphors for interacting with databases. *ACM SIGCHI Bulletin, 27*(2), 15-17.

Chen, H., Fuller, S. S., Friedman, C., & Hersh, W. (2005). *Medical Informatics: Knowledge Management and Data Mining in Biomedicine.* New York, NY: Springer.

Dionisio, J. D., Cardenas, A. F., Taira, R. K., Aberle, D. R., Chu, W. W., McNitt-Gray, M. F., et al. (1996). A unified timeline model and user interface for multimedia medical databases. *Comput Med Imaging Graph, 20*(4), 333-346.

Friedman, N., Linial, M., Nachman, I., & Pe'er, D. (2000). Using Bayesian networks to analyze expression data. *J Computational Biology, 7*(3-4), 601-620.

Friston, K. J., Penny, W., Phillips, C., Kiebel, S., Hinton, G., & Ashburner, J. (2002). Classical and Bayesian inference in neuroimaging: theory. *NeuroImage, 16*(2), 465–483.

Glynn, R. J., Schneeweiss, S., & Stürmer, T. (2006). Indications for propensity scores and review of their use in pharmacoepidemiology. *Basic Clin Pharmacol Toxicol, 98*(3), 253-259.

Hand, D. J. (1998). Intelligent data analysis: Issues and opportunities. *Intelligent Data Analysis, 2*(1), 67-79.

Heckerman, D. E., Horvitz, E. J., & Nathwani, B. N. (1992). Toward normative expert systems. Part I: the pathfinder project. *Methods Inf Med, 31*(2), 90-105.

Herskovits, E. H., & Gerring, J. P. (2003). Application of a data-mining method based on Bayesian networks to lesion-deficit analysis. *NeuroImage, 19*(4), 1664-1673.

Holmes, J. H., & Peek, N. (2007). Intelligent data analysis in biomedicine. *J Biomedical Informatics, 40*(6), 605-608.

Hsu, W., & Bui, A. A. (2006). A framework for visually querying a probabilistic model of tumor image features. In D.W. Bates (Ed.), *AMIA Annu Symp Proc*, 354-358.

Johnson, S. B. (1996). Generic data modeling for clinical repositories. *J Am Med Inform Assoc, 3*(5), 328-339.

Kahn, C. E., Roberts, L. M., Shaffer, K. A., & Haddawy, P. (1997). Construction of a Bayesian network for mammographic diagnosis of breast cancer. *Computers in Biology and Medicine, 27*(1), 19-29.

Kline, J. A., Novobilski, A. J., Kabrhel, C., Richman, P. B., & Courtney, D. M. (2005). Derivation and validation of a Bayesian network to predict pretest probability of venous thromboembolism. *Annals of Emergency Medicine, 45*(3), 282-290.

Lavrac, N., Kononenko, I., Keravnou, E., Kukar, M., & Zupan, B. (1998). Intelligent data analysis for medical diagnosis: Using machine learning and temporal abstraction. *AI Communications, 11*(3), 191-218.

Leibovici, L., Fishman, M., Schonheyder, H. C., Riekehr, C., Kristensen, B., Shraga, I., et al. (2000). A causal probabilistic network for optimal treatment of bacterial infections. *IEEE Transactions on Knowledge and Data Engineering, 12*(4), 517-528.

Lisboa, P. J. G. (2002). A review of evidence of health benefit from artificial neural networks in medical intervention. *Neural Networks, 15*(1), 11-39.

Lucas, P. J., van der Gaag, L. C., & Abu-Hanna, A. (2004). Bayesian networks in biomedicine and health-care. *Artif Intell Med, 30*(3), 201-214.

Marcus, A. (1998). Metaphor design for user interfaces. *Conference on Human Factors in Computing Systems*, 129-130.

McCormack, M.J., Kenney, A.R., Bryant C.W., Covington C.D., Dickinson, R.L., Coggins R.E. et al. (2007). Patent No. WO/2007/030696. Geneva: World Intellectual Property Organization.

Meyer, J., Phillips, M. H., Cho, P. S., Kalet, I., & Doctor, J. N. (2004). Application of influence diagrams to prostate intensity-modulated radiation therapy plan selection. *Physics in Medicine and Biology, 49*(9), 1637-1653.

Monti, S. (1999). *Learning hybrid Bayesian networks from data.* (Ph.D. Dissertation, University of Pittsburgh, 1999).

Monti, S., & Carenini, G. (2000). Dealing with the expert inconsistency in probability elicitation. *IEEE Transactions on Knowledge and Data Engineering, 12*(4), 499-508.

Murphy, K. P. (2002). *Dynamic Bayesian Networks: Representation, Inference and Learning.* (Ph.D. Dissertation, University of California, Berkeley, 2002).

Nadkarni, P. M., Marenco, L., Chen, R., Skoufos, E., Shepherd, G., & Miller, P. (1999). Organization of heterogeneous scientific data using the EAV/CR representation. *J Am Med Inform Assoc, 6*(6), 478-493.

Nikiforidis, G. C., & Sakellaropoulos, G. C. (1998). Expert system support using Bayesian belief networks in the prognosis of head-injured patients of the ICU. *Med Inform (Lond), 23*(1), 1-18.

Ogunyemi, O. (2006). Methods for reasoning from geometry about anatomic structures injured by penetrating trauma. *J Biomedical Informatics, 39*(4), 389-400.

Pearl, J. (1988). *Probabilistic Reasoning in Intelligent Systems: Networks of Plausible Inference.* San Francisco, CA: Morgan Kaufmann.

Pham, D. L., Xu, C., & Prince, J. L. (2000). Current methods in medical image segmentation. *Annual Review of Biomedical Engineering, 2*(1), 315–337.

Rubin, D. L., Shah, N. H., & Noy, N. F. (2008). Biomedical ontologies: a functional perspective. *Brief Bioinform, 9*(1), 75-90.

Sebastiani, P., Ramoni, M. F., Nolan, V., Baldwin, C. T., & Steinberg, M. H. (2005). Genetic dissection and prognostic modeling of overt stroke in sickle cell anemia. *Nature Genetics, 37*, 435-440.

Shwe, M. A., Middleton, B., Heckerman, D. E., Henrion, M., Horvitz, E. J., Lehmann, H. P., et al. (1991). Probabilistic diagnosis using a reformulation of the INTERNIST-1/QMR knowledge base. I. The probabilistic model and inference algorithms. *Methods Inf Med, 30*(4), 241-255.

Shyu, C. R., Brodley, C. E., Kak, A. C., Kosaka, A., Aisen, A. M., & Broderick, L. S. (1999). ASSERT: A physician-in-the-loop content-based retrieval system for HRCT image databases. *Computer Vision and Image Understanding, 75*(1), 111-132.

Wyatt, J. C., & Wright, P. (1998). Design should help use of patients' data. *Lancet, 352*(9137), 1375-1378.

Yu, J., Smith, V.A., Wang, P.P., Hartemink, A.J., & Jarvis, E.D. (2004). Advances to Bayesian network inference for generating causal networks from observational biological data. *Bioinformatics, 20*(18), 3594-3603.

Zou, Q., Chu, W. W., Morioka, C., Leazer, G. H., & Kangarloo, H. (2003). IndexFinder: A method of extracting key concepts from clinical texts for indexing. In M. Musen (Ed.), *AMIA Annu Symp Proc*, 763-767.

KEY TERMS

Intelligent Data Analysis: The use of statistical, pattern recognition, machine learning, data abstraction, and visualization tools for analysis of data and discovery of mechanisms that created the data.

Data Mining: The principle of sorting through large amounts of data and picking out relevant information.

Probabilistic Graphical Model: A graph that represents independencies among random variables by a graph in which each node is a random variable and missing edges represent conditional independencies.

Bayesian Belief Network: A directed acyclic graph that represents a set of variables and their probabilistic independencies.

Dynamic Bayesian Network: A directed graphical model of stochastic processes that generalize hidden Markov models and are typically used to model a time series.

Graphical Metaphor: Unique and identifiable visual representations of variables specified in the disease model.

Visual Query Interface: A tool that enables user to visually interact with the underlying graphical model and guides the user through the query formulation process by adapting the interface based on the structure of the model.

Chapter III
Analysis and Quantification of Motion within the Cardiovascular System:
Implications for the Mechanical Strain of Cardiovascular Structures

Spyretta Golemati
National Technical University of Athens, Greece

John Stoitsis
National Technical University of Athens, Greece

Konstantina S. Nikita
National Technical University of Athens, Greece

ABSTRACT

The estimation of motion of the myocardial and arterial wall is important for the quantification of tissue elasticity and contractility and has gained attention as a determinant of cardiovascular disease. In this chapter, a review is attempted regarding the analysis and quantification of motion within the cardiovascular system from sequences of images. The main sources of cardiovascular wall motion include blood pressure, blood flow and tethering to surrounding tissue. The most commonly applied techniques for cardiovascular motion analysis include feature-based and pixel-based methodologies; the latter further include block matching, optical flow and registration techniques. Two distinct paradigms based on these methodologies are highlighted, namely myocardium and carotid artery wall motion. The current status of research in these areas is reviewed and future research directions are indicated.

INTRODUCTION

Cardiovascular disease (CVD) is caused by disorders of the heart and blood vessels, and includes coronary heart disease (heart attacks), cerebrovascular disease (stroke), raised blood pressure (hypertension), peripheral artery disease, rheumatic heart disease, congenital heart disease and heart failure. According to the World Health Organization (World Health Organization website), CVD is the number one cause of death globally and is projected to remain the leading cause of death. An estimated 17.5 million people died from cardiovascular disease in 2005, representing 30% of all global deaths. Of these deaths, 7.6 million were due to heart attacks and 5.7 million were due to stroke. Around 80% of these deaths occurred in low- and middle-income countries. If appropriate action is not taken, by 2015, an estimated 20 million people will die from cardiovascular disease every year, mainly from heart attacks and strokes.-

Clinical diagnosis, treatment and follow-up of cardiovascular disease are greatly aided by a number of imaging techniques which provide qualitative and quantitative information about morphology and function of the heart and the blood vessels. Furthermore, advanced image processing methods can be used to extract features from digitized images and facilitate image interpretation and subsequent decisions on disease management. Among such features, the estimation of motion of the myocardial and arterial wall is important for the quantification of tissue elasticity and contractility and has gained attention as a determinant of cardiovascular disease. Myocardial and arterial wall elasticity is altered with age as well as in the presence of pathology (eg. myocardial infarction, atherosclerosis) mainly due to altered wall composition.

In this chapter, a review is attempted regarding the analysis and quantification of motion within the cardiovascular system from sequences of images. The main sources of cardiovascular wall motion are described, techniques for imaging tissue motion are reported and the most commonly applied methodologies for motion estimation based on temporal image sequences are discussed. Specific clinical applications of these methodologies for the analysis and quantification of motion of the myocardium and the carotid artery wall are also presented within this chapter.

BACKGROUND

Motion of the Myocardial and Arterial Wall

Throughout the cardiovascular system, tissue motion is caused by blood pressure, blood flow and tethering to surrounding tissue. Blood pressure, commonly expressed in terms of the transmural pressure (intramural minus extramural), causes tensile stress in the wall. As the transmural pressure rises, mechanical stresses are induced in all directions within the wall. Compressive stress may occur and is enhanced when the less compliant deeper wall layers prevent the surface layers from expanding, resulting in further compression. Stresses in the longitudinal and circumferential directions, on the other hand, are generally tensile in nature, leading to tissue lengthening.

Unlike orthogonal forces such as those induced by transmural pressure, fluid shear generated by friction or viscous drag due to blood flow acts tangentially upon the cardiovascular wall and endothelium. The magnitude of fluid shear depends on factors such as local geometry, local velocity of blood flow and the viscosity of blood as largely related to the haematocrit. In the heart, shear strain may be developed between the endocardium, the myocardium and the pericardium, whereas in arteries between neighboring arterial layers (intima, media, adventitia) and between arterial wall and surrounding tissue. In arteries, atherosclerotic plaques tend to occur where flow velocity and shear stress are reduced and flow departs from a laminar unidirectional pattern. The relationship is unclear and may reflect a direct effect of shear on the wall. Many features of endothelial cell biology, including production of nitric oxide, are modified by shear. Alternatively, low flow characteristics tend to increase the residence time of circulating particles in susceptible regions while particles are cleared rapidly from regions of relatively high wall shear stress and laminar unidirectional flow.

Tether, a term used to describe the constraint imposed on the wall from the tissues surrounding it and from arterial side branches, is another source of wall motion. Tethering reduces motion due to haemodynamic factors but can induce wall movement due to body motion.

Cardiovascular structures are characterized by a wide variability of their material properties: (1) they are distinctly anisotropic; (2) their elastic properties are nonlinear, becoming stiffer with higher degrees of strain; and (3) in the case of atherosclerotic plaques, stiffness also increases with increases in frequency of applied stress.

Altered motion patterns of the myocardial wall in the presence of disease (eg. heart infarcts) include reduced mobility of wall segments. Such segments are usually characterized as hypokinetic or akinetic.

Mechanical factors are more complicated in the case of diseased (atherosclerotic) arterial walls, where the presence of atheromatous plaque alters the local geometry and, subsequently, blood flow and mechanical forces acting on the wall. Intrinsic mechanical forces clearly contribute to plaque rupture and occurrence of vascular symptoms (Falk et al., 1995). It has also been demonstrated that reduction of arterial wall motion inhibits experimentally mediated atherosclerosis (Tropea et al., 2000). Plaque rupture, often with thrombosis superimposed, is a complication of the advanced atherosclerotic lesion (Falk, 1992). It occurs when the tension on a plaque exceeds its tensile strength and may lead to acute ischaemic events (McIsaac et al., 1993). Plaque composition, rather than plaque size, seems to determine the risk of plaque rupture (Falk, 1992). Histological features that characterise the unstable (rupture-prone) plaque include a thin, eccentric fibrous cap and a large necrotic core of lipid and cellular debris (Lee & Libby, 1997). This plaque configuration is particularly unstable because large mechanical stresses develop in the thinnest portions of the fibrous cap. The soft lipid core is unable to bear these mechanical forces and excess stresses are thus "concentrated" in the fibrous cap, particularly at the junction with the normal vessel, also called the "shoulder" region (Lee & Libby, 1997). Even in a mildly stenosed model of a patient-derived artery with compliant wall, the plaque shoulder exhibited raised internal stress, which along with reversed flow in the post-stenotic zone, is believed to be important for the continued development of the plaque and for potentially catastrophic events in the end stages of the disease (Lee et al., 2004).

Imaging Cardiovascular Tissue Motion

Although the title of the very first description of echocardiography by Edler and Hertz (1954) mentioned 'recording of the movements of heart walls' as its goal, the objective and quantitative measurement of cardiovascular wall motion has remained difficult in clinical practice. Modern imaging systems allow real-time imaging of moving structures as well as storage of temporal image sequences, or cine loops, for further processing. Tissue motion can be quantitatively estimated from these sequences provided they are acquired at sufficiently high frame rates. The major imaging modalities allowing recording of wall motion include ultrasound and magnetic resonance imaging (MRI).

Ultrasound imaging is widely used in the diagnosis of cardiovascular disease because it allows non-invasive assessment of disease severity and tissue morphology. M-mode and real-time

B-mode scanning, although developed in the 1960s and 1970s respectively, are still the most commonly applied methods for studying tissue motion (Anderson & McDicken, 1999). They are now used in combination whereby the B-mode depicts the motion of tissues in a two-dimensional (2D) image and the M-mode provides more detailed information on how some selected tissue parts in the image move with time, often over several cardiac cycles. Images of moving tissue may also be produced by modifying the filters used in Doppler blood flow imaging to reject the low amplitude blood echoes and retain the higher amplitude signals from tissue; the technique is known as tissue Doppler imaging (TDI) (Yu et al., 2007). A disadvantage of both M-mode and TDI is that they provide motion estimation in only one direction, i.e. along the ultrasound beam axis. A recently introduced approach to imaging mechanical properties of tissue is elastography (Ophir et al., 1999). The method consists in calculating 2D local tissue strain through cross-correlation of radio-frequency segments for the estimation of the time shift resulting from a small deformation. Because ultrasonic images are 2D tomograms, three-dimensional (3D) reconstruction can be readily achieved off-line from multiple image slices if the imaging planes are spatially encoded. 3D real-time imaging (Nelson et al., 1999) is a relatively new development in ultrasound that allows 3D quantitation of organ dynamic geometry.

MRI is an established, although still rapidly advancing, imaging modality providing accurate quantification of anatomy, function, flow and perfusion of the cardiovascular system at rest and under stress conditions (J Magn Reson Imag, 1999). Compared to ultrasound imaging, MRI offers a wider topographical field of view (window) and superior contrast resolution resulting in easy definition of anatomical information without the need for contrast medium or invasive techniques. An MRI technique suitable for non-invasive assessment of tissue motion is MRI tagging (van der Geest & Reiber, 1999). With the use of this technique, cine MR images are acquired with a superimposed parallel grid of dark saturation lines. These tagging lines are induced by a special pre-pulse sequence immediately following the R-wave of the ECG and can subsequently be followed over the cardiac cycle. Dedicated computer algorithms can subsequently be used to track the intersection points of the tagging lines automatically over the cardiac cycle, to quantify tissue deformations. Another well-known MRI method for measuring local motion is motion-encoded phase-contrast imaging. In contrast to the tagging that image longitudinal magnetization, the motion-encoding methods obtain information about tissue dynamics by phase encoding the velocity of transverse magnetization (Mc Veigh, 1996). Over the past decade, MR elastography (MRE) has emerged as a sensitive method for noninvasively evaluating the mechanical properties of biological tissues (Manduca et al., 2001). MRE enables direct quantification of the viscoelastic mechanical properties of tissue by dynamically imaging the propagation of cyclical shear deformations that are induced in a material.

Methods for Cardiovascular Tissue Motion Analysis from Sequences of Images

A number of approaches have been used to recover cardiovascular motion from sequences of images. They can be divided into two main categories: (i) feature-based methodologies, and (ii) pixel-based methodologies. Techniques of each category, with their relative advantages and limitations, can be used to investigate different aspects of the motion field. The principal characteristics of methodologies of each category are described below.

Feature-based methodologies. These rely on the estimation of movement of salient features in the imaged scene (Aggarwal & Nandhakumar, 1988). Features include lines, edges, object boundaries, corners, etc. To apply such methodologies, the images need first be segmented so as to extract the features to be followed throughout the sequence. Rigid body motion is usually assumed for the extracted features (Fig. 1). Deformable models, designed to track deformable object contours, are more appropriate for biological structures (McInerney & Terzopoulos, 1996). In addition to this, the Hough Transform (HT), which detects parametric curves in an image, may be applied to individual sequence images to track the location of straight lines, circles or ellipses, corresponding to anatomical structures of interest (Nash et al., 1997).

Pixel-based methodologies. These allow for motion estimation by studying displacement between frames at the pixel level. The most widely used pixel-based methodologies in medical image applications include block matching, optical flow and registration methods.

Block matching. Given a block of pixels, or reference block, in the first of two images, matching consists in finding the block in the second image that best matches the block in the first image, termed reference image (Dufaux & Moscheni, 1995) (Fig. 2a). This definition relies on the assumption that the reference block remains constant over time and motion which is valid if the frame rate is sufficiently high. The method requires a good measure of match. The value of such a measure should be large when the selected block and the interrogated image region coincide in intensity levels and small otherwise. The search for the best-matched block is typically constrained to a search window, the size of which has to be appropriately chosen because it may affect motion analysis results. A large search window allows accurate tracking of rapid movements that could be lost if the search widow was smaller, but increases the possibility for mismatch and the computational complexity of the algorithm. In conventional block matching methods, pixel velocities are considered constant within pixel blocks. To overcome this constraint, the affine block motion model (Fig. 2b) can be used to estimate the velocity field of a block that undergoes not only translation but also rotation and scaling (Glasbey & Madria, 1998).

Optical flow. Optical flow relies on the estimation of the spatiotemporal change of the intensities of individual pixels, rather than of blocks of pixels, throughout an image sequence (Dufaux & Moscheni, 1995). The result is a dense vector map where each pixel is represented by a vector corresponding to its velocity between two frames (Fig. 3). The assumption is made that the intensity of a given pixel is constant between two consecutive frames of the sequence. This assumption is true when the temporal separation between the two frames is small, or, in other words, when the frame rate is high.

Figure 1. Schematic illustration of feature-based motion analysis algorithm. (a) Reference image. (b) Interrogated (current) image.

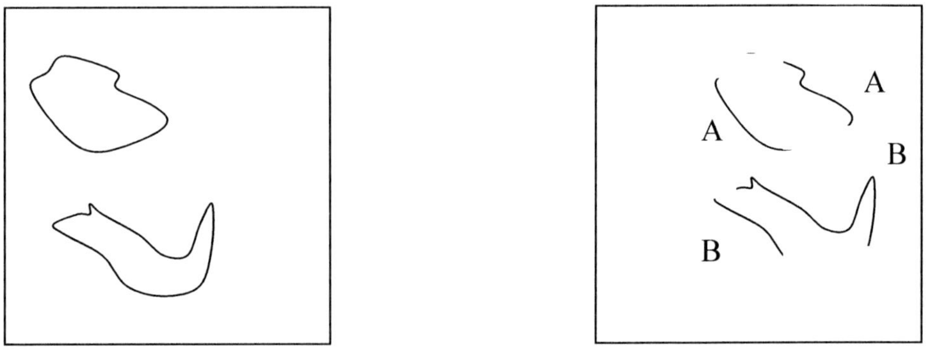

Figure 2. Schematic illustration of block matching algorithms. (a) Conventional block matching. Motion of a block of pixels is estimated by searching for the most similar block of pixels in a search window at subsequent frames. (b) Affine block matching. Motion of a block of pixels is estimated by wrapping the block at the current frame according to the affine parameters computed in the previous frame.

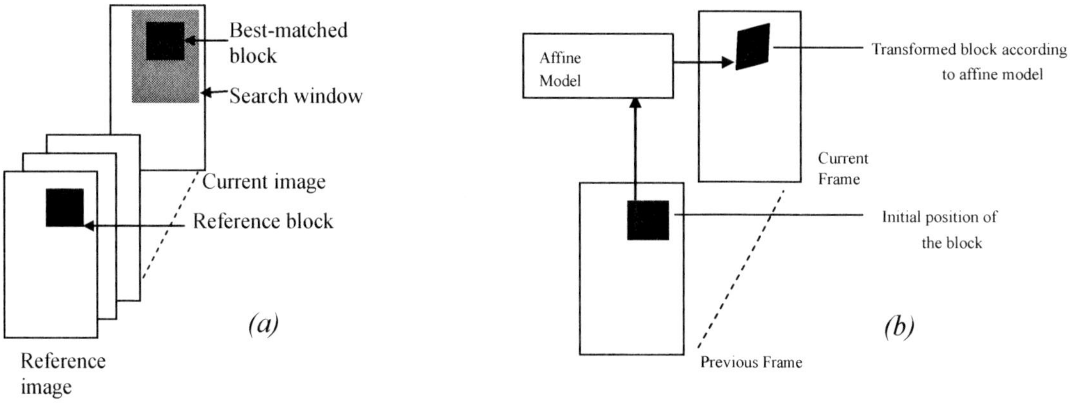

Figure 3. Schematic illustration of the optical flow algorithm. The optical flow at the pixel (x,y) is the 2D-velocity vector ($\frac{dx}{dt}, \frac{dy}{dt}$).

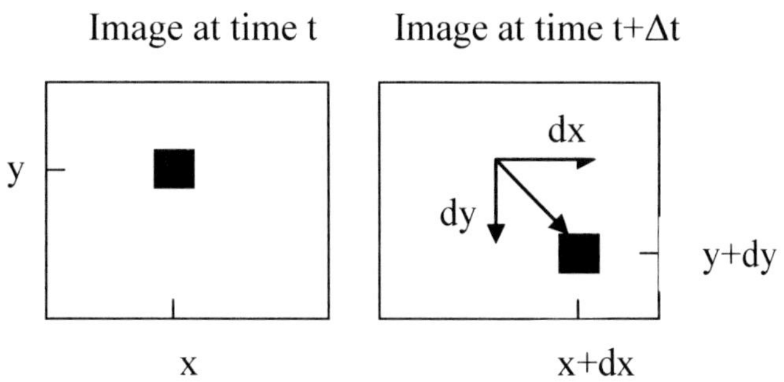

Registration. Image registration consists in finding a correspondence function (transformation) mapping coordinates from a reference image to coordinates of homologous point in a test image (Fig. 4). Registration methods are usually applied to data acquired at the same time point either to achieve multimodal integration or to compensate for small misalignments. Motion tracking applications of registration techniques have also been reported. Registration schemes may be rigid, when only translations and rotations are allowed, affine, when the transformation maps parallel lines onto parallel lines (Maintz & Viergever, 1998) or nonrigid, allowing for soft tissue deformation (Crum et al., 2004). Optical flow has been used in combination with registration approaches to enhance the efficiency of the latter.

The selection of the appropriate methodology to be used in a specific application depends on a number of factors, including (a) the type of motion information that is required, (b) the quality of the available images and (c) the merits and demerits of particular methods. Feature-based methodologies are suitable for applications in which feature segmentation is a feasible task; they may not be the optimal choice in cases where

Figure 4. Schematic illustration of image registration. The correspondence function, f(x,y), maps coordinates from a reference image (a) to coordinates of homologous points in the current image (b).

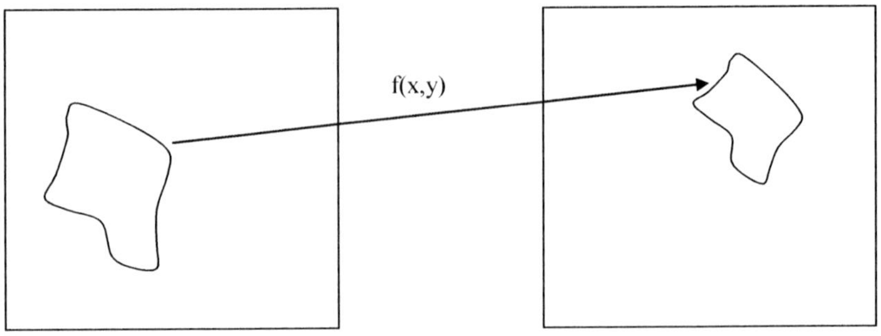

image features have a fuzzy appearance, as is the case of noisy ultrasound images. A limitation of these methodologies is the assumption of rigid body motion which may not be representative of anatomical structures. Pixel-based methodologies do not rely on such assumptions, but require that motion be smooth and small thus requiring high rates of image acquisition. In particular, a limitation of optical flow approaches is its sensitivity to noise due to its dependence on spatio-temporal gradients.

CLINICAL APPLICATIONS

A number of approaches based on the methods described in the previous section have been used to estimate different aspects of the displacement fields of the myocardial and arterial wall described in section II.A. In this section, examples of such applications are presented concerning the study of motion of the myocardium and arterial wall. These are the most studied anatomical structures of the cardiovascular system, probably because they are associated with the two main causes of death due to cardiovascular disease, namely heart attack and stroke, respectively.

Reliable analysis and quantification of tissue motion requires the use of (i) an appropriate imaging modality allowing the recording of temporal image sequences at sufficiently high frame rates and (ii) a robust technique for processing the acquired image sequences. The use of standardized procedures, in the form of a carefully designed protocol, is crucial not only for image recording but also for accurate interpretation of the motion analysis results. Technical issues related to constraints imposed by cardiovascular wall physiology and physical principles of the imaging modality should be taken into account in such protocols. More specifically, issues including the subject setup, the imaging angle of the anatomical structure of interest and the consideration of sources of displacement other than the cardiovascular forces, should be addressed in a clinical protocol. In addition to this, the settings of the imaging modality during the recording process should also be determined in the same protocol.

Myocardium

The estimation of cardiac motion contributes in identifying localized regions exhibiting movement abnormalities, which are indicative of the existence of ischemic segments caused by insufficient tissue microcirculation. A large number of approaches have been developed to describe and quantify heart motion. They may be divided into three main categories: (i) estimation of endocardial motion through image intensity changes, (ii) detection and tracking of boundary of anatomical structures (eg. ventricular wall) and (iii) tracking of anatomical, implanted or induced myocardial landmarks (Frangi et al., 2001).

Optical flow, block matching and registration methods have been applied to approximate motion estimation problems of the first category. Sühling et al. (2004) used multiscale motion mapping, a technique similar to optical flow, to determine motion and deformation at arbitrary locations of synthetic and real echocardiograms. The usefulness of the method was demonstrated in a series of complex motion analyses that included abnormal septal motion and analysis of myocardial twisting. Ledesma-Carbayo et al. (2005) proposed a novel spatio-temporal elastic registration algorithm to estimate myocardial displacement fields from 2D ultrasound sequences. The key feature of the algorithm consists in the use of an analytical representation of the displacement based on a semilocal parametric model of the deformation using B-splines. Application to real image sequences showed that displacement and strain parameters were significantly different for normal, hypokinetic and akinetic myocardial segments.

Curvature-matching has been used to find point correspondences in an attempt to automatically track nonrigid cardiac structures (Amini & Duncan, 1992; Benayoun & Ayache, 1998). Amini & Duncan (1992) presented a unified framework for motion tracking of curves and surfaces using elastic models of the objects and constraints on the types of motion. Potential applications of the methodology were illustrated in 3D MR and computed-tomography image sequences. More recently, a number of approaches have been proposed for automated detection and tracking of endocardial structures from 2D or 3D image sequences allowing measurement of global functional parameters (Angelini et al., 2005; Gérard et al., 2002; Zagrodsky et al., 2005). Most of these methodologies require a manual initialization step, thus compromising the reproducibility of the analysis. Zagrodsky et al (2005) proposed an automatic, registration-assisted, initialization which, however, suffers from being time-consuming. Alternative approaches to automated initialization for segmentation and tracking of the endocardial wall border included the use of the HT for circles in MR (van der Geest et al., 1997; Müller et al., 2005) and ultrasound images (Van Stralen et al., 2008). The methodology presented by van Stralen et al (2008) used the HT to detect candidate left ventricle center points subsequently used to detect the ventricle long axis by combining dynamic programming in 3D and 2D+time data. The demonstrated robustness, accuracy and low computational cost of the methodology make it a valuable starting point for various high-level segmentation techniques.

Landmark-based methods provide information on material point correspondence. Implanted markers suffer from being invasive, precluding their routine use in humans. Although they are regarded as the gold standard, there are some concerns in the literature about their effect on both image quality and modification of the motion patterns (Frangi et al., 2001). Among potential anatomical markers, coronary artery bifurcation points and the mitral valve annulus have been reported. Nevo et al. (2007) used multidimensional dynamic programming combined with apodized block matching to automatically track the mitral valve hinge points motion from echocardiographic images. For sequences of 20 patients with acute myocardial infarction, the automatic technique agreed well with results obtained manually and outperformed two commonly used tracking methods, namely forward tracking and minimum tracking.

Carotid Arteries

Motion of the normal and diseased carotid artery wall is important in the diagnosis of carotid atherosclerosis. The motion patterns of atheromatous plaques may be related to the risk for cerebrovascular complications, such as stroke. Studies on the analysis and quantification of motion of the carotid artery wall are relatively limited – especially when compared to those about myocardial wall motion – and are based on the processing of temporal sequences of 2D and 3D ultrasound images.

Block-matching-based techniques have been used to estimate arterial motion from B-mode (Golemati et al., 2003; Cinthio et al., 2005; Cinthio et al., 2006) and radiofrequency (Bang et al., 2003; Dahl et al., 2004) ultrasound images using high frame rates; 25 Hz in (Golemati et al., 2003) and 55 Hz in (Cinthio et al., 2005; Cinthio et al., 2006; Bang et al., 2003; Dahl et al., 2004). Golemati et al. (2003) estimated motion at the wall-lumen interface and within the tissue using block sizes of 3.2×2.5 mm and 6.3×2.5 mm, respectively, and the normalized correlation coefficient as the matching criterion. Measurements in 9 normal (non-atherosclerotic) adults showed that arterial wall distensibility in the radial direction was significantly higher than distensibility in the longitudinal direction (10.2±4.5% vs. 2.5±0.89%).

Cinthio et al (2005) designed and evaluated a novel non-invasive echo-tracking system based on block matching for measurement of radial and longitudinal motion of the arterial wall. They used a small block size, namely 0.7×0.7 mm, which allowed them to estimate motion of individual arterial layers. Reproducibility, or intra-rater variability, was determined in terms of the standard deviation of the measurements in in-vitro experiments using an agar phantom. Recordings including three periods of 0.5 Hz square wave movements of amplitudes ranging from 0.05 to 2 mm showed that reproducibility ranged from 0 to 8 μm for the radial direction and from 0 to 12 μm for the longitudinal direction. Experiments in 10 healthy humans showed a distinct bidirectional longitudinal movement of the intima-media complex during the cardiac cycle (Cinthio et al., 2006). More specifically, an antegrade movement, i.e., in the direction of the blood flow, in early systole was followed by a retrograde movement, i.e., opposite the direction of blood flow, later in systole and a second antegrade movement in diastole. The adventitial region showed the same basic pattern of longitudinal movement, but with lower magnitude; thereby introducing shear strain and, thus, shear stress within the wall.

Bang et al. (2003) studied motion dynamics of carotid plaques using a computerized method based on cross-correlation similar to that used by Golemati et al (2003). Their method produced a dense displacement vector map from which 29 parameters were estimated representing amplitude, stretch/compression and shear motion (Dahl et al., 2004). They made five independent recordings of two-three heart cycles each in 12 patients to study intra-operator variability between recordings and between heart cycles within individual recordings. Of the 29 motion parameters, 7 were found to reproduce well and their ability to discriminate between plaque types should be further investigated; these parameters describe tensional and torsional motion, in addition to mere velocity amplitude. With regard to the acquisition scheme, averaging of three repeated recordings, each covering at least two heart cycles, yielded acceptable accuracy.

An optical-flow-based approach was one of the first attempts to quantitatively analyze carotid artery motion (Chan, 1993). In that study, 2D motion analysis from ultrasound images was performed for low frame rates, namely 1 Hz, and a small number of tracked points. Meairs and Hennerici (1999) used optical flow to estimate carotid plaque surface motion from three-dimensional (3D) ultrasound image sequences obtained at a frame rate of 25 Hz. 13 symptomatic and 18 asymptomatic plaques with no significant differences in echogenicity or surface structure were investigated. Asymptomatic plaques had surface motion vectors of equal orientation and magnitude to those of the internal carotid artery, whereas symptomatic plaques demonstrated evidence of inherent plaque movement. Maximal surface velocity was not different between the two plaque types, but maximal discrepant velocity, defined as the maximal difference between maximal and minimal velocities, was significantly higher in symptomatic plaques. Mokhtari-Dizajl et al (2006) used an optical-flow-based motion analysis algorithm to estimate systolic and diastolic diameters of the right common carotid artery from sequences of colour Doppler ultrasound images acquired at a frame rate of 30 Hz. They subsequently calculated standard arterial stiffness indices, which were found to be significantly different in subjects with severe, i.e. greater than 40%, stenosis compared to subjects with mild or no stenosis.

Recently, Golemati et al (2007) used a feature-based methodology, namely the Hough Transform (HT), to automatically extract straight lines and circles from sequences of B-mode ultrasound images of longitudinal and transverse sections, respectively, of the carotid artery. Extracted features were further used to estimate vessel diameters as well as indices of arterial wall physiology, such as the intima-media thickness and the arterial distension waveform. The results were reasonably similar to those obtained using block matching; suggesting the possibility of using the HT to segment dynamic images of the carotid artery.

FUTURE TRENDS

The analysis and quantification of motion within the cardiovascular system is expected to provide valuable information about myocardial and arterial wall mechanics. Future trends in this challenging field include three major axes of potential research interest:

(1) The development, implementation and validation of a large number of motion estimation algorithms capable to efficiently quantify wall strain under a variety of clinical scenarios.

(2) The selection of appropriate methods from a pool of robust algorithms (see (a)) and their systematic application in large-scale clinical studies to demonstrate the usefulness of quantitatively assessed contractility as a determinant of cardiovascular disease.

(3) The combination of wall contractility indices with other clinical biomarkers of cardiovascular disease (eg. genetic, clinical, image-based) in an integrated diagnosis support system. This should allow global description of different disease patterns, characterized by different combinations of markers' values, and may contribute not only to early and valid diagnosis of cardiovascular disease but also to optimized selection of treatment schemes.

DISCUSSION AND CONCLUSION

Motion of the cardiovascular tissue, which may be used to quantify tissue elasticity and contractility and is considered a determinant of cardiovascular disease, can be efficiently estimated from temporal image sequences using a number of feature-based, pixel-based and registration methodologies. A carefully designed study protocol taking into account technical issues important for reliable image recording is crucial for valid interpretation of the motion analysis results.

An important step in the estimation of tissue motion is the validation of the motion analysis techniques. Validation may be achieved using either specially devised phantoms which simulate the properties of biological tissue or computer-generated images. Tissue-mimicking phantoms have proved useful in validation experiments (Cinthio et al., 2005; Bang et al., 2003; Dineley et al., 2006), but require specialized equipment which may not be easily available. Software programs capable of simulating medical images have been developed, which allow the evaluation not only of imaging modality settings but also of image processing methods. As an example, FIELD II, an ultrasound simulation package, was used to evaluate the accuracy of a spatio-temporal nonrigid registration algorithm for ultrasound cardiac motion estimation (Ledesma-Carbayo et al., 2005).

The motion field of the healthy and diseased cardiovascular wall remains to be studied in detail using one or more appropriate algorithms. Indices of motion may subsequently be combined with (i) other image-derived indices, including tissue echogenicity and (ii) clinical markers of disease, in an attempt to globally characterize the physiology of the cardiovascular tissue. Further in-depth investigation of the myocardial and arterial wall motion may provide useful insights into the mechanisms of cardiovascular disease and may assist in selection of optimal treatment.

REFERENCES

Aggarwal, J. K., & Nandhakumar, N. (1988). On the computation of motion from sequences of images – A review. *Proceedings of the IEEE*, *76*(8), 917-935.

Amini, A. A., & Duncan, J. S. (1992). Bending and stretching models for LV wall motion analysis from curves and surfaces. *Image and Vision Computing*, *10*(6), 418-430.

Anderson, T., & McDicken, W. N. (1999). Measurement of tissue motion. *Proceedings of the Institution of Mechanical Engineers*, *213*(3), 181-191.

Angelini, E. D., Homma, S., Pearson, G., Holmes, J. W., & Laine, A. F. (2005). Segmentation of real-time three-dimensional ultrasound for quantification of ventricular function: A clinical study on right and left ventricles. *Ultrasound in Medicine and Biology*, *31*(9), 1143-1158.

Bang, J., Dahl, T., Bruinsma, A., Kaspersen, J. H., Hernes, T. A. N., & Myhre, H. O. (2003). A new method for analysis of motion of carotid plaques from rf ultrasound images. *Ultrasound in Medicine and Biology*, *29*(7), 967-976.

Benayoun, S., & Ayache, N. (1998). Dense non-rigid motion estimation in sequences of medical images using differential constraints. *International Journal of Computer Vision*, *26*(1), 25-40.

Chan, K. L. (1993). Two approaches to motion analysis of the ultrasound image sequence of carotid atheromatous plaque. *Ultrasonics*, *31*(12), 117-123.

Cinthio, M., Ahlgren, A. R., Jansson, J. T., Eriksson, A., Persson, H. W., & Lindström, K. (2005). Evaluation of an ultrasonic echo-tracking method for measurements of arterial wall movements in two dimensions. *IEEE Transactions on Ultrasonics, Ferroelectrics and Frequency Control*, *52*(8), 1300-1311.

Cinthio, M., Ahlgren, A. R., Bergkvist, J., Jansson, T, Persson H. W., & Lindström, K. (2006). Longitudinal movements and resulting shear strain of the arterial wall. *American Journal of Physiology – Heart and Circulatory Physiology*, *291*(1), H394-H402.

Crum, W. R., Hartkens, T., & Hill D. L. (2004). Non-rigid image registration: theory and practice. *British Journal of Radiology*, *77*(2), S140-S153.

Dahl, T., Bang, J., Ushakova, A., Lydersen, S., & Myhre, H. O. (2004). Parameters describing motion in carotid artery plaques from ultrasound examination: a reproducibility study. *Ultrasound in Medicine and Biology*, *30*(9), 1133-1143.

Dineley, J., Meagher, S., Poepping, T. L., McDicken, W. N., Hoskins, P. R. (2006). Design and characterisation of a wall motion phantom. *Ultrasound in Medicine and Biology*, *32*(9), 1349-1357.

Dufaux, F., & Moscheni, F. (1995). Motion estimation techniques for digital TV: a review and a new contribution. *Proceeding of the IEEE*, *83*(6), 858-876.

Edler, I., & Hertz, C. H. (1954). The use of ultrasonic reflectoscope for the continuous recording of the movements of heart walls. *Kungl Fysiografiska Sällskapets i Lund Förhandlingar, 24*(5), 1-19.

Falk, E., Shah, P. K., & Fuster, V. (1995). Coronary plaque disruption. *Circulation, 92*(3), 657-671.

Frangi, A. F., Niessen, W. J., & Viergever, M. A. (2001). Three-dimensional modeling for functional analysis of cardiac images: a review. *IEEE Transactions on Medical Imaging, 20*(1), 2-25.

Gérard, O., Billon, A. C., Rouet, J. M., Jacob, M., Fradkin, M., & Allouche, C. (2005). Efficient model-based quantification of left ventricular function in 3-D echocardiography. *IEEE Transactions on Medical Imaging, 21*(9), 1059-1068.

Glasbey, C. A., & Madria, K. V. (1998). A review of image-warping methods *Journal of Applied Statistics, 25*(2), 155–171.

Golemati, S., Sassano, A., Lever, M. J., Bharath, A. A., Dhanjil, S., Nicolaides, A. N. (2003). Motion analysis of carotid atherosclerotic plaque from B-mode ultrasound. *Ultrasound in Medicine and Biology, 29*(3), 387-399.

Golemati, S., Stoitsis, J., Sifakis E. G., Balkizas, T., & Nikita K. S. (2007). Using the Hough Transform to segment ultrasound images of longitudinal and transverse sections of the carotid artery. *Ultrasound in Medicine and Biology, 33*(12), 1918-1932.

J Magn Reson Imag (1999). *Special issue: Cardiovascular MRI, 10*(5).

Ledesma-Carbayo, M. J., Kybic, J., Desco, M., Santos, A., Sühling, M., Hunziker, P., & Unser, M. (2005). Spatio-temporal nonrigid registration for ultrasound cardiac motion estimation. *IEEE Transactions on Medical Imaging, 24*(9), 1113-1126.

Lee, K. W., Wood, N. B., & Xu, X. Y. (2004). Ultrasound image-based computer model of a common carotid artery with a plaque. *Medical Engineering Physics, 26*(10), 823-840.

Lee, R. T., & Libby, P. (1997). The unstable atheroma. *Arteriosclerosis Thrombosis Vascular Biology, 17*(10), 1859-1867.

Maintz, J. B. A., & Viergever, M. A. (1998). A survey of medical image registration. *Medical Image Analysis, 2*(1), 1-36.

Manduca, A., Oliphant, T. E., Dresner, M. A., Mahowald, J. L., Kruse, S. A., Amromin, E., Felmlee, J. P., Greenleaf, J. F., & Ehman, R. L. (2001). Magnetic resonance elastography: noninvasive mapping of tissue elasticity. *Medical Image Analysis, 5*(4), 237-254.

McInerney, T., & Terzopoulos, D. (1996). Deformable models in medical image analysis: a survey. *Medical Image Analysis, 1*(2), 91-108.

McIsaac, A. I., Thomas, J. D., & Topol, E. J. (1993). Toward the quiescent coronary plaque. *Journal of the American College of Cardiology, 22*(4), 1228-1241.

Mc Veigh, E. R. (1996). MRI of myocardial function: motion tracking techniques. *Magnetic Resonance Imaging, 14*(2), 137-150.

Meairs, S., & Hennerici, M. (1999). Four-dimensional ultrasonographic characterization of plaque surface motion in patients with symptomatic and asymptomatic carotid artery stenosis. *Stroke, 30*(9), 1807-1813.

Mokhtari-Dizajl, M., Montazeri, M., & Saberi, H. (2006). Differentiation of mild and severe stenosis with motion estimation in ultrasound images. *Ultrasound in Medicine and Biology, 32*(10), 1493-1498.

Müller, A., Neitmann, A., Merkle, N., Wohrle, J., Hombach, V., & Kestler, H. A. (2005). Contour detection of short axis slice MR images for contraction irregularity assessment. *Computers in Cardiology, 32*, 21-24.

Nash, J. M., Carter, J. N., & Nixon, M. S. (1997). Dynamic feature extraction via the velocity

Hough transform. *Pattern Recognition Letters, 18*, 1035-1047.

Nelson, T. R., Downey, D. B., Pretorius, D. H., & Fenster, A. (1999). *Three-dimensional Ultrasound.* Philadelphia, PA: Lippincot, Williams & Wilkins.

Nevo, S. T., van Stralen, M., Vossepoel, A. M., Reiber, J. H. C., de Jong, N., van der Oteen, A. F. W., & Bosch, J. G. (2007). Automated tracking of the mitral valve annulus motion in apical echocardiographic images using multidimensional dynamic programming. *Ultrasound in Medicine and Biology, 33*(9), 1389-1399.

Ophir, J., Alam, S. K., Garra, B., Kallel, F., Konofagou, E. E., Krouskop, T., & Varghese, T. (1999). Elastography: ultrasonic estimation and imaging of the elastic properties of tissues. *Proceedings of the Institution of Mechanical Engineers, 213*(3), 203-233.

Sühling, M., Jansen, C., Arigovindan, M., Buser, P., Marsch, P., Unser, M., & Hunziker, P. (2004). Multiscale motion mapping – A novel computer vision technique for quantitative, objective echocardiographic motion measurement independent of Doppler – First clinical description and validation. *Circulation, 110*(19), 3093-3099.

Tropea, B. I., Schwarzacher, S. P., Chang, A., Asvar, C., Huie, P., Sibley, R. K., & Zarins, C. K. (2000). Reduction of aortic wall motion inhibits hypertension-mediated experimental atherosclerosis. *Arteriosclerosis Thrombosis Vascular Biology, 20*(9), 2127-2133.

Van der Geest, R. J., Buller, V. G., Jansen, E., Lamb, H. J., Baur, L. H., van der Wall, E. E., de Roos, A., & Reiber, J. H. C. (1997). Comparison between manual and semiautomated analysis of left ventricular volume parameters from short-axis MR images. *Journal of Computer Assisted Tomography, 21*(5), 756-765.

Van der Geest, R. J., & Reiber, J. H. C. (1999). Quantification in cardiac MRI. *Journal of Magnetic Resonance Imaging, 10*(5), 602-608.

Van Stralen, M., Leung, K. Y. E., Voormolen, M. M., de Jong, N., van der Steen, A. F. W., Reiber, J. H. C., & Bosch, J. G. (2008). Time continuous detection of the left ventricular long axis and the mitral valve plane in 3-D echocardiography. *Ultrasound in Medicine and Biology, 34*(2), 196-207.

Yu, C. M., Sanderson, J., E., Marwick, T. H., & Oh, J. K. (2007). Tissue Doppler imaging – A new prognosticator for cardiovascular diseases. *Journal of the American College of Cardiology, 49*(9), 1903-1914.

World Health Organization website, www.who.int/ncd/cvd.

Zagrodsky, V., Walimbe, V., Castro-Pareja, C. R., Qin, J. X., Song, J. M., & Shekhar, R. (2005). Registration-assisted segmentation of real-time 3-D echocardiographic data using deformable models. *IEEE Transactions on Medical Imaging, 24*(9), 1089-1099.

KEY TERMS

Tissue Motion Analysis: Detection and tracking of motion of manually or automatically selected tissue areas from temporal image sequences using appropriate image processing methodologies.

Tissue Motion Quantification: Extraction of indices characterizing tissue motion patterns. (Tissue motion patterns may have been estimated using tissue motion analysis – see above).

Imaging Modality: System making use of fundamental concepts of physical science (eg. acoustics, magnetic resonance, X-ray, nuclear physics) to provide images of biological tissues.

Cardiovascular Forces: Mechanical forces exerted on the myocardium and the arterial wall. They are due to blood pressure, blood flow and tethering to surrounding tissue. They are responsible for cardiovascular tissue strain, expressed through its motion pattern.

Feature-Based Methodologies (for motion analysis): Methodologies which rely on the identification and subsequent motion estimation of salient features in the imaged scene.

Pixel-Based Methodologies (for motion analysis): Methodologies which rely on the differences of pixel intensities between frames of a sequence.

Registration Methodologies (for motion analysis): Methodologies which rely on recovering a correspondence function mapping coordinates from a reference image to coordinates of homologous point in a test image.

Chapter IV
New Developments in Intracoronary Ultrasound Processing

Christos V. Bourantas
Michailideion Cardiology Center, Greece & University of Hull, UK

Katerina K. Naka
Michailideion Cardiology Center, Greece

Dimitrios I. Fotiadis
Michailideion Cardiology Center, Greece

Lampros K. Michalis
Michailideion Cardiology Center, Greece

ABSTRACT

Intracoronary Ultrasound (ICUS) imaging is an intravascular catheter-based technique which provides real-time, high resolution, cross-sectional images of coronary arteries. In these images the lumen, the media-adventitia border, the plaque burden and the composition of the plaque can be identified. Conventionally, ICUS border detection is performed manually. However, this process is laborious and time consuming. To enhance the clinical applicability of ICUS, several automated algorithms have been developed for fast ICUS segmentation and characterisation of the type of the plaque. In this chapter the authors present an overview on the developments in ICUS processing and they describe advanced methodologies which fuse ICUS and X-ray angiographic data in order to overcome indigenous limitations of ICUS imaging and provide complete and geometrically correct coronary reconstruction.

INTRODUCTION

Accurate assessment of luminal pathology is useful for the diagnosis and treatment of coronary artery disease. The traditional method used for the depiction of coronary artery morphology is coronary angiography, which provides two–dimensional (2-D) views of the luminal silhouette. Major limitation of this modality is its inability to provide information regarding the plaque burden and the composition of the plaque, data which are useful to guide treatment and estimate prognosis.

To overcome these limitations intracoronary ultrasound (ICUS) has been introduced. ICUS requires the insertion of a catheter, within the coronary artery. At the tip of the catheter there is a transducer which transmits ultrasound signal perpendicular to its axis. There are two types of ICUS systems: the "mechanical" and the "electronic" ICUS systems. In mechanical systems a single rotating transducer, at 1800 rpm (30 revolutions per second), sweeps a high frequency (20 – 40 MHz) ultrasound signal perpendicular to the axis of the catheter, while in electronic systems there is an array of small crystals which have been programmed so that one set of crystals to transmit and the other to receive simultaneously. In both systems cross–sectional images of the coronary artery are produced by detecting the reflections of the ultrasound signal while this is passing through the vessel. As the ICUS catheter is pulled–back (either manually or by a motorized pull–back device) a series of images is generated. In each image, the luminal border, the outer vessel wall border (in the text the term media–adventitia border is used), the stent border, the plaque and the composition of the plaque can be identified and accurate measurements can be obtained (Mintz et al., 2001).

In ICUS images there are often several artefacts which may reduce the ability to identify the regions of interest (Figure 1). These artefacts include: the non–uniform rotational distortion which appears only in the mechanical ICUS systems, the ring down artefact (a bright halo surrounding the transducer) that is due to a high amplitude of the ultrasound signal, the guide wire artefact, the near field artefact, the blood speckles artefact, etc. (Nissen et al., 1993).

Initially, ICUS border detection was performed manually. However, it became apparent that this process is laborious, time consuming and can be unreliable in the hands of inexperienced operators. Therefore, there was an emerging interest in the development of fast and accurate (semi-) automated segmentation algorithms which would enhance the clinical applicability of ICUS. These algorithms had to face several challenges mostly caused by the high noise content, the low image resolution, the non–uniform luminance and contrast as well as the presence of the above mentioned artefacts.

Another problem that needed to be addressed was the reliable identification of the type of the plaque as well as the integration of the detected ICUS borders into a 3-D object which would represent the coronary vessel. Some of the earlier work on the 3-D reconstruction and visualization of the ICUS sequence assumed that the vessels were straight. However, with this assumption, ICUS could not provide any information on the 3-D arterial geometry or the spatial orientation of the plaque onto the artery. To overcome these limitations fusion of biplane angiographic data and ICUS has been proposed.

In this chapter we attempt to present an overview of the developments in ICUS processing. This review is organised as follows: in the next section we describe the segmentation algorithms which have been introduced for ICUS border detection and plaque characterization. We also present methodologies which have been initially proposed for 3-D coronary reconstruction. In the main part of the chapter we describe novel techniques able to fuse ICUS and angiographic data in order to generate geometrically correct coronary segments. In addition, we present two advanced user–friendly systems, that incorporate these data fusion techniques and allow reliable and comprehensive coronary representation with the general goal to show future trends and interesting potentialities of these systems.

BACKGROUND

(Semi-) Automated Border Detection Algorithms

Over the last two decades a multitude of methodologies has been introduced for the segmentation of the ICUS images. The first semi–automated method was described by Dhawale et al. (1993). Their approach required an expert observer to approximate the regions of interest in each ICUS image. These estimations were then used to guide a 1-D dynamic search algorithm. Two years later, Sonka et al. (1995) developed a faster segmentation methodology. His approach incorporated *a priori* knowledge of the ICUS images' characteristics and utilised a minimum cost algorithm for border detection. In this method an expert observer had to approximate the regions of interest only in the first image and afterwards the algorithm found automatically the regions of interest in the next frames. Bouma et al. (1996) were the first to introduce a fully automated methodology for luminal border detection. This approach processed images obtained at the same coronary segment and at the same phase of the cardiac circle to detect the region with different luminosity. This region corresponded to the blood speckles and thus to the lumen. Even though this method was fully automated, it had limited clinical applicability since it failed to identify the media–adventitia border and required an increased number of ICUS frames.

Von Birgelen et al. (1996) developed a semi–automated, clinically applicable segmentation methodology. Their approach utilised a minimum cost algorithm for border detection. Initially, they modelled the ICUS sequence in a 3-D cylinder–like object. In a next step, a minimum cost algorithm was applied to identify the regions of interests in longitudinal cut planes of the object.

Figure 1. Structures and artefacts observed in an ICUS image

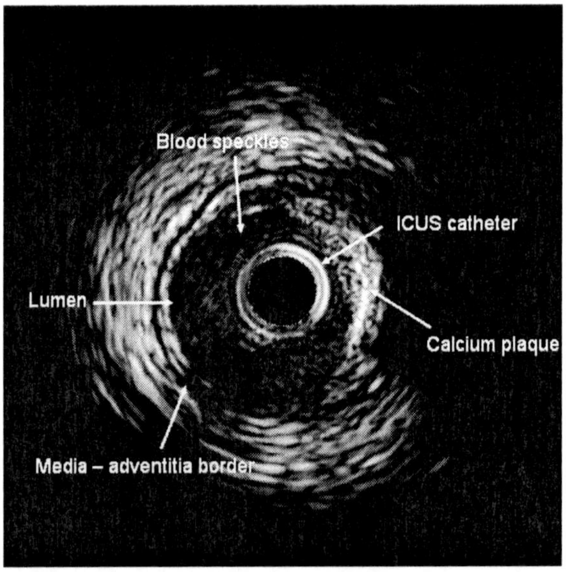

These borders were then transferred onto the ICUS images and used to guide the segmentation of each image.

Lobregt and Viergever (1995) suggested the use of deformable models (snakes) for ICUS border detection. Snakes are parametrical curves that are described by an energy function. In an ICUS image the deformable models have the ability to be attracted by the regions of interest which minimize their energy function. This desirable feature renders them useful in ICUS processing. Thus, over the last years many methodologies have incorporated deformable models for ICUS border detection (Plissiti et al., 2004; Giannoglou et al., 2007; Sanz-Requena et al., 2007). An interesting approach was introduced by Plissiti et al. (2004). In their method a Hopfield neural network was utilised to expedite the minimisation of the deformable model's energy function. They also incorporated efficient algorithms to overcome common artefacts observed in ICUS images (e.g. the blood speckle artefact and the guide wire artefact) and to address ordinary problems in ICUS segmentation such as the increased noise and the computation of the media–adventitia border in images where calcified lesions are present. In 1999 Shekhar et al. (1999) modelled the ICUS sequence into a 3-D cylinder–like object and then they used for first time a 3-D deformable model to identify the regions of interest. A year later Kovalski et al. (2000) suggested a modification in the energy function of the 3-D model introducing the balloon snakes while in 2002 Klingensmith and Vince (2002) proposed a segmentation approach based on 3-D B-spline surfaces.

Today, there is variety of segmentation algorithms and user–friendly systems (Koning et al., 2002) that are available for ICUS border detection. However, ICUS segmentation still remains a challenging and heated issue since none of the existed methodologies appears to be as reliable as the expert observers (Klingensmith et al., 2000; Bourantas et al., 2005). This is due to the fact that the increased noise and artefacts seen in ICUS frames often mislead these algorithms. Therefore, most systems require an expert observer to inspect the segmentation process, introduce the appropriate corrections whenever the method fails and restart the procedure from the corrected image.

Plaque Characterization Algorithms

There is direct and indirect evidence that the architecture and the histological characteristics of the atherosclerotic plaque play an important role in outcome and natural evolvement of the atherosclerotic process (Falk et al., 1995). Recognition of the type of the plaque may also be a key in the lesion–specific treatment strategy. Several studies have showed that ICUS can be a useful tool in assessing various morphologic features and identifying the composition of the plaque (Gussenhoven, 1989).

Traditionally, plaque's characterization was performed by expert observers. The categorization of an atheroma was depended on its echogenicity in ICUS frames. According to Mintz et al. (2001) an atheroma could be classified as: calcific (a bright echogenic plaque which obstructs the penetration of the ultrasound), soft (an echolucent plaque with high lipid content), fibrous (a plaque with intermediate echogenicity between soft and calcific) or mixed (a plaque including more than one acoustic subtype, e.g. fibrocalcific, fibrofatty etc.). Rasheed et al. (1995) and Zhang et al. (1998) developed the first computerized methods for plaque characterisation. Both they compared the gray–scale intensity of the plaque with the adventitial region of the artery to classify the plaque as calcified, mixed, or soft.

Nair et al. (2002) and Kawasaki et al. (2002) proposed more advanced methodologies to identify the type of the plaque. These approaches are called "virtual histology" and are superior to those introduced by Rasheed et al. (1995) and Zhang et al. (1998) since the latter often fail to differentiate the soft from the mixed plaque. Virtual histology today constitutes the gold standard for plaque characterisation and is based on spectral analysis of the radiofrequency back–scattered ICUS signals. In these methods the average power of the back–scattered signal from a small volume of tissue is calculated and used to identify the composition of the plaque which is then depicted in each ICUS image using a comprehensive colour–coded map.

3-D Reconstruction of ICUS Images

To visualize the vessel's morphology and to measure the plaque volume integration of the ICUS sequence into a 3-D object has been suggested. Conventional 3-D reconstruction methodologies stack all the ICUS frames to form a cylinder–shaped object (Rosenfield et al., 1991; Roelandt et al., 1994). However, this process did not take into account the luminal and outer vessel wall changes during the cardiac circle, resulting in a "sawtooth" artefact that was more prominent in normal vessels with increased diameter and preserved compliance. This problem was overcome by gating the image acquisition and selecting only the ICUS frames that corresponded to the same phase of the cardiac circle (e.g. to the end–diastolic phase). There are two methodologies for ICUS gating: the prospective electrocardiographic gating (Bruining et al., 1998) and the retrorespective gating (Zhang et al., 1998). In the first case the ICUS images are acquired only at a predefined phase of the cardiac circle (e.g. at the peak of R wave). After the acquisition of the first frame the catheter is pulled–back at a specific distance, by an automated ECG gated pull–back device, to acquire the next frame and so on. Thus, immediately after acquisition, a volumetric dataset is obtained, ready for volumetric analysis. In retrorespective gating the ICUS images are obtained continuously while the ICUS catheter is pulled–back at a constant speed (e.g. 0.5mm/sec or 1mm/sec) by an automated pull–back device. Then, the ICUS frames are selected on the basis of the electrocardiogram, to prepare the final volumetric dataset.

Even though these straight 3-D reconstruction methods managed to overcome the "sawtooth" artefact they still have two significant limitations. The first is that they fail to provide reliable information about the spatial orientation of the plaque onto the artery and the second is that they do not take into account the vessel curvature. These approximations may lead to miscalculation of the plaque volume especially in segments with increased curvature where the error can be up to 5% (Schuurbiers et al., 2000).

FUSION OF ICUS AND ANGIOGRAPHIC DATA

Developed Methodologies for Geometrically Correct Arterial Reconstruction

To overcome the above mentioned limitations reliable combination of the 3-D arterial geometry (obtained from biplane angiographic images) with the luminal and vessel wall data (obtained from ICUS images) has been proposed. The first methodology able to fuse ICUS and X–ray angiographic data was proposed by Klein et al. (1992). A limitation of this methodology was the fact that they used the vessels' midline to approximate the ICUS catheter path. In addition, Klein et al. did not estimate the spatial orientation of the ICUS images onto the reconstructed vessel. Three years later Lengyel et al. (1995) implemented a snake algorithm to extract the vessel's midline in a more accurate fashion. Lengyel et al. also proposed a methodology which used anatomical landmarks, that were visible in both ICUS and angiographic images (e.g. side branches, calcium plaques etc.), to estimate the spatial orientation of the ICUS images.

A different approach was introduced by Cothren et al. (2000) who used dynamic biplane angiographic images to reconstruct the pull–back of the ICUS catheter. In a next step, they placed the ICUS images onto the reconstructed path and then, they back–projected each frame onto the angiographic images to find its spatial orientation. Although, this approach appeared to provide geometrically correct coronary arteries it had limited clinical use since it required an increased number of biplane angiographic images to reconstruct the catheter path. In addition, it became apparent that the methodology used to identify the absolute orientation of the ICUS images was not accurate in the common cases of vessels' overlapping or angiographic artefacts. Finally, the validation of this method showed that the cardiac and respiratory movements reduce its accuracy.

These limitations were overcome by Slager et al. (2000) who developed a clinically applicable methodology. Slager et al. used a parametric 3-D curve to extract the ICUS catheter path from two biplane angiographic images. In a next step, they placed the ICUS images perpendicular onto the path. To find the spatial orientation of each frame they first determined their relative twist using the Frenet–Serret formula. Then, they back–projected the reconstructed artery onto the angiographic images and compared these projections with the outline of the artery as shown in biplane angiographies. Afterwards, they rotated the first frame around its axis and the angle of the first frame, at which these outlines best match, represented the correct absolute orientation. A similar reconstruction method was proposed by Wahle et al. (1999), while Bourantas et al. (2005) introduced a methodology which used B-spline surfaces to extract the ICUS catheter path in a more accurate fashion.

User–Friendly Systems for Geometrically Correct Arterial Reconstruction

In order to enhance the clinical and research applicability of the previously described data fusion techniques the development of user–friendly systems is required. These systems have to be fast, stable, and able to overcome common difficulties such as the presence of arterial overlapping or foreshortening or the partial visualisation of the ICUS catheter in the X–ray images. Moreover, they should not require visualisation of additional calibration objects to define image geometry and to correct distortion. Finally, they should include a visualisation platform for comprehensive representation of the final objects and a quantitative analysis sub–system which will provide the operator with accurate measurements.

Today, there are two systems available. The first was developed by Wahle et al. (2004). This includes the 3-D reconstruction methodology introduced by Wahle et al. (1999) which provides 3-D or 4-D (3-D + time) objects from ICUS and X–ray angiographic images. It also incorporates a module that can create a finite–element mesh into the final objects. This mesh is used to estimate the local plaque thickness and to compute the local haemodynamics.

To visualise the final objects, Wahle et al. used the standardised Virtual Reality Modelling Language (VRML). More specifically, the visualisation module utilised the 2-D texture mapping capabilities of VRML to render a 3-D volume as a set of 2-D surfaces. In these images the operator can see the luminal and the media–adventitia surface and visually assess the severity of the atherosclerosis since the plaque is depicted in a colour–coded map (where the blue corresponds to the low amount of plaque and the red to the increased amount, Figure 2A1). In addition, the system allows visual estimation of the vessel's local curvature showed in a colour–coded map (the red indicates the inner curvature while the blue indicates the outer curvature, Figure 2A2) and assessment of the correlation between the vessel's curvature and the plaque burden (Figure 2A3). Apart from the VRML 2-D texture mapping technique, a 3-D graphical user interface was incorporated that allows virtual endoscopy of the reconstructed vessel. Thus, the operator can see the coronary artery from inside, estimate the type of the plaque and the local shear stresses and assess in detail the extent of atherosclerosis (Figure 2B1, 2B2). The system introduced by Wahle et al. (2004) has features which render it as a practical tool in research but it has limited clinical applicability since it fails to provide arterial reconstruction in real time.

This limitation was addressed by Bourantas et al. (2008) who developed a novel system able to perform expedite coronary reconstruction. The fact that this novel system is fast and manages to provide all diagnostic data that are valuable for treatment planning, while the patient is in the catheterisation table, renders it useful in clinical practice. This system, named by the inventors ANGIOCARE, incorporates a well–established and validated methodology (Bourantas et al., 2005) for arterial reconstruction and a quantitative analysis sub–system able to process the detected ICUS borders and the final 3-D objects and to provide reliable measurements. ANGIOCARE operates in a user–friendly environment (Figure 3) facilitating fast learning by the operator and includes an advanced 3-D photorealistic visualisation environment which allows comprehensive 3-D representation of the final object. In this visualisation platform the operator can examine the arterial morphology and visually assess the distribution of the plaque (depicted in a colour–coded map, Figure 4A). In addition, he can interact with the

Figure 2. Image A shows a left coronary artery with part of the left main and a segment of the left anterior descending artery; the branch to the left circumflex artery (red line) has not been followed and was discarded: A1) Plaque thickness showed in a rainbow colour–map from low (blue) to high (red) amounts of plaque. The media–adventitia border is depicted with a grey colour; A2) representation of the local curvature in a colour–coded map. The red indicates "inner" curvature, the blue indicates "outer" curvature while the green marks the sides; A3) Correlation analysis between local vessel's curvature and circumferential plaque distribution: blue regions indicate a high correlation and red a low correlation. B1) Endoscopy of the reconstructed artery. ICUS data showed in semi–transparent fashion. In this images it is possible to look behind of the stenosis (arrow); B2) Reconstructed luminal surface of the same view with depiction of the shear stress in colour–coded fashion. The increased shear stresses correspond to the red areas while the low shear stresses to the dark blue. (From Wahle et al., 2004)

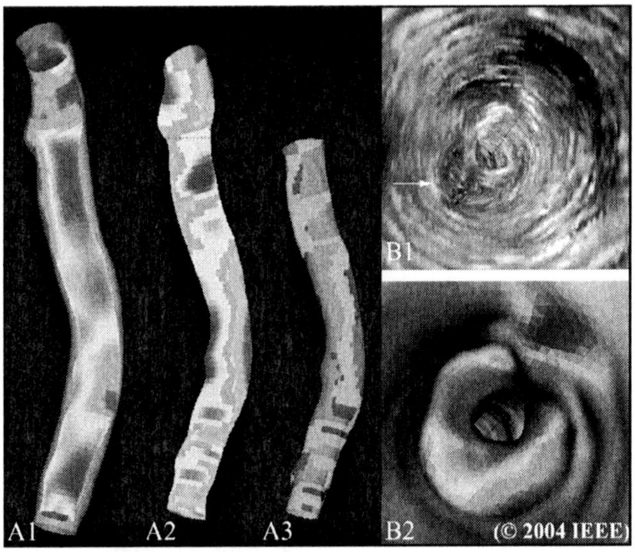

object in real time, select a segment of his interest and obtain quantitative measurements (Figure 4C). He can also back–project the object onto the angiographic images and assess the distribution of the plaque by performing virtual endoscopy (Figure 4D).

These two systems today constitute the gold standard in coronary imaging since they provide complete, accurate and comprehensive representation of coronary artery's morphology. The obtained 3-D objects are superior to those, derived by all the other systems which process data from different imaging modalities (e.g. X-ray angiography, multi slices computed tomography, magnetic resonance imaging) and allow more accurate assessment of plaque burden.

Figure 3. Snapshot of the user–friendly interface used for the extraction of the catheter path (A) and the segmentation of the ICUS images (B). (From Bourantas et al., 2008).

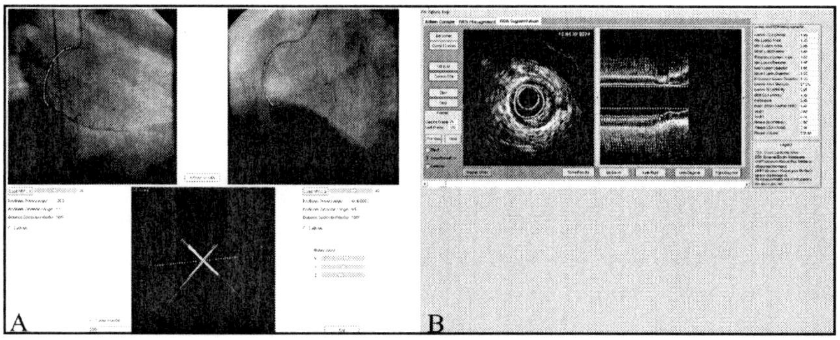

Figure 4. A) Luminal surface with colour–coded delineation of the plaque thickness (red indicates increased plaque while blue reduced); B) depiction of the luminal and the media–adventitia borders. The outer vessel wall is showed in a semi–transparent fashion; C) Quantitative measurements (displayed at the bottom-left side of the screen) from a segment with significant luminal stenosis; D) Virtual endoscopy of the reconstructed vessel. (From Bourantas et al., 2008).

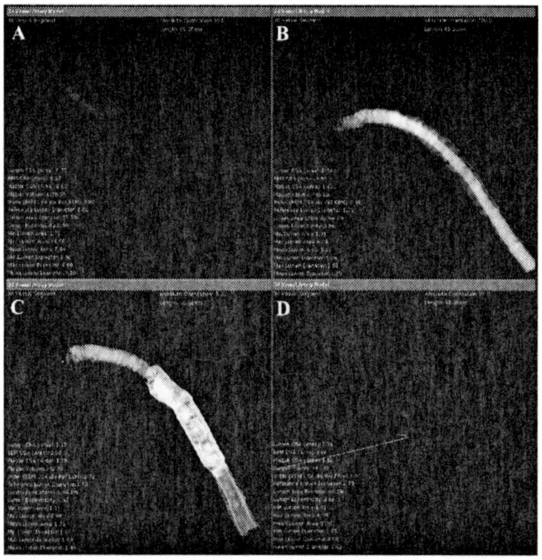

FUTURE TRENDS

Nowadays, there is an augmented interest in the role of blood flow in the atherosclerotic process since it seems that local haemodynamics create an environment which determines the behaviour of the endothelium and affects plaque's formation. The above mentioned systems can be used to further investigate this relationship. They can be utilised to implement complex haemodynamics, determine the local endothelial shear stress and predict changes in arterial morphology and blood flow after stent implantation. In addition, the already developed systems may be used to process data regarding the composition of the plaque (given by virtual histology) and create objects which will allow the identification of the vulnerable and ruptured plaque. These objects will provide information that is necessary to study in detail the role of local haemodynamics in the process of vulnerable plaque formation and rapture.

Finally, the present systems can be implemented to process other imaging modalities such as the optical coherence tomographic images (OCT). OCT images have higher resolution (axial capacity 15μm) than ICUS and allow the identification of neointimal coverage in stents (Takano et al., 2007). Data suggests that neointimal coverage is incomplete after drug eluting stent implantation resulting possibly in late thrombosis. Fusion of OCT and angiographic images will allow us to further understand the mechanisms that are involved in this process and decide about the type and duration of antiplatelet treatment.

CONCLUSION

New developments in ICUS processing allow fast, reliable and reproducible segmentation of the ICUS images and accurate quantification of the type of the plaque. Novel methodologies able to fuse X–ray and ICUS data provide fully and geometrically correct coronary representation and nowadays constitute the state of the art in arterial reconstruction. The newly developed user–friendly systems for 3-D reconstruction appear to have increased research applicability as they allow blood flow simulation and direct evaluation of the correlation between the local haemodynamics and the plaque thickness. In addition, these systems constitute a useful tool in clinical practice since they provide in real time comprehensive coronary representation and offer measurements useful to guide treatment.

REFERENCES

Bouma, C., Niessen, W., Zuiderveld, K., Gussenhoven, E., & Viergever, M. (1996). Automated lumen definition from 30MHz intravascular ultrasound images. *Med Imag Analysis, 1*(4), 363-377.

Bourantas, C. V., Kalatzis, F. G., Papafaklis, M. I., Fotiadis, D. I., Tweddel A. C., Katsouras, C. S, et al. (2008). ANGIOCARE: an automated system for fast three dimensional coronary reconstruction using angiographic and intracoronary ultrasound data. *Cathet Cardiovasc Inter, 72*(2), 166-175.

Bourantas, C. V., Kourtis, I. C., Plissiti, M. E., Fotiadis, D. I., Katsouras, C. S., Papafaklis, M. I., et al. (2005). A method for 3-D reconstruction of coronary arteries using biplane angiography and intravascular ultrasound images. *Comput Med Imaging Graph, 29*(8), 597-606.

Bourantas, C. V., Plissiti, M. E., Fotiadis, D. I., Protopappas, V. C., Mpozios, G. V., Katsouras, C. S., et al. (2005). In vivo validation of a novel semi-automated method for border detection in intravascular ultrasound images. *Br J Radiol, 78*(926), 122-9.

Bruining, N., von Birgelen, C., de Feyter, P. J., Ligthart, J., Li, W., Serruys, P. W., et al. (1998). ECG-gated versus nongated three-dimensional intracoronary ultrasound analysis: implications for volumetric measurements. *Cathet Cardiovasc Diagn, 43*(3), 254-60.

Cothren, R., Shekhar, R., Tuzcu, E., & Nissen, S. (2000). Three-dimensional reconstruction of the coronary artery wall by image fusion of intravascular ultrasound and bi-plane angiography. *Int J Card Imag, 16*, 69-85.

Dhawale, P., Rasheed, Q., Griffin, N., Wilson, D., & Hodgson, J. (1993). Intracoronary Ultrasound Plaque Volume Quantification. *In: Proc Comput Cardiol, Los Alamitos (CA),* IEEE Computer Society Press (pp.121-24).

Falk, E., Shah, P. K., & Fuster V. (1995) .Coronary plaque disruption. *Circulation, 92*(3), 657-71.

Giannoglou, G. D., Chatzizisis, Y. S., Koutkias, V., Kompatsiaris, I., Papadogiorgaki, M., Mezaris, V., et al. (2007). A novel active contour model for fully automated segmentation of intravascular ultrasound images: in vivo validation in human coronary arteries. *Comput Biol Med, 37*(9), 1292-302.

Gussenhoven, E. J., Essed, C. E., Lancée, C. T., Mastik, F., Frietman, P., van Egmond, F. C., et al. (1989). Arterial wall characteristics determined by intravascular ultrasound imaging: an in vitro study. *J Am Coll Cardiol, 14*(4), 947-52.

Kawasaki, M., Takatsu, H., Noda, T., Sano, K., Ito, Y., Hayakawa, K., et al. (2002). In vivo quantitative tissue characterization of human coronary arterial plaques by use of integrated backscatter intravascular ultrasound and comparison with angioscopic findings. *Circulation, 105*(21), 2487-92.

Klein, H. M., Gunther, R. W., Verlande, M., Schneider, W. D. Vorwerk, D., Kelch J., et al. (1992). 3D-surface reconstruction of intravascular ultrasound images using personal computer hardware and a motorized catheter control. *Cardiovasc Intervent Radiol, 15*(2), 97-101.

Klingensmith, J. D., Sheknar, R., Vince, D. G. (2000). Evaluation of three dimensional segmentation algorithms for the identification of luminal and medial-adventitial borders in intravascular ultrasound images. *IEEE Trans Med Imag, 19*, 996-1011.

Klingensmith, J. D., & Vince, D. G. (2002).B-spline methods for interactive segmentation and modeling of lumen and vessel surfaces in three-dimensional intravascular ultrasound. *Comput Med Imaging Graph, 26*(6), 429-38.

Koning, G., Dijkstra, J., Von Birgelen, C., Tuinenburg, J. C., Brunette, J., Tardif, J. C., et al. (2002). Advanced contour detection for three–dimensional intracoronary ultrasound: a validation in–vitro and in vivo. *Int J Cardiovasc Imag, 18*, 235-48.

Kovalski, G., Beyear, R., Shofti, R., Azhari, H. (2000). Three–dimensional automatic quantitative analysis of intravascular ultrasound images. *Ultrasound Med Biol, 26*(4), 527-537.

Lengyel, J., Greenberg, D. P., & Pop, R. (1995). Time–dependent three-dimensional intravascular ultrasound. In: Robert Cook, (Ed). *The SIGGRAPH 95 Conference on Comp Graphics*, (pp. 457-64).

Lobregt, S., & Viergever, M. A. (1995). Discrete dynamic control model. *IEEE Trans Med Imag, 14*, 12-24.

Mintz, G. S., Nissen, S. E., Anderson, W. D., Bailey, S. R., Elber, R., Fitzgerald, P. J., et al. (2001). American college of cardiology clinical expert consensus document on standards for acquisition, measurement and reporting of intravascular ultrasound studies: a report of the American College of Cardiology task force on clinical expert consensus documents (committee to develop a clinical expert consensus on standards for acquisition, measurement and reporting of intravascular ultrasound studies [IVUS]). *J Am Coll of Cardiol, 37*, 1478– 1492.

Nair, A., Kuban, B. D., Obuchowski, N., Vince, D. G. (2001). Assessing spectral algorithms to predict atherosclerotic plaque composition with normalized and raw intravascular ultrasound data. *Ultrasound Med Biol, 27*(10), 1319-31.

Nissen, S. E., Di Mario, C., & Tuzcu, E. M. (1998). Intravascular Ultrasound Angioscopy, Doppler and Pressure Measurements. In E. J. Topol (Ed.), *Comprehensive Cardiovascular Medicine* (pp. 2471-2501). Lippincott-Raven Publishers, Philadelphia.

Plissiti, M. E., Fotiadis, D. I., Michalis, L. K., Bozios, G. E. (2004). An automated method for lumen and media-adventitia border detection in a sequence of IVUS frames. *IEEE Trans Inf Technol Biomed, 8*(2), 131-41.

Rasheed, Q., Dhawale, P. J., Anderson, J., & Hodgson, J. M. (1995). Intracoronary ultrasound-defined plaque composition: computer-aided plaque characterization and correlation with histologic samples obtained during directional coronary atherectomy. *Am Heart J, 129*(4), 631-7.

Roelandt, J. R., di Mario, C., Pandian, N. G., Wenguang, L., Keane, D., Slager, C. J., et al. (1994). Three-dimensional reconstruction of intracoronary ultrasound images. Rationale, approaches, problems, and directions. *Circulation, 90*(2), 1044–55.

Rosenfield, K., Losordo, D. W., Ramaswamy, K., Pastore, J. O., Langevin, R. E., Razvi, S., et al. (1991). Three dimensional reconstruction of human coronary and peripheral arteries from images recorded during two-dimensional intravascular ultrasound examination. *Circulation, 84*(5), 1938-56.

Sanz-Requena, R., Moratal, D., García-Sánchez, D. R., Bodí, V., Rieta, J. J., Sanchis, J. M. (2007). Automatic segmentation and 3D reconstruction of intravascular ultrasound images for a fast preliminar evaluation of vessel pathologies. *Comput Med Imaging Graph, 31*(2), 71-80.

Schuurbiers, J. C., Von Birgelen, C., Wentzel, J. J., Bom, N., Serruys, P. W., De Feyter, P. J., et al (2000). On the IVUS plaque volume error in coronary arteries when neglecting curvature. *Ultrasound Me Biol, 26*(9), 1403-11.

Shekhar, R., Cothern, R. M., Vince, D. G., Chandra, S., Thomas, J. D., & Cornhill, J. F. (1999). Three–dimensional segmentation of luminal and adventitial borders in serial intravascular ultrasound images. *Comput Med Imag Graph, 23*, 299 –309.

Slager, C. J., Wentzel, J. J., Schuurbiers, J. C. H., Oomen, J. A. F., Kloet, J., Krams, R., et al. (2000). True 3-Dimensional reconstruction of coronary arteries in patients by fusion of angiography and IVUS (ANGUS) and its quantitative validation. *Circulation, 102*, 511-16.

Sonka, M., Zhang, X., Siebes, M., Bissing, M., DeJong, S., Collins, S., & McKay, C. (1995). Segmentation of Intravascular Ultrasound Images: A knowledge-Based approach. *IEEE Trans Med Imag, 14*(4), 719-732.

Takano, M., Inami, S., Jang, I. K., Yamamoto, M., Murakami, D., Seimiya, K., et al. (2007). Evaluation by optical coherence tomography of neointimal coverage of sirolimus-eluting stent three months after implantation. *Am J Cardiol, 99*(8), 1033-8.

Von Birgelen, C., van der Lugt, A., Nicosia, A., Mintz, G. S., Gussenhoven, E. J., de Vrey, E., et al. (1996). Computerized assessment of coronary lumen and atherosclerotic plaque dimensions in three-dimensional intravascular ultrasound correlated with histomorphometry. *Am J Cardiol, 78*(11), 1202-9.

Wahle, A., Prause, G. P. M., DeJong, S. C., & Sonka, M. (1999). Geometrically correct 3-D reconstruction of intravascular ultrasound images by fusion with biplane angiography–methods and validation. *IEEE Trans Med Imag, 18*(8), 686-98.

Wahle, A., Olszewski, M. E., & Sonka, M. (2004). Interactive virtual endoscopy in coronary arteries based on multimodality fusion. *IEEE Trans Med Imag, 23*(11), 1391-403.

Zhang, X., McKay, C. R., & Sonka, M. (1998). Tissue characterization in intravascular ultrasound images. *IEEE Trans Med Imag, 17*(6), 889-99.

KEY TERMS

B-Splines: Parametrical curves which are described by the following formula:

$$C\ (u) = \sum_{i=0}^{n} N_{i,p}(u) P_{A,i}\,, \qquad 0 \le u \le 1 \qquad 4.10$$

where, u is B-spline's $C\ (u)$ knot vector, $N_{i,p}(u)$ is B-spline's basis functions and $P_{A,i}$ is the sum of the control points that have been used to approximate spline's morphology.

Frennet–Serret Formula: A mathematical formula developed by Jean Frédéric Frenet and Joseph Alfred Serret to calculate the curvature and torsion of a 3-D curve.

Neural Network: A modelling technique based on the observed behaviour of biological neurons and used to mimic the performance of a system. It consists of a set of elements (neurons) that start out connected in a random pattern, and, based upon operational feedback, are modelled into the pattern required to generate the optimal results.

Neointima Coverage: A new or thickened layer of arterial intima formed especially on a prosthesis (e.g. stents) by migration and proliferation of cells from the media.

Optical Coherence Tomography: Intravascular imaging modality which provides cross–sectional images of the vessel. It is similar to ICUS since it requires the insertion of a catheter within the artery, which transmits infrared light. The light is back–reflected as passing through the vessel. These reflections are obtained and analysed to finally generate high resolution cross–sectional images.

Drug Eluting Stent: A metal tube, which is placed into diseased vessels to keep them open and releases a drug that blocks cells' proliferation

Vulnerable Plaque: Atherosclerotic plaque which is prone to thrombosis or has high probability of undergoing rapid progression and causing coronary events.

Chapter V
Diagnostic Support Systems and Computational Intelligence:
Differential Diagnosis of Hepatic Lesions from Computed Tomography Images

Stavroula G. Mougiakakou
National Technical University of Athens, Greece

Ioannis K. Valavanis
National Technical University of Athens, Greece

Alexandra Nikita
University of Athens, Greece & DIAKENTRO, Diagnostic Imaging Center for the Woman and the Child, Greece

Konstantina S. Nikita
National Technical University of Athens, Greece

ABSTRACT

Recent advances in computer science provide the intelligent computation tools needed to design and develop Diagnostic Support Systems (DSSs) that promise to increase the efficiency of physicians during their clinical practice. This chapter provides a brief overview of the use of computational intelligence methods in the design and development of DSSs aimed at the differential diagnosis of hepatic lesions from Computed Tomography (CT) images. Furthermore, examples of DSSs developed by our research team for supporting the diagnosis of focal liver lesions from non-enhanced CT images are presented.

INTRODUCTION

Hepatic diseases, including disorders that cause the liver to function improperly or cease its function (e.g. hepatitis and cirrhosis), are one of the most common diseases all over the world. According to the National Center for Health Statistics, the American Liver Foundation, and the United Network for Organ Sharing over 26.000 people in the United States die each year from chronic liver disease and cirrhosis, while according to the Office for National Statistics in the United Kingdom, liver disease is now the fifth most common cause of death after heart disease, stroke, chest disease and cancer. Hepatic cancer is one of the fastest growing cancers in the United States, while the number of Hepatocellular Carcinomas (HCC), type of primary liver cancer and one of the top eight most common cancers in the world, is rising worldwide. HCC is much more common outside the United States, representing 10% to 50% of malignancies in Africa and parts of Asia. Advances in imaging technologies permit the non-invasive detection and diagnosis of liver of both diffuse hepatic disease, like hepatitis and cirrhosis, and focal liver lesions like cysts, hemangiomas and HCC. The diagnosis can be performed through a wide array of medical imaging techniques including Ultrasonography (US), Magnetic Resonance (MR) imaging, and Computed Tomography (CT) with or without contrast agents. The choice of imaging test depends on the clinical question, availability of the test, patient's condition and clinician's familiarity with the test. US imaging is inexpensive, widely available, can easily detect cysts, but its diagnostic accuracy depends strongly on the operator and his/her experience. CT and MR imaging are more sensitive in detecting focal liver lesions. MR imaging although accurate in detecting and differentiating liver lesions, is very expensive and therefore not very popular. The most commonly used image-based detection method of liver lesions is CT due to its short acquisition time, wide imaging range, high spatial resolution, and relatively low cost. Although the quality of liver images has lately improved, it is difficult even for an experienced clinician to discriminate various types of hepatic lesions with high accuracy and without the need for diagnosis confirmation by means of contrast agents (related with renal toxicity or allergic reactions).

Rapid development of computer science permitted the design and development of computerized systems able to assist radiologists in the interpretation, early detection and diagnosis of abnormalities from hundreds of medical images every day. These systems are known as Diagnostic Support Systems (DSSs). Recent advances in DSSs demonstrated that the application of digital image processing techniques along with advanced Computational Intelligence (CI) methods increase the efficiency, diagnostic confidence and productivity of radiologists, acting as a "second" opinion to the clinician.

The main areas of computerized analysis of liver images are: i) general image preprocessing in order to improve the quality of hepatic images; ii) registration of images in case of multi data sets; iii) manually, semi- or fully-automatic segmentation of Regions of Interest (ROIs) corresponding to anatomical structures and/or liver lesion; iv) visualization into two- and/or three-dimensional (2D and/or 3D) space of liver lesions for diagnosis, surgery, radiation therapy planning, quantitative studies and final presentation purposes; v) image analysis for the detection of an abnormality and its classification into one out of several types of liver tissues. Generally, a DSS includes tools based on image processing techniques in order to support all the above mentioned techniques of computerized analysis, while the intelligence is provided through the usage of CI based algorithms embedded into the DSS. CI algorithms belong to Artificial Intelligence (AI) methods and are able to handle complex data characterized by non-linearities.

It is worth mentioning that a DSS can be combined with computer based medical image archiving and management systems following certain information protocols, e.g. DICOM and HL7. Furthermore, a DSS can support telematic technologies, in order to permit the remote diagnosis and tele-consultation between health care professionals, and can be integrated with the electronic medical patient record (Mougiakakou, to appear).

This chapter presents an overview of advanced computer analysis methods used to provide intelligent diagnostic support in the assessment of focal liver lesions from CT images. Furthermore, specific DSS architectures, developed by the Biomedical Simulations and Imaging (BIOSIM) Laboratory, aimed at supporting the diagnosis of focal liver lesions from non-enhanced CT images, are presented. Some future perspectives in the area of DSSs and concluding remarks are also given.

BACKGROUND

In the following, the fundamentals for the development of a DSS for liver diseases are given, along with examples of DSSs already published in the literature.

DSS General Architecture

A general architecture of a DSS is presented in Figure 1. Typically a DSS for diagnosis of liver lesions consists of the following modules: (1) image preprocessing; (2) registration; (3) segmentation; (4) visualization; and (5) image analysis supporting tools for feature extraction, selection, and classification (Stoitsis, 2006).

1. **Image preprocessing:** The image preprocessing module improves the quality of the images through the application of image

Figure 1. General architecture of a DSS for CT liver lesions

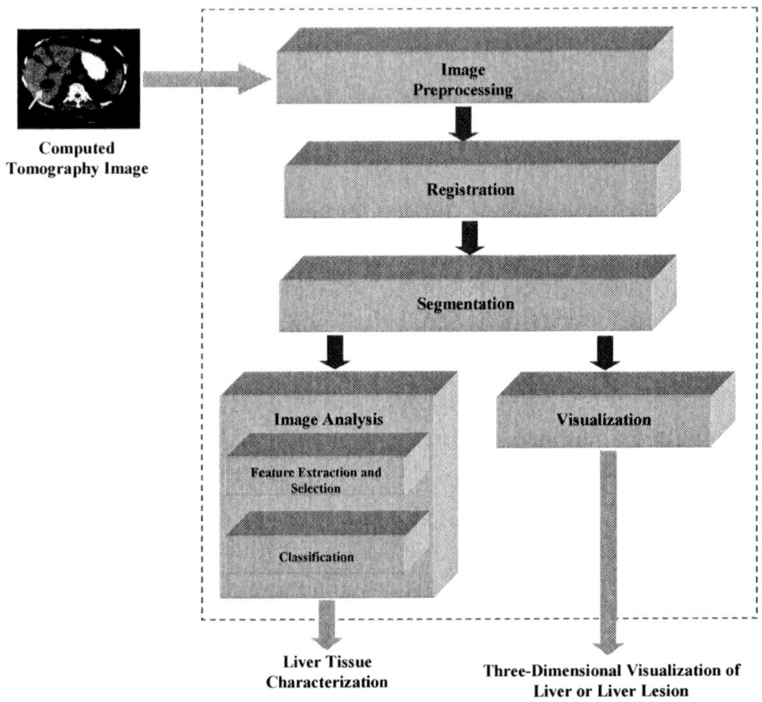

processing algorithms that perform noise removal, contrast enhancement and edge sharpening. Noise removal is done mainly through the application of simple filtering methods (average, median, Gaussian) (Russ, 1992). Since these low-pass filtering methods perform edge smoothing, edge-preserving noise reduction methods have also been proposed, e.g. bilateral filtering (Tomasi, 1998) and anisotropic diffusion (Perona, 1990) was used prior to liver segmentation (Eibenberger, 2008). Local or global histogram equalization can be used for further enhancing the image (Gonzales, 2002). Histogram based manipulation can be used to improve the contrast of the hepatic image and reveal originally unapparent textural information, e.g. global histogram equalization was successfully used prior to extraction of textural features and rendered conspicuous texture (Huang, 2006).

2. **Registration:** In the case of multi image data sets or multimodal images, the application of registration (or matching) algorithms is needed, in order to avoid misalignments among images. Registration is used to compare two or more medical images, to discover difference between them or to combine information aiming to reveal information not accessible from individual images. Medical image registration methods can be distinguished into intensity-based registration and feature-based registration (Wang, 2005). For liver images many registration algorithms have been proposed, but the most promising are based on Free Form Deformation (FFD) (Masutani, 2006).
3. **Segmentation:** In the segmentation module, the whole liver and/or sub-areas corresponding to normal or abnormal ROIs are extracted. Liver segmentation is a difficult task due to the diversity and complexity of its anatomical structure. Therefore, conventional segmentation methods cannot be applied in clinical practice. Segmentation can be performed using manual, semi-automatic or fully-automatic methods. In general, liver segmentation methods include (i) intensity-based e.g. thresholding, (ii) deformable model-based, e.g. snake algorithms and level-set techniques, and (iii) statistical model-based approaches (Lee, 2007). Figure 2 presents examples of liver segmentation using a semi-automatic method based on the seeded region growing technique optimized by the self-similar mapping method (Mougiakakou, to appear).
4. **3D Visualization:** For the 3D visualization of the organ and/or the segmented ROI(s), surface rendering and volume rendering techniques are usually applied. For 3D visualization from CT images, a modified version of the Marching Cubes (MC) algorithm, which belongs to surface rendering algorithms, has been also proposed (Mougiakakou, to appear), as presented in Figure 3.
5. **Image analysis:** Each of the extracted ROIs is fed to the image analysis module where (i) feature extraction, (ii) feature selection and (iii) classification, are performed. More specifically, for each ROI, a set of features is estimated, usually by means of texture analysis. First Order Statistics (FOS) and the Spatial Gray Level Dependence Matrix (SGLDM) method are the most widely used methods for texture analysis. FOS calculate simple characteristics using the ROI intensity function, e.g. mean value, contrast, angular second moment (Haralick, 1992). The elements of the SGLDM (Haralick, 1973; Haralick, 1992) represent the values of the probability function P_{ij}, which measure the normalized frequency in which all pixel pairs consisting of pixels with interpixel distance d along a direction θ and with gray level values i and j, respectively, appear in the ROI. Several features can be obtained

Figure 2. Examples of segmented liver from non-enhanced CT image data using (a) the seeded region growing technique, and (b) after the application of the self-similar mapping method

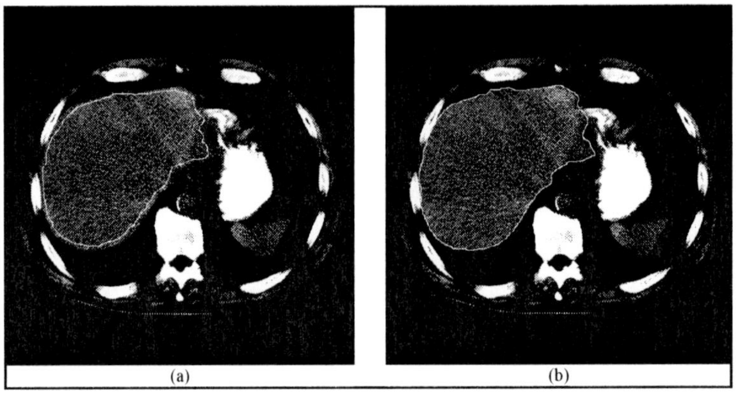

Figure 3. Three-dimensional visualization of liver from CT data

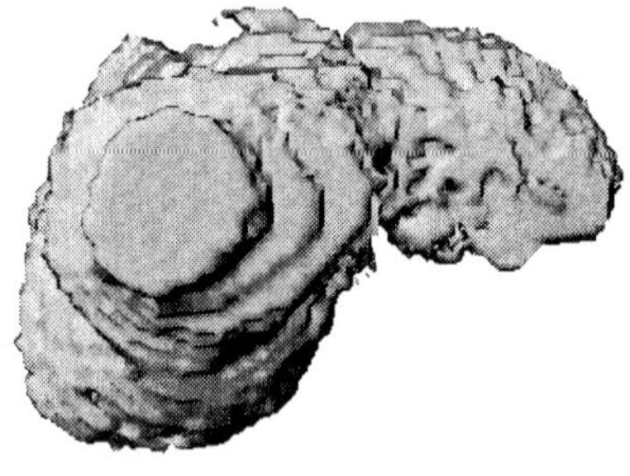

from SGLDM elements, e.g. correlation and contrast. Similarly, textural features can be obtained using the Gray Level Difference Matrix (GLDM) (Wezka, 1976), whose elements represent the probability that a particular absolute difference in grey level appear within an interpixel distance d along a direction θ. Gray Level Run Length Method (GLRLM) identifies paths of pixels with the same gray level within the ROI and extracts features based on the identified paths, e.g. short run length emphasis, long run length emphasis, run length distribution (Mir, 1995). Convolving the ROI with Laws' masks and calculating the so-called energy statistics on the resulted image comprises another way for analyzing a hepatic tissue image (Laws, 1980). The use of Gabor filters at different orientations and frequencies and extraction of features of the resulted image after convolving the ROI with these filters (mean, standard deviation, energy) have been also used (Lee, 2006; Dettori, 2007). Auto-covariance coefficients that reflect the interpixel correlation within an image have been used as texture measurements of hepatic tissue images (Huang, 2006). Fractal dimension measurements capture the roughness of a ROI and have been used successfully for texture analysis of liver images (Sariyanni, 2001).

Once the initial feature set from a hepatic ROI has been obtained, it is desirable to select the most robust features in order to provide input to the classification module where the computerized diagnosis is performed. Since an exhaustive search in the feature space is impossible due to computational cost, sub-optimal methods can be applied. Thus, a forward feature selection method was proposed to select the features used to classify liver tissue based on the texture of US images (Sun, 1996). Statistical approaches have also appeared in literature. Specifically, the f-ratio obtained using analysis of variance was proposed to select the best texture features derived from vascular US images (Stoitsis, 2006), while the Fischer criterion was also proposed to compare texture features obtained using Gabor filters on a set of test images (Grigorescu, 2002). The evolutionary strategy of Genetic Algorithm (GA) (Goldberg, 1989) based feature selection seems promising for identifying the most robust texture features obtained from hepatic CT images (Gletsos, 2003). GAs follow the evolutionary model of Darwin and select the most informative subset starting from an initial population of random feature subsets (chromosomes) that are evaluated by a fitness function. All chromosomes exchange genetic material, mate, depending on their fitness and mutate within a number of generations that GA runs for. When the pre-defined number of generations has been executed, the algorithm returns the best subset of features according to the used fitness function that corresponds to the chromosome that has evolved from the optimization process.

Finally, the features selected in the previous step are fed to a classifier. The classifier decides on the type of hepatic tissue that the ROI under examination corresponds to, and actually provides a second opinion to the physician. The classifier comes usually from the fields of machine learning and statistics. Most of the times the classifier is a supervised one, i.e. the classifier has been trained offline and can generalize to unknown data. The generalization ability of the classifier is usually measured using resampling techniques during training and evaluation process, e.g. bootstrapping and cross-validation (Efron, 1982). The most popular classifiers belong to the class of Artificial Neural Networks or Neural Networks (NNs), e.g. multi-layer perceptron NNs (Gletsos, 2003, Hein, 2005) or probabilistic NNs (Chen, 1998). Support Vector Machines (SVMs) is a state-of-the-art technique for constructing optimal separating hyperplanes in feature space by mapping the input vector to a space of higher dimensionality using a non-linear mapping. They have been successfully applied for the discrimination of liver tissue using texture features (Huang, 2006; Lee, 2006; Lee, 2007). Nearest-neighbor classifiers decide on the type of hepatic lesion according to a distance-based similarity metric of the query feature vector among feature vectors that correspond to already known types of tissue (Kyriakou, 1997; Mougiakakou, to appear). Finally, a fuzzy c-means clustering algorithm has been used to discriminate hepatic lesions using fractal measurements (Sariyanni, 2001). Given that the feature space has been defined, all known classifiers can be used for the discrimination of liver tissue. However, one should be careful when constructing the classifier, e.g. training it with a partition of the available data, in order to obtain an acceptable generalization ability. Lately, the use of ensembles of classifiers has gained interest in the field of computer aided diagnosis (Christodoulou, 2003; Jerebko, 2003) and they can also be applied within DSSs for the discrimination of hepatic lesions from CT (Mougiakakou, 2007).

Examples of DSS for Liver Diseases from CT Images

The above mentioned modules are common to the majority of the available intelligent DSS for liver diagnosis from US (Asvestas, 1998; Kadah, 1996; Sujana, 1996; Sun, 1996), MR (Zhang, 2005) and CT imaging modalities. In the following paragraphs, intelligent systems for the diagnosis of liver diseases from CT images are presented.

A DSS able to identify automatically the liver boundary from CT images and distinguish the extracted ROI into normal liver, hepatoma and hemageoma has been proposed by Chen (1998). The system is based on the concept of the normalized fractional Brownian motion model to find an initial liver boundary and then uses a deformable contour model to precisely delineate the liver boundary. For each segmented ROI, a set of texture features based on SGLDM is estimated providing input to a probabilistic NN for the characterization of the hepatic tissue. The system results to a classification performance of the order of 83%.

Additionally, a DSS for the classification of hepatic tissue from non-enhanced CT images into four categories has been proposed by Gletsos (2003). The system consists of two modules: the feature extraction and the classification modules. The feature extraction module calculates the average gray level and 48 texture characteristics, which are derived from the SGLDM, obtained from the free-hand ROIs, as delineated by an experienced radiologist. The classifier module consists of three sequentially placed feed-forward NNs. The first NN classifies into normal or abnormal liver regions. The abnormal liver regions are characterized by the second NN as cyst or "other disease". The third NN classifies "other disease" into hemangioma or hepatocellular carcinoma. Furthermore, GA-based feature selection is applied in order to select the most robust features and improve the classification performance. An overall classification performance of the order of 97% was achieved.

Huang (2006) has proposed a system able to differentiate benign from malignant hepatic tumors from non-enhanced CT images. Suspicious tumor regions were delineated in CT images by an experienced radiologist. For each region autocovariance texture features have been estimated providing input to a SVM for discriminating the various types of hepatic tumors.

Furthermore, the use of a wide set of image derived features (e.g. size, shape, diffuse of liver disease) has been proposed for the development of statistical prediction rules into a computer model, in order to discriminate benign from malignant and hepatocyte-containing vs non–hepatocyte tissue (Seltzer, 2002). The features have been derived from non-enhanced MR, contrast material-enhanced CT and contrast enhanced MR images.

Hein (2005) has investigated the applicability of a modified NN training algorithm (based on simulated annealing with a logarithmic cooling schedule) in the detection of pathological focal liver lesions. More specifically, square ROIs of contrast-enhanced CT images have been used as input to the algorithm, which uses the entire ROI information and not the information from extracted features. The accuracy of the algorithm in evaluating liver CT images showing either normal findings or hypovascularized focal liver lesions was of the order of 99%.

Shimizu (2005) has proposed a DSS for early and late phase three dimensional CT images of liver cancer obtained with a multi-detector row CT scanner. First, registration of two phase images using FFD has been applied and liver regions including malignant and cystic lesions have been extracted. Then malignant liver regions were enhanced and candidate regions were determined using region growing and level set methods. Finally, for each candidate region three features - selected by means of a forward stepwise selection method - corresponding to shape and gray values in and around the candidates, were fed to an SVM for the classification into normal and malignancy.

DIAGNOSIS OF FOCAL LIVER LESIONS FROM NON-ENHANCED CT IMAGES

DSS architectures developed by the BIOSIM Laboratory aimed at the computerized diagnosis of CT focal liver lesions have been based on the use of several texture features sets combined with

Ensembles of Classifiers (ECs). Several intelligent DSS architectures that use FOS, SGLDM, GLDM, Texture Energy Measurements (TEM) and Fractal Dimension Measurements (FDM) as texture descriptors of hepatic images and an EC have been comparatively assessed (Mougiakakou, 2007). The best performing architecture for the discrimination of liver tissue ROIs into four categories, namely normal tissue (C1), cyst (C2), hemangioma (C3) and hepatocellular carcinoma (C4) has been defined and is presented in the present chapter (Figure 4).

The selected architecture uses a fused optimal feature set of texture measurements of ROIs extracted using FOS, SGLDM, GLDM, TEM and FDM and an ensemble of five statistical and machine-learning based classifiers. In the following, the image acquisition, feature extraction, selection and classification sub-modules of the DSS are presented and its performance in the discrimination of the liver tissue ROIs is discussed. Furthermore, the discriminative ability of all feature sets to detect each type of hepatic tissue was assessed in terms of area (A_Z) under Receiver Operating Characteristic (ROC) curves and results are reported (Valavanis, 2007).

Image Acquisition

Abdominal non-enhanced CT images with a spatial resolution of 512×512 pixels and 8-bit gray-level at the W150+60 window were taken from both patients and healthy controls. A total of 147 ROIs 76 of which corresponded to C1, 19 to C2, 28 to C3, and 24 to C4 were identified by the radiologist (Figure 5). The diagnosed hepatic lesions from patients with C2, C3, and C4, were validated by needle biopsies, density measurements, and the typical pattern of enhancement after the intravenous injection of iodine contrast.

Feature Extraction

For each ROI a set of 89 texture features are extracted initially using the methods of FOS, SGLDM, GLDM, TEM and FDM:

First order Statistics: For each ROI, six features are obtained from FOS (Haralick, 1992) using the image intensity function. These features correspond to average gray level (*avg*), standard deviation (*sd*), entropy (*ent*), coefficient of variance (*cv*), skewness (*sk*), and kurtosis (*kur*).

Spatial Gray-Level Dependence Matrix: Eight texture features can be calculated from the SGLDM of each ROI. These correspond to angular second moment (*asm*), contrast (*con*), correlation (*corr*), sum of squares (*ss*), inverse difference moment (*idm*), entropy (*ent*), homogeneity (*hg*), cluster tendency (*clt*) and depend on intersample spacing and angular direction (Haralick, 1973; Haralick, 1992). The SGLDM features are calculated for six different values of the interpixel

Figure 4. Proposed DSS for the characterization of liver tissue from non-enhanced CT images

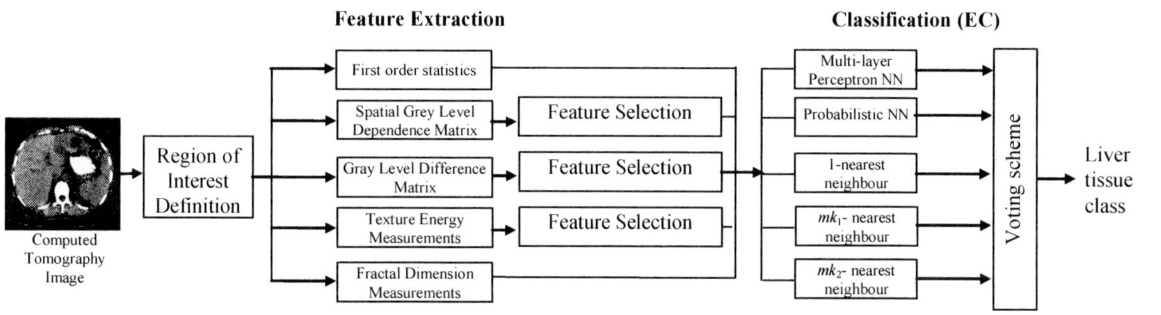

distance d: d=1, 2, 4, 6, 8, 12 pixels. For each value of d, the values are computed by averaging over four uniformly distributed angular directions, 0°, 45°, 90°, and 135°. Thus, a total of 48 texture characteristics are obtained.

Gray-Level Difference Matrix: Application of the GLDM to each ROI results to a set of 20 texture features. These are derived using the gray level difference density function (Wezka, 1976) and correspond to values of contrast (*con*), mean (*mn*), entropy (*ent*), inverse difference moment (*idm*), and angular second moment (*asm*) for interpixel distance d=1, 2, 3, 4. For each d, the feature values are calculated as the mean value of the feature estimations for the directions (0, d), ($-d$, d), (d, 0), ($-d$, $-d$).

Texture Energy Measurements: The TEM features are extracted after the application of Laws masks which are originally derived from the vectors $L3$={1, 2, 1}, $E3$={-1, 0, 1}, and $S3$={-1, 2, -1} (Laws, 1980). Convolving these vectors with themselves or with one another, vectors of length five can be derived. In the current study the following vectors were calculated: $L5$={1, 4, 6, 4, 1}, $S5$={-1, 0, -2, 0, -1}, $E5$={-1, -2, 0, 2, 1} and $R5$={1, -4, 6, -4, 1}. Multiplication of the column vectors of length 5 with the row vectors of the same length results in 5x5 Laws' masks. In this study the following Laws' masks were considered: $L5^TE5$, $L5^TS5$, $-E5^TS5$, and $R5^TR5$. After the convolution of each mask with the ROIs, texture statistics are applied, estimating absolute sum / # of pixels (*as*), sum of squares / # of pixels (*ss*), and entropy (*ent*). Thus, the resulting feature vector contains twelve texture features.

Fractal Dimension Measurements: In order to extract more information on a ROI, a feature extraction method based on the concepts of the Fractional Brownian Motion (FBM) model and multiple resolution imagery was employed (Wu,

Figure 5. Regions of Interest (ROIs) identified by an experienced radiologist on CT images from (a) normal hepatic parenchyma, (b) cyst, (c) hemangioma, and (d) hepatocellular carcinoma.

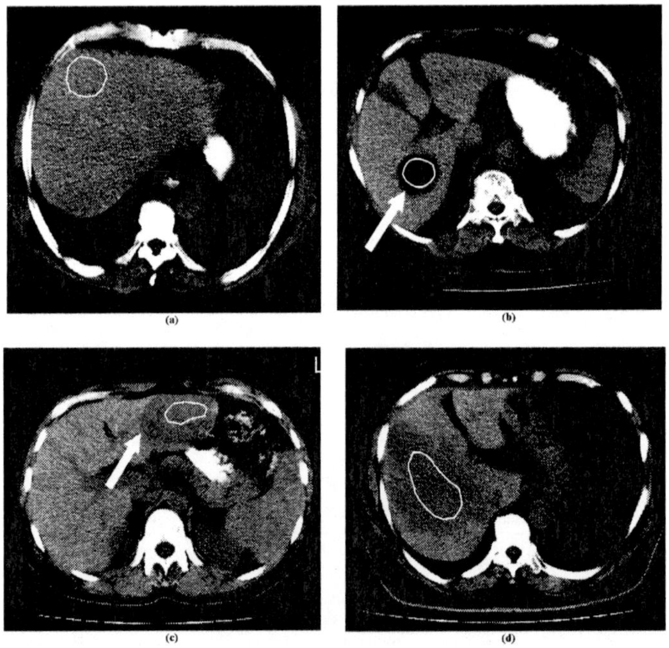

1992). The roughness of a surface of the ROI, naturally occurring as the end result of random walks, can be characterized by its Fractal Dimension (FD), $FD = H - 3$, according to the FBM model developed by Mandelbrot (Mandelbrot, 1983). The values $H^{(k)}$, which correspond to the H value of the image computed for an image resolution k, can provide more texture information, i.e. for the lacunarity or the regularity of the ROI. The original image corresponds to a k=1 resolution, the original image reduced to a half-sized image corresponds to a k=2 resolution, etc. Here, we calculated 3 FDM features that correspond to $H^{(1)}$, $H^{(2)}$, and $H^{(3)}$.

Feature Selection

Feature selection based on a GA (Goldberg, 1989) has been applied to the subsets of the texture features extracted in order to get the most informative ones for discriminating the four liver tissue types. More specifically, feature selection was applied offline to feature vectors estimated from SGLDM, GLDM and TEM, in order to produce the parsimonious feature vectors with dimensionality lower than ten (Gletsos, 2003). The features that were selected from the original SGLDM, GLDM and TEM feature sets are presented in Table 1.

Feature Sets Evaluation using ROC

Both full FOS, SGLDM, GLDM, TEM, FDM and reduced SGLDM, GLDM, and TEM features sets have been thoroughly evaluated using ROC curves generation for all binary classification tasks in the discrimination of four liver tissue types (Valavanis, 2007). Thus, ROC curves for all binary tasks, namely "C1 vs all", "C2 vs all", "C3 vs all", "C4 vs all" were generated using a multilayer perceptron NN as classifier and measurements of area under curve A_z values were obtained. Furthermore, total area under curve measurements (total A_z) were calculated in order to evaluate each

Table 1. The selected features from the SGLDM, GLDM and TEM feature sets fed into EC of DSS

SGLDM	GLDM	TEM
idm_{SGLDM} $(d = 1)$	idm_{GLDM} $(d = 1)$	as_{TEM} (*Mask: $L5^TE5$*)
ent_{SGLDM} $(d = 1)$	asm_{GLDM} $(d = 1)$	ss_{TEM} (*Mask: $L5^TE5$*)
clt_{SGLDM} $(d = 1)$	ent_{GLDM} $(d = 2)$	ent_{TEM} (*Mask: $L5^TE5$*)
cor_{SGLDM} $(d = 2)$	$mean_{GLDM}$ $(d = 4)$	ss_{TEM} (*Mask: $-E5^TS5$*)
idm_{SGLDM} $(d = 2)$	idm_{GLDM} $(d = 4)$	ent_{TEM} (*Mask: $-E5^TS5$*)
con_{SGLDM} $(d = 4)$		ss_{TEM} (*Mask: $L5^TS5$*)
cor_{SGLDM} $(d = 8)$		ent_{TEM} (*Mask: $L5^TS5$*)
con_{SGLDM} $(d = 12)$		ss_{TEM} (*Mask: $R5^TR5$*)

feature set in the multi-class problem. Results show that FOS feature set outperforms all other full or reduced feature sets in all binary decision cases and in the total A_z measurement (0.802 ± 0.08). The second best performing feature set in terms of total A_z measurement is the TEM set in its full (0.754 ± 0.063 using twelve features) or reduced version (0.765 ± 0.066 using eight features). SGLDM and GLDM feature sets seem to follow in total performance with rather small differences in total A_z measurements (mean A_z within the range [0.67 0.72]), whereas FDM is the worst performing feature set (total A_z: 0.613±0.059 using only three features). It has to be noted that the application of feature selection keeps the high A_z measurements of TEM feature set, thus providing an equally performing set of lower dimensionality (eight out of 12 features were selected). Total A_z measurements imply the same for SGLDM set (eight out of 48 features were selected). A moderate reduce in total A_z measurement was observed for the reduced GLDM set (five out of 20 features were selected). Finally, A_z values for the binary decisions show that C3 is the most difficult case to discriminate using the texture features used in this study. On the other hand, C2 is the easiest to discriminate with the maximum A_z value of all other liver tissue types (0.996 ± 0.016 obtained using FOS features).

ROI Classification

The 30-dimensional feature vector resulted after the combination of full FOS, FDM and reduced SGLDM, GLDM and TEM texture features is fed to an EC that classify the ROI into one of the four classes (C1, C2, C3 or C4). The EC consists of one multi-layer perceptron NN (MLP-NN) (Haykin, 1999), one probabilistic NN (P-NN) and three k-nearest neighbour classifiers (k-NN) (Kadah, 1996). Once the five primary classifiers have been generated, a weighed voting scheme (Jerebko, 2003) is used to combine their outputs.

DSS Evaluation

In order to obtain reliable results on the performance of the DSS, the design, implementation and evaluation of both the primary classifiers and the EC was undertaken 50 times according to the resampling technique of bootstrapping (Efron, 1982; Mougiakakou, 2007). The EC achieved a classification accuracy 84.96% ± 5.67%. The EC has been evaluated in the bootstrap testing sets using the one-versus-all comparisons (Patel, 2005) in order to get sensitivity and specificity when discriminating one type of liver tissue from the remaining three. The resulted sensitivities and specificities, in terms of mean values and corresponding standard deviations, are presented in Table 2. It can be observed that the EC is characterized by high sensitivity and specificity in the diagnosis of C1, C2, and C4, while a significantly lower sensitivity is achieved in the case of C3 due to misclassification of C3 into C1 and C4. This can be explained by the similar texture values of the ROIs belonging to classes C1, C3 and C4, thus making the discrimination difficult for the EC.

The presented DSS has been integrated into the pilot version of DIAGNOSIS (Mougiakakou, to appear), a telematics-enabled system for the archiving and management of medical images and assistance of diagnosis. The system is now under evaluation at the Radiological Department of Euginidion Hospital, Athens, Greece.

FUTURE TRENDS

Focusing on diagnosis support of liver diseases, full automation in the detection of hepatic lesions is the ultimate goal in the design and development of DSSs for the characterization of liver tissue from CT images. To this end, further research is needed towards the optimization of the registration methods and the improvement of segmentation algorithms for both segmentation of the liver and

Table 2. Sensitivity and specificity measurements for all one-vs-all comparisons in the bootstrap testing sets (mean value ± standard deviation)

	Sensitivity	Specificity
C1-vs-all	95.83 ± 5.45	81.93 ± 10.66
C2- vs-all	98.60 ± 5.63	100.00 ± 0.00
C3-vs-all	44.44 ± 26.60	97.14 ± 3.22
C4-vs-all	81.57 ± 16.43	96.19 ± 3.82

detection of suspicious ROIs. Furthermore, the application of feature selection methods in order to obtain highly informative and parsimonious feature sets seems to reduce the computational complexity, while the combination of classifiers into an ensemble can improve the final performance. Furthermore, FOS texture features were found in our studies to provide superior informative content on the texture of focal liver lesions. Additionally, the use and optimal tuning of kernel-based classifiers, e.g. SVMs, for a specific hepatic tissue classification problem and the employment of new strategies in constructing ECs, e.g. genetic programming, may comprise the next steps towards the improvement of the image analysis module.

An important issue in the design and development of DSSs is the reliable evaluation of their performance. This can be done using evaluation methods such as the leave-one-out, cross-validation, hold-out, and bootstrapping. These techniques have become lately valuable when classification techniques are applied in biomedical engineering studies, since small-sized samples often used in these studies can lead to biased evaluation results.

Future work in the field of DSSs for hepatic lesions may include the use of information extracted from 3D CT images and multimodal imaging modalities, as well. The latter would permit assisting a physician during the diagnosis of a wider range of hepatic diseases.

In general, DSSs are estimated to become part of clinical work in the characterization of various lesions in the next years. They promise to increase the efficiency of health care professionals during the diagnostic examinations in daily clinical work, while increasing accuracy in medical diagnosis.

CONCLUSION

In this chapter state-of-the-art DSSs for the computerized diagnosis of liver diseases from CT images have been presented. Image preprocessing, registration and segmentation algorithms, visualisation techniques, as well as image texture descriptors and classifiers from the fields of computational intelligence and statistics have been described and are widely used in order to produce a "second" opinion and assist the procedure of diagnosis. Finally, DSSs designed and developed by our research team for the differential diagnosis of focal liver lesions from non-enhanced CT images have been presented.

ACKNOWLEDGMENT

The design and development of the DSS of focal liver lesions from CT images was the result of the collaboration with the 2nd Department of Radiology, Medical School, University of Athens (Prof. D. Kelekis, Dr. A. Nikita), which was supported in part by the General Secretariat for Research and Technology of the Greek Ministry of Development under the 96SYN20 project.

REFERENCES

Asvestas, P., Matsopoulos, G. K., & Nikita, K. S. (1998). A power differentiation method of fractal dimension estimation for 2-D signals. *Journal of Visual Communication and Image Representation, 9*(4), 392-400.

Chen, E. L., Chung, P. C., Chen, C. L., Tsa, H. M., & Chang, C. I. (1998). An automatic diagnostic system for CT liver image classification. *IEEE Transactions on Biomedical Engineering, 45*(6), 783-794.

Christodoulou, C. I., Pattichis, C. S., Pantziaris, M., & Nicolaides, A. (2003). A Texture-based classification of atherosclerotic carotid plaques. *IEEE Transactions on Medical Imaging, 22*(7), 902 - 912.

Dettori, L., & Beshir, A. (2007). Texture classification of normal tissues in computed tomography using Gabor filters. In J. P. W. Pluim, J. M. Reinhardt (Ed), *SPIE Medical Imaging: Vol. 6512*, (6512Q).

Dhawan, A. P., Chitre, Y., Kaiser-Bonasso, C., & Moskowitz, M. (1996). Analysis of mammographic microcalcifications using gray-level image structure features. *IEEE Transactions on Medical Imaging, 15*(3), 246-259.

Efron, B. (1982). *The jackknife, the bootstrap, and other resampling plans*, Philadelphia, CBMS-NSF Regional Conf. Series in Applied Mathematics, Society for Industrial and Applied Mathematics (SIAM).

Eibenberger, E., Borsorf, A., Wimmer, A., & Hornegger, J. (2008). Edge-Preserving Denoising for Segmentation in CT-Images, In T. Tolxdorff, J. Braun, T. M. Deserno, H. Handels, A. Horsch, H. P. Meinzer (Ed.) *Bildverarbeitung für die Medizin 2008 - Algorithmen, Systeme, Anwendungen* (pp. 257-261). Springer-Verlag.

Gletsos, M., Mougiakakou, S. G., Matsopoulos, G. K, Nikita, K. S., Nikita, A., & Kelekis, D. (2003). A computer-aided diagnostic system to characterize CT focal liver lesions: Design and optimization of a neural network classifier. *IEEE Transactions on Information Technology in Biomedicine*, *7*(3), 153-162.

Goldberg, D. (1989). *Genetic algorithms in search, optimization and machine learning.* Boston, MA. Addison-Wesley.

Gonzalez, R. C., & Woods, R. E. (2002). Image Enhancement in the Spatial Domain. In *Digital image processing* (pp. 75-146). Reading, MA. Addison-Wesley.

Grigorescu S., Petkov N., & Kruizinga P. (2002). Comparison of Texture Features Based on Gabor Filters. *IEEE Transactions on Image Processing, 11*(10), 1160-1167

Haralick, R. M., & Shaphiro L. G. (1992), *Computer and Robot Vision.* vol. I., Boston, MA. Addison-Wesley.

Haralick, R. M., Shanmugan, K., & Dinstein, I. (1973). Textural features for image classification. *IEEE Transactions on Systems, Man and Cybernetics, 3*(6), 610-622.

Haykin, S. (1999). *Neural Networks: A Comprehensive Foundation*, NJ. Prentice-Hall.

Hein, E., Albrecht, A., Melzer, D., Steinhöfer, K., Rogalla, P., Hamm, B., & Taoupitz, M. (2005). Computer-assisted diagnosis of focal liver lesions on CT images: Evaluation of the perceptron algorithm. *Academic Radiology. 12*(9), 1205-1210.

Huang, Y. L., Chen, J. H., & Shen, W .C. (2006). Diagnosis of hepatic tumors with texture analysis in non-enhanced computed tomography images. *Academic Radiology, 13*(6), 713-720.

Jerebko, A. K., Malley, J. D., Franaszek, M., & Summers, R. M. (2003). Multiple neural network classification scheme for detection of colonic polyps in CT colonography data sets. *Academic Radiology, 10*(2), 154-160.

Kadah, Y. M., Frag, A. A., Zurada, J. M., Badawi, A. M., & Youssef, A.B. M. (1996). Classification algorithms for quantitative tissue characterization of diffuse liver disease from ultrasound images. *IEEE Transactions on Medical Imaging, 15*(4), 466-478.

Kyriacou, E., Pavlopoulos, S., Koutsouris, D., Zoumpoulis, P., & Theotokas, I. (1997). Computer assisted characterization of liver tissue using image texture analysis techniques on B-scan images. In *19th Annual International Conference of the IEEE Engineering in Medicine and Biology Society. Vol. 2.* (pp. 806-809).

Laws, K. I. (1980) Rapid texture identification, In *SPIE Conference for Missile Guidance. Vol. 238.* (pp. 376-380).

Lee, C. C., Chen, S. H., Tsai, H. M., Chung, P. C., & Chiang, Y. C. (2006). Discrimination of liver diseases from CT images based on Gabor filters. In *19th IEEE International Symposium on Computer-Based Medical Systems. Vol. 1.* (pp.203-206)

Lee, C. C, Chen, S. H., & Chiang, Y. C. (2007). Classification of liver disease from CT images using a support vector machine. *Journal of Advanced Computational Intelligence and Intelligent Informatics, 11*(4), 396-402.

Lee, J., Kim, N., Lee, H., Seo, J. B., Won, H. J., Shin, Y. M., Shin, Y. G., & Kim, S.H. (2007). Efficient liver segmentation using level-set method with optimal detection of the initial liver boundary from level-set speed images. *Computer Methods and Programs in Biomedicine, 88*(1), 26-38.

Mandelbrot, B. B. (1983). *Fractal geometry of nature*. NY. W. H. Freeman and Co.

Masutani, Y., Uozumi, K., Akahane, M., & Ohtoo, K. (2006). Liver CT image processing: A short introduction of the technical elements. *European Journal of Radiology, 58*(2), 246-251.

Mir, A. H., Hanmandlu M., & Tandon S. N. (1995). Texture analysis of CT images. *IEEE Engineering in Medicine and Biology Magazine, 14*(6), 781-786.

Mougiakakou, S. G., Valavanis I. K., Nikita A., & Nikita K. (2007). Differential diagnosis of CT focal liver lesions using texture features, feature selection and ensemble driven classifiers. *Artificial Intelligence in Medicine, 41*(1), 25-37.

Mougiakakou, S. G., Valavanis, I. K., Mouravliansky, N. A., Nikita, A., & Nikita K. S. (in press). DIAGNOSIS: A telematics enabled system for medical image archiving, management and diagnosis assistance. *IEEE Transactions on Instrumentation and Measurements.*

Patel, A. C, & Markey, M. K. (2005) Comparison of three-class classification performance metrics: A case study in breast cancer CAD. In M. P. Eckstein, Y. Jiang Y (Ed.), *SPIE Medical Imaging 2005: Image Perception, Observer Performance, and Technology Assessment. Vol.* 5749. (pp. 581-589).

Perona, P., & Malik. J. (1990). Scale space and edge detection using anisotropic diffusion. *IEEE Transactions on Pattern Analysis and Machine Intelligence, 12*(7), 629-639.

Russ, J. C. (1992). *The image processing handbook*. FL. Boca Raton CRC.

Sariyanni, C. P. A., Asvestas P., Matsopoulos, G. K., Nikita, K. S., Nikita, A.S., & Kelekis, D. (2001). A Fractal Analysis of CT Liver Images for the Discrimination of Hepatic Lesions: A Comparative Study. In *23rd Annual EMBS International Conference. Vol. 2.* pp.1557-1560.

Schmitt, M., Teodorescu, H. N., Jain, A., Jain, S., & Jain, L. (2002). *Computational intelligence processing in medical diagnosis.* NY. Physica-Verlag.

Seltzer, S. E., Getty, D. J., Pickett, R. M., Swets, J. A., Sica, G., Brown, J., Saini, S., Mattrey, R.F., Harmon, B., Francis, I. R., Chezmar, J., Schnall, M. O., Siegelman, E. S., Ballerini, R., & Bhat, S. (2002). Multimodality diagnosis of liver tumors: Feature analysis with CT, Liver-specific and Contrast-enhanced MR, and a computer model. *Academic Radiology, 9*(3), 256-259.

Shimizu, A., Kawamura, T., & Kobatake, H. (2005). Proposal of computer-aided detection system for three dimensional CT images of liver cancer. *International Congress Series, 1281*, 1157-1162.

Stoitsis, J., Golemati, S., & Nikita K. S. (2006). A modular software system to assist interpretation of medical images - Application to vascular ultrasound images. *IEEE Transactions on Instrumentation and Measurement, 55*(6), 1944-1952.

Stoitsis, J., Valavanis, I., Mougiakakou, S. G., Golemati, S., Nikita, A., & Nikita, K. S. (2006). Computer aided diagnosis based on medical image processing and artificial intelligence methods. *Nuclear Instruments & Methods in Physics Research A, 569*(2), 591-595.

Sujana, H., Swarnamani, S., & Suresh, S. (1996). Application of artificial neural networks for the classification of liver lesions by image texture parameters. *Ultrasound in Medicine and Biology, 22*(9), 1177-1181.

Sun, Y. N., Horng, M. H., Lin, X. Z., & Wang, J. Y. (1996). Ultrasound image analysis for liver diagnosis: A noninvasive alternative to determine liver disease. *IEEE Engineering in Medicine and Biology Magazine*, 93-101.

Tomasi, C., & Manduchi, R. (1998). Bilateral filtering for gray and color images. In *6th IEEE International Conference on Computer Vision.* (pp. 839-846).

Valavanis, I. K, Mougiakakou, S. G., Nikita, A., & Nikita, K. S. (2007). Evaluation of texture features in hepatic tissue tissue discrimination. In *29th IEEE Conference in Engineering in Medicine and Biology.* (pp. 3741-3744).

Wang, X.Y., & Feng, D. D. (2005). Biomedical image registration for diagnostic decision making and treatment monitoring. In F. Dong, G. Ghinea and S. Y. Chen (Ed.), *User Centered Design for Medical Visualization* Premier Reference Source.

Weszka, J. S., Dryer, C. R., & Rosenfeld A. (1976). A comparative study of texture measures for terrain classification. *IEEE Transactions on Systems, Man and Cybernetics, 6*, 269-285.

Wu, C. M, Chen, Y. C., & Hsieh, K. S. (1992). Texture features for classification of ultrasonic liver images. *IEEE Transactions on Medical Imaging, 11*(2), 141-151.

Wu, Y., Ianakiev. K., & Govindaraju, V. (2002). Improved k-nearest neighbor classification, *Pattern Recognition, 35*(10), 2311-2318.

Zhang, X., Fujita, H., Kanematsu, M., Zhou, X., Hara. T., Kato, H., Yokoyama, R., Hoshi, H. (2005). Improving the classification of cirrhotic liver by texture features. In *27th IEEE Conference of Engineering in Medicine and Biology.* (pp. 867-870).

KEY TERMS

Diagnostic Support Systems: Computer programs that assist a physician or a health professional during the diagnostic process.

Computational Intelligence: A branch of computer science that develops algorithms and techniques to imitate some cognitive abilities, like recognition, learning and evolution.

Artificial Neural Networks: Information processing systems with interconnected components analogous to neurons that mimic biological nervous systems and the ability to learn through experience.

Genetic Algorithms: Algorithms which vary a set of parameters and evaluate the quality or "fitness" of the results of a computation as the parameters are changed or "evolved".

Texture Features: Numerical descriptors calculated from the intensity of pixels in a given image region that characterize the texture (roughness) of this region.

Feature Selection: Strategy for selecting a sub-set of variables from an initial set towards reducing the dimensionality of input vector to a classifier and building more robust learning models.

Ensemble of Classifiers: A set of classifiers whose individual predictions are fused through a combining strategy.

Non-Enhanced CT Images: CT images obtained without administration of contrast agents.

Chapter VI
Significance Estimation in fMRI from Random Matrices

Marotesa Voultsidou
University of Crete, Greece

J. Michael Herrmann
University of Edinburgh, UK

ABSTRACT

Indicative features of an fMRI data set can be evaluated by methods provided by theory of random matrices (RMT). RMT considers ensembles of matrices and yields statements on the properties of the typical eigensystems in these ensembles. The authors have studied the particular ensemble of random correlation matrices that can be used as a noise model for the empirical data and that allows us thus to select data features that significantly differ from the noisy background. In this sense RMT can be understood as offering a systematic approach to surrogate data. Interestingly, also the noise characteristics change between different experimental conditions. This is revealed by higher-order statistics available from RMT. The authors illustrate the RMT-based approach by an exemplary data set for the distinction between a visuomotor task and a resting condition. In addition it is shown for these data that the degree of sparseness and of localization can be evaluated in a strict way, provided that the data are sufficiently well described by the pairwise cross-correlations.

The aim of art is to represent not the outward appearance of things, but their inward significance. — Aristotle

INTRODUCTION

In order to reveal features of interest in empirical data there is often no other option than a comparison to the corresponding quantities in surrogate data, that is, shuffled, boosted, randomized or otherwise rearranged data of the same kind. Surrogate data (Theiler, Eubank, Longtin, Galdrikian, & Farmer, 1992) provide a contrast or a baseline against which relevant data features are to be compared, while the actual generation process of surrogate data that provide the desired contrast remains a matter of an on-going debate. Not only may the shuffling of the data cause a level of randomness against which any feature appears significant, but also may the surrogate data in a high-dimensional problem become sparse and thus not sufficiently representative for the underlying distribution. By reference to random matrices we suggest a more systematic framework for providing baselines to data features of potential interest. This framework does not necessarily include the discrimination of artifacts from intrinsic features. It will, however, systematically reduce the data space such that later other methods may be invoked in order to further analyze the data. It will further provide sensitive means for the distinction of various scenarios at which seemingly similar data were obtained. If for a certain quantity a prediction from Random Matrix Theory (RMT) exists then it is possible to rate the difference between two data sets relative to their respective distance to the theoretical value. Of particular interest is, furthermore, that RMT provides descriptions of spatial properties of the data. These can be used for the discrimination of active and non-active brain voxels which forms an essential step in the analysis of fMRI data. Thus, suggestive data properties such as sparseness and localization of features can be expressed as well by quantities which are meaningful in the theory of random matrices.

Random matrix theory studies ensembles of matrices. An ensemble is a distribution over the set of all matrices. In the limit of high dimensions all matrices of the ensemble are similar in the sense that they share certain properties regardless of the dynamical principles or the interactions underlying the system. In this sense the properties of the ensemble are universal. In this way a random matrix approach to data processing does not only study a few sets of surrogate data, but allows us in principle to compare the given data set to a set of all possible surrogate samples.

BACKGROUND

Dimension Reduction

A main objective of fMRI analysis is to discriminate between brain voxels that are active or non-active for a specific stimulus or task. Because of noise originating from the scanning equipment, movements of the subject and the hemodynamic processes the discrimination is ambiguous and noise removal remains a key step in the analysis of the data. Independent Component Analysis (ICA) or clustering methods (Voultsidou, Dodel, & Herrmann, 2005; Dodel, Herrmann, & Geisel, 2002) have been proposed in order to detect the informative components underlying the data. Noise removal can be interpreted as the problem of estimating the intrinsic dimensionality of the data, that is the number of variables that is required for a faithful representation of the relevant processes. For this purpose, often a cutoff in the eigenvalue spectrum of the data covariance matrix is employed, which defines the dimensionality of the signal and noise space. The most simplistic approach in estimating the model order is Principal Component Analysis (PCA) of the sample covariance matrix, where a cutoff can be defined by any abrupt change in the sequence of the eigenvalues.

In order to extract interesting components from fMRI data, Hansen et al. (1999) suggested the use of the estimated generalization error for finding the optimal number of principal components while further components can be safely ignored. Likewise in ICA, the predicted sum of squares was used (M. J. McKeown, 2000). Cordes and Nandy (2006) assumed correlated Gaussian noise that satisfies an auto-regressive model the coefficients of which were estimated by maximizing the quality of fit of the model with respect to the data and were used as well to indicate the number of relevant eigenvalues. Other approaches are based on information-theoretic criteria such as Minimum Description Length (M. H. Hansen & Yu, 2001), Akaike Information Criterion, Bayesian Information Criterion (Schwarz, 1978), and Probabilistic Principal Component Analysis (PPCA) (Minka, 1999). By explicitly incorporating Gaussian noise to the model, Everson and Roberts (2000) used a Bayesian framework to estimate the eigenvalues and the rank of the covariance matrix while Beckmann and Smith (2004) used a PPCA scheme to estimate the number of activation and non-Gaussian noise sources before applying ICA. Here it is the theory of random matrices that provides us with a measure of the dimensionality of the data such that must not use a map that actually performs the reduction of the data.

RMT for Data Processing

Although RMT has been originally established in physics (Wigner, 1967; Brody, Flores, French, Mello, Pandey & Wong, 1981; Mehta, 1991) it has turned out to be applicable successfully to a number of phenomena such as the stock market (Plerou et al., 2002) and EEG studies (Šeba, 2003) because it permits the identification and subsequent suppression of features which are universally present in large classes of systems (Brody et al., 1981). In physics such features are considered as a direct characterization of the system. In the present context, however, they will serve as a baseline against which the significance of those that deviate from universality can be estimated. More specifically, by comparing the properties of the data correlation matrix with the generic properties of random matrices we aim at separating the contributions to it into two groups, namely (i) the part that conforms to the universal properties of random matrices and is interpreted as "noise" and (ii) the part that deviates from the RMT predictions and can hence be interpreted as the informative part. This separation becomes evident by studying the statistical properties of the eigenvalues of the correlation matrix and in particular the eigenvalue distribution, the level space distribution and the number variance, as well as the localization properties of the corresponding eigenvectors.

Data Correlation Matrices

The data from an fMRI experiment are given as an $(M \times T)$-matrix $\mathbf{X}$ where M denotes the number of voxels in one (volume) image and T is the length of the trial measured by the number of time steps. The correlation matrix requires centering and normalization of the data. If X_i is the time series of activities of voxel i, and X_{it} is the intensity of voxel i at time t then

$$D_i = \frac{(X_{it} - \frac{1}{T}\sum X_{it})}{\sqrt{\frac{1}{T}\sum (X_{it} - \frac{1}{T}\sum X_{it})^2}} \tag{1}$$

is its centered and variance-normalized version. The data correlation matrix is given by the matrix product $\mathbf{C} = \mathbf{D}\mathbf{D}^T$, where $\mathbf{D}$ consists of the columns $\mathbf{D}_i$ (1). In order to obtain the eigenvalues and the eigenvectors of $\mathbf{C}$ we performed a Singular Value Decomposition on the data matrix $\mathbf{D}$ such that $\mathbf{D} = \mathbf{U}\mathbf{S}\mathbf{V}^T$. The eigenvalues of $\mathbf{C}$ are the non-zero entries of the diagonal matrix $\mathbf{S}_C = \mathbf{S}\mathbf{S}^T$ while its eigenvectors form the columns of $\mathbf{U}$. The temporal average in Eq. 1 may as well be replaced by a spatial average (Dodel, Geisel & Herrmann, 2000) in order to obtain spatial correlation matrices of the form $\mathbf{C}' = \mathbf{D}'^T\mathbf{D}'$ with $\mathbf{D}'$ being the corresponding spatially centered data.

The Ensemble of Random Correlation Matrices

A typical ensemble in RMT is the Gaussian Orthogonal Ensemble (GOE), a set of matrices with entries drawn independently from a fixed Gaussian distribution. In the context of data analysis, the correlation matrices are characterized by non-negativity and bounded entries. In order to satisfy this property an ensemble of random correlation matrices (RCE) is defined. Matrices **C** in RCE can be obtained from matrices **B** by $\mathbf{C} = \mathbf{B}\mathbf{B}^T$, where **B** is a matrix of random elements with zero mean and unit variance. While the RCE is naturally better suited as a comparator to the data, the GOE is used as a reference. Theorems in RMT usually hold for matrices of infinite size. Although in many cases finite-size corrections are available (Izrailev, 1990), we will include also numerics on the finite size effects for comparison to the standard RMT results.

RMT-BASED DATA CHARACTERIZATION

Eigenvalue Distribution

An early result of RMT is the Wigner semi-circle law describing the normalized spectrum of a matrix that contains independently Gaussian distributed elements by the density of eigenvalues μ

$$p(\mu) = \frac{2}{\pi}\sqrt{1-\mu^2} \tag{2}$$

where the width of the distribution is scaled to [−1, 1]. Since we are interested in correlation matrices, the law assumes a modified form. Correlation matrices are positive semi-definite, (i.e. all of their eigenvalues $\lambda_n \geq 0$), and can thus be represented as $\mathbf{C} = \mathbf{A}\mathbf{A}^T$, where **A** can be chosen as a symmetric matrix. If $\lambda = \mu^2$ is an eigenvalue of **C** then μ is an eigenvalue of **A**. In the place of the semi-circle law now a quarter-circle law is considered:

$$p(\lambda) = \frac{2}{\pi}\sqrt{\frac{1}{\lambda} - 1} \tag{3}$$

The integrated form

$$P(\lambda) = \int_0^{\lambda} p(\lambda')d\lambda' = \frac{2}{\pi}\left(\lambda\sqrt{1-\lambda^2} + \arcsin(\lambda)\right) \tag{4}$$

is statistically more reliable and thus often practically preferable. Its inverse function is also known as *level distribution* and can be compared with empirical data. It is given by

$$P^{-1}\left(\frac{n}{N}\right) = \lambda_n \tag{5}$$

where λ_n, $n \in \{1,2,\ldots,N\}$, are the non-zero eigenvalues of the correlation matrix **C** and N is the total number of eigenvalues.

In order to compare Eq. 4 with the corresponding one for experimental data, the function

$$N_C(\lambda_n) = n \tag{6}$$

is defined on the discrete set of empirical eigenvalues $\{\lambda_1,\ldots,\lambda_N\}$. For the comparison the scaling of the spectrum to unity length is necessary as assumed in Eq. 3. Because the scaling depends on the extreme eigenvalues such that the applicability of RMT will not become visible, we proceed by restricting the fit to a part of the spectrum while minimizing at the same time the number of points which are excluded from the fit.

In place of Eq. 4 a more general fitting function is considered, which allows for shifts a and scaling along both axis by means of b and c,

$$P(\lambda)=\frac{2c}{\pi}\left(\left(\frac{\lambda-\alpha}{b}\right)\sqrt{1-\left(\frac{\lambda-\alpha}{b}\right)^2}+\arcsin\left(\frac{\lambda-\alpha}{b}\right)\right) \tag{7}$$

The fit is performed by gradient descent with respect to α, b, and c on the squared fitting error

$$E_{n_0}(\alpha,b,c)=\sum_{n=n_0}^{n_1}(P(\lambda_n)-N_C(\lambda_n))^2 \tag{8}$$

where $n_0 \geq 0$ large eigenvalues and $N\text{-}n_1$ small eigenvalues are excluded, while for the analysis of errors the locally resolved version of Eq. 8 for a particular n_0

$$E_{n,n_0}=(P(\lambda_n)-N_C(\lambda_n))^2 \tag{9}$$

is considered. The eigenvalues that when are excluded from the fitting process in the course of the minimization of the fitting error are considered to form the informative part of the data and are thus assigned to the signal space.

Four cases can be distinguished in a typical quality of fit. In the first case the semi-circle law is well obeyed. In the second one the quality of the fit is drastically reduced. In the third case the scaling in the optimized fitting function is such that the test values fall outside the domain of definition (arcsin!). A fourth case is characterized by very large extrapolation errors, which indicate clearly that the large eigenvalues do not obey RMT and thus are considered to reflect non-random processes underlying the data.

Unfolding the Spectrum

Universality of the results from RMT is revealed only after a normalization procedure.

This unfolding procedure (Brody et. al. 1981) transforms the envelope of the spectral density to uniformity such that only local differences are left for further analysis, that is, the smooth part of the cumulative spectral function is extracted and only the fluctuations of the eigenvalues (or "*levels*") are considered. The integrated density of states

$$N(\lambda)=\int_{-\infty}^{\lambda}\sum_i\delta(\lambda'-\lambda_i)d\lambda'=\sum_i\theta(\lambda'-\lambda_i) \tag{10}$$

with δ being the Dirac delta function and θ the Heaviside step function is of staircase-shape.

Several approaches have been proposed to smooth $N(\lambda)$. Polynomial fitting of Eq. 10 works well for systems with level density as smooth as a polynomial. Another widely used method is replacing the δ-functions in Eq. 10 by Gaussian functions of standard deviation σ which can be a constant for the whole spectrum or be adapted to the local variability of the spectrum. The most common approach to unfold the spectrum is the so called local unfolding. The unfolded eigenvalues ε are calculated by

$$\varepsilon_{i+1}=\varepsilon_i+\frac{\lambda_{i+1}-\lambda_i}{K_i} \tag{11}$$

where K_i is the local mean level space

$$K_i=\frac{1}{2k+1}\sum_{j=i-k}^{i+k}(\lambda_{j+1}-\lambda_j) \tag{12}$$

and the number of consecutive level spaces $2k$ in the running average is the free parameter of the model.

Level Space Distribution

A simple statistical quantity that is studied in RMT is the (nearest-neighbor) level space distribution $P(s)$, that relates to the distance $s_i=\varepsilon_{i+1}-\varepsilon_i$ between the unfolded eigenvalues. $P(s)$ provides information on short range spectral correlations. For the GOE it is known to obey the Wigner surmise (Wigner, 1967):

$$P(s)=\frac{\pi}{2}se^{-\pi s^2/4} \tag{13}$$

Instead of calculating the level space distribution directly, the more robust, integrated form

$$N(s) = \int P(s)ds \qquad (14)$$

is usually preferred, which leads to $N_{RMT}(s) = 1 - e^{-\pi s^2/4}$. Finite-size results differ from the theoretical value, as shown in Fig. 1(a).

The Number Variance

Higher-order information is contained in the number variance $\Sigma^2(L)$ which is defined as the variance of the number of unfolded eigenvalues in an interval of length L:

$$\Sigma^2(L) = \langle N^2(L,\varepsilon_0)\rangle - \langle N(L,\varepsilon_0)\rangle^2 \qquad (15)$$

where $N(L,\varepsilon_0)$ counts the number of levels in the interval $[\varepsilon_0, \varepsilon_0 + L]$ of unfolded eigenvalues and the averages are over ε_0. Usually, $\Sigma^2(L)$ is defined by an additional average over the ensemble. For a GOE the number variance in the limit of large matrix size is given by (Brody et al., 1981):

$$\Sigma^2(L) = 2\pi^2\left(\ln(2\pi L) + 1.5772 - \frac{\pi^2}{8}\right) \qquad (16)$$

The number variance for the GOE and the RCE samples is shown in Fig. 2(a). Apart from a scaling factor that compensates for finite size effects, $\Sigma^2(L)$ saturates as L increases and especially as it approaches the width of the unfolding procedure k, allowing thus no statements for L above that value. In the following, comparisons based on $\Sigma^2(L)$ will be therefore restricted to L values below k.

Statistical Analysis of Eigenvectors

Entropy Localization Length

RMT provides also a natural way to study the localization of activity. The concepts of the entropy localization length and the width of an eigenvector cover two main aspects, namely the sparsity of the eigenvectors and the relative location of their largest components, respectively. The entropy localization length is based on Shannon entropy (Izrailev, 1990; Luna-Acosta, Méndez-Bermúdez, & Izrailev, 2001) which is defined as

$$H_N^{(n)} = -\sum_{i=1}^{N} w_i^n \ln(w_i^n) \qquad (17)$$

where $w_i^n \equiv (u_i^n)^2$ and u_i^n denotes the ith component of the nth normalized eigenvector, $(n = 1, \ldots, N)$ of the data correlation matrix **C**. The entropy $H_N^{(n)}$ gives a measure of the number of components in an eigenvector that are significantly large. In the case of extreme localization $w_i^n = (0,\ldots,0,1,0,\ldots,0)$ and $H_N^{(n)} = 0$, while the most extended eigenvectors is $w_i^n = (1/N,\ldots,1/N)$ with $H_N^{(n)} = \ln(N)$.

The entropy localization length l_H^n is defined as

$$l_H^n = Ne^{\left(H_N^{(n)} - \overline{H}_N\right)} \qquad (18)$$

where, $\overline{H}_N$ introduces a normalization factor for a finite basis such that in the case of a fully extended eigenvectors the value l_H^n equals the size of the basis N.

Width of an Eigenvector

The entropy localization length (Eq. 18) represents the effective number of large components of an eigenvector, however, without any information about their location. Eigenvectors of the same length may have different structure depending on the location of the large or small components. Additional information can be expressed by the mean square root (or *width of an eigenvector*) l_c (Luna Acosta et al., 2001), which is defined by introducing the center of mass of an eigenvector

$$l_c^{(n)} = \left\{ \sum_{i=1}^{N} w_i^n \left[\left(i_x - n_{cx}(n)\right)^2 + \left(i_y - n_{cy}(n)\right)^2 \right] \right\}^{12} \qquad (19)$$

where i_x, i_y denote the position of a voxel i in the image and n_{cx}, n_{cy} denote the corresponding center of mass. Small values of l_c imply localization while large values indicate extendedness.

Contrast in an Illustrative Data Set

The applicability of RTM to fMRI analysis can be demonstrated by studying the differences between correlation matrices obtained from the experimental data and from the random ensembles. By construction the sets have the same number of eigenvalues as the data correlation matrix **C** such that a direct comparison of the statistical properties is possible even in the finite-dimensional case. The fMRI data, consisting of six layers each, were recorded under two conditions. The first has been captured while the subject was in resting state (REST) while in the second the subject was engaged into a visuomotor task (TASK). The integrated level space distribution (14) does not indicate a significant deviation from the surrogate data (RCE and GOE, cf. Fig. 1). This observation confirms earlier findings in EEG data (Šeba, 2003) and suggested to consider more complex statistical quantities.

The two fMRI data sets differ from the synthetic sets with respect to the number variance, while the artificial matrices produced very similar results (see Fig. 2(a)). In addition, the number variance of the TASK data set deviates more from the GOE/RCE sets than the REST set which is mainly caused by differences among the largest eigenvalues or more specifically by the fact that the eigenvectors representing stimulus-related activity are more prominent in the TASK data.

Figure 1. Integrated level space distribution for the GOE (a), the RCE (b) and the two fMRI data sets (REST (c) and TASK (d)) In the insets the differences from the theoretical prediction are shown.

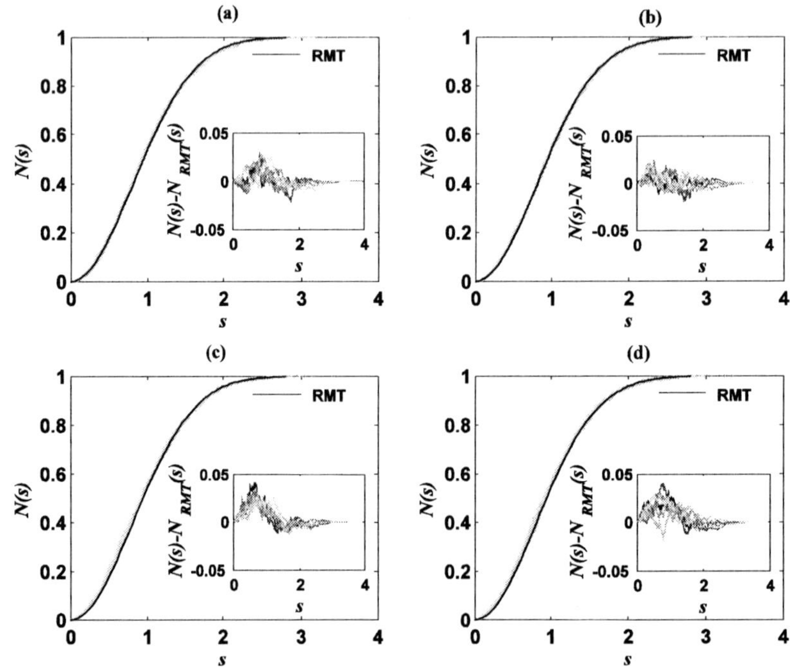

A number of eigenvectors that correspond to the largest eigenvalues are responsible for the deviations from the random behavior and can be characterized as significant data features. This can be seen if a number N_l of the largest eigenvalues are discarded from the analysis. Figs. 2(b), (c) demonstrate the process of approaching the universal behavior described by RMT as N_l increases. If a number $N_l = 10$ of the largest eigenvalues are discarded from the analysis then the REST results converge to the GOE/RCE behavior while the TASK results are affected when the random "bulk" is more exposed after removal of $N_l = 20$ eigenvalues. By continuously increasing N_l one expects the difference in $\Sigma^2(L)$ between the fMRI data sets and the synthetic ones to vanish. The REST data set shows no substantial difference when N_l increases further but shows a sub-Gaussian behavior which implies that the bulk of the REST spectrum is more "rigid" than the GOE/RCE ones.

Exclusion of an increased number of large eigenvalues from the analysis of the TASK data set shows a tendency to reach the GOE/RCE curve but the procedure is extremely slow (Fig. 2(b),(c)). This suggests that the rest of the spectrum still carries information that cannot be separated by second order statistics used in this approach.

The differences in $\Sigma^2(L)$ between the two fMRI data sets as a function of the number of excluded eigenvalues N_l can be measured in terms of standard deviation (Fig. 2(d)). For the six layers we calculate the mean Σ^2 and the corresponding standard deviation for each value of L, to obtain the mean standard deviation (MSD) of the two sets. Their difference averaged over L is then defined

Figure 2. (a) Number variance for the fMRI data sets (REST and TASK) and the GOE and RCE sets. The theoretical prediction is also shown. (b) ,(c) Number variance for the fMRI and the synthetic data sets after exclusion of some of the largest eigenvalues (N_l=10 in (b) and N_l=20 in (c)). (d) Mean $\Sigma^2(L)$ difference between the TASK and the REST data set in units of mean standard deviation as a function of the number of omitted largest eigenvalues

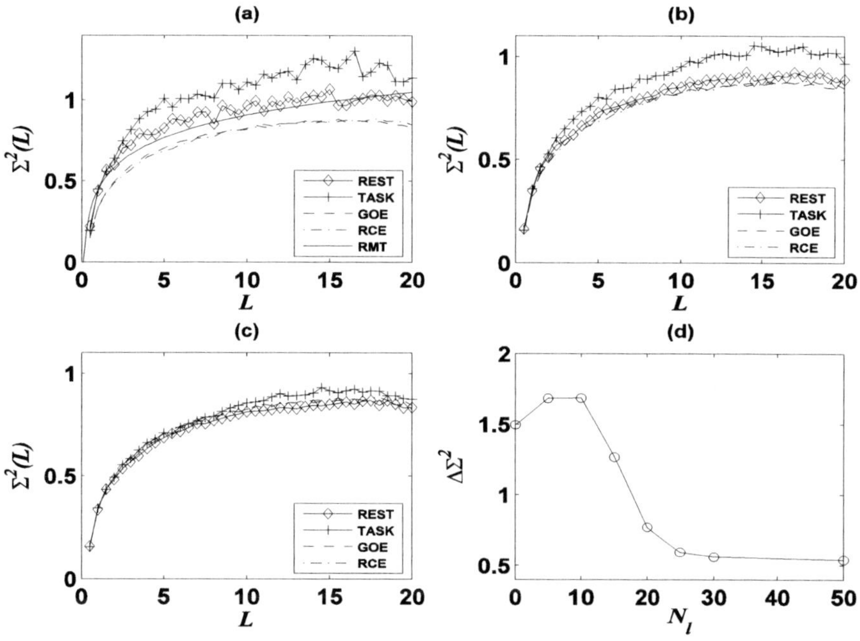

as $\Delta\Sigma^2 = \left(\Sigma_T^2 - \Sigma_R^2\right)/MSD$ where Σ_T^2 and Σ_R^2 hold for the TASK and the REST data set respectively. A further exclusion of eigenvalues does not lead to a further decay of $\Sigma^2(L)$, implying that traces of the stimulus are no longer noticeable in this way.

The relevant eigenvectors of the empirical correlation matrices can be identified by comparing their spatial properties to the random ensembles in terms of entropy localization length and widths of the eigenvectors (Fig. 3). For the GOE sample, neither l_H nor l_c show a systematic dependency on the eigenvalue number. The entropy localization length l_H and the width of the eigenvector l_c of both fMRI data sets deviate from the GOE case, as is shown in Fig. 3(c) and 3(d), respectively. The eigenvectors with the highest eigenvalues exhibit small values of l_H and thus contain a small number of relative high components. The largest l_H value corresponds to the eigenvector with the largest eigenvalue and indicates global activation. Towards the center of the spectrum the eigenvectors tend to show similar behavior as the random vectors, because l_H is close to the number of components.

The width l_c of the eigenvectors provides additional information. Neighboring eigenvectors in particular those with the largest eigenvalues exhibit different degrees of sparsity. Although their entropy localization length is smaller than that of the rest of the spectrum their effective components are distributed from high localization to high extendedness. We propose to combine information from the entropy localization length l_H and the width of the eigenvectors l_c to

Figure 3. Entropy localization length of the eigenvectors of a GOE-like matrix (a) and of the eigenvectors of a correlation matrix of fMRI data (c). In (a) the mean l_H (white line) is very close to the total number of eigenvectors N indicating that the eigenvectors are extended. In (b) and (d) the width of the eigenvectors of a GOE-like matrix and those of a covariance matrix of fMRI data is shown respectively. The index n of the eigenvectors is given in descending order according to the corresponding eigenvalue. Black dots correspond to the REST data set while gray to the TASK data set.

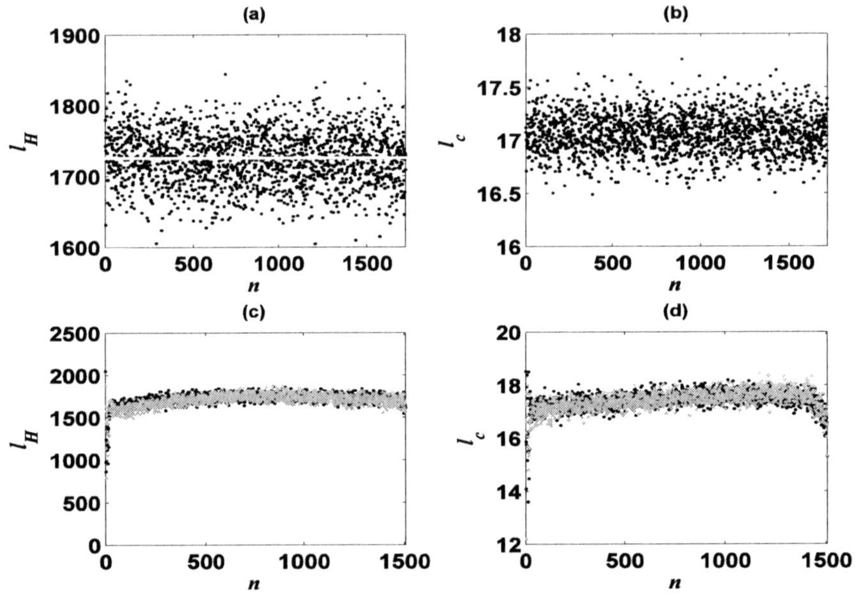

Figure 4. Entropy localization length l_H, as a function of the width of the eigenvectors l_c for a slice of fMRI data (upper left corner) and a GOE-like matrix (upper right corner). The height of vertical lines represents the eigenvalues of the corresponding eigenvectors. In the bottom row a localized eigenvector with small l_H, small l_c and large eigenvalue (left) and an extended eigenvector with relatively high l_H and l_c from the bulk of the spectrum (right) are shown.

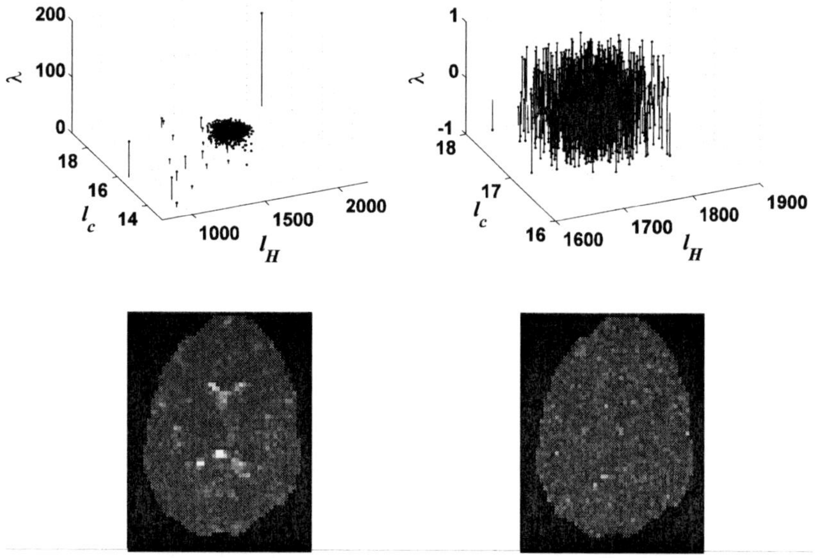

select potentially interesting eigenvectors. The candidates are chosen from a limited number of large components and are represented by small l_H. Then these eigenvectors are characterized by small l_c values. Because such features might be present as well for small eigenvalues, the variance of the eigenvalues must be also taken into account. Fig. 4 illustrates this concept for the eigenvectors of the correlation matrix of one slice from the fMRI data and from a GOE-like matrix for comparison.

The RMT approach in feature selection in fMRI is conceptualized in Fig. 5. Deviations from the universal properties described by RMT can be interpreted as data features that can be considered significant. These can be obtained by studying the statistical properties of the eigenvalues and the eigenvectors of the data correlation matrix. In particular the investigation of the eigenvalue distribution and statistical quantities such as the level space distribution and the number variance of neighboring eigenvalues can provide the corresponding eigenvectors of potential interest. Furthermore by studying the entropy localization length and the width of the eigenvectors, significant eigenvectors can be distinguished from the unstructured noise-like random vectors.

FUTURE TRENDS

We have presented methods derived from RMT that express rather abstract features of the data. This is expected to enable comparisons of data sets that include different trials, sessions and subjects, and establishes thus an important precondition for the meta-analysis of families of data sets. While the identification of more practical features might

Figure 5. Schematic overview of the described RMT methods for the analysis of fMRI data.

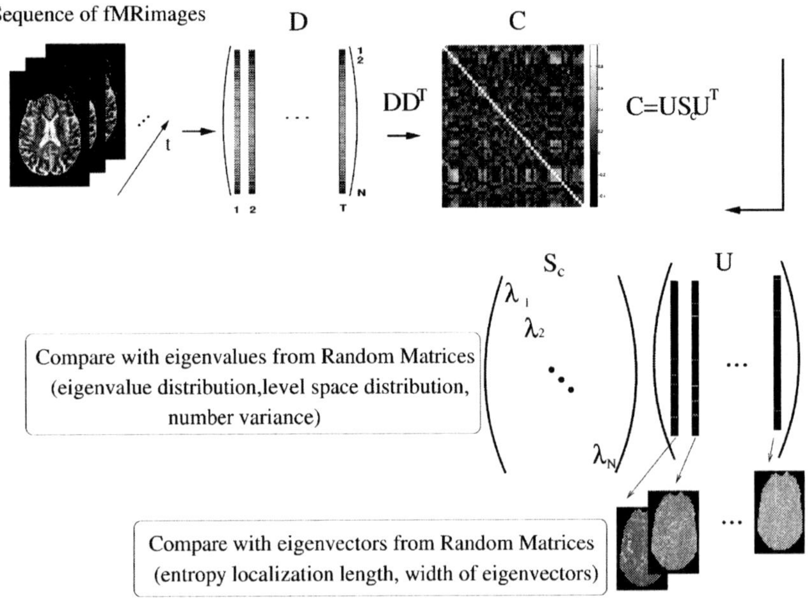

still be problematic it seems realistic to compose a noise model by a combination of noise-like eigenvectors from various data sets, which can be used as a significance threshold for relevant features such as the foci of activation.

It should be also noted that while we were using temporal PCA, an implementation based on spatial PCA is easily possible. To proceed further, one may also consider extensions to ensembles of mixing matrices such those obtained by ICA or to matrices that are studied in linear dynamic models of fMRI activity.

A further drawback of the present approach may be seen in its apparent linearity. Although it is clear that the extraction of spatial or temporal non-linearities in the data is possible, it might be interesting to combine the present statistical approach with the computationally more handy non-linear methods from the theory of neural networks. Voultsidou, Dodel & Herrmann (2005) have considered but the simplest properties, but also higher order structures can be revealed in correspondingly higher-order neural networks. In the same direction points a natural extension that has been achieved by local RMT (cf. Leitner and Wolynes, 1997), which in principle allows the definition of matrix ensembles for particular spatial or temporal ranges and thus a more focus analysis.

The potential of RMT is certainly not exhausted and the last few years have brought about a large number of papers on this theory and its application to all branches of the study of complex systems. Although in brain theory RMT is unlikely to occur as a self-contained theory, it can be used as a preprocessing or complementary tool to other statistical approaches.

DISCUSSION AND CONCLUSION

We have presented a technique based on random matrix theory to analyze the cross-correlations of fMRI data that will allow the selection of the number of relevant eigenvectors. The technique was demonstrated on two fMRI data sets. The first data set contains records from a resting subject while the second one was obtained under a visuomotor task.

At the first stage of the approach we have employed a Principal Component Analysis in order to find the eigenvectors and the eigenvalues of the fMRI correlation matrices, the statistical properties of which we investigated. The eigenvectors of the correlation matrix describe distributed patterns of functional connectivity while the eigenvalues represent their corresponding prevalence. After unfolding, a required procedure for testing the statistical properties of the eigenvalues and their deviations from the RMT predictions, the physical meaning of the transformed eigenvalues is not necessarily interpreted as before. Regarding the statistical properties of the eigenvalues, two of the most common quantities have been studied, namely the level space distribution and the number variance. The level space distribution appeared to be insensitive in stimulus presentation as it was also shown in a similar study of an EEG experiment under visual stimulation (Šeba, 2003). On the other hand, $\Sigma^2(L)$ turned out to be the main indicator of the significance of the important features in the data. The number variance of both data sets deviates from the RMT predictions, but is much more prominent to the data set that corresponds to recordings under stimulation. These deviations are due to the largest eigenvalues. While in the case of resting condition the largest eigenvalues may correspond to heart beat and respiratory effects, stimulus effects also contribute in the case of task condition data. Excluding a number of the largest eigenvalues results in a decrease of Σ^2 difference between the two fMRI data sets as well as between the fMRI data sets and the GOE/RCE ensembles providing a first evidence of the number of stimulus related eigenvalues and their corresponding eigenvectors.

We also investigated the statistical properties of the eigenvectors. In particular we studied the entropy localization length which gives the number of effective components in an eigenvector. The width of the eigenvectors distinguishes between localized and extended ones. Stimulus related eigenvectors are expected to be of a limited number of high valued components and gathered in localized regions. The combination of the entropy localization length and the width of the eigenvectors offer an additional criterion for selecting the appropriate number of potentially interesting eigenvectors.

REFERENCES

Beckmann, C. F., & Smith, S. M. (2004). Probabilistic independent component analysis for functional magnetic resonance imaging. *IEEE Trans. Med. Imaging*, *23*(2), 137-152.

Brody, T. A., Flores, J., French, J. B., Mello, P. A., Pandey, A., & Wong, S. S. M. (1981). Random-matrix physics: spectrum and strength fluctuations. *Rev. Mod. Phys.*, *53*(3), 385-479.

Cordes, D., & Nandy, R. R. (2006). Estimation of the intrinsic dimensionality of fMRI data. *Neuroimage*, *29*, 145-154.

Dodel, S., Herrmann, J. M., & Geisel, T. (2002). Functional connectivity by cross-correlation clustering. *Neurocomputing,* 44-46, 1065-1070.

Dodel, S., Geisel, T., & Herrmann. J. M. (2000). Comparison of temporal and spatial ICA in fMRI data analysis. *Proc. ICA 2000*, Helsinki, Finland, 543-547.

Everson, R., & Roberts, S. (2000). Inferring the eigenvalues of covariance matrices from limited, noisy data. *IEEE Trans. Signal Processing*, *48*(7), 2083-2091.

Hansen, L., Larsen, J., Nielsen, F. A., Strother, S., Rostrup, E., Savoy, R., et al. (1999). Generalizable patterns in neuroimaging: How many principal components? *NeuroImage*, *9*, 534-544.

Hansen, M. H., & Yu, B. (2001). Model selection and the principle of minimum description length. *J. Am. Stat. Assoc.*, *96*(454), 746-774.

Izrailev, F. M. (1990). Simple models of quantum chaos:spectrum and eigenfunctions. *Phys. Rep.*, *196*, 299-392.

Leither, D. M., & Wolynes, P.G. (1997) Vibrational mixing and energy flow in polyatomics: quantitative prediction using local random matrix theory. *J. Phys. Chem. A*, *101*, 541-548.

Luna-Acosta, G. A., Méndez-Bermúdez, J. A., & Izrailev, F. M. (2001). Periodic chaotic billiards: Quantum-classical correspondence in energy space. *Phys. Rev. E*, *64*, 036206+18.

McKeown, M. J. (2000). Detection of consistently task-related activations in fMRI data with hybrid independent component analysis. *Neuroimage*, *11*, 24-35.

Mehta, M. L. (1991). Random matrices. Boston: *Academic Press.*

Minka, T. (1999). Automatic choice of dimensionality for PCA. *MIT, Technical Report, 514.*

Plerou, V., Gopikrishnan, P., Rosenow, B., Amaral, L. A. N., Guhr, T., & Stanley, H. E. (2002). Random matrix approach to cross correlations in financial data. *Phys. Rev. E*, *65*, 066126+18 .

Schwarz, G. (1978). Estimating the dimension of a model. *Annals of Statistics*, *6*(2), 461-464.

Šeba, P. (2003). Random matrix analysis of human EEG data. *Phys. Rev. Lett.*, *91*(19), 198104+4.

Theiler, J., Eubank, S., Longtin, A., Galdrikian, B., & Farmer, J. D. (1992). Testing for nonlinearity in time series: The method of surrogate data. *Physica D*, *58*, 77-94.

Voultsidou, M., Dodel, S., & Herrmann, J. M. (2005). Neural networks approach to clustering of activity in fMRI data. *IEEE Trans. Med. Imaging*, *12*(8), 987-996.

Wigner, E. P. (1967). Random matrices in physics. *SIAM Rev.*, *9*, 1-23.

KEY TERMS

functional Magnetic Resonance Imaging (fMRI): A non invasive neuroimaging technique that studies neural activity based on metabolic changes in the brain under the subject's stimulation or task performance.

Model Order Selection: The proper selection of the number of effective features underlying the data.

Principal Component Analysis (PCA): A linear orthogonal transformation that transforms the data to a new coordinate system such that the new directions point to the maximal variance of multivariate data. The objectives of PCA are 1) to identify meaningful underlying variables and 2) to possibly reduce the dimensionality of the data set.

Independent Component Analysis (ICA): A computational method for separating statistically independent sources that are linearly mixed.

Random Matrix Theory (RMT): Concerned with questions about the statistical properties of the eigenvalues and eigenvectors of large matrices of various ensembles which are determined by certain symmetries such as real symmetric, Hermitian matrices etc.

Universality: In statistical mechanics refers to the observation that a large class of systems share properties that are independent of their dynamics.

Shannon Entropy: Or information entropy is a measure of the uncertainty associated with a random variable. It quantifies the amount of information conveyed per message.

AUTHOR NOTE

Please send any comments to marotesa@physics.uoc.gr. The authors would like to thank the NMR GmbH Göttingen and J. B. Poline for providing us with the data, and S. Dodel, T. Geisel, G. Lohmann, G. Tsironis and T. Kottos for very inspiring discussions as well as the chapter reviewers for their comments. This work has been supported by EU and the Greek Ministry of Education (ΕΠΕΑΕΚ II) and by the Marie Curie program. J.M.H. is PI of the BCCN Göttingen and is affiliated to the Max Planck Institute for Dynamics and Self-Organization, Bunsenstraße 10, 37073 Göttingen, Germany.

Chapter VII
Optimal Diffusion Encoding Strategies for Fiber Mapping in Diffusion MRI

Dimitrios C. Karampinos
University of Illinois at Urbana-Champaign, USA

Robert J. Dawe
Illinois Institute of Technology, USA

Konstantinos Arfanakis
Illinois Institute of Technology, USA

John G. Georgiadis
University of Illinois at Urbana-Champaign, USA

ABSTRACT

Diffusion Magnetic Resonance Imaging (diffusion MRI) can provide important information about tissue microstructure by probing the diffusion of water molecules in a biological tissue. Although originally proposed for the characterization of cerebral white matter connectivity and pathologies, its implementation has extended to many other areas of the human body. In a parallel development, a number of diffusion models have been proposed in order to extract the underlying tissue microstructural properties from the diffusion MRI signal. The present study reviews the basic considerations that have to be taken into account in the selection of the diffusion encoding parameters in diffusion MRI acquisition. Both diffusion tensor imaging (DTI) and high-order schemes are reviewed. The selection of these parameters relies strongly on requirements of the adopted diffusion model and the diffusion characteristics of the tissue under study. The authors review several successful parameter selection strategies for the imaging of the human brain, and conclude with the basics of parameter optimization on promising applications of the technique on other tissues, such as the spinal cord, the myocardium, and the skeletal muscles.

INTRODUCTION

Diffusion Magnetic Resonance Imaging (diffusion MRI) based on the H^1 signal is a unique noninvasive imaging technique that can be used to probe the intrinsic diffusion properties of free water in deep tissues. Motivated by the idea of probing molecular diffusion with NMR, diffusion MRI was first applied *in vivo* in the 1980s (Le Bihan, Breton, & Lallemand, 1986; Moseley, Cohen, & Kucharcyzk, 1990). As the explosive growth of diffusion MRI literature indicates, the technique has been used extensively for the noninvasive characterization of tissue structure and function. Since water diffusion is restricted by morphological transport barriers, the technique has been extremely useful in the early clinical diagnosis of certain pathologies such as stroke and brain trauma (Moseley, Cohen, & Mintorovitch, 1990). In terms of characterizing tissue histoarchitecture, one prevalent application of diffusion MRI is to probe the integrity and the connectivity of white matter in the central nervous system (Arfanakis, Haughton et al., 2002).

In order to translate the diffusion MRI measurements into mass transport barrier geometry information and ultimately morphological tissue properties, several different models of the underlying diffusion process have been proposed to accurately represent the characteristics of the tissue microstructure. Numerous review papers have been published covering the various aspects of diffusion MRI. Some have focused on the theoretical foundations of the various diffusion models (Minati & Weglarz, 2007), and others on the comparison of the performance of the various techniques (Alexander, 2005). The present review is oriented towards selecting experimental parameters for the available basic and advanced diffusion encoding techniques to image the human brain. The basic elements of the various diffusion models proposed are briefly reviewed in a unified way based on the "q-space formalism", with a particular focus on ways to optimize the diffusion encoding schemes in order to maximize the precision of fiber mapping. The challenges arising from the application of these schemes in tissues other than the brain are also discussed.

DIFFUSION ENCODING FORMULATION

We introduce below the q-space formalism to describe the evolution of the transverse magnetization of the spins of protons of the water molecules. The prototypical diffusion MRI experiment is based on the pulsed-gradient spin-echo (PGSE) sequence, which uses two identical gradient pulses inserted on both sides of the 180° refocusing pulse of a conventional spin-echo sequence, following the formulation of Stejskal-Tanner (Stejskal & Tanner, 1965). A schematic of the PGSE sequence is given in Figure 1. The diffusion gradient is labeled $\boldsymbol{g}$, the diffusion gradient duration δ, and the spacing between the diffusion gradients Δ. Since the diffusion gradient constitutes a vector quantity, it can be further described by the product of its amplitude g and a unit vector $\hat{\boldsymbol{g}}$.

Based on the assumption that the diffusion gradient pulses are sufficiently narrow, we can neglect spin motion during δ (short pulse approximation). A spin located at position $\boldsymbol{r}$ at time $t = 0$ will gain phase equal to $\gamma\delta\boldsymbol{g}\boldsymbol{r}$ following the application of the first diffusion gradient pulse. If we assume that the molecule has moved to a position $\boldsymbol{r}'$ during time Δ and just before the second (refocusing) gradient pulse is applied, the spin phase will change by $-\gamma\delta\boldsymbol{g}\boldsymbol{r}'$ after the application of the second diffusion gradient pulse. The net phase shift will be finally $\gamma\delta\boldsymbol{g}(\boldsymbol{r} - \boldsymbol{r}')$. If $P(\boldsymbol{r}' \mid \boldsymbol{r}, \Delta)$ represents the probability of a spin to be located at position $\boldsymbol{r}'$ at time $t = \Delta$, given that it was at position r at time $t = 0$, then the normalized amplitude of the echo (echo amplitude with diffusion weighting over echo amplitude without diffusion weighting) for a uniform spin density is (Callaghan, 1991):

Figure 1. Schematic representation of the pulsed-gradient spin-echo sequence.

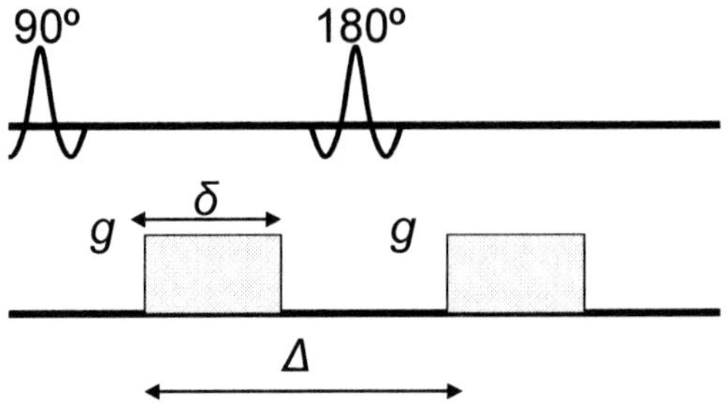

$$E(\boldsymbol{q},\Delta) = \int\int P(\boldsymbol{r}'|\boldsymbol{r},\Delta)\exp\left[i2\pi\boldsymbol{q}(\boldsymbol{r}'-\boldsymbol{r})\right]\mathrm{d}\boldsymbol{r}'\mathrm{d}\boldsymbol{r}$$

where $\boldsymbol{q} = (2\pi)^{-1}\gamma\delta\boldsymbol{g}$ defines the reciprocal space of spin displacements. In the case when $P(\boldsymbol{r}'|\boldsymbol{r},\Delta)$ is independent of the starting position $\boldsymbol{r}$ and depends only on the net displacement $\boldsymbol{R} = \boldsymbol{r}' - \boldsymbol{r}$, we can define the ensemble average propagator:

$$\overline{P}(\boldsymbol{R},\Delta) = \int P(\boldsymbol{r}+\boldsymbol{R}|\boldsymbol{r},\Delta)\mathrm{d}\boldsymbol{r}$$

We can then rewrite the expression for the echo signal:

$$E(\boldsymbol{q},\Delta) = \int\overline{P}(\boldsymbol{R},\Delta)\exp\left[i2\pi\boldsymbol{qR}\right]\mathrm{d}\boldsymbol{R}$$

The above expression indicates that the diffusion MRI signal is the Fourier transform of the ensemble average propagator. For Gaussian diffusion with a constant diffusion coefficient D, the normalized signal becomes $E(b) = \exp(-bD)$, where $b = \gamma^2\delta^2 g^2\left(\Delta - \frac{\delta}{3}\right)$ is the variable most commonly used to quantify the amount of diffusion weighting in a diffusion MRI experiment.

In the case of crossing fibers, information about the angular structure of the ensemble average propagator is sought in terms of the orientation distribution function, defined as the radial projection of propagator:

$$ODF(\boldsymbol{u}) = \int_0^{+\infty}\overline{P}(r\boldsymbol{u})r^2\mathrm{d}r$$

The extraction of the tissue diffusion properties relies on the ability to recover accurately the ensemble average propagator from the MRI signal. As the above analysis indicates, the signal intensity is obtained in terms of the spin displacement $\boldsymbol{R} = \boldsymbol{r}' - \boldsymbol{r}$ rather than in a physical absolute space coordinates (Callaghan, 1991). Blumich (Blumich, 2003) points out that the increased resolution of methods based on this formalism (~ 100 μm) is derived from the fact the signal is averaged over an ensemble of similar structures. Therefore the success of such methods in resolving the microstructure is based on the presence of short range spatial order in each voxel and on the effectiveness in the *q*-space sampling to adequately represent this order. Focusing on tissues in the central nervous system and especially white matter provides this short range order. Neural tracts correspond to multiple diverging and crossing bundles of myelinated axons. In healthy living neural tissue, each axon consists of an aqueous core (with a diameter of a few microns) surrounded by a tubular sheath of myelin that is less permeable to water than the intra-axonal space. We should note in passing that in the following text, as well as in the relevant literature, the term "crossing fibers" is employed for simplicity to refer to crossing fiber bundles, rather than to crossing individual axons. The latter feature is not consistent with human histology and anatomy.

Different diffusion models have been proposed in order to assure efficient signal acquisition and accuracy in the quantification of the tissue microstructure properties, such as the mean spatial correlation length or fiber orientation. These models have been based either on q-space or displacement-space formulations. Techniques based on q-space formulations use *a priori* information of the underlying diffusion process to model the diffusion MRI signal. Techniques working in displacement-space can directly measure characteristics of the propagator without using a priori information of the tissue diffusion properties.

Several reviews have appeared in the MRI literature comparing the performance of diffusion MRI techniques in mapping cerebral neuronal fiber networks. Instead of comparing the advantages and the disadvantages of the various previously proposed methods, the goal of the present review is to focus on the optimal diffusion encoding strategies for certain classes of these techniques. We will start from the most basic diffusion model and then proceed with high order models. We will also extend our discussion to the selection of optimal parameters, in tissues other than the brain, where diffusion MRI has been applied.

OPTIMIZATION OF DIFFUSION ENCODING STRATEGIES

In diffusion MRI, noise that is present in the raw diffusion-weighted images is propagated to the final calculations of the diffusion propagators and their associated scalar quantities (e.g. mean diffusion coefficient and anisotropy metrics). Therefore, much effort in recent years has been focused on optimization of diffusion acquisition schemes, with the aim of reducing the inherent errors in raw data acquisition as well as their propagation to the final diffusion propagator estimation. The optimization of the diffusion encoding strategies involves the selection of the variables related to the q-space coverage (Figure 2) which includes the number of the diffusion encoding directions (N_{dir}), the number of b-values (N_{b}), the number of averages with and without diffusion-weighting ($N_{\mathrm{av,b}}$ and $N_{\mathrm{av,b=0}}$), and the optimum choice of the set of b-values. The selection of the aforementioned parameters depends strongly on the adopted diffusion model and the measurement noise characteristics.

Signal-Based Diffusion Models

Diffusion Tensor Imaging

Diffusion Tensor Imaging (DTI) was introduced in 1990s (Basser, Mattiello, & Le Bihan, 1994) and constitutes the basic diffusion model for characterization of the anisotropic diffusion properties of a tissue. In DTI, anisotropic diffusion is described by a 2nd rank tensor $\boldsymbol{D}$. The corresponding expressions for the ensemble average propagator and the diffusion MRI signal are:

$$\overline{P}(\boldsymbol{R},\Delta)=\frac{1}{\sqrt{|\boldsymbol{D}|(4\pi\Delta)^{3}}}\exp\left(-\frac{\boldsymbol{R}^{T}\boldsymbol{D}^{-1}\boldsymbol{R}}{4\Delta}\right)$$

$$E(b,\hat{\boldsymbol{g}})=\exp\left[-b\hat{\boldsymbol{g}}^{T}\boldsymbol{D}\hat{\boldsymbol{g}}\right]$$

If $\lambda_1, \lambda_2, \lambda_3$ are the eigenvalues of the diffusion tensor, we can define the mean diffusivity and the fractional anisotropy (FA) metrics:

$$\overline{\lambda}=\frac{\mathrm{Trace}(\boldsymbol{D})}{3}=\frac{\lambda_1+\lambda_2+\lambda_3}{3}$$

$$\mathrm{FA}=\sqrt{\frac{3}{2}}\sqrt{\frac{\left(\lambda_1-\overline{\lambda}\right)^2+\left(\lambda_2-\overline{\lambda}\right)^2+\left(\lambda_3-\overline{\lambda}\right)^2}{\lambda_1^2+\lambda_2^2+\lambda_3^2}}$$

There have been a significant number of previous studies focusing on the optimization of

Figure 2. Basic q-space sampling parameters: N_{dir} points distributed on each of the N_b spherical shells.

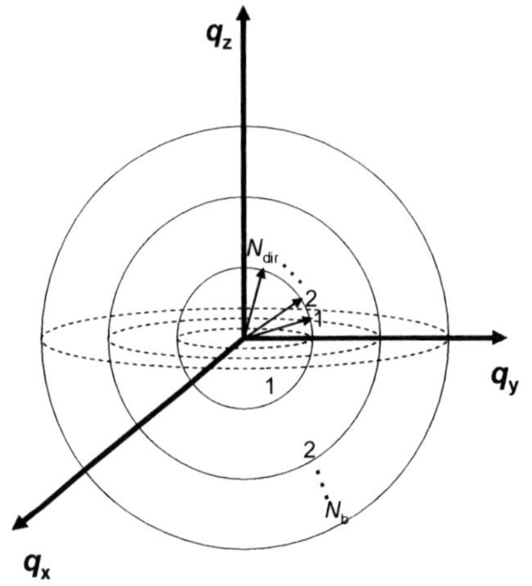

DTI acquisition schemes exploring the number of gradient diffusion encoding directions, the orientation of diffusion directions, and the amount of diffusion weighting (*b*-values).

Number of Diffusion-Encoding Directions

The estimation of the diffusion tensor requires a minimum of six diffusion-weighted measurements along six non-collinear directions, and a b=0 s/mm^2 measurement. In order to increase the accuracy in the estimation of the diffusion tensor, more than seven signals in total are typically acquired. In that case, the problem becomes over-determined, and various approaches can be used for tensor estimation. However, for a given total imaging time, it is possible to repeat multiple times, $N_{av,b}$, the acquisition of data along few diffusion directions, N_{dir}, or to acquire data along many directions, N_{dir}, without repeating any acquisition ($N_{av,b}$=1). For example, data for six diffusion directions could be acquired twice, or data for 12 directions could be acquired once in the same imaging time.

In-vivo experiments suggest that accuracy in the estimation of the diffusion tensor in anisotropic systems increases when diffusion-weighted signals are acquired along as many different directions as possible, rather than repeating measurements in only a few directions. In one study, FA maps from the brain of healthy human volunteers exhibited higher SNR and improved contrast between white matter structures and the surrounding brain tissue when more diffusion directions were employed (Jones, Horsfiled, & Simmons, 1999). Similarly, another study reported greater contrast-to-noise ratio (CNR) in FA maps between white and gray matter for an increasing number of diffusion directions (Arfanakis, Cordes, Haughton, Carew, & Meyerand, 2002) (Figure 3). In this study, schemes with N_{dir}=6, 11, 23, and 46 directions were investigated, while the total imaging time was held approximately constant by repeating the acquisition for schemes with fewer directions. The CNR increased quite rapidly between the 6- and 11-direction schemes (0.08 to 0.15), as well as between the 11- and 23-direction schemes (0.15 to 0.17), but appeared to reach a plateau between 23 and 46 directions (Figure 3).

For a small number of diffusion-encoding directions, the accuracy in estimating the eigenvalues of the diffusion tensor and quantities based on the eigenvalues of the tensor, such as the commonly used FA parameter, is highly dependent upon the orientation of the tensor in relation to the diffusion directions. For example, a scheme with three of its diffusion directions perfectly aligned with the principle axes of the tensor (defined by the three eigenvectors of the tensor) would yield a more accurate estimate of the eigenvalues and FA than a scheme whose directions were not aligned with the tensor axes, since the former scheme directly measures the tensor eigenvalues. However, *a priori* information regarding the exact tensor orientations *in vivo* is generally not available. In this case, the dependence of the noise in the eigenvalues on tensor orientation can be minimized by selecting a scheme with a relatively large number of uniformly distributed diffusion directions. Skare et al. (Skare, Hedehus, Moseley, & Li, 2000) have shown that for just six directions, the noise of FA is dependent on tensor orientation (Figure 4a). For 30 uniformly distributed directions (Jones et al., 1999), the noise in FA is low and rotationally invariant (Skare et al., 2000) (Figure 4b). Therefore, also taking into consideration the findings discussed above, schemes that include at least N_{dir}=30 uniformly distributed directions, approximately, are desirable for performing DTI of the human brain, which normally contains the full range of tensor orientations, as shown in Figure 5.

Distribution of Diffusion-Encoding Directions in Three-Dimensional (3D) Space

The advantages of using a large number of diffusion directions can not be fully realized unless their orientations are optimized. For anisotropic systems in which no *a priori* information is available regarding the local orientations of the tensors, the diffusion directions should be distributed as uniformly as possible in three-dimensional space. Toward this end, the diffusion-weighted directions have been defined based on one of three types of schemes: heuristic, geometric polyhedra, and numerically optimized.

Heuristic schemes consist of diffusion directions defined by vectors that originate at the center of an imaginary cube and point to the cube's vertices, face centers, and edge bisectors (Hasan, Parker, & Alexander, 2001). Heuristic schemes with up to 13 directions have been devised, but it is important to note that these directions have not been uniformly distributed according to any

Figure 3. Contrast-to-noise ratio (CNR) between gray and white matter of a single subject, for acquisition schemes with 6, 11, 23 and 46 diffusion directions. CNR increases when more DW gradient orientations are used. A plateau is achieved for approximately 30 diffusion directions.

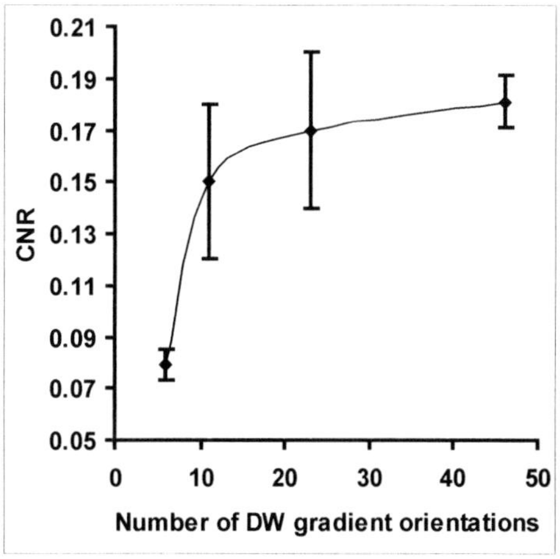

quantitative criteria. As such, these schemes are not expected to be optimal.

Similarly, schemes based on geometric polyhedra also consist of diffusion directions defined by the vertices of various solids (Hasan et al., 2001). Unlike the heuristic schemes, however, the polyhedra have at least 12 faces, and the resulting schemes appear to possess optimality, as discussed later. The regular icosahedron provides a framework for the minimum six diffusion directions that are required for tensor estimation. This polyhedron consists of 20 equilateral triangle faces, with 5 faces meeting to form each vertex. Lines connecting each vertex to its counterpart on the opposite side of the icosahedron are used to define the six diffusion directions of the ICOSA6 scheme (Hasan et al., 2001). The dual of the icosahedron is the dodecahedron, which consists of

Figure 4. Standard deviation of FA of a simulated cylindrical tensor as a function of the orientation of the primary eigenvector, for (minimum energy) schemes with 6 (a) and 30 (b) diffusion directions, respectively. θ and φ are the azimuth and zenith angles respectively. The standard deviation of FA varies significantly with tensor orientation when a scheme with few diffusion directions is used, and is almost independent of tensor orientation when many diffusion directions are used.

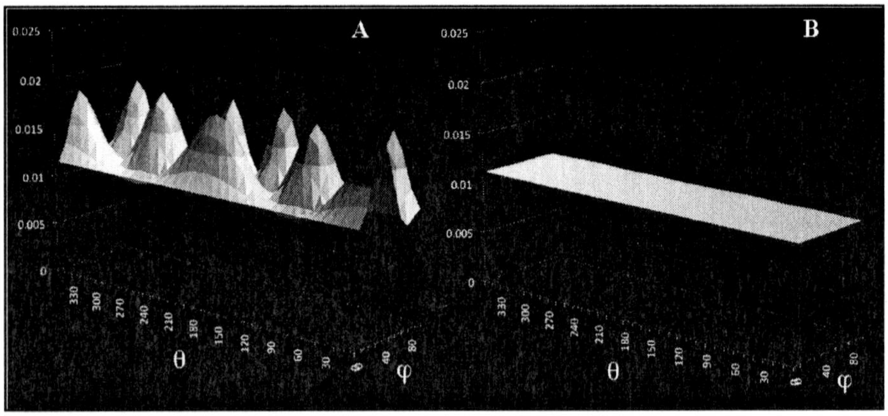

Figure 5. (a) Uniform distribution of tensor orientations in 3D space. (b) Distribution of the orientation of all white matter tensors of a single human subject. θ and φ are the azimuth and zenith angles respectively.

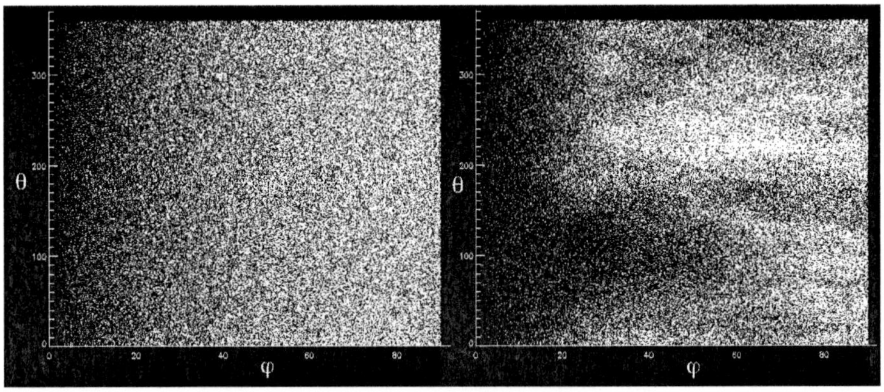

12 pentagonal faces and 20 vertices, allowing for the definition of 10 unique diffusion directions. An obvious disadvantage of relying on polyhedra for defining diffusion directions is the fact that only schemes with a "magic number" of directions can be formed. For instance, Hasan's family of "icosahedron polyhedra" can provide schemes with number of directions equal to $5n^2 + 1$ for $n = 1, 2, 3$, etc. Although a variety of other polyhedra can be used to obtain diffusion direction sets, the fact remains that geometric polyhedra schemes do not allow ultimate flexibility in the number of directions employed.

The most flexible and optimal sets of diffusion directions appear to be those constructed using numerical optimization. One of several quantities can be used for the minimization criterion, including the total variance of the diffusion tensor and the inverse pseudo-determinant or condition number of the diffusion encoding matrix (Hasan et al., 2001; Skare et al., 2000). In addition, Jones et al. (Jones et al., 1999) described the use of a "minimum force" criterion for achieving uniformly distributed diffusion directions in three dimensions. In this scheme, unit charges are placed on the surface of a sphere and arranged to minimize the force exerted between the charges (Figure 6). Since antiparallel diffusion directions are equivalent, there is an added constraint that each charge must pair with a complementary charge on the exact opposite surface of the sphere. The diffusion directions are then defined as vectors pointing from the center of the sphere to one charge from each pair. The minimum energy criterion is similar to the minimum force scheme, except that the total Coulombic energy is minimized instead of the force. The numerically optimized schemes described here can accommodate any number of diffusion directions.

After correcting for unequal imaging times, the icosahedral schemes and most of the numerically optimized schemes were shown to be equivalent (Hasan et al., 2001). The schemes that were found to be suboptimal were heuristic schemes and those based on minimization of the condition number of the diffusion-encoding matrix.

Diffusion Weighting: b-Values

Another important aspect in the development of optimal DTI acquisition schemes is the selection of diffusion weighting and the number of measurements at different *b*-values. Although multiple *b*-values can be used to probe diffusion in multiple compartments, the use of a single *b*-value in addition to b=0 s/mm^2, yields information that is usually most valuable for the range of diffusion coefficients found in the human brain. The optimal value of the diffusion-weighting (*b*-value) depends on the tissue under investigation, and more specifically on the tissue's microstructural boundaries to diffusion, as well as on the noise levels of the DTI experiment. Employing *b*-values that are too low will fail to detect anisotropic diffusion characteristics, while *b*-values that are too high will lead to significantly low diffusion-weighted signals, comparable to the noise floor. Given a priori knowledge of the trace of the diffusion tensor, the optimum *b*-value can be chosen to be approximately $1.11 \times 3 / Tr(\boldsymbol{D})$, where $Tr(\boldsymbol{D})$ is the trace of the diffusion tensor (Jones et al., 1999). Using this method with $Tr(\boldsymbol{D}) = 3.0 \times 10^{-3}$ mm^2/s ($\bar{\lambda} = 1.0 \times 10^{-3}$ mm^2/s), the *b*-value becomes 1110 s/mm^2. The situation is more complex *in vivo*, however, since the chosen *b*-value must be sensitive to $\bar{\lambda}$ values ranging from about 0.3 to 3.0×10^{-3} mm^2/s at different locations within the human brain (Armitage & Bastin, 2001). This problem has been addressed by Armitage and Bastin, who have defined the diffusion-to-noise ratio (DNR) as the SNR of the calculated diffusion tensor trace map. This quantity is the product of the SNR of the low *b*-value image and a factor that describes the sensitivity of the high *b*-value to a given rate of diffusion. Adjusting the high *b*-value can make the acquisition optimally sensitive to various ranges of $\bar{\lambda}$ by ensuring that the DNR remains above a desired threshold of 20 or

Figure 6. Each vertex of this polyhedron represents the location of a charge from a set of 46 equal charges, positioned on the surface of a sphere in such a manner that the total energy is minimized. Each pair of vertices on exact opposite locations on the surface of the sphere define a diffusion-encoding direction for a scheme with 23 directions total.

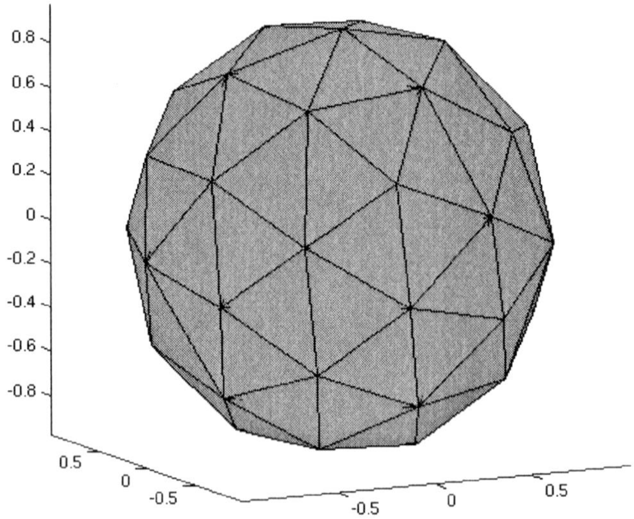

greater (Armitage & Bastin, 2001). A range of b-values from approximately 900 to 1000 s/mm^2 have been found to be appropriate for conventional DTI acquisitions in the human brain (Armitage & Bastin, 2001; Jones et al., 1999). Finally, an appropriate ratio of the number of measurements at the high b-value to the number of measurements at low b-value (typically $b \approx 0$ s/mm^2) for DTI is between 6 and 9 (Jones et al., 1999).

Diffusion Tensor Imaging constitutes the basic diffusion model employed in clinical research. Nevertheless, in a typical diffusion MRI experiment, the imaging voxel is millimeter sized, which is several orders of magnitude larger than the cell (e.g. axon) diameter. The MRI voxel can therefore accommodate multiple bundles of axonal fibers with different orientations. In such cases, the simple DTI model has to be refined to accommodate the multiple fiber orientations that can potentially exist within each voxel. Several higher order models of the diffusion signal have been proposed to account for these complications, and they are discussed in detail below.

Multiple Compartments Models

The simplest modification of the basic DTI model in order to account for intravoxel fiber crossings is by modeling the signal as a linear weighted sum of multiple exponentials. If $\hat{\boldsymbol{g}}$ is the unit vector along a diffusion direction, then for M crossing-branching fibers the normalized diffusion signal is:

$$E(b,\hat{\boldsymbol{g}}) = \sum_{i=1}^{M} f_i \exp[-b\hat{\boldsymbol{g}}^T \boldsymbol{D}_i \hat{\boldsymbol{g}}]$$

Alexander and Barker (2005) used Monte Carlo simulations to estimate the optimal value for b in a diffusion MRI experiment to determine fiber orientations using the multi-exponential model and q-space sampling on a single spherical shell.

For the two fiber directions case they show that the main variable that has a strong effect on the optimal setting of b is the mean diffusivity. Specifically, for typical values of mean diffusivities in the brain, they find that the optimal b values for estimating two fiber orientations are in the range between 2200 and 2800 s/mm^2. They also show that the optimal setting is largely independent of the total number of measurements $N_{av,b=0}+N_{dir}$ with $N_{dir}/N_{av,b=0}$ fixed.

More elaborate models haven been proposed based on the assumption of non-interacting multiple compartments and involve elaborate analytical expressions describing diffusion inside cylindrical fibers, as in CHARMED (Assaf, Freidlin, Rohde, & Basser, 2004) and in QUAQ (Raguin et al., 2006). These models further compartmentalize the signal in terms of intracellular and extracellular space. They use multiple shells in q-space and can therefore afford optimal accuracy for one- and two-fibers reconstruction for the same b-value range. Specifically, Assaf and Basser (2005) follow an interesting approach for optimizing the q-space sampling strategy by increasing the number of directions at higher b values. This is consistent with the fact that high angular resolution is needed at higher b-values in order to detect the angular dependence of the signal.

ADC Modeling Techniques

A second class of diffusion methods models the angular pattern of the diffusion coefficient along each diffusion encoding direction which is defined by the unit vector $\hat{\mathbf{g}}(\varphi,\theta) = [\sin(\varphi)\cos(\theta); \sin(\varphi)\sin(\theta); \cos(\varphi)]$ based on the equation:

$$D_{ap}(\hat{\mathbf{g}}(\varphi,\theta)) = -\frac{1}{b}\ln(E(b,\hat{\mathbf{g}}(\varphi,\theta)))$$

where θ, φ are the azimuth and zenith angles, respectively. The measurement of diffusion coefficient along a large number of diffusion gradient directions is referred as high angular resolution diffusion imaging (HARDI).

The first proposed technique of this kind is the spherical decomposition method proposed by Alexander et al. and Frank (Alexander, Barker, & Arridge, 2002; Frank, 2002), which is based on the decomposition of the apparent diffusion coefficient in terms of real-valued spherical harmonics:

$$D_{ap}(\hat{\mathbf{g}}(\varphi,\theta)) = \sum_{l=0}^{\infty}\sum_{m=-l}^{l}\alpha_{lm}S_l^m(\varphi,\theta)$$

Terms up to second order originate from single fiber populations, whereas terms of fourth order or higher represent the effect of crossing fibers. The spherical harmonics decomposition scheme uses q-values distributed over a single spherical shell and a high number of diffusion directions which depends on the highest order of coefficients needed to describe the underlying diffusion process. Specifically, a rotation-invariant spherical harmonic decomposition (Zhan, Stein, & Yang, 2006) shows that for N_{dir}>90 and SNR>60 for the reference image the results are consistent for the coefficients up to the 4th order in phantom simulations. For for N_{dir}>128 and SNR>80 for the reference image the results are consistent for the coefficients up to the 6th order.

Another application of the spherical harmonics set is based on the expression of the normalized signal as the direct spherical convolution of the response function for a single axially symmetric fiber aligned with the z-axis with the orientation distribution function, decomposed on spherical harmonics (Tournier, Calamante, Gadian, & Connelly, 2004):

$$E(b,\hat{\mathbf{g}}(\theta,\phi)) = E_o(b,\theta) \otimes ODF(\hat{\mathbf{g}}(\theta,\phi))$$

Tournier et al investigated the effect of the b value on the performance of the spherical deconvolution method concluding that intermediate b values should be preferred to allow adequate angular dependency on the signal without attenuating the signal down to the noise level. For SNR=30 for the reference image, their results reveal an optimal b value in the 3000-4000 s/mm^2 range.

Diffusion circular spectrum mapping (DCSM) methods (Zhan, Gu, Silbersweig, Stern, & Yang, 2003; Zhan, Stein, & Yang, 2004) used the angle ψ between the applied diffusion direction and the primary fiber direction to represent angular deviation results for the apparent diffusion coefficient profile:

$$D_{CS}(\psi) = \frac{\beta - 1}{2}\lambda_1 \cos(2\psi) + \frac{\beta + 1}{2}\lambda_1$$

Zhan and Yang (2006) show that b-value has little effect on the angular deviation of the DCSM method for the two fibers case for the noise-free case. When noise effects are included, the results for b=2000 s/mm^2 are more robust than the results with b=5000 s/mm^2.

Finally, a generalized DTI method has been proposed (Ozarslan & Mareci, 2003), using b>1000 s/mm^2 and a number of diffusion directions comparable to spherical harmonics decomposition:

$$D(\hat{g}) = \sum_{i_1=0}^{3}\sum_{i_2=0}^{3}\cdots\sum_{i_l=1}^{3} D_{i_1 i_2 \ldots i_l} g_{i_1} g_{i_2} \cdots g_{i_l}$$

An extensive analysis of the optimal diffusion encoding parameters for the generalized DTI is lacking, but these parameters should follow the general rules like the spherical harmonics decomposition scheme, since there is a well understood equivalency between the two methods (Ozarslan & Mareci, 2003).

Propagator-Based Diffusion Models

All the methods described up to this point model the diffusion signal. Another family of methods extracts information for the fiber orientation based on the propagator characteristics. The reconstruction of the ensemble average propagator by means of the Fourier transform of the diffusion normalized signal is referred to as diffusion spectrum imaging (DSI) (Wedeen et al., 2000). The extraction of the propagator is possible either by three-dimensional Fourier transform of the diffusion signal on a cartesian lattice (Lin, Wedeen, Chen, Yao, & Tseng, 2003), or by one-dimensional Fourier transform of the diffusion signal along each direction to retrieve radial components of the propagator (Cohen & Assaf, 2002).

Assuming that the diffusion gradient vectors are distributed isotropically over a sphere, the nominal angular resolution of DSI (in radians) is inversely proportional to the square root of the number of directions (Wedeen, Hagmann, Tseng, Reese, & Weisskoff, 2005). The fiber orientation separation power depends strongly on the maximal sampling radius (b value). While extending the maximal sampling radius above b-values of 18000 s/mm^2 is not expected to improve accuracy, not going far enough in q-space will limit the angular contrast. Wedeen et al (Wedeen et al., 2005) showed that a maximal b-value of 12000-18000 is adequate to resolve well known areas of crossing fiber, such as in the brainstem and the *centrum semiovale* using 515 q-space samples.

Since information about the angular structure of the diffusion spectrum is sought, researchers focused on techniques for direct measurement of the orientation distribution function (ODF). Tuch (Tuch, 2004) showed that the Funk-Radon transform, which is a generalization of the Radon transform to spherical coordinates, can be used to extract ODF from measurements taken on a sphere corresponding to a single q value in a method called q-ball imaging (QBI):

$$ODF(\boldsymbol{u}) = \int_{\boldsymbol{q}\perp\boldsymbol{u}} E(\boldsymbol{q})\mathrm{d}\boldsymbol{q}$$

The initial implementation of q-ball imaging was done a single q-value and was able to resolve fiber crossings with b values between 2500 and 4000 s/mm^2. A recent generalization of q-ball imaging fusing the diffusion signal from different diffusion wavevectors (labeled as multiple wavevector fusion, or MWF) has shown that the q-space sampling efficiency of q-ball imaging can be significantly boosted by employing samples in two q-space shells (Klachaturian, Wisco, & Tuch, 2007). They show that the combination of samples at b=700 s/mm^2 and b=3200 s/mm^2 can induce a reduction in the number of required q-space samples from 322 to 193. The improved accuracy of MWF can be explained by the fact that the low b value samples provide the low angular resolution characteristics of the propagator while the high b value samples enhance the high angular resolution information.

Finally, Zhan and Yang (2006) performed a systematic study on the effect of b value and SNR for DSI and QBI methods. Their noise-free results show that DSI and QBI methods should be used for b>1000 s/mm^2. When they considered the effect of noise, the angular deviation in the prediction of the fiber angles was higher for b=5000 s/mm^2 than for b=2000 s/mm^2.

Hybrid Diffusion Models

Wu and Alexander (2007) have recently introduced a comprehensive diffusion encoding and analysis approach, labeled hybrid diffusion imaging (HYDI), to assess the complementary information provided from the various diffusion models. In the proposed q-space sampling scheme, multiple shells are used with an increasing number of diffusion encoding directions per encoding shell as the diffusion-weighting increases. The most interior shells are then used for diffusion tensor analysis, the outermost shell is used for QBI processing and the all the shells may be used for implementing DSI.

DISCUSSION

We have pointed out earlier that the success of diffusion weighted MRI is based on the presence of short range spatial order in the tissue microstructure contained in each voxel and on the optimization of the q-space sampling in order to adequately represent this microstructure. The emphasis of the present chapter is on the second aspect, which hinges on selecting a subvoxel diffusion model. We can broadly classify diffusion models into diffusion tensor schemes and high-order schemes. DTI constitutes the most basic diffusion model and the family of high-order models includes multiple compartments models, ADC modeling techniques, propagator-based diffusion models and hybrid methods. As the previous discussion indicates, the majority of the studies available in the literature related to the optimization of diffusion encoding parameters have focused on DTI schemes. Although several high order diffusion models have been proposed in order to resolve crossing and branching neuronal fiber structures, a systematic investigation of the effect of the main diffusion encoding parameters on the extracted results for many of these techniques is currently lacking for many high-order schemes. This is mostly related to the complexity of its implementation and the requirement to first validate each technique with either simulations or phantoms or studies involving (post mortem) histological analysis performed in tandem with MRI, before the optimization step. However, optimization of the diffusion encoding parameters is not only related to the improvement of outcome in terms of increased SNR or spatial resolution, but it is also connected to the total acquisition time, with long imaging protocols constituting a major obstacle in the clinical implementation of many high-order schemes.

A significant number of human brain studies have been conducted in an effort to determine the DTI acquisition strategy that provides unbiased estimation and desirably low noise properties of the diffusion tensors. In brief, a diffusion weighting (b-value) of 900-1000 s/mm^2 (Armitage & Bastin, 2001; Jones et al., 1999), a ratio of high b-value images to low b-value images between 6 and 9 (Armitage & Bastin, 2001; Jones et al., 1999; Skare et al., 2000), an SNR of the b=0 map of 20 or greater (Armitage &

Bastin, 2001), and a set of diffusion directions uniformly distributed in 3D space (Hasan et al., 2001), such as those provided by the "minimum energy" or "icosahedral" schemes, are some of the essential characteristics of a DTI acquisition scheme that provides high quality DTI measurements. Furthermore, for a specified total imaging time, measuring DW signals in multiple diffusion directions, instead of acquiring multiple copies of few DW images, increases the contrast to noise ratio in FA maps (Arfanakis, Cordes et al., 2002; Jones et al., 1999). In addition, for anisotropic diffusion, using acquisition schemes with less than approximately 30 diffusion directions causes the noise of the diffusion tensor to become dependent on the orientation of the primary eigenvector of the tensor (Skare et al., 2000). For approximately 30 diffusion directions, the noise of the diffusion tensor becomes rotationally invariant.

Although quantitative studies for optimizing diffusion encoding strategies in numerous high-order diffusion schemes employed for fiber mapping are lacking, we are presenting here a qualitative comparison of the main experimental parameters of these schemes. Table 1 summarizes some of the employed diffusion encoding parameters for *in vivo* brain measurements using the high-order diffusion schemes discussed above.

In terms of the level of the employed diffusion-weighting, all of these methods require higher *b*-values (b>1000 s/mm^2) than DTI acquisitions so that the sensitivity of the signal to higher angular resolution structures is maximized. DSI techniques rely on sampling up to very high *b*-values (b up to 17000 s/mm^2) to assure high angular contrast on the derived orientation distribution function. Both ADC modeling techniques and QBI rely also on *q*-space data acquired on shells with higher *b*-values (b=2000-4000 s/mm^2) than DTI in order to characterize regions of complex histoarchitecture with crossing white matter tracts. One important issue related to the selection of *b*-value, is the need of avoiding signal levels near the "noise-floor". Some high-order schemes employ *b*-values of the order of 6000-10000 s/mm^2 for the outer shells. The signal level for this strong diffusion-weighting can become comparable to the noise level for some of the diffusion encoding directions. The extraction of the diffusion parameters in these cases can be potentially improved using Rician noise models.

Considering the required number of diffusion encoding shells and directions per shell, the optimum angular sampling on each shell is uniform, and the number of shells depends on the characteristics of the model. ADC modeling techniques use experimental data on a single shell with a number of directions higher than 30 (as proposed for DTI) but in general lower than 100. Diffusion spectrum imaging is the most demanding method in terms of *q*-space coverage, since it relies on the 3-dimensional inverse Fourier transform of the echo attenuation signal. The QBI technique, as originally proposed, requires sampling on a single shell with a high number of diffusion encoding directions (> 100). New techniques have been proposed based on optimizing the *q*-space coverage depending on the specific application and the information that is sought (Klachaturian et al., 2007; Wu & Alexander, 2007). By using variable number of sampling points on different *q*-space cells, these techniques are effectively introducing new ideas for *q*-space sampling that is more efficient than that for QBI and DSI, but they have not yet been optimized.

FUTURE TRENDS

The application of diffusion weighted MRI to areas other than the brain focuses on tissues which are mainly characterized by locally oriented fibrous microstructure. Diffusion tensor imaging is the main method employed for fiber mapping in areas outside the brain. Applications of DTI in areas with a preferred orientation, such as the spinal cord (Summers, Staempfli, Jaermann, Kwiecinski, & Kollias, 2006), the skeletal muscle (Sinha, Sinha,

Table 1. Summary of basic q-space sampling parameters for the various high order diffusion encoding schemes.

High-order diffusion models	N_{dir}	N_b	b (s/mm²)	$N_{av,b=0}$	$N_{av,b}$
Multiple compartments techniques					
Bi-exponential model (Alexander & Barker, 2005)	28-246	1	2200-2800	$\sim N_{dir}/9$	1
CHARMED model (Assaf & Basser, 2005)	6-30	10	714-10000	1	1
ADC modeling techniques					
Spherical harmonics descomposition (Frank, 2002)	43	1	3000	20	20
Spherical harmonics descomposition (Alexander et al., 2002)	60	1	1000	3	1
Spherical harmonics deconvolution (Tournier et al., 2004)	60	1	2971	18	3
Diffusion circular spectrum mapping (Zhan et al., 2003)	90	1	3076	6	6
Generalized diffusion tensor imaging (Ozarslan & Mareci, 2003)	81	1	1050	1	1
Propagator-based techniques					
Diffusion spectrum imaging (Wedeen et al., 2005)	515 points on a cubic lattice of 5 lattice units in radius with b_{max} = 17000			1	1
q-ball imaging (Tuch, 2004)	253	1	4000	1	1
Multiple wavevector fusion (Klachaturian et al., 2007)	60 directions at b_1=700 and 123 directions at b_2=3200			10	1
Hybrid techniques					
Hybrid diffusion imaging (Wu & Alexander, 2007)	3-50	5	375-9375	-	-

& Edgerton, 2006), and the peripheral nerves (Skorpil, Karlsson, & Nordell, 2004), could potentially use a lower number of directions, which could be further optimized if there is a priori knowledge of that preferred orientation (Peng & Arfanakis, 2007; Skorpil, Engstroem, & Nordell, 2007). The corresponding b value also has to be modified according to the mean diffusion coefficient of the tissue (i.e. b=500-600 s/mm² in the case of skeletal muscle). More elaborate muscle architecture, such as in the tongue (Wedeen et al., 2005), can be potentially resolved with high order diffusion models. Finally, further optimization of the diffusion encoding parameters is needed in tissues involving secondary structures and additional morphometric parameters defined by the secondary and tertiary eigenvectors of DTI, as is the case for the myocardium (Helm, Tseng, Younes, McVeigh, & Winslow, 2005), and the skeletal muscle (Karampinos, King, Sutton, & Georgiadis, 2007).

CONCLUSION

In summary, diffusion MRI constitutes a valuable tool towards the *in vivo* characterization of tissue microstructure, such as in the human central nervous and skeletal systems. However, the extraction of parameters of physiological relevance relies on the interpretation of the measured diffusion MR signal, which is not straightforward and depends on the complexity of the underlying mass transport process. Numerous diffusion models have been proposed to quantify this transport process. Each method imposes different requirements for optimizing the diffusion encoding acquisition, depending on the employed q-space coverage. The distribution and the number of diffusion encoding directions, the number of shells and the level of diffusion-weighting are the main diffusion encoding parameters that have to be determined. The selection of the above parameters is strongly related to the employed diffusion encoding scheme and is ultimately determined by the information sought by the radiologist, the physiologist, or the MR physicist. The optimization of the parameters basically relies on the need for minimizing noise while keeping the acquisition time reasonably short and should be always addressed with considerable attention. As the application of diffusion MRI penetrates deeper into the clinical practice, the blending of diffusion modeling and imaging will generate more insight for the optimization of the diffusion MRI encoding strategies under clinical settings.

REFERENCES

Alexander, D. C. (2005). Multiple-fiber reconstruction algorithms for diffusion MRI. *Annals of the New York Academy of Sciences, 1064*, 113-133.

Alexander, D. C., & Barker, G. J. (2005). Optimal imaging parameters for fiber-orientation estimation in diffusion MRI. *Neuroimage, 27*, 357-367.

Alexander, D. C., Barker, G. J., & Arridge, S. R. (2002). Detection and modeling of non-gaussian apparent diffusion coefficient profiles in human brain data. *Magnetic Resonance in Medicine, 48*, 331-340.

Arfanakis, K., Cordes, D., Haughton, V. M., Carew, J. D., & Meyerand, M. E. (2002). Independent component analysis applied to diffusion tensor MRI. *Magnetic Resonance in Medicine, 47*, 354-363.

Arfanakis, K., Haughton, V. M., Carew, J. D., Rogers, B. P., Dempsey, R. J., & Meyerand, M. E. (2002). Diffusion tensor MR imaging in diffuse axonal injury. *American Journal of Neuroradiology, 23*, 794-802.

Armitage, P. A., & Bastin, M. E. (2001). Utilizing the diffusion-to-noise ratio to optimize magnetic resonance diffusion tensor acquisition strategies for improving measurements of diffusion anisotropy. *Magnetic Resonance in Medicine, 45*, 1056-1065.

Assaf, Y., & Basser, P. J. (2005). Composite hindered and restricted model of diffusion (CHARMED) MR imaging of the human brain. *Neuroimage, 27*, 48-58.

Assaf, Y., Freidlin, R. Z., Rohde, G. K., & Basser, P. J. (2004). A new modeling and experimental framework to characterize hindered and restricted diffusion in brain white matter. *Magnetic Resonance in Medicine, 52*, 965-978.

Basser, P. J., Mattiello, J., & Le Bihan, D. (1994). MR diffusion tensor spectroscopy and imaging. *Biophysical Journal, 66*, 259-267.

Blumich, B. (2003). *NMR imaging of materials.* New York: Oxford University Press.

Callaghan, P. H. (1991). *Principles of magnetic resonance microscopy.* Oxford, UK: Oxford University Press.

Cohen, Y., & Assaf, Y. (2002). High *b*-value *q*-space analyzed diffusion-weighted MRS and MRI in neuronal tissues- a technical review. *NMR in Biomedicine, 15*, 516-542.

Frank, L. R. (2002). Characterization of anisotropy in high angular resolution diffusion-weighted MRI. *Magnetic Resonance in Medicine, 47,* 1083-1099.

Hasan, K. M., Parker, D. L., & Alexander, A. L. (2001). Comparison of gradient encoding schemes for diffusion-tensor MRI. *Journal of Magnetic Resonance Imaging,* 769-780.

Helm, P. A., Tseng, H.-J., Younes, L., McVeigh, E. R., & Winslow, R. L. (2005). Ex vivo 3D diffusion tensor imaging and quantification of cardiac laminar structure. *Magnetic Resonance in Medicine, 54,* 850-859.

Jones, D. K., Horsfiled, M. A., & Simmons, A. (1999). Optimal strategies for measuring diffusion in anisotropic systems by magnetic resonance imaging. *Magnetic Resonance in Medicine, 42,* 515-525.

Karampinos, D. C., King, K. F., Sutton, B. P., & Georgiadis, J. G. (2007). *In vivo study of cross-sectional skeletal muscle fiber asymmetry with diffusion-weighted MRI.* Paper presented at the IEEE Engineering in Medicine and Biology Conference, Lyon, France.

Klachaturian, M. H., Wisco, J. J., & Tuch, D. S. (2007). Boosting the sampling frequency of *q*-ball imaging using multiple wavevector fusion. *Magnetic Resonance in Medicine, 57,* 289-296.

Le Bihan, D., Breton, E., & Lallemand, D. (1986). MR imaging of intravoxel incoherent motions: application to diffusion and perfusion in neurologic disorders. *Radiology, 161,* 401-407.

Lin, C.-P., Wedeen, V. J., Chen, J.-H., Yao, C., & Tseng, W. I. (2003). Validation of diffusion spectrum magnetic resonance imaging with manganese-enhanced rat optic tracts and *ex vivo* phantoms. *Neuroimage, 19,* 482-495.

Minati, L., & Weglarz, W. P. (2007). Physical foundations, models and methods of diffusion magnetic resonance imaging of the brain: a review. *Concepts in Magnetic Resonance A, 30,* 278-307.

Moseley, M. E., Cohen, Y., & Kucharcyzk, J. (1990). Diffusion-weighted MR imaging of anisotropic water diffusion in cat central nervous system. *Radiology, 176,* 439-445.

Moseley, M. E., Cohen, Y., & Mintorovitch, J. (1990). Early detection of regional cerebral ischemic injury in cats: evaluation of diffusion and T2-weighted MRI and spectroscopy *Magnetic Resonance in Medicine, 14,* 330-346.

Ozarslan, E., & Mareci, T. H. (2003). Generalized diffusion tensor imaging and analytical relationships between diffusion tensor imaging and high angular resolution diffusion imaging. *Magnetic Resonance in Medicine, 50,* 955-965.

Peng, H. L., & Arfanakis, K. (2007). Diffusion tensor encoding schemes optimized for white matter fibers with selected orientations. *Magnetic Resonance Imaging, 25,* 147-153.

Raguin, L. G., Hernando, D., Karampinos, D. C., Ciobanu, L., Sutton, B. P., Liang, Z.-P., et al. (2006). *Quantitative analysis of q-space MRI data: theoretical and experimental validation.* Paper presented at the International Society of Magnetic Resonance in Medicine (ISMRM), 14th Scientific Meeting, Seattle, WA, USA.

Sinha, S., Sinha, U., & Edgerton, V. R. (2006). In vivo diffusion tensor imaging of the human calf muscle. *Journal of Magnetic Resonance Imaging, 24,* 182-190.

Skare, S., Hedehus, M., Moseley, M. E., & Li, T. Q. (2000). Condition number as a measure of noise performance of diffusion tensor data acquisition schemes with MRI. *Journal of Magnetic Resonance, 147,* 340-352.

Skorpil, M., Engstroem, M., & Nordell, A. (2007). Diffusion-direction-dependent imaging: a novel MRI approach for peripheral nerve imaging. *Magnetic Resonance Imaging, 25,* 406-411.

Skorpil, M., Karlsson, M., & Nordell, A. (2004). Peripheral nerve diffusion tensor imaging. *Magnetic Resonance Imaging, 22*, 743-745.

Stejskal, E. O., & Tanner, T. E. (1965). Spin diffusion measurements: spin echoes in the presence of a time-dependent field gradient. *Journal of Chemical Physics, 42*, 288-292.

Summers, P., Staempfli, P., Jaermann, T., Kwiecinski, S., & Kollias, S. (2006). A preliminary study of the effects of trigger timing on diffusion tensor imaging of the human spinal cord. *American Journal of Neuroradiology, 27*, 1952-1961.

Tournier, J. D., Calamante, F., Gadian, D. G., & Connelly, A. (2004). Direct estimation of the fiber orientation density distribution function from diffusion-weighted MRI data using spherical deconvolution. *Neuroimage, 23*, 1176-1185.

Tuch, D. S. (2004). *q*-ball imaging. *Magnetic Resonance in Medicine, 52*, 1358-1372.

Wedeen, V. J., Hagmann, P., Tseng, W. I., Reese, T. G., & Weisskoff, R. M. (2005). Mapping complex tissue architecture with diffusion spectrum magnetic resonance imaging. *Magnetic Resonance in Medicine, 54*, 1194-1206.

Wedeen, V. J., Reese, T. G., Tuch, D. S., Weigel, M. R., Dou, J.-G., Weisskoff, R. M., et al. (2000). *Mapping fiber orientation spectra in cerebral white matter with Fourier-transform MRI.* Paper presented at the International Society for Magnetic Resonance in Medicine (ISMRM), Denver, CO.

Wu, Y.-C., & Alexander, A. L. (2007). Hybrid diffusion imaging. *Neuroimage, 36*, 617-629.

Zhan, W., Gu, H., Silbersweig, D. A., Stern, E., & Yang, Y. (2003). Circular spectrum mapping for intravoxel fiber structures based on high angular resolution apparent diffusion coefficients. *Magnetic Resonance in Medicine, 49*, 1077-1088.

Zhan, W., Stein, E. A., & Yang, Y. (2004). Mapping the orientation of intravoxel crossing fibers based on the phase information of diffusion circular spectrum. *Neuroimage, 23*, 1358-1369.

Zhan, W., Stein, E. A., & Yang, Y. (2006). A rotation-invariant spherical harmonic decomposition method for mapping intravoxel multiple fiber structures. *Neuroimage, 29*, 1212-1223.

Zhan, W., & Yang, Y. (2006). How accuately can the diffusion profiles indicate multiple fiber orientations? A study on general fiber crossings in diffusion MRI. *Journal of Magnetic Resonance, 183*, 193-202.

KEY TERMS

Apparent Diffusion Coefficient (ADC): Diffusion coefficient derived from the normalized diffusion signal along a specific encoding direction.

***b* Value:** Variable expressing the amount of diffusion-weighting on a diffusion MRI experiment.

Diffusion Spectrum Imaging (DSI): Method for the reconstruction of ensemble average propagator based on the 3D inverse Fourier transform of the complex echo attenuation signal in 3D *q*-space.

Diffusion Tensor Imaging (DTI): Basic diffusion model representing tissue diffusion as an anisotropic Gaussian diffusion process described by a second rank tensor.

Fractional Anisotropy (FA): Metric of the anisotropy of the diffusion tensor in DTI.

High Angular Resolution Diffusion Imaging (HARDI): Measurement of diffusion coefficient along a large number of non-collinear directions.

Pulsed-Gradient Spin-Echo (PGSE) Sequence: The basic diffusion-weighted spin-echo sequence employing two identical gradient pulses on both sides of the refocusing pulse.

***q*-Ball Imaging (QBI):** Method for the reconstruction of the orientation distribution function from diffusion measurements taken on a sphere in *q*-space based on the Funk-Radon transform.

***q*-Space:** Reciprocal vector space of average spins displacement.

Chapter VIII
Segmentation of Cardiac Magnetic Resonance Images

Dimitrios G. Tsalikakis
University of Ioannina, Greece

Petros S. Karvelis
University of Ioannina, Greece

Dimitrios I. Fotiadis
University of Ioannina, Greece

ABSTRACT

Segmentation plays a crucial role in cardiac magnetic resonance imaging (CMRI) applications, since it permits automated detection of regions of interest. In this chapter we review semi-automated and fully automated cardiac MRI segmentation techniques and discuss their advantages. We classify those segmentation methods as classical and model-based.

INTRODUCTION

The structure and the size of the left ventricle (LV) are important indicators for the primary diagnosis of several cardiovascular diseases. LV contraction, capacity and wall thickness play a key role in the absorption and transportation of blood to the cardiac tissue(ischemia), while a decrease in LV output or the ejection fraction (EF), causes fatal consequences (hypertension) (Reeder et al. 2001). The rapid development of medical imaging techniques makes possible the acquisition of cardiac anatomy images. These images come from a variety of medical imaging methodologies, including X-ray, X-ray Computed Tomography (CT), MRI, and ultrasound. However, segmentation of Cardiac Magnetic Resonance (CMR) images faces several difficulties. First, the inadequate edge information in the image between the myocardium and the surrounding anatomical structure makes the detection of epicardium a difficult task. Second, the detection of the endocardium boundary is not easy, because cavity heterogeneities usually include wrong contours (Rogowska, 2000). In this chapter we review recent CMRI automated segmentation techniques and discus their advantages.

BACKGROUND

CMRI can be acquired from several views. Long-axis (LA) and short-axis (SA) views of the heart are obtained routinely since random imaging planes can be selected. Figure 1 demonstrates the most common selected MRI views in a typical cardiovascular MR examination. CMRI mages are used to assess global and regional, RV and LV function as represented by systolic volume (SV), ejection fraction (EF), LV mass (Lorenz et al. 1999), wall-thickening (Vallejo et al. 2000), myocardial motion (Buckberg et al. 2007), and circumferential shortening of myocardial fibers (Tseng et al. 2003).

Segmentation is the process of partitioning an image into regions which are homogeneous, related to one or more characteristics or features (Castleman, 1996). For the estimation of several cardiac functions during a CMRI examination, the boundaries of the LV, RV and epicardium need to be accurately determined. Thus, edge detection and image segmentation must be performed in

Figure 1. Horizontal LA multi-segmented cine MR images during: (a) the end–diastolic phase and (b) the end–systolic phase. Vertical LA multi–segmented cine MR images during: (c) the end–diastolic phase and (d) the end–systolic phase. SA multi–segmented cine MR images during: (e) the end–diastolic phase and (f) the end–systolic phase.

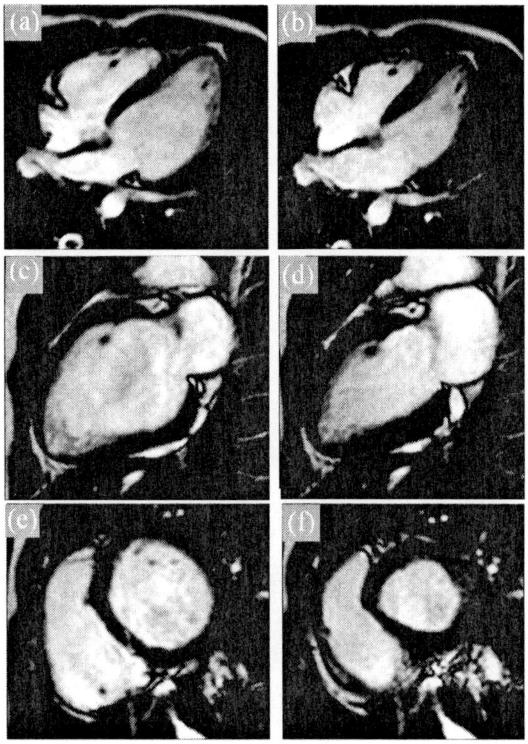

order to generate topologically correct cardiac surfaces from image data with minimum human effort and user interaction.

The mathematical description for the segmentation problem is: Consider an image I which is assumed to have N regions $S_k \subset I$, k=1…N, such that the union of all those regions is the entire image I:

$$I = \bigcup_{k=1}^{N} S_k \tag{1}$$

and these regions are disjoint:

$$S_i \cap S_j = \varnothing \tag{2}$$

Thus, segmentation is defined as the procedure to find all the disjoint regions S_k (Sonka et al. 1998).

In the literature, several works have been published introducing techniques for the segmentation for several imaging modalities (MRI, CT, echocardiograph, etc.). For each modality the problems are different and the methods are tailored to each modality.

In addition, segmentation methods can be classified in many ways:

- Manual, semi-automatic, fully automatic
- Pixel-based (local methods) and region-based (global methods)
- Manual depiction, low level segmentation (thresholding, region growing, etc.) and model-based segmentation (deformable contours, statistical shape models, etc.)
- Classical (thresholding, region-based, edge-based) and model-based segmentation (deformable contours, statistical shape models, active appearance models (AAMs), active shape models (ASMs))

The segmentation methods for CMRI published up to 2000, have been extensively reviewed in (Pham et al. 1998; Suri, 2000; Suri et al. 2002).

Manual detection of boundaries is difficult and time consuming. The problem becomes more intensive when the amount of images grows. Manual methods are inferior to inter- and intra- observer variability and are out of the scope of this chapter. The elementary semi-automated techniques, such as thresholding or region growing are not sophisticated (Adams & Bischof, 1994; Zhu & Yuille, 1996; Hojjatoleslami & Kittler, 1998). Those techniques are used to detect simple boundaries and they require high quality of images. The current trend is to move to fully automated segmentation of cardiac structure (Hautvast et al. 2006; Pednekar et al. 2006; Lynch et al. 2006). Semi-automated methods utilize the extracted boundary results (generated by sophisticated automatic algorithms) as initial guess, and then allow the user to draw the required boundaries manually. Usually, it is required from the operator to place an initial contour around the desired area or move the cursor around this area. These methods still need expert knowledge by the user, but reduce significantly the effort (Waiter et al. 1999; Gerard, 2002).

In this chapter we discuss the most common used semi-automatic and fully automatic segmentation methods which have been employed in CMRI. We classify those methods as classical and model-based.

CLASSICAL SEGMENTATION METHODS

Classical segmentation methods for CMRI are categorized into two classes. The first refers to region-based methods, which rely on the homogeneity of spatially localized features. The second is based on boundary finding, using discontinuity information. Homogeneity is the characteristic of a region and discontinuity is the characteristic of the boundary of a region. Region-based approaches include region growing, thresholding and watershed methods. Boundary-based approaches include edge detection and edge linking methods.

Thresholding Methods

It is the simplest segmentation technique and it is an effective tool to separate out structures which have different intensity ranges. Two of the most commonly used techniques for determining the threshold value in an image are: the intensity histogram and the Otsu's method (Otsu, 1978). A survey of these methods can be found in (Saho, 1988). Thresholding methods are: global (single threshold) or local threshold (depending on the position in the image), multi- thresholding and adaptive thresholding (Sonka et al. 1998). Thresholding methods are applied in several cardiac image modalities to separate the LV, by finding the minimum between the two modes in a grey scale histogram. Those are semi-automated and provide limited accuracy and low reliability in extracting the boundaries (Suri, 2000). For the segmentation of LV and RV in CMRI, Weng et al. proposed an extension of the thresholding algorithm (Weng, 1997). A preliminary global threshold value is determined, by performing an analysis of the intensity histogram. This threshold value is adapted dynamically to subsequent steps of the algorithm by fine-tuning it using feedback from a learned-likelihood measure. Recently, Lynch (2006) has also utilized intensities in an unsupervised threshold clustering technique. The procedure started with an edge preserving filter followed by an adapted k-means clustering algorithm to successfully segment the LV cavity from the SA CMRI.

In general, threshold-based methods are not suitable for segmenting CMRI because of their sensitivity to noise. They are very susceptible to noise in low contrast images and produce scattered groups of pixels rather than connected regions.

Edge Detection Methods

Those are not segmentation methods but the obtained results of the edge detection can be used as a pre-processing stage in segmentation. Morphological operators are used to extract edges: Roberts, Prewitt, Kirch, Robinson, Frei-Chen and Sobel. A review of those operators is available in (Sonka et al. 1998; Rogowska, 2000). One of the most commonly used edge detectors, which perform well in a variety of medical modalities, is the Canny edge detector (Canny, 1986). Since first and second derivatives are very sensitive to the existence of noise, those methods might fail. One straightforward solution is to remove noise from the images. Pratt (1991) describes noise-removing image filters, such as the median filter, the low pass filter and the Wiener filter. Wu (1997) published applications of 3D edge detection methods in combination with matched filters for the segmentation of cardiac CT and MRI data using the Laplacian and Gaussian operators.

Edge detection is not commonly used in CMRI segmentation. In (Zhang, 1999), the author pointed out that the Sobel edge detector failed to detect continuous epicardium boundary, and failed to detect LV and RV boundaries. However, the Canny edge detector succeeded in detecting the epicardium and the LV boundary, but failed to detect the RV boundary. A semi-automated edge-detection procedure was used by Waiter (1999) to exctract the endocardial and epicardial borders of the LV in SA cine-MRI scans. The semi-automated approach started with an estimation by the user for the epicardial and endocardial borders.

A similar method to edge detection is the boundary tracing. In the boundary-based segmentation, the boundary is represented as a collection of ordered points, which lie between areas of the image with different intensity values. Each point on the boundary is locally the maximum of the gradient magnitude of the image intensity. Boundary or edge extraction can be treated as a two-step process: edge detection and edge linking (Canny, 1986; Cox et al. 1993; Zhang, 1999). In Figure 2, an example of edge detection in SA CMRI is shown.

The intensity of an image provides only partial and uncertain information about the edges location. This is due to the existence of noise introduced in the imaging process and the fact that any measurement device is imperfect. This means that edge detection methods are in general ill-posed

Region-Based Methods

Those are techniques which extract regions within an image. A region is an area within an image which is connected based on a predefined criterion. A simple approach is to start with some user-selected pixels (seeds) representing distinctive image regions and to grow them until the area around them is covered.

Concerning CMRI region growing methods have either become obsolete (Balzer et al. 1998) or are used with others (Cassen et al. 2001; Jolly, 2006). Cassen (2001) suggest a combination of a region growing method, which is based on a split and merge algorithm, and active contours. His algorithm integrates the topological and geometrical characteristics of the LV in CMRI over time. Recently, a region-based segmentation method has been proposed by Jolly (2006). It uses the expectation-maximization (EM) algorithm to fit a mixture of three Gaussians to the histogram. They create a myocardium response image by computing the probability that a pixel belongs to the middle Gaussian distribution which corresponds to the myocardium. In Figure 3, the histogram of the CMRI that was used by (Jolly, 2006) is shown.

Watershed Segmentation

The watershed transform was originally proposed by Digabel (1978). In this transformation, an image can be viewed as a 3D surface with its grey-levels determining the height of the surface at any point. The lighter the shade of grey value at a point in the image, the higher will be the altitude of the cor-

Figure 2. Examples of edge detection and edge linking: (a) An intensity SA CMRI, (b) The edge detection result. Bright pixels are the detected boundary pixels, (c) The edge linking result. The red line denotes the epicardium boundary and the blue lines denote the endocardium boundaries and, (d) Image segmentation result, a binary image with the boundaries superimposed (Zhang, 1999).

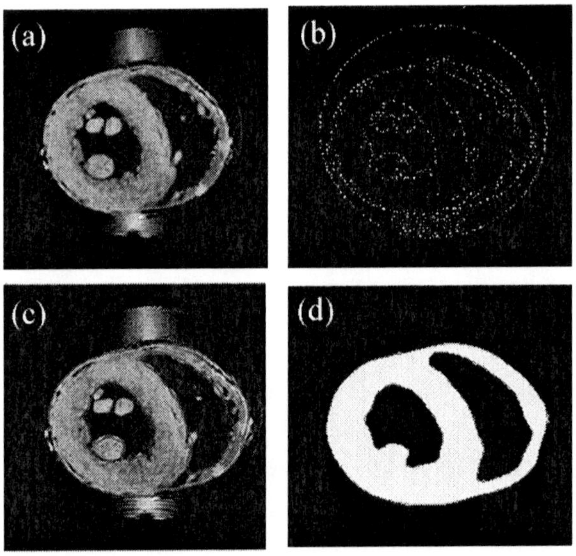

Figure 3. Region-based segmentation for CMRI: (a) Input image, (b) Histogram, (c) Myocardium response image (Jolly, 2006).

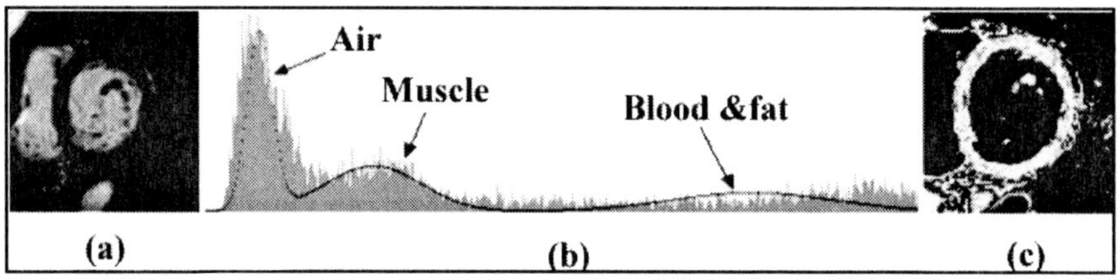

responding point on the surface. Thus, an image can be thought as a topographical relief containing valleys (minimas) and peaks (maximas). Grau (2004), proposed an improvement of the watershed transformation, which makes it more suitable for use in medical images. The improved algorithm enables the usage of prior information-based different functions for each object to be segmented, instead of the usual gradient calculation which watershed algorithms normally use.

Interactive Watershed Transform (IWT) is applied by Hahn (2003), to efficiently segment multidimensional grayscale images and CMRI. The application of IWT on CMRI, using a single marker on an arbitrary slice and phase with an appropriate "preflooding" height, was enough to segment the LV on all slices and phases. The latest work in this field came by Hamarneh (2007). He proposed a method to enhance watershed segmentation utilizing prior shape and appearance knowledge. His method iteratively alligned a shape histogram with the result of an improved k-means clustering algorithm of the watershed segments. Figure 4 demonstrates the application of the improved k-means clustering to a watershed segmentation of a SA CMRI.

Watershed segmentation has several disadvantages. It is sensitive to noise: each noisy pixel corresponds to a catchment basin, which causes the watershed algorithm to segment it. Besides, it is also limited when regions with low contrast boundaries are detected.

Model-Based Segmentation Methods

Inherent difficulties (image artefacts, noise and motion) impose the use of prior knowledge in order to improve CMRI segmentation performance. Methods based on *a priori* models of cardiac geometry, known as deformable models, have retained attention and obtained a provided high accuracy results.

Active Contours or "Snakes"

Those are special cases of the deformable models. They were first introduced by Kass (1988) and they are energy-minimizing models. The energy to be minimized is an aggregate of the internal, image and external forces of a contour (snake). The internal energy imposes a piecewise smoothness constraint and the image forces push the snake towards salient features in an image such as edges, lines and subjective contours (Kass et al. 1988). The external forces, such as those coming from a user interacting with the snake, are responsible for reaching the snake towards a local minimum.

Geometrically, the snake is a parametric contour embedded in a 2D image plane $(x, y) \in \mathbb{R}^2$. The snake can be represented parametrically by $v(s) = (x(s), y(s))^T$ where x and y are coordinate functions and $s \in [0,1]$ is the parametric domain. Thus, the energy equation which must be minimized is:

Figure 4. LV segmentation using the watershed algorithm: a) Original MR cardiac image, b) Watershed transformation of the image, c) Coalesced watershed segments resulting from improved k-means clustering and d) The initial segmentation estimate (Hamarneh & Li, 2007).

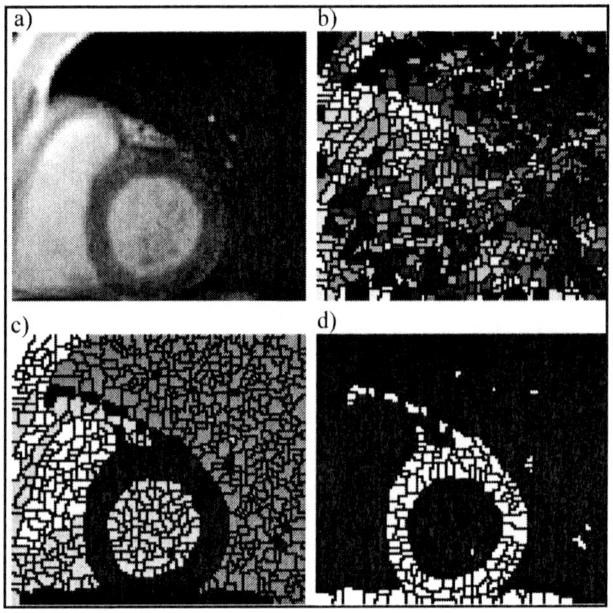

$$E_{snake} = \int_0^1 E_{\text{int}}\big(v(s)\big) + E_{image}\big(v(s)\big)ds + \int_0^1 E_{ext}\big(v(s)\big)ds \qquad (3)$$

A review of the active contour models in medical image analysis can be found in (McInerney & Terzopoulos, 1996). In the last ten years, many researchers have employed active contours to segment CMRI. In most of them, the interest was on the LV due to the nature of its shape in SA CMRI slices. The performance of active contours was the subject of research in numerous extensions to the original snake formulation. These extensions are classified in three main categories: geometrical representations, optimization algorithms and external force extensions. Extended geometrical representation include B-spline snakes (Brigger et al. 2000), T-snakes (McInerney & Terzopoulos, 2000), and Fourier parametering (Staib & Duncan, 1992). The most well-known applicable external force extensions include the pressure force (Cohen, 1991), the gradient-vector-flow (GVF) (Xu & Prince, 1998; Santarelli et al. 2003) and the distance potential force (Cohen L. & Cohen I., 1993).

Santarelli (2003) obtained good agreement between manual and automatic LV volume estimation with the use of a non-linear anisotropic filtering and a GVF snake. The introduction of the GVF field into the traditional snake permitted the progressive growth of a deformable contour in homogeneous regions extending the capturing range over that of a traditional snake. Spreeuwers (2003) proposed a coupled active contour approach which is based on the fact that the epicardial and endocardial boundaries are not independent and extract both contours simultaneously.

A new external force for the active contour model, which is based on the orientation gradient of three-dimensional velocity vector fields from cardiac phase contrast MRI is introduced in (Cho et al. 2003). Velocity images together with the magnitude images were used for the segmentation of myocardial boundaries. A tensor-based orientation gradient force and the seed contour tracking scheme for the generalized active contour model were developed to improve the accuracy of semi-automated segmentation of the myocardium throughout the entire cardiac cycle.

Extending the snake theory, Lorenzo et. al. (2004), designed a probabilistic atlas of manually segmented temporally aligned data. Automatic segmentation was achieved by registering the atlas on the data, using this as the initial guess for the EM algorithm. The EM algorithm iterates until convergence and this is followed by the application of a final classification step, where the Markov random fields (MRF) and connected components (CC) are employed to refine the initial segmentation.

Recently, Pluempitiwiriyawej (2005) have developed a novel stochastic active contour scheme (STACS) for cardiac image segmentation. They choose an energy minimization approach which combines characteristics of curve evolution theory and statistical modeling of the images to segment a homogeneous object (the heart and its structures) from the background (chest wall or other anatomy). They also compared three different active contour algorithms (Xu & Prince, 1998; Chan & Vese, 2001) with the proposed active contour and a manual LV segmentation (Figure 5).

A modification of the active contour model, which tends to maintain a constant contour environment by matching gray values in profiles perpendicular to the contour, it is introduced in (Hautvast et al. 2006). The contours must maintain a constant position with respect to neighboring anatomical structures, such as the resulting contours reflect the preferences of the user.

Figure 5. Comparing the segmentation results of a CMRI using different algorithms. Initial contours are the dashed lines; the final contours are the solid lines: (a) Xu and Prince's GVF snake algorithm, (b) Chan and Vese's active contour algorithm, (c) STACS and (d) Contour traced manually by an expert. (Pluempitiwiriyawej et al. 2005).

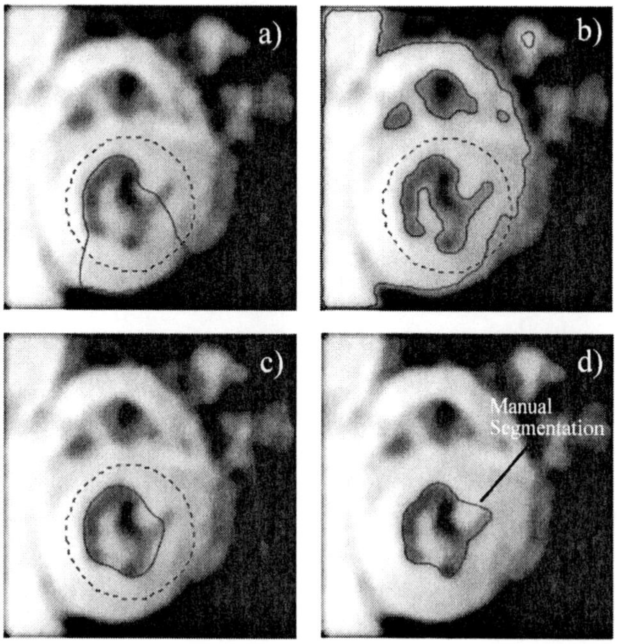

Nguyen (2007) published a comparative study on the external force extensions of the active contour model and filtering techniques usually used to improve CMRI quality. The segmentation performances were established for a GVF snake, a pressure force-based snake and a guided pressure force-based snake in comparison to the traditional snake formulation. They clearly pointed out, that the local assessment of segmentation accuracy showed a number of segmentation difficulties in both endocardial and epicardial levels, despite the proposed extensions of the traditional snake formulation.

Active Shape Models

Active Shape Model (ASM) is a statistical model which encodes shape variability across a training set of an object of interest. It was first proposed by Cootes (1994). Recently, many studies on ASMs for cardiac segmentation have been published (Shen & Davatzikos, 2000; Shen & Davatzikos, 2001; De Bruijne et al. 2003; Davatzikos et al. 2003; Frangi et al. 2003; van Assen et al. 2003; van Assen et al. 2006; Nain et al. 2006).

Once a training set has been acquired, the next step is to landmark the training set. Landmarking is the process of determining and locating a set of corresponding points across a training set of images. The cardiac shape includes two anatomical landmarks: the points where the RV border meets the epicardial called anterior and inferior junction as it is shown in Figure 6.

Figure 6. Basic anatomical landmarks of a cardiac MR image shape: Anterior and inferior junctions between RV and LV.

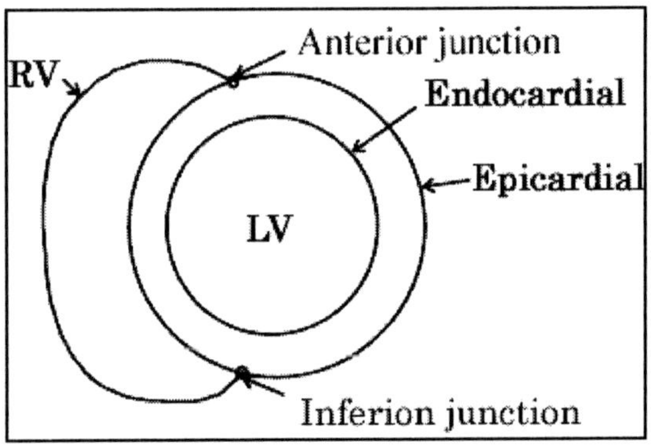

Kaus (2004) proposed an approach to automatically segment the LV in SA an LA CMR images. He integrated diverse sources of prior knowledge learned from annotated images into the deformable surface model as in (Kass et al. 1988; Montagnat et al. 1998). Those sources of prior information include inter- and intra-subject shape variability, surface features and spatial relationships between the endocardium and epicardium. Prior knowledge such as intra- and inter-subject variability is modeled using a Point Distribution Model (PDM) which is embedded into the deformable model as an ASM, as described in (Weese et al. 2001). The surfaces features are modeled using a k-means clustering scheme. In addition to this, the spatial relationship of the epicardium and endocardium is modeled to prevent the two separate meshes from intersecting with each other due to attraction to missing or false features.

Ordas (2003) proposed an extension of the ASM framework making use of a non-linear appearance model as in the Optimal Features ASMs (OF-ASMJ approach by van Ginneken (2002)) and incorporated a reduced set of differential Cartesian invariant features as local image descriptors. Results depict that both optimal features algorithms have barely the same performance. Statistical properties of the wavelet transform of cardiac shape, were introduced by Davatzikos (2003), making the shape deformation more global and, thus, getting better results for small training sets. This allowed to have a robust ASM, improving the segmentation of CMRI. A methodology for incorporating more knowledge about cardiac structure through the use of level set methods and ASMs, and could potentially offer a robust approach to CMRI segmentation is presented in (Rousson et al. 2004).

A 3D statistical shape model of the heart (atria, ventricles and epicardium) was developed by Lotjonen (2004), combining information from both LA and SA CMRIs. The shape variations were modeled in two ways: using Principal Component Analysis (PCA) and Independent Component Analysis (ICA) based shape models with non-parametric distributions. Delhay (2005) presented a 3D surface model which also considers a temporal constraint to increase the accuracy of the segmentation. Fritz (2006) proposed an automatic cardiac segmentation procedure with minimal user interaction. It is based on a combined bi-temporal statistical model of the LV and RV using PCA, as well as, ICA to model global and local shape variations. Recently, Renno (2006) designed a software to automate the steps in ASM training. ASMs were constructed from manually segmented ventricular models, allowing the user to cite entire datasets for processing using a GVF-based landmarking procedure and PCA to construct the statistical shape model. In Figure 7 a comparison of manual segmentation of SA CMRI with automatic segmentation using PCA models derived from landmarked templates is shown.

Active Appearance Models

Active Appearance Models (AAMs) were introduced as a learning-based method of registration and interpretation of face images (Edwards et al. 1988; Cottes et al. 1998). These models were built based on a set of order-less annotated images. Cootes (2001) presented a review of AAMs applications in medicine. An AAM can be applied to detect automatically a contour in CMRI by minimizing the difference between the model and the image, where the model is constrained to 'statistically plausible' organ appearances (Figure 8).

Several authors have proposed methods based on the AAM including extensions to 3D [Steven et al. 2002], 2D + time [van der Geest et al. 2004], or 3D + time [Stegmann, 2001]; also called active appearance motion models (AAMMs). AAMMs represent the contours for the whole cardiac cycle simultaneously, and they are suitable for full-cycle contour detection. AAMMs have the advantage that the detected contours change smoothly over time, omitting discontinuities inherent to conventional 2D frame-by-frame contour detection techniques.

Figure 7. Comparison of: (a) manual segmentation with automatic segmentation using PCA derived from landmarked templates (ASMs), with (b) 25, (c) 50, (d) 100 decimations and (e) PCA restriction for the template with 100 decimations at the same slice (Renno et al. 2006).

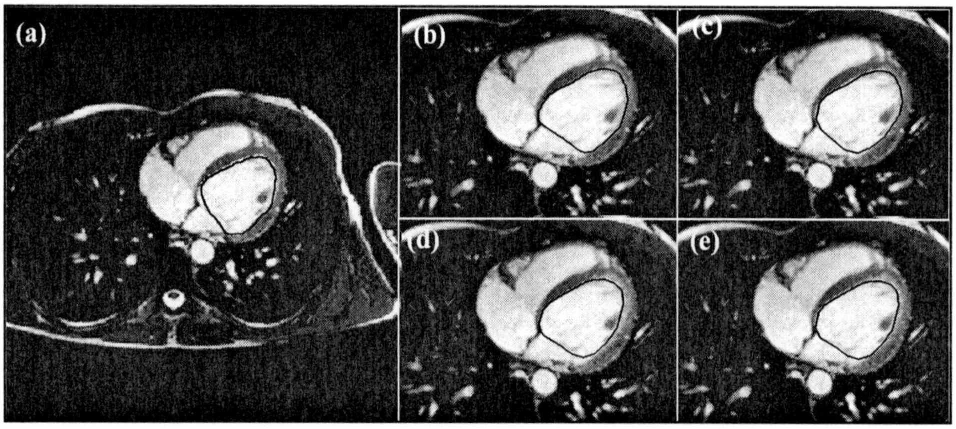

Figure 8. Two examples (top and bottom row) of an AAM for simultaneous contour detection in: (a), (d) four chamber, (b), (e) SA and (c), (f) two chamber CMRI views.

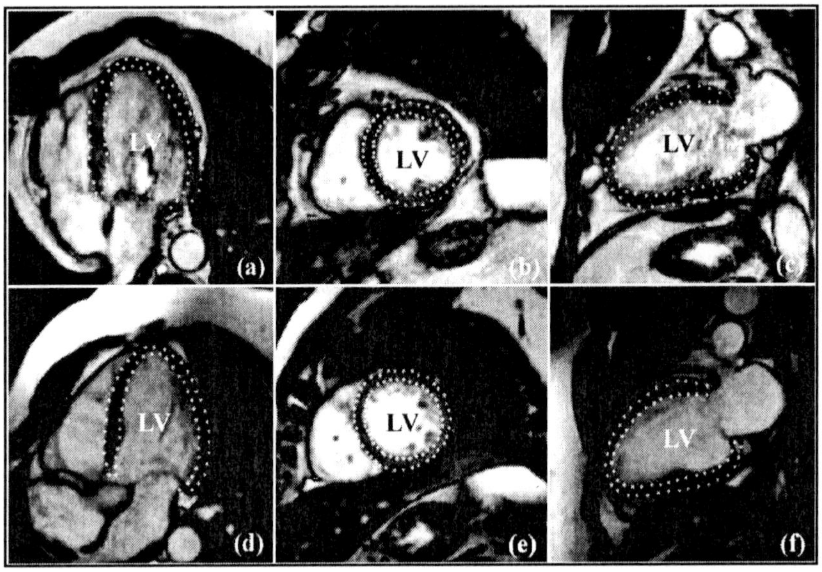

Mitchell (2001) applied a hybrid ASM and an AAM model matching scheme to SA CMR slices of the LVs and RVs. He argues that conventional AAM approach failss to produce precise borders in the segmentation of SA cardiac MR data. This is since AAM is optimized for global appearance and so it is less sensitive to local structures and boundary information. However, since the heart is a three-dimensional organ and the CMRI data is three-dimensional as well, the 2D AAM was extended to 3D in (Mitchell et al. 2002). In Figure 9, an application of a 3D AAM for the segmentation of the LV is shown.

Stegmann (2004) further extended the AAM towards 3D + time by coupling the 3D detection in the end-diastolic and end-systolic frames in one model. They further improved Mitchell's (2002) work by introducing an improvement on the solution of breath holding problem. The comparison of the segmentation results, after the utilization of ICA and PCA in AAM, was presented by Uzumcu (2003). Since the introduction of the PCA is followed by global shape variations which can lead to unsatisfying segmentation results, Suinesiaputra (2004) use the ICA in order to handle local shape variations by the minimization of statistical dependence of the components of the shape representation. The approach is applied to CMRI for the detection of abnormalities in the context of infracted myocardial areas. Extending his previous work, Stegmann (2005) introduced a bi-temporal AAM of the LV. He simply combined the end-diastolic and end-systolic landmarks into one feature vector and thus created a bi-temporal AAM representation. Zambala (2006) presented a two-component model extension based on AAMs and its integration into a software tool for heart function analysis. The proposed system provides automatic segmentation and visualization of important data such as wall thickening and EF. Andreopoulos (2008) proposed a framework for the analysis of SA CMRI, using statistical models of shape and appearance. They introduced an algorithm for fitting 3D AAMs on SA CMRI and a hierarchical 2D + time ASMs which integrates temporal constraints and simultaneously improves the 3D AAM segmentation results.

The basic difference between ASMs and AAMs lies in the mechanism fitting the model to the image data, which is based on locally updating surface points for the ASMs, instead of using the complete volume for the AAMs. An advantage of ASMs over AAMs is the fact that they can be applied to 3D processing of sparse MR data, such as the LA and SA views.

FUTURE TRENDS

To develop successfully robust automated contour detection in CMRI, it is clear that a priori knowledge of cardiac image is needed. This knowledge is related to cardiac shape, motion, image characteristics or spatial context. Because of their integral knowledge about organ shape and image characteristics, model-based methods are more efficient in solving a variety of difficult cardiac contour detection problems. In addition systems in 3D+time dimension will be proven more efficient.

CONCLUSION

Segmentation of CMRI remains a challenging filed in medical image analysis. The need for semi- or fully-automatic methods to extract useful clinical measurements from CMRI has led to the development of various techniques. In this chapter, we reviewed the most significant segmentation methods, both classical and models-based. Classical methods are not efficient in segmenting CMRI since they are sensitive to noise and intensity inhomogeneity. Even, noise can be treated using various filters those do not stand alone but work in combination with other methods.

Figure 9. (a) Three-dimensional AAM determined segmentation of the LV, (b) The result of the application of a 3-D AAM in several views of a CMRI dataset (Mitchell et al. 2002).

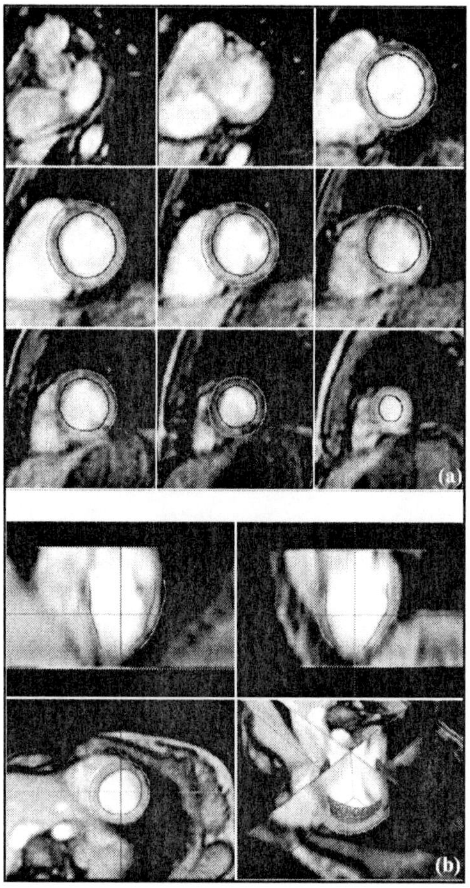

REFERENCES

Adams, R., & Bischof, L. (1994). Seeded Region Growing. *IEEE Transactions on Pattern Analysis and Machine Intelligence*, *16*(6), 641-647.

Andreopoulos, A., & Tsotsos, J. K. (2008). Efficient and generalizable statistical models of shape and appearance for analysis of cardiac MRI. *Medical Image Analysis*, (in press)

Balzer, P., Furber, A., Cavaro-Menard, C., Croue, A., Tadei, A., Geslin, P., & Jallet, P. (1998). Le Jeune L Simultaneous and correlated detection of endocardial and epicardial borders on short-axis MR images for the measurement of left ventricular mass. *Radiographics, 18*, 1009–1018.

Brigger, P., Hoeg, J., & Unser, M. (2000). B-Sline Snakes: a flexible tool for parametric contour detection. *IEEE Transactions on Image Processing, 9*(9), 1484–1496.

Buckberg, G. D., Mahajan, A., Jung, B., Markl, M., Hennig, J., & Ballester-Rodes, M. (2006). MRI myocardial motion and fiber tracking: A confirmation of knowledge from different imaging modalities, *European journal of cardio-thoracic surgery*, 29, 165-177.

Canny, J. (1986). A computation approach to edge detection. *IEEE Transactions on Pattern and Machine Intelligence*, *8*(6), 679-698.

Cassen, C., Domenger, J. P., Braquelaire, A., & Barat, J. L. (2001). Left ventricular segmentation in MR images. *Proceedings of ISPA*, (pp. 244–249).

Castleman, K. R. (1996). *Digital Image Processing.* Upper Saddle River, Prentice Hall.

Chan, T. F., & Vese, L. A. (2001). Active contours without edges. *IEEE Transactions on Image Processing, 10*(2), 266–277.

Cho, Brummer, M., & Benkeser, P. J. (2003). Velocity-aided Cardiac Segmentation. *IEEE Proceedings of EMBS*, (pp. 17-21).

Cohen, L., & Cohen, I. (1993). Finite-element methods for active contour models and balloons for 2-D and 3-D images. *IEEE Transactions on Pattern Analysis and Machine Intelligence*, *15*(11), 1131–1147.

Cohen, L. (1991). On active contour models and balloon. *CVGIP: Image Understanding, 53*(2), 211-218.

Cootes, T., Taylor, C., Hill, A., & Halsm, J. (1994). The use of active shape model for locating structures in the medical image. *Image and Vision Computing, 12*(6), 355–366.

Cootes, T. F., Edwards, G. J., & Taylor, C. J. (1998). Active appearance models, *In Proceedings of European Conference on Computer Vision, 2*, 484–498.

Cootes, T. F., Edwards, G. J., & Taylor, C. J. (2001). Active appearance models. *IEEE Transactions on Pattern Analysis and Machine Intelligence, 23*(6), 681–685.

Cox, I., Rehg, J., & Hingorani, S. (1993). A bayesian multiple-hypothesis approach to edge grouping and contour segmentation. *International Journal of Computer Vision, 11*(1), 5-24.

Davatzikos, C., Tao, X., & Shen, D. (2003). Hierarchical active shape models using the wavelet transform. *IEEE Transactions on Medical Imaging, 22*(3), 414–422.

De Bruijne, M., van Ginneken, B., Viergever, M., & Niessen, W. (2003). Adapting active shape models for 3D segmentation of tubular structures in medical images, *Proceedings on Information Processing in Medical Imaging*, (pp. 136–147).

Delhay, B., Lotjonen, J., Clarysse, P., Katila, T., & Magnin, I. (2005). A dynamic 3D cardiac surface model from MR images. *IEEE Proceeding of CINC,* (pp. 423- 426).

Digabel, H., & Lantuejoul, C. (1978). Iterative algorithms. *In Actes du Second Symposium Européen' Analyse Quantitative des Microstructures en Sciences des Matériaux*. Biologie et Médecine, Caen.

Edwards, G. J., Taylor, C. J., & Cootes, T. F. (1998). Interpreting face images using active appearance models. *IEEE Proceedings of Automatic Face and Gesture Recognition*, (pp. 300-305).

Frangi, A. F., Rueckert, D., Schnabel, J. A., & Niessen, W. J. (2003). Automatic construction of multiple-object three-dimensional statistical shape models: application to cardiac modeling. *IEEE Transaction on Medical Imaging*, 21, 1151–1166.

Fritz, D., Rinck, D., Dillmann, R., & Scheuering, M. (2006). Segmentation of the left and right cardiac ventricle using a combined bi-temporal statistical model. *Proceedings of the SPIE, 6141*, 605-614.

Gerard, O., Deschamps, T., Greff, M., & Cohen, L. (2002) Real-time interactive path extraction with on-the-fly adaptation of the external forces, *European Conference on Computer Vision,* (pp. 239-266).

Gonzalez, R. C., & Woods, R. E. (2002). *Digital Image Processing.* Prentice Hall.

Grau, V., Mewes, U. J., & Alcanz, M. (2004). Improved watershed transform for medical image segmentation using prior information. *IEEE Transactions on Medical Imaging, 23*(4), 447- 458.

Hahn, H. K., & Peitgen, H. O. (2003). IWT - Interactive watershed transform: A hierarchical method for efficient interactive and automated segmentation of multidimensional gray-scale images. *Proceedings of SPIE, 5032*, 643-653.

Hamarneh, G., & Li, X. (2007). Watershed segmentation using prior shape and appearance knowledge. *Image and Vision Computing*, (in press).

Hautvast, G., Lobregt, S., Breeuwer, M., & Gerritsen, F. (2006) Automatic contour propagation in cine cardiac MRI. *IEEE Transactions on Medical Imaging, 25*(11), 1472-1482.

Hilger, K. B., Stegmann, M. B., & Larsen, R. (2002). A noise robust statistical model for image representation. *Proceedings of MICCAI, 2488*, 444–451.

Hojjatoleslami, S. A., & Kittler, J. (1998). Region growing: A new approach. *IEEE Transactions on Image Processing*, *7*(7), 1079–1084.

Jolly, M. P. (2006). Automatic segmentation of the left ventricle in cardiac MRI and CT images. *International Journal of Computer Vision, 70*, 151-163.

Kass, M., Witkin, A., & Terzopoulos, D. (1988). Snakes: Active contour models. *International Journal of Computer Vision*, *1*(4), 321–331.

Kaus, M. R., von Berg, J., Weese, J., Niessen, W., & Pekar, V. (2004) Automated segmentation of the left ventricle in cardiac MRI. *Medical Image Analysis*, *8*, 245–254.

Laarse, A., Bruschke, V. G., Reiber, J. H. C., van der Wall, E. E., Holman, E. R., Buller, V. G. M., de Roos, A., van der Geest, R. J., Baur, L. H. B., & van der Detection, A. (1997). Quantification of dysfunctional myocardium by magnetic resonance imaging: A new three-dimensional method for quantitative wall. *Thickening Analysis Circulation, 95*(4), 924 - 931.

Lelieveldt, B., van der Geest, R., Mitchell, S. C., Bosch, J., Sonka, M., & Reiber, J. (2002). 3D active appearance models: Fully automatic detection of endo- and epicardial contours in short-axis cardiac MR data. *Proceedings of ISMRM, 2*, 1668.

Lorenz, C. H., Walker, E. S., Morgan, V. L., Klein, S. S., & Graham, T. P. (1999). Normal human right and left ventricular mass, systolic function, and gender differences by cine magnetic resonance imaging. *Journal of Cardiovascular Magnetic Resonance*, *1*(1), 7–21.

Lorenzo-Valdes, M., Sanchez-Ortiz, G. I., Elkington, A. G., Mohiaddin, R. H., & Rueckert, D. (2004). Segmentation of 4D cardiac MR images using a probabilistic atlas and the EM algorithm. *Medical Image Analysis*, *8*(3), 255-65.

Lotjonen, S., Kivist, O., Koikkalainen, J., Smutek, D., & Lauerma, K. (2004). Statistical shape model of atria, ventricles and epicardium from short- and long-axis MR images. *Medical Image Analysis*, *8*, 371–386.

Lynch, M., Ghita, O., & Whelan, P. F. (2006). Automatic segmentation of the left ventricle cavity and myocardium in MRI data. *Computers in Biology and Medicine*, *34*(4), 389-407.

Markus, S., Yan Shang, R., Sweeney, J., & Dössel, O. (2006). Segmentation of 4D cardiac images: investigation on statistical shape models. *IEEE Proceedings of EMBS,* (pp. 3086-3089).

McInerney, T., & Terzopoulos, D. (1996). Deformable Models in Medical Image Analysis: A Survey. *Medical Image Analysis*, *1*(2), 91-108.

McInerney, T., & Terzopoulos, D. (2000). T-snakes: topology adaptive snakes. *Medical Image Analysis*, *4*, 73–91.

Mitchell, S., Lelieveldt, B., Geest, R., Schaap, J., Reiber, J., & Sonka, M. (2000). Segmentation of cardiac MR images: An active appearance model approach. *Proceedings of SPIE*, *1*, 224–234.

Mitchell, S. C., Bosch, J. G., Lelieveldt, B. P. F., van der Geest, R. J., Reiber, J. H. C., & Sonka, M. (2002). 3D Active Appearance Models: segmentation of cardiac MR and ultrasound images. *IEEE Transactions on Medical Imaging, 21*, 1167–1178.

Mitchell, S. C., Lelieveldt, B. P. F., van der Geest, R. J., Bosch, H. G., Reiber, J. H. C., & Sonka, M. (2001). Multistage hybrid active appearance model matching: Segmentation of left and right ventricles in cardiac MR images. *IEEE Transactions on Medical Imaging, 20*(5), 415–423.

Montagnat, J., & Delingette, H. (1998). Globally constrained deformable models for 3D object reconstruction. *Signal Process*, *71*(2), 173– 186.

Nain, D., Haker, S., Bobick, A., & Tannenbaum, A. (2006) Shape-driven 3D segmentation using spherical wavelets. *Proceedings of the MICCAI*, (pp. 66-74).

Nguyen, D., Masterson, K., & Vallée, J-P. (2007) Comparative evaluation of active contour model extensions for automated cardiac MR image segmentation by regional error assessment. Magnetic *Resonance Material in Physics Biology and Medicine*, *20*, 69–82.

Ordas, S., Biosrobert, L., Huguet, M., & Frangi, A. F. (2003). Active shape models with invariant optimal features (IOF-ASM) application to cardiac MRI segmentation. *IEEE Proceeding of CINC*, *30*, 633-636.

Otsu, N. (1978). A threshold selection method from gray-level histogram. *IEEE Transaction on Systems, Man and Cybernetics, 9*, 62-66.

Pednekar, A., Kurkure, U., Muthupillai, R., Flamm, S., & Kakadiaris, I.A. (2006) Automated left ventricular segmentation in cardiac MRI. *IEEE Transactions on Biomedical Engineering, 53*(7), 1425-1428.

Pham, D. L., Xu, C., & Prince, J. L. (1998). *A survey of current methods in medical image segmentation.* The John Hopkins University, Baltimore.

Pham, D. L., Xu, C., & Prince, J. L. (2000). A survey of current methods in medical image segmentation. *Annual Review of Biomedical Engineering*, *2*, 315-337.

Pluempitiwiriyawej, C., Moura, J. M. F., Yi-Jen, L. W., & Chien, H. (2005). STACS: new active contour scheme for cardiac MR image segmentation. *IEEE Transaction on Medical Imaging, 24*(5), 593-603.

Pratt, W. K. (1991). *Digital Image Processing.* Wiley.

Reeder, S., Du, Y. P., Lima, J. A. C., & Bluemke, D. A. (2001). Advanced cardiac MR imaging of ischemic heart disease. *Radiographics, 21*, 1047–1074.

Renno, M. S., Shang, Y., Sweeney, J., & Dossel, O. (2006). Segmentation of 4D cardiac images: investigation on statistical shape models. *Proceedings of IEEE EMBS*, 3086-3089.

Rogowska, J. (2000). *Overview and Fundamentals of Medical Image Segmentation in the Handbook of Medical Imaging.* Academic Press.

Rousson, M., Paragios, N., & Deriche, R. (2004). Implicit active shape models for 3D segmentation in MRI imaging. *Proceedings of the MICCAI*, (pp. 209-216).

Sahoo, P. K., Soltani, S., & Wong, A. K. C. (1998). A Survey of thresholding techniques. *Computer Vision, Graphics and Image Processing, 41*, 233-260.

Santarelli, M. F., Positano, V., Michelassi, C., Lombardi, M., & Landini, L. (2003). Automated cardiac MR image segmentation: theory and measurement evaluation. *Medical Engineering & Physics, 25*(2), 149–159.

Shen, D., & Davatzikos, C. (2000). An adaptive-focus deformable model using statistical and geometric information. *IEEE Transactions on Pattern Analysis and Machine Intelligence, 22*(8), 906–913.

Shen, D., & Davatzikos, C. (2001). An adaptive-focus statistical shape model for segmentation and shape modeling of 3D brain structures. *IEEE Transactions on Medical Imaging, 20*(4), 257–270.

Sonka, M. (2002). Segmentation of cardiac MR volume data using 3D active appearance models. *Proceedings of SPIE,* (pp. 433-443).

Sonka, M., Hlavac, V., & Boyle, R. (1998). *Image Processing, Analysis and Machine Vision.* Chapman and Hall Computing.

Spreeuwers, L., & Breeuwer, M. (2003). Detection of left ventricular epi- and endocardian borders using coupled active contours. *International Congress Series, 1256*, 1147- 1152.

Staib, L., & Duncan, J. (1992). Boundary finding with parametrically deformable models. *IEEE Transactions on Pattern Analysis and Machine Intelligence, 14*(11), 1061–1075.

Stegmann, M. (2001). Analysis of 4D cardiac MRI. *Journal of the Danish Optical Society, 4*, 38-39.

Stegmann, M. B., & Pedersen, D. (2005). Bi-temporal 3D active appearance models with applications to unsupervised ejection fraction estimation. *Proceedings of SPIE, 5747*, 336-350.

Stegmann, M. B. (2004). *Generative interpretation of medical images.* PhD Thesis, University of Denmark, Denmark.

Stegmann, M. B., Ersboll, B. K., & Larsen, R. (2003). FAME – a flexible appearance modeling environment. *IEEE Transactions on Medical Imaging, 22*, 1319– 1331.

Steven, C. M., Bosch, J. G., Lelieveldt, P. F., van der Geest, R. J., Reiber, J. H. C., & Sonka, M. (2002). 3D active appearance models: segmentation of cardiac MR and ultrasound images. *IEEE Transactions on Medical Imaging, 21*(9), 1167-78.

Suinesiaputra, A., Uzumcu, M., Frangi, A., Kaandorp, T. A. M., Reiber, J. H. C., & Lelieveldt, B. P. F. (2004). Detecting regional abnormal cardiac contraction in short-axis MR images using independent component analysis. *Proceedings of MICCAI*, (pp. 737–744).

Suri, J. S. (2000). Computer vision, pattern recognition and image processing in left ventricle segmentation: The Last 50 Years. *Pattern Analysis and Applications, 3*, 209-242.

Suri, J. S., Setarehdan, S. K., & Singh, S. (2002). *Advanced Algorithmic Approaches to Medical*

Image Segmentation: State-of-the-Art Applications in Cardiology, Neurology, Mammography and Pathology. Springer, Berlin.

Tseng, W-Y.I., Van Wedeen, J., Reese, T. G., Smith, R. N., Elkan, F., & Halpern, E. F. (2003). Diffusion tensor MRI of myocardial fibers and sheets: Correspondence with visible cut-face texture. *Journal of Magnetic Resonance Imaging, 17*(1), 31-42.

Uzumcu, M., Frangi, A., Sonka, M., Reiber, J., & Lelieveldt, B. (2003). ICA vs. PCA active appearance models: Application to cardiac MR segmentation. *Proceedings of MICCAI,* (pp. 451–458).

Vallejo, E., Dione, D. P., Bruni, W. L., Constable, R. T., Borek, P. P., Soares, J. P., Carr, J. G., Condos, S. G., Wackers, F. J. Th., & Sinusas, A. J. (2000). Reproducibility and accuracy of gated SPECT for determination of left ventricular volumes and ejection fraction: Experimental validation using MRI. *The Journal of Nuclear Medicine, 41*(5), 874-882.

Van Assen, H. C., Danilouchkine, M. G., Behloul, F., Lamb, H. G., van der Geest, R. G., Reiber, G. H. C., & Lelieveldt, B. P. F. (2003). Cardiac LV segmentation using a 3D active shape model driven by fuzzy inference. *Proceedings Of MICCAI,* (pp. 533–540).

Van Assen, H. C., Danilouchkine, M. H., Frangi, A. F., Ordas, S., Westenberg, J. J., Reiber, J. H. & Lelieveldt, B. P. (2006). SPASM: a 3D-ASM for segmentation of sparse and arbitrarily oriented cardiac MRI data. *Medical Image Analysis, 10,* 286–303.

Van der Geest, R. J., Lelieveldt, B. P. F., Angelie, E., Danilouchkine, M., Sonka, M., & Reiber, J. H. C. (2004). Evaluation of a new method for automated detection of left ventricular contours in time series of magnetic resonance images using an active appearance motion model. *Journal of Cardiovascular Magnetic Resonance, 6,* 609–617.

Van Ginneken, B., Frangi, A. F., Staal, I. I., ter Haar-Romeny, B. M., & Viergever, M. A. (2002). Active shape model segmentation with optimal features. *IEEE Transactions on Medical Imaging, 21*(8), 924-933.

Waiter, G. D., McKiddie, F. I., Redipath, T. W., Semple, S. I. K., & Trentt, R. (1999). Determination of normal regional left ventricular function from cine-MR images using a semi-automated edge detection method. *Journal of Magnetic Resonance Imaging, 17,* 99-107.

Weese, J., Kaus, M., Lorenz, C., Lobregt, S., Truyen, R., & Pekar, V. (2001). Shape constrained deformable models for 3D medical image segmentation. *Proceedings on Information Processing in Medical Imaging,* (pp. 380-387).

Weng, J., Singh, A., & Chiu, M. Y. (1997). Learning-based ventricle detection from cardiac MR and CT images. *IEEE Transactions on Medical Imaging, 16*(4), 378-391.

Wu, G. (1997). *3-D segmentation-based image sequence processing.* PhD thesis, University of California, California.

Xu, C., & Prince, J. (1998). Snakes, shapes and gradient vector flow. *IEEE Transactions on Image Processing, 7*(3), 359-369.

Zambala, S., Hladůvka, J., & Bühler, K. (2006) Improving Segmentation of the Left Ventricle using a Two- Component Statistical Model. *Proceedings of MICCAI,* (pp. 151-158).

Zhang, J. (1999). *MR-based reconstruction of cardiac geometry.* MS thesis, The Johns Hopkins University, Baltimore.

Zhu, S., & Yuille, A. (1996). Region competition: Unifying snakes, region growing, and bayes/mdl for multi-band image segmentation. *IEEE Transactions on Pattern Analysis and Machine Intelligence, 18*(9), 884–900.

KEY TERMS

Classification: The process of deriving a mathematical function that can predict the membership of a class based on input data.

Expectation-Maximization (EM) Algorithm: It is used in statistics for finding maximum likelihood estimates of parameters in probabilistic models, where the model depends on unobserved latent variables.

Gaussian Distribution: Also called the standard normal distribution, is the normal distribution with mean zero and variance one.

Image Intensity: An image is defined as a two-dimensional function $f(x, y)$ the amplitude of f at any pair of coordinates (x, y) is called the intensity or gray level of the image at that point.

K-Means Algorithm: The k-means algorithm is an algorithm to cluster n objects based on attributes into k partitions, $k \leq n$. The algorithm minimizes the total intra-cluster variance or the squared error function.

Laplacian Operator: The Laplacian operator is a second order differential operator in the n-dimensional Euclidean space, defined as the divergence of the gradient.

Chapter IX
Image Registration Algorithms for Applications in Oncology

Katia Marina Passera
Politecnico di Milano, Italy

Luca Tommaso Mainardi
Politecnico di Milano, Italy

ABSTRACT

Image registration is the process of determining the correspondence of features between images collected at different times or using different imaging modalities. A wide range of registration algorithms was proposed in literature for solving this task. In this chapter the focus will be on oncology applications, where registration is the prior step of: i) subtraction imaging (to emphasize hyper (or hypo) enhanced structures), ii) fusion imaging (to integrate anatomical and functional information about lesions) and iii) serial imaging comparison (to monitor the progression/regression of a disease). These applications are of great relevance in tumors diagnosis, staging and treatment planning. The goal of this chapter is to provide an overview of registration algorithms considering these different applications in oncology. We discuss the advantages/disadvantages of each algorithm, the results gained and the possible future developments to comply with new requirements.

INTRODUCTION

The role of imaging in oncology has increased in the last few years, both for identification and staging of the primitive tumors and for re-evaluation of patients during chemotherapy or radiotherapy.

Often, clinical and therapeutic decisions are taken from the comparison of information extracted by images acquired using different modalities (*multimodal analysis*) or by a single modality at different time instants (*multitemporal analysis*).

Typical examples are the integration of anatomical information of CT and functional information of PET, the analysis of contrast-enhanced images for identification and characterization of lesions or the comparison of images acquired at different stages of a treatment (chemotherapy or radiotherapy).

For many of these tasks, image registration is a crucial step to recover the geometric relationship between corresponding points in multiple images of the same scene (Figure 1) which allows a direct, immediate point-to-point analysis.

Literature provides a wide range of articles and reviews treating the problem of image registration in biomedical applications (Maintz, 1998; Fitzpatrick, 2000; Zitova, 2003), some of them dedicated to a particular organ like heart (Makela, 2002) and brain (Toga, 2001; Thompson, 2000) or to a particular imaging modality like nuclear medicine (Hutton, 2002) or digital angiography (Meijering, 1998).

The goal of this chapter is to provide an overview of registration algorithms for applications in oncology and in particular for the diagnosis, staging and monitoring of tumors.

The chapter is organized as follows: after a brief recall of general concepts about image registration techniques, we will introduce three applications of registration procedure in oncology (image subtraction, image fusion and serial imaging comparison) and we will describe the registration algorithms that better suit with each particular task. In addition, we will discuss open issues and future trends of this topic.

BACKGROUND

Registration can be achieved by different methods that take into account different aspects. Maintz (1998) has suggested a nine dimensionality scheme to classify registration methods that Fitzpatrick (2000) has condensed in eight. For our purposes, the most useful classifications are with respect to (1) registration basis (i.e. the aspect/feature used to achieve the registration) and (2) geometrical transformation.

Registration Basis

According to registration basis, algorithms can be classified as being point-based, surface-based, or intensity-based.

In point-based methods, registration can be achieved by selecting a transformation that aligns a set of corresponding point pairs identifiable in the images to be aligned. Then, interpolation is used to infer correspondence throughout the rest of the image volume in a way consistent with the matched points.

Surface-based image registration methods involve determining corresponding surfaces in different images (and/or physical space) and computing the transformation that best aligns

Figure 1. Registration of one image (A) to the coordinate system of another image (B) by a transformation, T: $(x,y,z) \mapsto (x', y', z')$

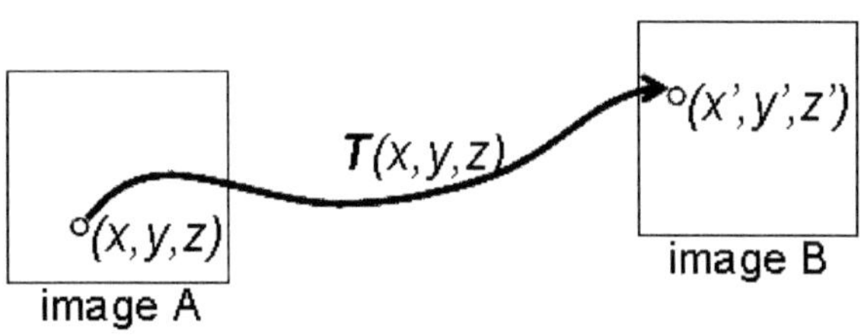

these surfaces. Intensity-based methods involve calculating a transformation between two images using the pixel (voxel) values only. They have recently become the most widely used registration methods. A major attraction of these algorithms is that the amount of pre-processing or user-interaction required is lower than for point-based or surface-based methods. In addition, feature calculation is straightforward or even absent when only grey-values are used, such that accuracy is not limited by segmentation errors as in point or surface based methods.

Intensity approaches match intensity patterns among images using mathematical or statistical criteria. They define a measure of similarity between the two images and adjust the transformation until this measure is maximized. They assume that the images will be most similar at the correct registration. The most used measures of similarity include: (1) squared differences in intensities, (2) correlation coefficient and (3) information-theoretic measures such as mutual information (Crum, 2004).

The first two similarity measures are suitable for mono-modal registration where the intensity characteristics are very similar in the images. For multi-modal registration, similarity measures have been developed, which define weaker relationships between intensities to reflect the different intensity scaling of the imaging modalities.

The most widely employed measure is *mutual information* (MI), or relative entropy, a basic concept of information theory, which can be considered a nonlinear generalization of cross-correlation. It was first proposed for medical image registration in 1995, independently by Viola and Wells (1995) and by Collignon (1995).

Given two images A and B, the definition of the mutual information MI (A, B) of these images is

$$MI(A,B) = H(A) + H(B) - H(A,B) \qquad (1)$$

with $H(A)$ and $H(B)$ the entropies of the images A and B, respectively, and $H(A,B)$ their joint entropy. The joint entropy $H(A,B)$ measures the dispersion of the joint probability distribution $p(a,b)$: the probability of the occurrence of intensity value a in image A and intensity value b in image B (at the same image position), for all a and b in the overlapping part of A and B. The joint probability distribution should have fewer and sharper peaks when the images are matched than for any case of misalignment. At misregistration, noncorresponding combinations of a and b will be aligned, causing dispersion in the distribution and hence a higher entropy value.

Therefore, to register images means to maximize mutual information that is equal to minimize joint entropy.

However, mutual information measure is dependent on the extension of overlap between images, since the joint histogram, and therefore the probability distributions, are computed only for the overlapping part of the images. In order to reduce the dependency of the overlapping area, normalized mutual information measures have been proposed, such as the entropy correlation coefficient ECC by Maes (1997),

$$ECC = \frac{2 \cdot H(A,B)}{H(A) + H(B)} \qquad (2)$$

and the normalized mutual information by Studholme (1999),

$$NMI = \frac{H(A) + H(B)}{H(A,B)} \qquad (3)$$

NMI and ECC are obviously related being $ECC = 2 - 2 \cdot NMI$.

The maximization of MI has become the method of choice for multimodal registration in a wide range of applications. Maes (2003) states that this success can be explained by the fact that it gets rid of the need for image segmentation or preprocessing as required with previous registration algorithms and that it allows for completely automated registration without need for user interaction, making the method very well suited for application in clinical practice.

Geometrical Transformation

A geometrical transformation maps points from space X of one image (*floating* image) to the space Y of the other image (*reference* image). The transformation T applied to a point in X represented by the column vector **x** produces a transformed point **x'**,

$$\mathbf{x}' = T(\mathbf{x}) \quad (4)$$

If the point $\mathbf{y} \in Y$ corresponds to **x**, then a successful registration will make **x'** equal, or approximately equal, to **y**. Any nonzero displacement T(**x**)-**y** is a registration error.

Fiztpatrick (2000) divides the set of all possible T into rigid and nonrigid transformations with the latter further divided into many subsets (scaling, affine, projective, perspective and curved). In medical applications, the most important classes are rigid, affine and curved transformations.

1. **Rigid:** In a rigid registration the misalignment correction involves only translations and rotations. This suffices to register images of rigid objects (like bones). In addition, rigid registration was also used to approximately align images that show small changes in object shape (for example serial MR images of the brain during contrast injection).
2. **Affine:** The affine transformation preserves the parallelism of lines, but not their lengths or their relative angles. It extends the degrees of freedom of the rigid transformation with a scaling factor for each image dimension, and, additionally, a shearing in each dimension. It is an appropriate transformation class when the image may have been skewed during acquisition as, for example, when the CT gantry angle is incorrectly recorded (Fitzpatrick, 2000).
3. **Curved (or non-linear):** This type of transformation allows the mapping of straight lines to curves. A detail review of this class of algorithms may be found in Crum (2004).

Deformation can be either free-form (any deformation is allowed) or guided by an underlying physical model of material properties, such as tissue elasticity or fluid flow.

Transformations used in curved registration range from smooth regional variation described by a small number of parameters to dense displacement fields defined at each voxel (Crum, 2004). One of the most important transformations is the family of *splines*. Spline-based registration algorithms use corresponding ("control") points, in the source and target image and a spline function to define correspondences away from these points. The two main categories are "thin-plate" spline and B-spline. Each control point belonging to a thin-plate spline has a global influence on the transformation: if its position is perturbed, all other points in the transformed image change. This can be a disadvantage because it limits the ability to model complex and localized deformations and because, as the number of control points increases, the computational cost associated with moving a single point rises steeply. By contrast, B-splines are only defined in the surrounding area of each control point; perturbing the position of one control point only affects the transformation in the neighbourhood of the point. Because of this property, B-splines are often referred to as having "local support". B-spline based non-linear registration techniques (Rueckert, 1999; Schnabel 2001) are popular due to their general applicability, transparency and computational efficiency. Their main disadvantage is that special measures are sometimes required to prevent folding of the deformation field and these measures become more difficult to enforce at finer resolutions.

Other approaches involve the use of elastic or viscous fluid models. Elastic models (Bajcsy, 1989) treat the source image as a linear, elastic solid and deform it using forces derived from an image similarity measure.

Replacing the elastic model by a viscous fluid model (Christensen,1996) allows large and highly localized deformations, but the higher flexibility increases the opportunity for misregistration.

Another technique, the "demons" algorithm (Thirion, 1998), can be thought of as an approximation to fluid registration.

Finite element (FE) models allow more principled control of localized deformations and have been mainly applied in surgical scenarios (Hagemann, 1999). These models divide the image into cells and assign to these cells a local physical description of the anatomical structure. Such approaches tend to be used where there are strong biomechanical constraints in operation, i.e. they are appropriate for serial registration of images of brains undergoing some mechanical intervention but not appropriate for intersubject registration.

Where registration speed is important some researchers (Dougherty, 1999) have applied optical flow techniques that were originally developed in the computer vision and artificial intelligence community. Some adaptation has been required for medical applications because the "constant intensity" assumption is usually broken in serial medical images and optical flow methods have not been widely adopted.

A number of strategies are employed to improve the speed of processing. The use of coarse-to-fine (multi-resolution, pyramidal) methods provides not only a means to gradually match finer and finer details but also faster initial estimates (Maes, 1999, Rueckert, 1999). In addition, most similarity measures do not require measurement at all points in order to determine the optimal transformation of the image. It is, therefore, quite common to sub-sample the image volume, at least during early iterations, increasing the sampling as the algorithm gets closer to the final solution.

Finally, recently some phase-based methods that are able to register images by simple analytical calculations (no iterations are required) have been introduced (Mainardi, 2006; Mainardi, 2008).

APPLICATIONS IN ONCOLOGY

The different categories of applications in oncology in which registration has a relevant role can be roughly divided in subtraction imaging, fusion imaging and serial imaging comparison.

Subtraction Imaging

In the last years, contrast-enhanced imaging, in particular Dynamic Contrast-Enhanced Magnetic Resonance Imaging (DCE-MRI) has gained attention in the early diagnosis of malignancies of different organs, in particular of breast and liver.

In a typical examination, a patient is scanned prior to and immediately after the intravenous injection of the contrast agent (usually chelates of Gadolinium). Post-contrast scans are performed repeatedly and the resulting MR image consists of a set of images of parallel tissue slices.

Subtraction of unenhanced images from gadolinium-enhanced images has been pursued in an attempt to maximize the qualitative recognition of lesion enhancement. In fact, the application of a technique to subtract pre- from post-contrast images makes it easier to pick out and characterize lesions, by eliminating common background signals and emphasizing hyper (or hypo) enhanced structures.

However, during MR dynamic acquisitions (which usually lasts a few minutes), any motion by the patient, even mere respiration activity, may induce changes in the shape of the breast and misalignment between pre-contrast and post-contrast volumes. Volumes matching is usually required to improve accuracy and efficiency of lesion detection.

Recently, dynamic subtraction MRI was used to characterize lesions in cirrhotic patients although small lesions were not shown optimally (Yu, 2005). The authors concluded that misregistration limited the qualitative assessment of lesions <2 cm in size.

In the subtraction of dynamic imaging of soft tissue organs like breast and abdominal organs the main requirements that registration algorithms should comply with are: (1) to be non-rigid, (2) pixel-independence and (3) computational efficiency.

Several registration methods have been proposed in literature for solving the specific problem of breast MRI registration (Mainardi, 2008; Pluim, 2003; Davis, 1997; Hayton, 1997; Hayton, 1999; Rueckert, 1999; Rohlfing, 2003; Lucht, 2000; Denton, 1999) using rigid and non-rigid transformations as well as different figures of merit. Intensity-based algorithms carry out alignment by the calculation of information-theoretic measures, such as Joint Entropy (JE), Mutual Information (MI) and Normalised Mutual Information (NMI) which are independent from pixel intensity. But these algorithms are usually limited to rigid or affine transformation (Pluim, 2003). Conversely a non-linear registration algorithm based on elastic deformation using physical models (Davis, 1997) assumes that the intensity of tissue between images remains constant.

An attempt to realise a non-linear transformation taking into account pixel intensity variation was proposed by Hayton (1997) who introduced a pharmacokinetic model to describe changes in pixel values. However, the need to select the model of the different tissues and lesions may limit the performance of the method. A different solution was proposed by Rueckert (1999) and later by Rohlfing (2003). The authors obtained a non-linear registration by combining an affine transformation for the global motion of the breast and a free-form deformation (FFD) based on B-splines for the local breast motion. The method iteratively minimises a cost function which represents a combination of the cost associated with the smoothness of the transformation and a measure of similarity (NMI).

Finally an approach including automatic feature extraction and realignment based on corresponding features between pre and post-contrast images was proposed (Lucht, 2000). In (Denton, 1999) the superiority of a non-linear registration method in respect to rigid or affine ones, was demonstrated. Anyway these last methods, although very attractive, are iterative and often very time consuming for a direct clinical application.

In order to speed up registration, Mainardi (2008) proposed a slice-to-slice registration (therefore 2D) of breast images (Figure 2) using a method (fully automatic) based on a multiresolution, phase-based motion estimation procedure performed through Complex-Discrete Wavelet Transform (CDWT).

This method is also applied to liver images by adding a first 3D rigid registration step before the slice-to-slice non rigid CDWT registration, in order to take into account the cranio-caudal excursion of liver (Mainardi, 2006).

Fusion Imaging

Different imaging modalities bring complementary information that can be advantageously used in the area of cancer diagnosis and treatment and many applications in clinical practice benefit from an integrated visualization and combined analysis of such multimodal images.

Image fusion in oncology raises clinical value of PET (Pattichis, 2001). PET scans combined with CT and MRI enable the visualization of functional and anatomic data, minimizing misinterpretations especially in the case of adjacent and very small tissues structures.

Early detection of brain tumors is possible on MRI and CT but tumor grading remains a difficult task, that can be better performed using PET images.

Figure 2. A case of multicentric lesion in the breast. MIP (maximum intensity projection) reconstruction of the subtraction image after (a) no registration, (b) rigid registration, (c) affine registration, (d) CDWT registration. The arrow shows a small medial lesion in the left breast.

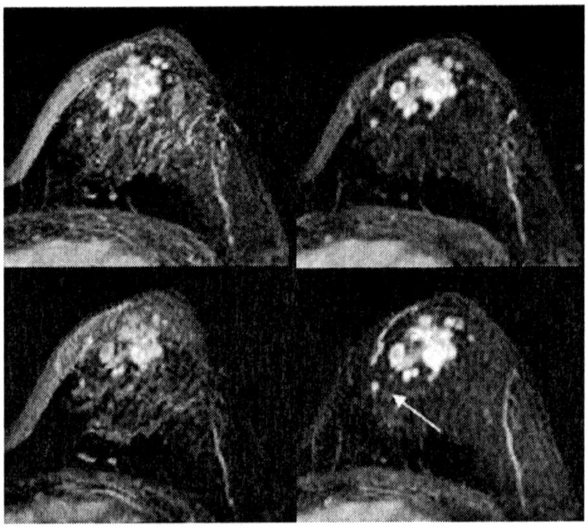

Nelson (1997) demonstrated the value of registering MRI and PET in the evaluation of patients with brain tumors. In fact, active tumor may not enhance on MRI but may be metabolically active on PET: PET may distinguish active tumor from radiation necrosis but without an exact localization that may be provided by MRI.

PET/CT fusion is also useful in planning radiation therapy of lung tumors (Driver, 2004). Moreover, PET is the most accurate procedure for the assessment of liver metastasis in liver surgery, linked with its fusion of CT and MRI (Pattichis, 2001).

Despite these advantages, there are some limiting factors to use image fusion in clinical practice that Pattichis (2001) underlined. About these, there are the cost intensive investment in hardware and software and the time-consuming fusion procedure.

The first problem related with the fact that exist hybrid scanners using PET and CT imaging and therefore this means very high costs. However, these scanners although very useful, don't solve the problem of soft tissue organ that can shift or deform anyway during the two consecutive but not simultaneous scans.

In terms of registration problem, there are differences with respect to an intramodality registration. The main difference is that it is not possible to assume that image intensities are linearly correlated and using some global measure such as absolute difference between image intensities of corresponding voxels or cross-correlation of intensities (Maes, 1997).

In this context, the main requirements are therefore: i) non linear measures of similarity, ii) correction of sharing and scaling due to different scanners iii) correction of large displacements iv) for soft tissue organs correction of deformations (curved transformations). In addition, the speed of calculating the final registration of two volumes is crucial for clinical usability.

Therefore, the most suitable registration algorithms in this case seem again intensity-based methods and especially those based on the information theoretic approach.

In fact, the matching of geometrical features of images, such as edges (Maintz, 1995) and ridges (van den Elsen, 1995) lead to have a very peaked optimum at the registration solution and be rather insensitive to misregistration at larger distances, as all nonedge or nonridge voxels correlate equally well. In addition, feature extraction involves extra time and may introduce geometrical errors.

Therefore, another approach has been proposed by Woods (1993) and by Hill (1993). They measure the dispersion of the 2-D histogram of the image intensities of corresponding voxel pairs and assume the minimum as the registered position. Unfortunately, Hill's criterion requires segmentation of specific regions to make the method work, while Wood's method assumes relationship between the grey-values in the different modalities, which reduces its applicability to some very specific multimodality combinations (PET/MR).

However, thanks to the work of Woods and Hill, other authors recognized that this particular registration problem may be better solved using the information theory and they arrive to introduce NMI maximization criterion (Viola, 1995; Collignon, 1995). This immediately attracted a lot of interest from the research community and a lot of authors recently use it for multimodal registration (Rizzo, 2005; Klein, 2007; Sundar, 2007; Loeckx, 2007). In Figure 3, an example of the effect of registration in fusion imaging is shown.

Figure 3. Registered and reformatted CT and MR images of the brain of a patient showing a lesion (Maes, 2003): (a) CT. (b) MR. (c) Blending of the skull from CT with the brain tissues from MR demonstrates the high quality of the registration result. (© 2003 IEEE)

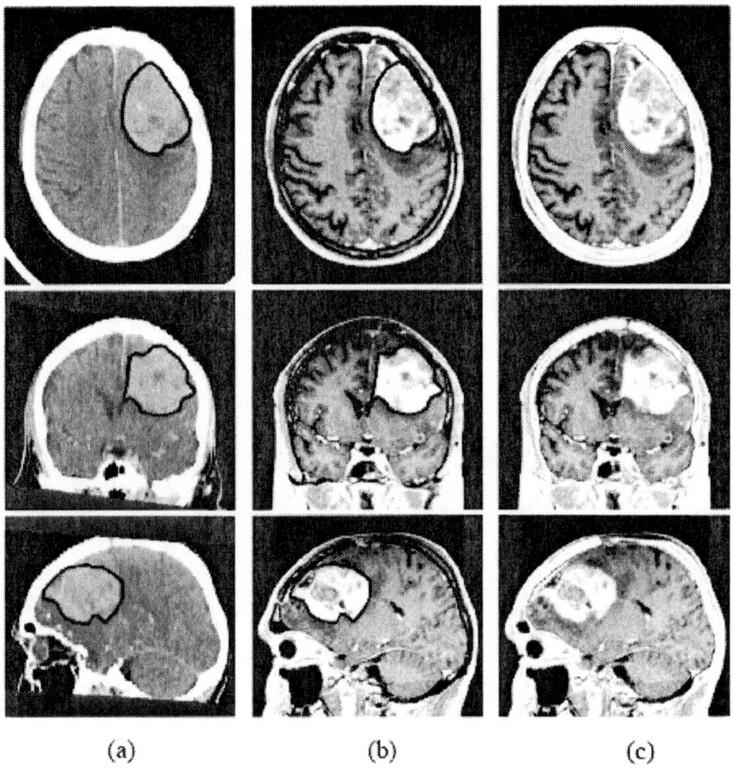

Serial Imaging Comparison

One of the most obvious clinical applications of registration is in the area of serial imaging. Comparison of scans from a given patient acquired over various time intervals can be routinely performed to follow disease progression and response to treatment.

A direct comparison between successively scanned images is generally not possible (Bosc, 2003): patient position is never identical and a variety of complex global or local deformations of anatomical structures may be observed.

In Patriarche (2004) it may be found a very detailed review of automated detection of change in serial MR imaging studies of the brain. A lot of different techniques were introduced in order to approach the problem of detection of change in brain tumors. The most common approach for the detection of change in imaging studies is visual inspection. The main problem of this approach is the huge amount of data presented to radiologist. Therefore, some authors proposed to use a registration-subtraction method in order to enhance changes in an unique image. In this case, registration aims to correct position (translation) and orientation (rotation) differences and geometrical distortions due to scanner (scaling and shearing). Classical intensity-based methods limited to rigid (or affine) alignment were used (Hajnal, 1995), while other authors used surface-based methods (Ettinger, 1994).

However, these methods don't provide a quantitative measure of change and to quantitatively assess brain deformations, non-linear registration algorithms may be applied (Figure 4).

There are a number of problems with using non-linear registration for change detection. One is that non-linear registration is underconstrained. For a given pair of acquisitions, there are an infinite number of displacement fields that will yield a match. This problem is typically partly addressed by specifying the constraints under which the displacement field will be derived, by using continuum mechanical models (Freeborough, 1998).

In addition, in tumor progression and regression, a given region of tissue can not only change position or deform, it can change also character: white matter can become enhancing or edematous; enhancing tumor can become necrotic, etc. Infiltration and expansion can coexist with this change of character as well. However, some non-linear algorithms are based on the assumption

Figure 4. Two serial MR transversal slices of a patient at different times aligned by a 3D affine registration. In each of them the segmentation of tumor is shown (a, b). In (c) synchronous views of the segmentation lesion and the displacement field obtained by non-rigid registration. Affine and non-rigid registration were obtained using b-spline method (ITK Rueckert software).

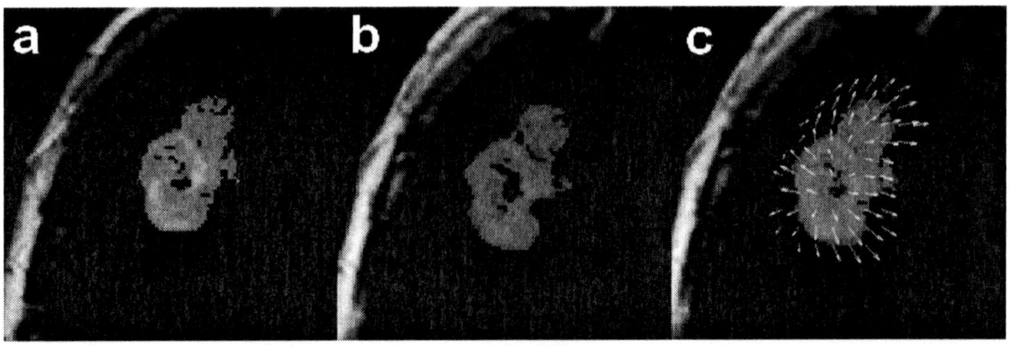

that a particular region of tissue exists in both acquisitions (and appears identical in terms of intensity) and has simply moved.

In order to solve this problem, a first solution is to use non linear registration algorithms based on information theory and thereof not influenced of intensity changes.

An approach that attempts to accomplish this disambiguation of frank growth from tissue character change has been described by Thirion (1999). The central theme provided by these authors is that if new tissue is being deposited (as in the case of tumor growth), then mass effect will be present in adjacent structures. Therefore, they use a warping algorithm to develop a vector displacement field from the serial imaging studies in neighbourhood tissues and arrive, in turn, to derive changes in tumors.

Another type of serial imaging widely used in cancer diagnosis and treatment is DCE-MRI. During DCE-MRI, a contrast agent (CA), such as Gd-DTPA, is introduced into the bloodstream and diffuses between the blood vessels and the interstitial spaces of the tissues. If a sufficient number of temporal acquisitions is used, it is possible to describe this process by deriving a contrast agent concentration time course and fitting a tracer kinetic model within each voxel in a volume of interest (VOI) (Jackson, 2005).

The quantitative, model-based, analysis of contrast agent uptake kinetics in DCE-MRI at high temporal resolution allows to estimate the magnitude and spatial distribution of physiological kinetic parameters such as the volume transfer coefficient of contrast agent between capillaries and the extravascular extracellular space (K_{trans}). These parameters provide useful information on microvascular status for studies of tumors and inflammatory conditions (Padhani, 2001). Potential clinical applications include screening for malignant disease, lesion characterization, monitoring of lesion response to treatment, and assessment of residual disease.

Unfortunately, the voxel signal profile will in general be corrupted by motion (Figure 5), and this should be corrected to ensure the highest levels of model parameter precision.

In this case, registration are two main requirements: (1) similarity index independence of signal intensity as DCE-MRI has the goal to distinguish different tissues by their different CA uptake characteristics, which leads to non-stationary contrast properties and (2) more important, computational time, being the set of serial images characterized by 50 and more acquisitions.

Buonaccorsi (2007) stated that conventional motion correction (e.g. registering each image volume in the time series to the time series mean) has limited success because the passage of the contrast agent introduces new image features. In addition, the resulting time-varying information content is problematic even for inter-modal cost functions (e.g. mutual information, correlation ratio), which are most effective with a consistent information content between the input and reference images. If computational cost is a must, registration algorithms should be limited to a ROI.

Some investigators have registered pre-contrast to post-contrast images and incorporated a simplified tracer kinetic model directly into a registration cost function (Hayton, 1997), but it has not yet been practicable to register an entire DCE-MRI time-series at high temporal resolution using a more detailed physiological model of enhancement in abdominal tumors.

In order to address the above issues, Buonaccorsi (2007) proposed a tracer-kinetic model driven registration method with a more detailed models of contrast agent kinetics. The iterative registration procedure is focused on a tumor volume of interest (VOI), employing a threedimensional (3D) translational transformation that follows only tumor motion.

The method was showed to be fast enough for routine use (it takes on the order of 2 hours to analyze a data set with 75 time-point image

Figure 5. Comparison of the contrast agent concentration time series and model-fit results for a single voxel within the tumor rim pseudotissue of the SNR 10 motion-corrupted software phantom (Buonaccorsi, 2007), before and after tracer kinetic model–driven registration. (Reprinted with permission of Wiley-Liss, Inc., a subsidiary of John Wiley & Sons, Inc, © 2003 Wiley-Liss).

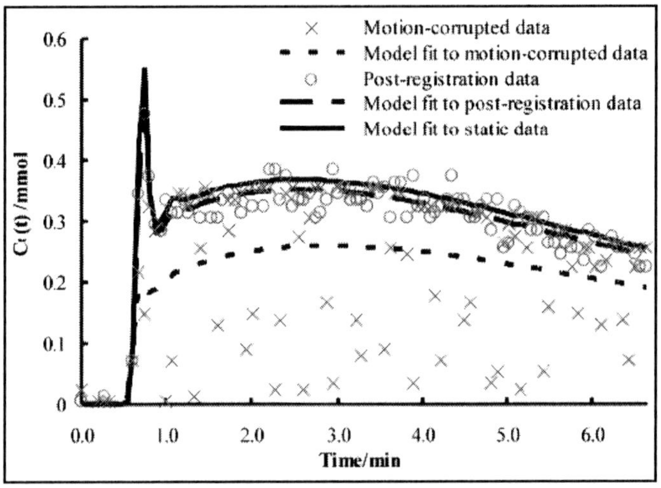

volumes) and it addresses the problems of rapidly varying signal intensity and the appearance of new features that confound conventional registration methods.

FUTURE TRENDS

Image registration is one of the most important tasks in oncology for integrating and analyzing information from various sources. In fact, there are a lot of techniques, among these subtraction imaging, fusion imaging, serial imaging analysis that are not feasible without a prior registration.

Although a lot of work has been done, automatic image registration still remains an open problem.

One of the most challenging tasks is the correction of soft tissues deformations. Although a lot of non-linear registration methods were introduced there is a conceptual question that should be addressed: how to distinguish between image deformations and real change in the scene.

In multimodal medical imaging registration, MI technique has become a standard reference. However, the MI criterion has some limitations. To overcome them, it is possible to combine the MI with other methods, such as feature-based methods in order to gain higher robustness and reliability.

Therefore, the future development on this field could pay more attention to the feature-based methods, where appropriate invariant and modality-insensitive features can provide good platform for the registration.

Another question is the computational cost and fastness. To speed up the computation, different authors often employed multiresolution along with fast optimization algorithms. Unfortunately, when the images have significant rotation and/or scaling differences, these methods either fail or become extremely time expensive.

In the case of serial imaging comparison, mainly for DCE-MRI, registration is a very demanding task due to high temporal resolution data (more than 50 temporal acquisitions to align).

Although the speed of computers has been growing, the need to decrease the computational time of methods persists. The complexity of methods as well as the size of data still grows (the higher resolution, higher dimensionality, larger size of scanned areas). Moreover, the demand for higher robustness and accuracy of the registration usually enforces solutions utilizing the iterations or backtracking, which also produces increase of computational complexity of the method.

One important improvement in the future could be to incorporate more knowledge and create expert systems able to recognize the type of given task and to decide by itself about the most appropriate solution.

CONCLUSION

This chapter gives a survey of the classical and up-to-date registration methods in oncology, underlying the requirements for each particular application (image subtraction, image fusion and change detection). These clinical applications can aid in diagnosis, treatment and therapy phases. The main problems to solve for applications in oncology are pixel intensity independence and fastness. Although, many authors have contributed to solve these issues, a final solution has not been yet reached. The future trends will be to include more information in the registration problem and the use of dedicated expert systems.

REFERENCES

Bajcsy, R., & Kovacic, S. (1989). Multiresolution elastic matching. *Computer vision, graphics, and image processing, 46,* 1–21.

Bosc, M., Heitz, F., Armspach, J. P., Namer, I., Gounot, D., & Rumbachc, L. (2003). Automatic change detection in multimodal serial MRI: application to multiple sclerosis lesion evolution. *Neuroimage 20,* 643-656.

Buonaccorsi, G., O'Connor, J. P. B., Caunce, A., Roberts, C., Cheung, S., Watson, Y., Davies, K., Hope, L., Jackson, A., Jayson, G. C., & Parker, G. J. M. (2007). Tracer Kinetic Model–Driven Registration for Dynamic Contrast-Enhanced MRI Time-Series Data. *Magnetic Resonance in Medicine, 58,* 1010–1019.

Christensen, G. E., Rabbitt, R. D., & Miller, M. I. (1996). *Multiresolution elastic matching. IEEE Transaction on Image Processing, 5,* 1435–1447.

Collignon, A., Maes, F., Delaere, D., Vandermeulen, D., Suetens, P., & Marchal, G. (1995). Automated multi-modality image registration based on information theory. In *Proceedings of the International Conference on Information Processing in Medical Imaging (IPMI),* Ile de Berder, France, June 1995 (pp. 263-274). Kluwer: Yves Bizais (Ed.).

Crum ,W. R., Hartkens, T., & Hill, D. L. G. (2004). Non-rigid image registration: theory and practice. *The British Journal of Radiology, 77,* S140–S153.

Davis, M. H., Khotanzad, A., Flamig, D. P., & Harms, S. E. (1997). A Physic-Based Coordinate Transformation for 3-D Image, Matching. *IEEE Transactions on Medical Imaging, 16(3),* 317–328.

Denton E. R. E., Sonoda, L. I., Rueckert, D., Rankin, S. C., Hayes, C., Leach, M. O., Hill, D. L. G., & Hawkes, D. J. (1999). Comparison and Evaluation of Rigid, Affine, and Nonrigid Registration of Breast MR Images. *Journal ofComputer Assisted Tomography, 23(5),* 800-805

Dougherty, L, Asmuth, J. C., Blom, A. S., Axel, L., & Kumar R. (1999). Validation of an optical flow method for tag displacement estimation. *IEEE Transaction on Image Processing, 18,* 359–363.

Driver, D., & Dobbs, H. J. (2004). Improvements in radiotherapy practice: the impact of new imaging technologies. *Cancer Imaging, 4,* 142-150.

Ettinger, G. J., Grimson, W. E., Lozano–Perez, T., Wells, W. M., III, White, S. J., & Kikinis, R. (1994). Automatic registration for multiple sclerosis change detection. In *Proceedings of the IEEE Workshop on Biomedical Image Analysis*, Seattle, WA, USA, 24-25 June 1994 (pp. 297-306)

Fitzpatrick, J. M., Hill, D. L. G., & Maurer, C. R. (2000). Image registration. In *Handbook of Medical Imaging, Volume 2: Medical Image Processing and Analysis* (pp. 451-507). Bellingham, WA: SPIE.

Freeborough, P. A., & Fox, N. C. (1998). Modeling brain deformations in Alzheimer disease by fluid registration of serial 3D MR images. *Journal of Computer Assisted Tomography, 22,* 838-843.

Hagemann, A., Rohr, K., Stiehl, H. S., Spetzger, U, & Gilsbach, J. M. (1999). Biomechanical modeling of the human head for physically based, nonrigid image registration. *IEEE Transaction on Image Processing, 18,* 875–884.

Hajnal, J. V., Saeed, N., Soar, E. J., Oatridge, A., Young, I. R., & Bydder, G. M. (1995). A registration and interpolation procedure for subvoxel matching of serially acquired MR images. *Journal of Computer Assisted Tomography, 19,* 289- 296.

Hayton, P. M., Brady, M., Tarassenko, L., & Moore, N. (1997). Analysis of dynamic breast images using a model of contrast enhancement. *Medical Image Analysis, 1(3),* 207-224.

Hayton, P. M., Brady, M., Tarassenko, L, & Moore, N. (1999). A non-rigid registration algorithm for dynamic breast MR images. *Artificial Intelligence 114,* 125-156

Hill, D. L. G, Hawkes, D. J., Harrison, N. A., & Ruff, C. F. (1993). A strategy for automated multimodality image registration incorporating anatomical knowledge and imager characteristics. In H. H. Barrett and A. F. Gmitro (Eds.) *Proc. 13th Int. Conf. Information Processing in Medical Imaging; Lecture Notes in Computer Science 687, June 1993* (pp. 182-196). New York: Springer-Verlag

Hutton, B. F., Braun, M., Thurfjell, L., & Lau, D. Y. H. (2002). Image registration: an essential tool for nuclear medicine. *European Journal of Nuclear Medicine and Molecular Imaging, 29,* 559–77.

Jackson, A., Buckley, D., & Parker, G. J. M. (2005). *Dynamic contrast-enhanced magnetic resonance imaging in oncology.* Springer-Verlag Berlin Heidelberg.

Klein, S., Staring, M., & Pluim, J. P. (2007). Evaluation of optimization methods for nonrigid medical image registration using mutual information and B-splines. *IEEE Trans Image Process, 16(12),* 2879-2890.

Loeckx, D., Slagmolen, P., Maes, F., Vandermeulen, D., & Suetens, P. (2007). Nonrigid image registration using conditional mutual information. In *Proceedings of the International Conference on Information Processing in Medical Imaging (IPMI),* The Netherlands, July 2-6, 2007 (pp. 725-37).

Lucht, R., Knopp, M. V., & Brix, G. (2000). Elastic Matching of Dynamic MR Mammographic Images. *Magnetic Resonance in Medicine, 43,* 9-16

Maes, F., Collignon, A., Vandermeulen, D., Marchal, G., & Suetens, P. (1997). Multimodality image registration by maximization of mutual information. *IEEE Transaction on Medical Imaging, 16,* 187–198.

Maes, F., Vandermeulen, D., & Suetens, P. (1999). Comparative evaluation of multiresolution optimization strategies for multimodality image registration by maximization of mutual information. *Medical image analysis, 3,* 373-377.

Maes, F., Vandermeulen, D., & Suetens, P. (2003). Medical Image Registration Using Mutual Information. *Proceedings of the IEEE, 91(10),* 1699-1722.

Mainardi L. T., Passera K. M., Lucesoli A., Vergnaghi D., Trecate G., Setti E., Musumeci R., & Cerutti S. (2008). A non-rigid registration of MR breast images using complex-valued Wavelet Transform. *Journal of Digital Imaging, 21(1),* 27-36.

Mainardi, L. T., Passera, K. M., Lucesoli, A., Potepan, P., Setti, E., & Musumeci, R. (2006). A method for dynamic subtraction mr imaging of the liver. *BMC Medical Imaging, 6,* 5.

Maintz, A. J. B., & Viergever, M. A. (1998). An overview of medical image registration methods. *Med. Image Anal., 2,* 1–37.

Maintz, J. B. A., van den Elsen, P. A., & Viergever, M. A. (1995). Comparison of feature-based matching of CT and MR brain images. In N. Ayache, (Eds.) *Proc. 1st Int. Conf. Computer Vision, Virtual Reality and Robotics in Medicine; Lecture Notes in Computer Science 905,* Nice, France, April 1995, (pp. 219-228) New York, Springer-Verlag

Makela, T., Clarysse, P., Sipila, O., Pauna, N., Pham, Q. C., Katila, T., & Magnin, I. E. (2002). A review of cardiac image registration methods. *IEEE Transactions on Medical Imaging, 21,* 1011–1021.

Meijering, E. H. W., Niessen, W. J., & Viergever, M. A. (1999). Retrospective motion correction in digital subtraction angiography: a review. *IEEE Transactions on Medical Imaging, 18,* 2–21.

Nelson, S. J., Day, M. R., Buffone, P. J., Wald, L. L., Budinger, T. F., Hawkins, R., Dillon, W. P., Huhn, S., Prados, M.D., Chang, S., & Vigneron, D. B.(1997). Alignment of volume MR images and high resolution [18F]fluorodeoxyglucose PET images for the evaluation of patients with brain tumors. *Journal of Computer Assisted Tomography, 21(2),* 183-91.

Padhani, A. R., & Husband, J.E. (2001). Dynamic contrast-enhanced MRI studies in oncology with an emphasis on quantification, validation and human studies. *Clinical Radiology, 56,* 607–620.

Patriarche, J., & Erickson, B. (2004). A Review of the Automated Detection of Change in Serial Imaging Studies of the Brain. *Journal of Digital Imaging, 17(3),*158-174.

Pattichis, C. S., Pattichis, M. S., & Micheli-Tzanakou, E. (2001). Medical Imaging Fusion Applications: An Overview. In *Proc. of the 35th Asilomar Conference on Signals, Systems, and Computers,* Pacific Grove, California (USA), November 2001 (pp. 1263-1267), IEEE Signal Processing Society Staf.

Pluim, J. P. W., Maintz, J. B. A., & Viergever, M. A. (2003). Mutual Information Based Registration of Medical Images: A Survey. *IEEE Transactions on Medical Imaging 22(8),* 986-1004.

Rizzo, G., Castiglioni, I., Arienti, R., Cattaneo, G. M., Landoni, C., Artioli, D., Gilardi, M. C., Messa, C., Reni, M., Ceresoli, G. L., & Fazio, F. (2005). Automatic registration of PET and CT studies for clinical use in thoracic and abdominal conformal radiotherapy. *Quarterly Journal of Nuclear Medicine and Molecular Imaging, 49(3),* 267-279.

Rohlfing, T., & Maurer, C. R. Jr (2003). Volume–Preserving Nonrigid Registration of MR Breast Images Using Free-Form Deformation With an Incompressibility Constraint. *IEEE Transactions on Medical Imaging, 22(6),* 730 – 741.

Rueckert D., Sonoda, L. I., Hayes, C., Hill, D. L. G., Leach, M. O., & Hawkes, D. J. (1999). Nonrigid registration using free-form deformation: application to breast MR images. *IEEE Transactions on Medical Imaging, 18(8),* 712-721

Schnabel, J. A., Rueckert, D., Quist, M., Blackall, J. M., Castellano Smith, A. D., Hartkens, T., Penney, G. P., Hall, W. A., Liu, H., Truwit, C. L., Gerritsen, F. A., Hill, D. L. G., & Hawkes, D. J. (2001). A Generic Framework for Non-Rigid Registration Based on Non-Uniform Multi-Level Free-Form Deformations. In *Proceedings of Medical Image Computing and Computer-Assisted Intervention (MICCAI)*, Utrecht, The Netherlands, 14-17 October 2001 (pp. 573-581).

Studholme, C., Hill, D. L. G., & Hawkes, D. J. (1999). An overlap invariant entropy measure of 3-D medical image alignment. *Pattern Recognition, 32,* 71–86.

Sundar, H., Shen, D., Biros, G., Xu, C., & Davatzikos, C. (2007). Robust computation of mutual information using spatially adaptive meshes. In *Proceedings of Medical Image Computing and Computer-Assisted Intervention (MICCAI)*, Brisbane, Australia, October 29 - November 2, 2007 (pp. 950-958)

Thirion, J. P. (1998). Image matching as a diffusion process: an analogy with maxwell's demons. *Med Image Analysis, 2,* 243–260.

Thirion, J. P., & Calmon, G. (1999). Deformation analysis to detect and quantify active lesions in three-dimensional medical image sequences. *IEEE Transactions on Medical Imaging, 18,* 429- 441.

Thompson, P. M., Woods, R. P., Mega, M. S., & Toga, A. W. (2000). Mathematical/computational challenges in creating deformable and probabilistic atlases of the human brain. *Human Brain Mapping, 9,* 81–92.

Toga, A. W., & Thompson, P. M. (2001). The role of image registration in brain mapping. *Image Vision Comput, 19,* 3–24.

van den Elsen, P. A., Pol E-J. D., Sumanaweera, T. S., Hemler, P. F., Napel S., & Adler, J. (1994). Grey value correlation techniques used for automatic matching of CT and MR brain and spine images. In R. A. Robb, (Ed.), *Proc. of SPIE, Visualization in Biomedical Computing, September 1994, 2359* (pp. 227–237)

van den Elsen, P. A., Maintz, J. B. A., Pol, E-J. D., & Viergever M. A. (1995). Automatic registration of CT and MR brain images using correlation of geometrical features. *IEEE Transactions on Medical Imaging, 14(2),* 384 - 396.

Viola, P. (1995). *Alignment by maximization of mutual information* (Tech. Rep. No. 1548). Massachusetts Institute of Technology.

Woods, R. P., Mazziotta, J. C., & Cherry, S. R. (1993). MRI-PET registration with automated algorithm, *Journal of Computer Assisted Tomography, 17(4),* 536–546

Yu, J.S., Kim, Y. H., & Rofsky, N. (2005). Dynamic subtraction magnetic resonance imaging of cirrhotic liver: assessment of high signal intensity lesions on nonenhanced T1-weighted images. *Journal of Computer Assisted Tomography, 29(1),* 51-58.

Zitova, B., & Flusser, J. (2003). Image registration methods: a survey. *Image and Vision Computing, 21,* 977–1000.

KEY TERMS

Contrast Enhancement: An image processing technique aiming at enhancing global or local contrast of an image. In MR or CT imaging, in order to characterize different types of lesions contrast is augmented by intravenous injection of a contrast agent.

Image Fusion: The process of combining relevant information from two or more images into a single image. The resulting image will be more informative than any of the input images.

Image Registration: The task of finding a correspondence function mapping coordinates from a reference image to coordinates of homologous points in a test image.

Image Subtraction: A technique that permits to emphasize hyper (or hypo) enhanced structures by subtracting pre- from post-contrast images in MR or CT imaging.

Mutual Information: In probability theory and information theory, the mutual information of two random variables is a quantity that measures the mutual dependence of the two variables.

Oncology: The branch of medicine that deals with tumors, including study of their development, diagnosis, treatment, and prevention.

Serial Imaging: Consists of the sequential acquisitions over time of images of the same patient to monitor changes of a pathological area and effects of therapies/treatments.

Chapter X
Computer-Aided Diagnosis in Breast Imaging:
Trends and Challenges

Lena Costaridou
University of Patras, Greece

Spyros Skiadopoulos
University of Patras, Greece

Anna Karahaliou
University of Patras, Greece

Nikolaos Arikidis
University of Patras, Greece

George Panayiotakis
University of Patras, Greece

ABSTRACT

Breast cancer is the most common cancer in women worldwide. Mammography is currently the most effective modality in detecting breast cancer, challenged by the presence of dense breast parenchyma, with relatively low specificity in distinguishing malignant from benign lesions. Breast ultrasound and Magnetic Resonance Imaging (MRI) are significant adjuncts to mammography providing additional diagnostic information. Various Computer-Aided Diagnosis (CADx) schemes have been proposed across modalities, acting as clinical tools that provide a "second opinion" to assist radiologists in the diagnostic task of lesion characterization by means of quantitative image feature extraction and classification methods. The advent of multimodality imaging broadens the role of CADx, in terms of complementary tissue properties analyzed. In this chapter, major stages of CADx schemes in breast imaging are reviewed, while challenges and trends are discussed and highlighted by corresponding application examples of CADx methodologies for microcalcification clusters in mammography and masses in Dynamic Contrast-Enhanced MRI.

INTRODUCTION

Breast cancer is the most common cancer in women worldwide and the second leading cause of cancer deaths after lung cancer. Lifetime risk of developing invasive breast cancer is approximately 1 in 8 women. Screen-Film Mammography (SFM), providing structural tissue properties by means of X-ray attenuation differences, is currently the most effective modality in detecting breast lesions such as masses, microcalcification (MC) clusters and architectural distortions.

SFM, although characterized by high spatial resolution (25 μm pixel size), is challenged by the relatively low image contrast, especially in case of dense breast parenchyma. Limitations of SFM are attributed to 3D information loss, due to projection geometry, and the sigmoid response curve (characteristic curve) of the screen-film, as image detector.

A natural extension of SFM is achieved by Full-Field Digital Mammography (FFDM) overcoming screen-film response limitation by the linear and broader characteristic curve of direct or indirect digital detectors (Williams et al., 2006). At present, the only technical limitation of FFDM is spatial resolution (40 μm pixel size). The higher detection accuracy of FFDM is demonstrated in screening of dense breasts (Pisano et al., 2005). Up to date, eight FFDM units have been approved by FDA[1]. Detection performance of FFDM is further enhanced by the capability to manipulate lesion-to-background contrast with image processing tools offered by viewing mammograms in softcopy display workstations. Recently, in an attempt to deal with 3D information loss, often resulting in misdetection of lesions obscured by overlapping dense parenchyma, Digital Breast Tomosynthesis has been introduced (Park et al., 2007). This is achieved by acquiring a small number of 2D projection images and adequately reconstructing tomographic images (slices) with respect to breast depth (z-axis).

When biological processes underlying disease are not captured by X-ray imaging, insight to additional structural and functional tissue properties as well as 3D imaging is exploited by modalities adjunct to mammography, such as Ultrasound (US) and Magnetic Resonance Imaging (MRI).

MRI acquires the nuclear magnetic resonance signal from hydrogen nuclei of tissue. By applying 3D encoded magnetic fields, time constants T1 and T2, characterizing the recovery of longitudinal and transverse magnetization respectively, provide unique biophysical properties used to differentiate contrast among tissues. In addition to 3D spatial information of anatomical structures, Dynamic Contrast-Enhanced MRI (DCE-MRI) offers a functional approach to imaging based on differentiation of malignant from benign tissue with respect to cellular composition, permeability and microvessel density. DCE-MRI data captures kinetics of contrast agents in targeted tissues (Wu & Markey, 2006).

Computer-Aided Detection and Diagnosis (CADe and CADx) schemes have been proposed across breast imaging modalities, acting as clinical tools that provide a "second opinion" to radiologists, with mammography being the most successful paradigm (Sampat et al., 2005).

CADe systems have been developed to improve radiologists' performance in detecting breast lesions, by identifying suspicious regions of masses and MC clusters. CADe methodologies employed and performances achieved are provided in excellent reviews (Tourassi, 2005; Chan et al., 2005; Sampat et al., 2005). High performance mammographic CADe schemes have been incorporated in commercially available, FDA approved systems[2]. The impact of CADe systems, i.e. significant increase of breast cancers detected with an acceptable increase of recall rate, is reported in peer-reviewed retrospective and prospective studies, although with some criticism (Fenton et al., 2007).

CADx systems in breast imaging aim to assist radiologists in the diagnostic task of lesion characterization (malignancy *vs.* benignity), thus affecting patient management (follow-up *vs.* biopsy). The development of CADx systems is still ongoing in breast imaging (Suri et al., 2006). The advent of intra- and inter-modality computerized analysis broadens the role of CADe/CADx schemes both in terms of image feature fusion and/or image data fusion.

BACKGROUND

By definition, CADx systems in breast imaging are fully automated computer vision algorithms developed to improve radiologists' performance in characterizing breast lesion status (malignant *vs.* benign), by providing probability estimates of malignancy of lesions. Specifically, CADx schemes are targeted to increase diagnostic specificity (i.e. fraction of benign lesions correctly characterized by the system), while maintaining high sensitivity (i.e. fraction of malignant lesions correctly characterized by the system). This presupposes a near perfect performance of CADx schemes dealing with the large variability of lesion appearance and low conspicuity (Giger et al., 2000). The major steps of a CADx scheme are illustrated in Figure 1.

Initialization of a CADx scheme requires identification of a lesion Region Of Interest (ROI) or Volume Of Interest (VOI) provided either by a radiologist or by the output of a CADe scheme. This step benefits from enhancement and/or denoising, segmentation and registration algorithms (Giger et al., 2000).

Lesion segmentation is critical for lesion morphology analysis, while in texture and pattern analysis this step can be omitted (Sampat et al., 2005).

Feature extraction aims at quantification of image content by means of computer algorithms to capture tissue alterations, due to underlying biological processes reflected either as morphology or as texture variations, mimicking or complementing radiologist interpretation. Feature extraction may also benefit from spectral and multiscale (frequency band) analysis. In addition to structural information, mainly provided

Figure 1. Flowchart of a typical CADx scheme. Optional steps are indicated by dashed lines.

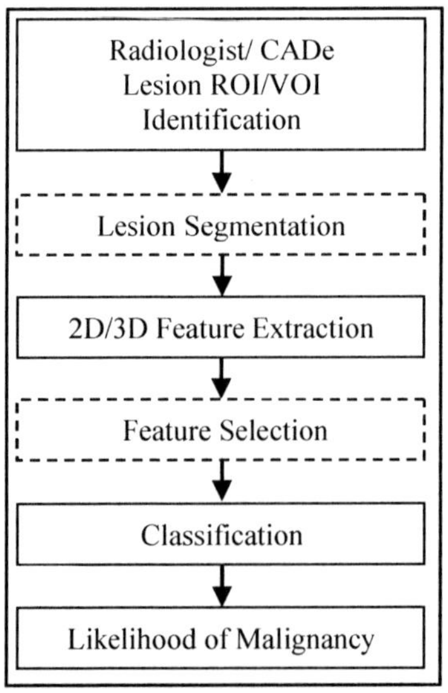

by mammography, functional tissue properties provided by 3D US and MRI data are also exploited. A second category of CADx schemes employing qualitative observer ratings of lesion characteristics as inputs to classification schemes are not subject of this review.

In case of highly dimensional feature spaces combined with small training datasets, a feature selection strategy is preferred to avoid overtraining. Depending on the feature selection method and the criterion used, a set of the most discriminant features can be defined to obtain improvements in classification accuracy.

Classification algorithms are utilized to partition the data in two or more classes. Classification performance depends on size and difficulty of the case sample, as well as evaluation methodology used, so that special care must be taken in study design (Suri et al., 2006).

The performance of CADx schemes is evaluated by metrics such as sensitivity and specificity or area under the ROC (Receiver Operating Characteristic) curve (Az). ROC curve expresses Sensitivity as a function of 1-Specificity. To satisfy high specificity while maintaining high sensitivity, the partial ROC curve (e.g. $^{0.9}$Az, defined as the area under the ROC curve above sensitivity threshold of 0.9) is suggested (Jiang et al., 1996).

CADX SCHEMES IN BREAST IMAGING

CADx Schemes in Mammography

The reported CADx schemes in mammography have dealt with both masses and MC clusters. CADx schemes have obtained high performance for masses (Sampat et al., 2005; Tourassi, 2005), while MCs remain a challenge (Cheng et al., 2003; Sampat et al., 2005).

Morphology-Based CADx Schemes for MC Clusters

Morphology analysis is a major approach for diagnosis of MCs, according to BIRADS lexicon. A wide range of individual MC morphology and intensity properties have been utilized:

- Area, perimeter, elongation, circularity, compactness, eccentricity, moment ratio, axis ratio, concavity index, effective thickness and volume, shape signature.
- Mean and standard deviation of intensity, mean and standard deviation of exterior intensity (background), MC contrast, edge strength (boundary sharpness).

CADx schemes that classify MC clusters are based on two categories of cluster features:

i. **Category I:** Features based on descriptive statistics of individual MC morphology and intensity properties (average, standard deviation, coefficient of variation, maximum, median, range).
ii. **Category II:** Features describing cluster morphology, intensity and individual MC distribution within a cluster, considering the cluster as an entity:
    - Area, diameter, perimeter, circularity, eccentricity, elongation, solidity.
    - Mean and standard deviation of background intensity.
    - Number of MCs, proximity to the nearest MC (mean number of nearest neighbours, distance to nearest neighbour), cluster density (mean distance between MCs), distance to pectoral and breast edge.

To avoid classifier overtraining in case of many features used, selection methods such as root-mean-square error, Karhunen-Loeve Transform and Principal Component Analysis have been utilized (Tsujii et al., 1999; Kallergi, 2004; Papadopoulos et al., 2005). However, such an approach does not highlight specific MC properties. Table I summarizes CADx schemes incorporating feature selection methods, providing discriminant MC cluster features.

Shape estimation of individual MCs at 100 μm spatial resolution is difficult, due to quantification errors, especially for small size MCs (Jiang et al., 1999). Even at 50 μm resolution, Betal et al. (1997) extracted individual MC features only from the three largest MCs within the cluster. Another limitation of morphology analysis is its dependence on the accuracy of the segmentation algorithm (Veldkamp & Karssemeijer, 1998). MC size and shape variability, superimposed surrounding tissues and high frequency noise challenge segmentation accuracy (Cheng et al., 2003; Sampat et al., 2005), and thus development of MC segmentation methods is currently ongoing.

Segmentation of individual MCs has employed grey-level based methods with empirically defined parameters, such as region growing (Chan et al., 1998; Jiang et al., 1999) and grey-level thresholding on pre-processed ROIs (Leichter et al., 2000a; Buchbinder et al., 2002; Kallergi, 2004). More sophisticated methods have been proposed, such as morphologic operations (Tsujii et al., 1999; Soltanian-Zadeh et al., 2004; Papadopoulos et al., 2005), watershed algorithms (Betal et al., 1997; Paquerault et al., 2004), Bayesian pixel classification combined with Markov Random Field models (Veldkamp et al., 2000) and radial gradient-based methods (Paquerault et al., 2004; Arikidis et al., 2008).

As observed in Table 1, morphology-based CADx schemes achieved high performance when the number of MCs (category II) was used as a feature. This observation is consistent with the fact that variability in morphology of individual MCs within the cluster is a strong indicator of malignancy. Leichter et al. (2000a) demonstrated that heterogeneity of individual MC morphology-based features outperforms features related to the distribution of MCs within the cluster (category II). On the other hand, many features of category I contribute to high performance, based however on segmentation methods with empirically set parameters (Chan et al., 1998; Leichter et al., 2000a; Buchbinder et al., 2002; Kallergi, 2004).

Recently, a parameter-free segmentation method was introduced, validated by a CADx scheme utilizing category I MC morphological properties (area, length and relative contrast). The method relies on implementation of active rays (polar-transformed active contours) within the B-spline wavelet representation, to initially provide point estimates of the MC contour. Subsequently, a region growing method constrained by the MC contour point estimates is utilized, to finally delineate individual MC contours (Arikidis et al., 2008). An application example of the method is provided for an individual MC (Figure 2) and for an MC cluster (Figure 3).

Texture-Based CADx Schemes for MC Clusters

Another approach that overcomes limitations associated to segmentation issues is texture analysis applied on ROIs containing MC clusters. This approach is based on the hypothesis that malignancy (as indicated by MCs) would cause changes in the texture of tissue surrounding it (Sampat et al., 2005). Aiming at capturing such tissue texture alterations, CADx schemes have exploited various texture feature sets as well as feature selection and classification algorithms (Cheng et al., 2003), summarized in Table 2. Since a direct comparison is not feasible, due to the heterogeneous datasets analyzed, in the following paragraphs existing trends in MC cluster texture analysis is provided.

The Grey Level Co-occurrence Matrix (GLCM) characterizes the spatial distribution of grey levels in an image (Haralick et al., 1973). Features extracted from GLCMs provide texture heterogeneity and coarseness, which is not nec-

Table 1. Morphology-based CADx schemes for MC clusters

Study	Discriminant Features	Feature Selection / Classifier	Performance (Az)
Betal et al., 1997	[I]Percentage of irregular and round MCs, inter-quartile range of MC area. [II]Number of MCs.	Exhaustive search / k-nearest-neighbour	0.84 (patient)
Chan et al., 1998	[I]Coefficient of mean density variation, moment ratio variation and area variation, maximum moment ratio and area.	Genetic algorithm and stepwise LDA / LDA	0.79 (cluster)
Jiang et al., 1999	[I]Mean area and effective volume, SD of effective thickness and effective volume, 2nd highest MC-shape-irregularity measure. [II]Number of MCs, circularity, area.	Qualitative correlation with radiologist's experience / NN	0.92 (patient) 0.83 (cluster)
Veldkamp et al., 2000	[I]SD of individual MC area, orientation and contrast, mean of individual MC area and orientation, cluster area. [II]Number of MCs, distance to pectoral edge and breast edge.	Sequential forward feature selection / *k*-nearest-neighbour	0.83 (patient) 0.73 (cluster)
Sklansky et al., 2000	[I]Mean area, aspect ratio and irregularity. [II]Number of MCs.	Genetic algorithm / NN	0.75 (cluster)
Leichter et al., 2000a	[I]Mean shape factor, SD of shape factor, brightness and area [II]Mean number of neighbours, mean distance to the nearest MC.	Stepwise LDA / LDA	0.98 (cluster)
Buchbinder et al., 2002	[I]Average of length extreme values.	Stepwise LDA / LDA	0.81 (cluster)
Paquerault et al., 2004	[I]Mean area and effective volume, relative SD of effective thickness and effective volume, 2nd highest MC-shape-irregularity. [II]Number of MCs, circularity, area.	Qualitative correlation with radiologist's experience / LDA and Bayesian NN	0.86 (LDA, patient) 0.82 (LDA, cluster)
Arikidis et al., 2008	[I]SD of length extreme values.	Exhaustive search / LSMD	0.86 (patient) 0.81 (cluster)

*SD: Standard Deviation; I: category I; II: category II; NN: Neural Network; LDA: Linear Discriminant Analysis; LSMD: Least Square Minimum Distance

essarily visually perceived. The discriminating ability of GLCMs features, as extracted from original image ROIs containing MCs, has been demonstrated by most studies (Dhawan et al., 1996; Kocur et al., 1996; Chan et al., 1997, 1998; Kramer & Aghdasi, 1999; Soltanian-Zadeh et al., 2004), with specific GLCMs feature combinations achieving an Az of 0.88 (Chan et al., 1997). In addition, GLCM-based features have shown to be more effective than morphology analysis (Chan et al., 1998), while their combination can provide an even higher classification performance. Soltanian-Zadeh et al. (2004) demonstrated that GLCMs extracted from ROIs containing the MCs were superior to GLCMs extracted from segmented MCs and suggested that "there may be valuable texture information concerning the benignity or malignancy of the cluster in those areas that lie outside the MCs".

Aiming at capturing tissue texture alterations in multiple scales, First Order Statistics (FOS) (i.e. energy, entropy and square root of the coefficients norm) extracted from wavelet or multi-wavelet transform subimages have been exploited. Wavelet/multi-wavelet FOS have shown to be more effective than GLCMs features (Kocur et al., 1996) and shape features (Soltanian-Zadeh et al., 2004), suggesting the advantages offered by the multiscale/multiresolution representation.

An obvious extension of wavelet FOS is the computation of co-occurrence matrix features from wavelet decomposed subimages to describe coefficients second order statistics. Kramer and Aghdasi (1999) demonstrated that co-occurrence matrices features extracted from wavelet decomposed subimages were superior to GLCMs and wavelet FOS.

Figure 2. B-spline active rays' segmentation method. (a) Individual MC of the cluster, depicted at Figure 3. (b) Dots indicate the initial estimate of the MC contour, 'x' the seed pixel and the solid line the final MC contour.

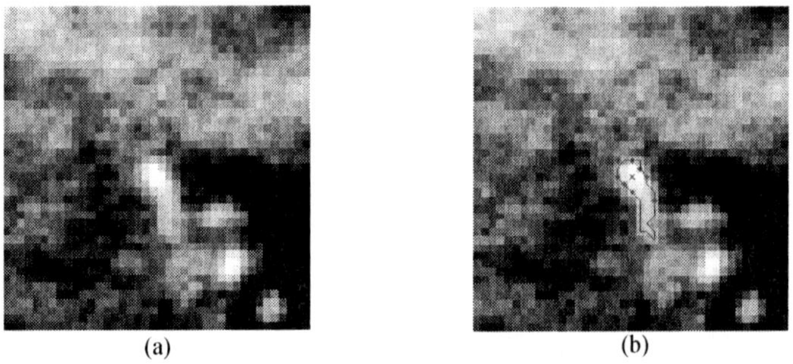

Figure 3. (a) Original ROI depicting pleomorphic MC cluster (DDSM_C_0309_1.RIGHT_CC). (b) Segmented individual MCs.

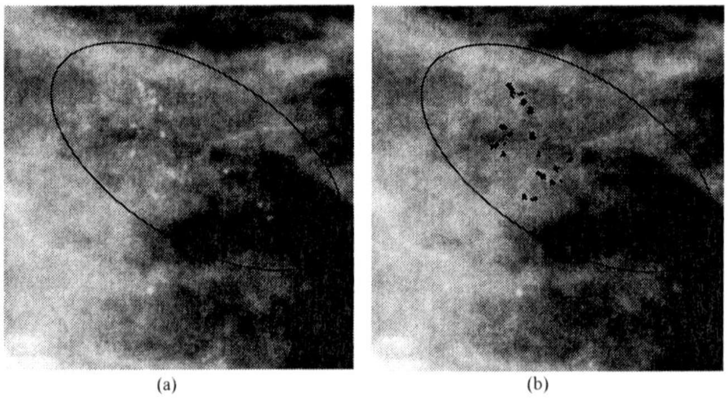

Another texture-based approach for classification of MC clusters focuses on analyzing texture of the tissue surrounding MCs (Thiele et al., 1996; Karahaliou et al., 2007, 2008a) rather than ROIs containing MCs. The rationale of this approach is based on the fact that the MC, a tiny deposit of calcium in breast tissue, can neither be malignant nor benign. This characterization refers rather to the MC surrounding tissue that is also the one subjected to pathoanatomical and immunochemistry analysis to derive a benign or a malignant outcome.

Recently, the surrounding tissue analysis approach was investigated in screening mammograms (Karahaliou et al., 2007, 2008a) to aid radiologists in decisions concerning follow-up and biopsy. Tissue surrounding MCs was defined on both original and wavelet decomposed images provided by Mallat's redundant dyadic wavelet transform, assuming a coarse MC segmentation step (Figure 4). Both grey level texture and wavelet coefficient texture features at three decomposition levels were extracted from surrounding tissue ROIs. The discriminating ability of each feature set was investigated using a Probabilistic NN (PNN). Classification outputs of most discriminating feature sets were combined using a majority voting rule. In a dataset of 100 MC clusters (54 malignant, 46 benign) originating from 85 dense mammographic images, the combined scheme demonstrated the highest performance (Az=0.989).

The main advantage of texture-based schemes is that they overcome increased accuracy demands of MC segmentation algorithms, employed in morphology-based schemes. In case of ROI analysis containing MCs, the MC segmentation step is completely omitted; while in the MC surrounding tissue approach only a coarse MC segmentation step is required.

The approach of surrounding tissue analysis on mammograms aims at analyzing the tissue that generates the MCs (the cause) rather the MC itself (the result). Whether this approach is just "the easy way" or the "correct way" is not clear yet. The surrounding tissue hypothesis has to be further investigated with respect to features and pattern classification methodologies, as well as correlation of extracted image features with pathoanatomical findings.

CADX SCHEMES IN BREAST MRI

The following section summarizes CADx approaches for diagnosis of breast lesions in DCE-MRI, thoroughly described in detail in recent reviews (Wu & Markey, 2006; Meinel & Reinhardt, 2006; Behrens et al., 2007; Eyal & Degani, 2007), with emphasis on quantification of lesion contrast uptake heterogeneity, a current trend.

DCE-MRI, in addition to 3D spatial information of anatomical structures, provides functional information of the tissue by recording the distribution of contrast agents over time (dynamic data).

Due to its high sensitivity in detecting malignant lesions even in presence of dense parenchyma, DCE-MRI is increasingly used as an adjunct to mammography or for imaging high risk women and for assessing tumor response to therapy. However, reported specificity values in discriminating malignant from benign tissue are highly varied (35%-85%).

Breast lesion diagnosis in DCE-MRI is achieved by assessment of morphological properties, requiring high spatial resolution imaging protocols, and analysis of contrast-enhancement kinetics, requiring high temporal resolution imaging protocols (Schnall & Ikeda, 1999).

Analysis of contrast-enhancement kinetics is achieved by generation of a kinetic curve (signal intensity *vs.* time) conventionally computed from a user defined ROI, either covering the entire lesion or placed within the lesion, and subsequent categorization of the kinetic curve into persistent, plateau or washout (Kuhl et al., 1999). This approach quantifies average local contrast uptake ignoring however uptake heterogeneity.

While the combined assessment of morphological/architectural characteristics and average contrast kinetics has shown to improve DCE-MRI specificity (Schnall et al., 2001), the increased inter- and intra-observer variability in interpretation of DCE-MRI data, mainly due to ROI-based kinetics analysis (Stoutjesdijk et al., 2005), has motivated the development of CADx schemes.

CADx methodologies based on average contrast kinetics combined with either qualitative morphological features (Kinkel et al., 2000; Vomweg et al., 2003) or with computer extracted morphological features (Meinel et al., 2007) have demonstrated a positive impact on radiologists' diagnostic performance.

In order to take into account lesion uptake heterogeneity, CADx schemes have focused on pixel- or voxel-wise analysis of kinetics data (Lucht et al., 2001; Subramanian et al., 2004; Twellmann et al., 2005; Chen et al., 2006) in combination with quantitative morphology descriptors (Gilhuijs et al., 2002; Chen et al., 2004; Deurloo et al., 2005) or on pixel-wise parametric modelling of lesion kinetics and subsequent spatial color mapping (Eyal & Degani, 2007).

While the impact of breast DCE-MRI CADx schemes in the clinical environment is under investigation (Wiener et al., 2005), several schemes have obtained FDA approval[3].

Table 2. Texture-based CADx schemes for MC clusters

Study	Features	Feature Selection / Classifier	Performance *
Dhawan et al., 1996	GLCMs features Entropy, Energy (Decomposition: wavelet packets; Filters: Daubechies 6/20; Levels: 0, 1) Cluster features	Multivariate Cluster Analysis, Genetic Algorithm-based method / Backpropagation Neural Network, Linear classifier, k-Nearest Neighbor	Combined feature space: 0.86
Kocur et al., 1996	SRN (Decomposition: DWT; Filters: Daubechies4 & Biorthogonal 9.7; Levels: 0-5) GLCMs feature (angular second moment). Eigenmasses (Karhunen-Loeve coefficients)	Neural Network, Decision Boundary Analysis / Multilayer Perceptron Neural Network	Wavelet-based: 88%
Thiele et al., 1996**	GLCMs features Fractal Geometry based features	Linear and Logistic Discriminant Analysis	Combined feature space: 85%
Chan et al., 1997	GLCMs features	Stepwise Linear Discriminant Analysis / Neural Network	0.88
Chan et al., 1998	GLCMs features Cluster features (Morphological)	Genetic Algorithm, Stepwise Linear Discriminant Analysis / Linear Discriminant Analysis	Combined feature space: 0.89 (0.93, patient-basis)
Kramer & Aghdasi, 1999	GLCMs features Entropy, Energy, SRN (Decomposition: DWT; Filters: Daubechies 4/6/20 & Biorthogonal 2.8; Levels: 0-4) Co-occurrence based (Decomposition: DWT; Filters: Daubechies 4/6/20 & Biorthogonal 2.8; Levels: 1-4)	Sequential Forward Selection / Neural Network, k-Nearest Neighbor	Combined feature space: 94.8%
Soltanian-Zadeh et al., 2004	GLCMs features from segmented MCs and from ROIs containing the MCs Entropy, Energy (Decomposition: wavelet packets; Filters: Daubechies 6/10/12; Levels: 1, 2 Entropy, Energy (Decomposition: multi-wavelet (3 Filters); Levels: 1, 2) Cluster features (shape)	Binary and Real valued Genetic Algorithm / k-Nearest Neighbor	Multi-wavelet features: 0.89
Karahaliou et al., 2008a**	First order statistics GLCMs features Laws' texture energy measures Energy, Entropy (Decomposition: redundant DWT; Filter: B-spline; Levels: 1-3) Co-occurrence based (Decomposition: redundant DWT; Filter: B-spline; Levels: 1-3)	Exhaustive search per feature set (with respect to highest classification accuracy and minimum # of features) / Probabilistic Neural Network	Combined scheme: 0.989

*Performance on a cluster-basis in terms of Az index or % overall classification accuracy. Patient-basis performance is further provided for Chan et al. (1998).
**Studies analyzing tissue surrounding MCs.
SRN: Square Root of the Norm of coefficients; DWT: Discrete Wavelet Transform

The significance of quantifying lesions' kinetics heterogeneity and its potential both in cancer diagnosis and in evaluation of anticancer therapy has been recently highlighted (Jackson et al., 2007). Following, studies having focused on quantifying breast lesion kinetics heterogeneity are reviewed.

Issa et al. (1999) quantified heterogeneity of breast lesions expressed on exchange rate parameter maps provided by pixel-wise compartmental

Figure 4. (a) 600x600 pixels ROI depicting a MC cluster (DDSM_B_3406, RIGHT_CC). Surrounding tissue ROI (area outside the segmented MCs) depicted on original (b), approximation 1st scale (c), approximation 2nd scale (d), gradient magnitude 2nd scale (e), and gradient magnitude 3rd scale (f) subimage (128x128 pixel ROI).

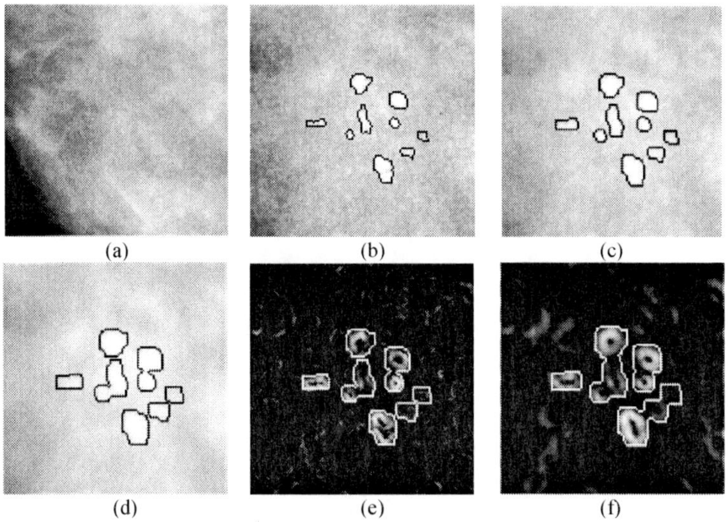

pharmacokinetic modelling on semi-automatically delineated ROIs. Heterogeneity was quantified by statistical moments (mean and standard deviation) of 10 different segments of the lesion parameters distribution. A specificity of 88% with sensitivity 88% was achieved in classification of 50 breast lesions (25 malignant, 25 benign), suggesting the ability of lesion heterogeneity quantification metrics in breast lesion differentiation.

Gibbs & Turnbull (2003) also investigated GLCMs features extracted from a rectangular ROI containing the lesion on a representative post-contrast slice. Using LRA, a 3 texture parameter model achieved an Az of 0.80±0.07 in discriminating malignant from benign lesions. When combining texture features with lesion size, patient age and time-to-peak enhancement diagnostic accuracy was increased to 0.92±0.05. These results are consistent with the fact that benign lesions present more homogeneous uptake patterns, while malignant lesions demonstrate more heterogeneous patterns.

Chen et al. (2007) extended the approach of contrast uptake heterogeneity quantification for breast cancer diagnosis by investigating 3D GLCMs features. The proposed volumetric texture analysis, applied on automatically segmented 3D breast lesions by fuzzy c-means clustering, was tested on a dataset of 121 breast lesions (77 malignant, 44 benign), and further compared to a 2D texture analysis. The 3D texture analysis yielded significantly higher classification performance over the 2D texture analysis suggesting its potential in computer-assisted diagnosis of breast lesions in MRI.

Woods et al. (2007) employed a 4D co-occurrence texture analysis on DCE-MRI data to distinguish between non-malignant and malignant breast tissue. The algorithm employs a back-propagation NN to label each voxel into "malignant" or "non-malignant" type based on local spatial and temporal voxel intensity variations. The method was tested on dataset 8 breast lesions (4 malignant, 4 benign) and achieved an

Figure 5. (a) Color-coded ROI depicting invasive ductal carcinoma. (b) Gradient of color-coded ROI. (c) Delineated lesion boundary (boundary pixels are assigned white grey level) on the gradient color-coded ROI. (d) Wash Out map. (e) Time-to-Peak Enhancement map. (f) Peak Enhancement map.

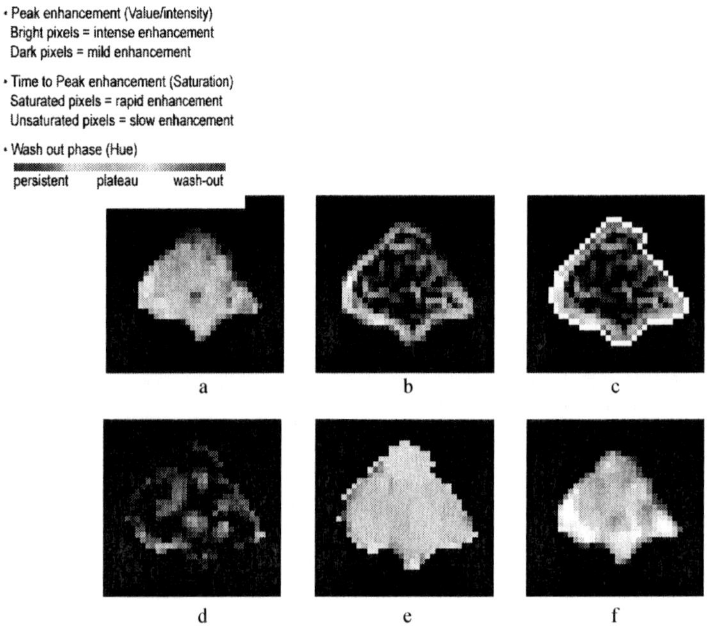

Az=0.998 in correctly classifying breast lesion voxels, suggesting its potential in segmenting malignant lesions in DCE-MRI.

Recently, a texture analysis approach in DCE-MRI was introduced (Karahaliou et al., 2008b) aimed at quantifying heterogeneity of lesions not only with respect to contrast uptake (Peak Enhancement) but also with respect to Time-to-Peak Enhancement and Post-Initial Enhancement (Wash out). This is achieved by fitting a linear-slope model pixel-wise to a representative lesion slice time series and using fitted parameters to create three kinetic maps. Maps are converted to a single HSV color-coded image, subsequently used for delineating lesion uptake boundary, by grey level thresholding followed by morphological operations, on the gradient of color-coded ROI (Figure 5a-c). The delineated boundary is then used to define corresponding areas on each kinetic map (Figure 5d-f). Kinetic maps are treated as grey level images and subjected to texture analysis by means of FOS and GLCMs features. The most discriminating subset of features (combination of 2-5 features) was selected per map, via exhaustive search, using PNN and leave-one-out training-testing methodology. Final classification was obtained by combining classification outputs of most discriminating feature subsets from the three maps, via majority voting. Performance evaluation of individual maps classifications and of the combined scheme was achieved by ROC analysis, on a dataset of 57 breast lesions (30 malignant, 27 benign). The combined scheme achieved the highest performance (0.978±0.017) and statistically significantly ($p<0.05$), as compared to individual maps classification. Texture features extracted from the Wash Out map outperformed (0.902±0.040) features extracted from the other two individual maps.

Results suggest that quantification of breast lesion kinetics heterogeneity is a highly promising approach that has to be further exploited in the frame of DCE-MRI CADx systems.

FUTURE TRENDS

The advantages offered by the various CADx schemes across breast imaging modalities have been exploited and well recognized (Leichter et al., 2000b; Horsch et al., 2004, Sahiner et al., 2007; Behrens et al., 2007).

A "unimodal" CADx scheme can objectively "diagnose" a breast lesion either by mimicking some of the radiologists' interpretation criteria as specified by BIRADS lexicon per imaging modality or by offering information that cannot be visually perceived. In addition, recently reported unimodal CADx schemes have tried to take advantage of information offered by multiple views based on feature fusion, i.e. combination of features from two or more images of the same modality (Huo et al., 2001; Gupta & Markey, 2005; Timp et al., 2007). However, in case of not conclusive information provided by a single modality, the effectiveness of unimodal CADx schemes is limited. In order to mimic radiologists' work-up flow in such cases, integration of diagnostic information provided by adjunct modalities is required.

Multimodality image fusion (Behrenbruch et al., 2004) and multimodality CADx schemes (Giger, 2004; Drukker et al., 2005; Horsch et al., 2006) account for emerging and highly promising technologies in breast cancer diagnosis, by exploiting complementary tissue properties as provided by imaging modalities. Recently, "bimodal" CADx schemes (i.e. mammography and US) have been reported based either on feature fusion (Drukker et al., 2005) or on decision fusion (Jesneck et al., 2006), demonstrating the increased potential of the multimodality approach.

Recently, Content-Based Image Retrieval (CBIR) systems based on knowledge obtained from "similar" confirmed cases, employing various similarity indices for retrieval, have been proposed for mass diagnosis in mammography and US imaging (Giger, 2004). "Interactive CADx" schemes, also exploiting CBIR technologies and enabling relevance feedback (Tourassi, 2005) are suggested as alternative to "silent CADx readers".

Emerging molecular imaging involving MRI, PET and optical imaging are expected to offer new insights in capturing altered physiology or cellular metabolism of breast tissue, eventually affecting future CADx schemes (Suri et al., 2006).

CONCLUSION

One approach of improving interpretation accuracy of breast imaging is to increase radiologists' confidence levels regarding breast lesion detection and diagnosis, especially in cases of early or occult disease, by means of image processing and analysis methods.

Following the successful paradigm of CADe systems in the clinical environment, CADx schemes are aimed at assisting radiologists in the diagnostic task, by providing estimates of probability of malignancy by means of quantitative image feature extraction and classification methods.

The classification performance of such schemes depends on tissue properties captured by various modalities (structural and/or functional), as well as by optimizing all stages of a CADx scheme such as segmentation, feature spaces exploited, as well as feature selection and classification methods employed to deal with high dimensional spaces.

Combining complementary multimodal information in comprehensive environments is expected to further enhance diagnostic accuracy of CADx schemes, by providing a more realistic simulation of clinical work-up flow.

Although, stand alone evaluation of CADx schemes, by means of ROC analysis, is limited by the size and quality of case sample analyzed up to now, the true impact is expected to be derived from large scale prospective clinical studies.

ACKNOWLEDGMENT

Part of this work is supported by the Caratheodory Programme (C.183) of the University of Patras, Greece.

REFERENCES

Arikidis, N., Skiadopoulos, S., Karahaliou, A., Likaki, E., Panayiotakis, G., & Costaridou, L. (2008). B-spline active rays segmentation of microcalcifications in mammography. *Medical Physics, 35*(11), 5161-5171.

Behrenbruch, C. P., Marias, K., Armitage, P. A., Yam, M., Moore, N. R., English, R. E., Clarke, P. J., Leong, F. J., & Brady, J. (2004). Fusion of contrast-enhanced breast MR and mammographic imaging data. *The British Journal of Radiology, 77*(2), S201-208.

Behrens, S., Laue, H., Althaus, M., Boehler, T., Kuemmerlen B., Hahn, H. K., & Peitgen, H. O. (2007). Computer assistance for MR based diagnosis of breast cancer: Present and future challenges. *Computerized Medical Imaging and Graphics, 31*(4-5), 236-247.

Betal, D., Roberts, N., & Whitehouse, G. H. (1997). Segmentation and numerical analysis of microcalcifications on mammograms using mathematical morphology. *The British Journal of Radiology, 70*(837), 903-917.

Buchbinder, S. S., Leichter, I. S., Lederman, R., Novak, B., Bamberger, P. N., Coopersmith, H., & Fields, S. I. (2002). Can the size of microcalcifications predict malignancy of clusters at mammography? *Academic Radiology, 9*(1), 18-25.

Chan, H.-P., Sahiner, B., Petrick, N., Helvie, M. A., Lam, K. L., Adler, D. D., & Goodsitt, M. M. (1997). Computerized classification of malignant and benign microcalcifications on mammograms: Texture analysis using an artificial neural network. *Physics in Medicine and Biology, 42*(3), 549-567.

Chan, H.-P., Sahiner, B., Lam, K. L., Petrick, N., Helvie, M. A., Goodsitt, M. M., & Adler, D. D. (1998). Computerized analysis of mammographic microcalcifications in morphological and texture feature spaces. *Medical Physics, 25*(10), 2007-2019.

Chan, H.-P., Sahiner, B., Petrick, N., Hadjiiski, L., & Paquerault, S. (2005). Computer-aided diagnosis of breast cancer. In: L. Costaridou (Ed.), *Medical Image Analysis Methods*, (pp. 1-49). Boca Raton: Taylor & Francis Group, CRC Press.

Chen, W., Giger, M. L., Lan, L., & Bick, U. (2004). Computerized interpretation of breast MRI: Investigation of enhancement-variance dynamics. *Medical Physics, 31*(5), 1076-1082.

Chen, W., Giger, M. L., Bick, U., & Newstead, G. M. (2006). Automatic identification and classification of characteristic kinetic curves of breast lesions on DCE-MRI. *Medical Physics, 33*(8), 2878-2887.

Chen, W., Giger, M. L., Li, H., Bick, U., & Newstead, G. M. (2007). Volumetric texture analysis of breast lesions on contrast-enhanced magnetic resonance images. *Magnetic Resonance in Medicine, 58*(3), 562-571.

Cheng, H. D., Cai, X., Chen, X., Hu, L., & Lou, X. (2003). Computer-aided detection and classification of microcalcifications in mammograms: A survey. *Pattern Recognition, 36*(12), 2967-2991.

Deurloo, E. E., Muller, S. H., Peterse, J. L., Besnard, A. P., & Gilhuijs, K. G. (2005). Clinically and mammographically occult breast lesions on MR images: Potential effect of computerized assessment on clinical reading. *Radiology, 234*(3), 693-701.

Dhawan, A. P., Chitre, Y., Kaiser-Bonasso, C., & Moskowitz, M. (1996). Analysis of mammographic microcalcifications using gray-level image structure features. *IEEE Transactions on Medical Imaging, 15*(3), 246-259.

Drukker, K., Horsch, K., & Giger, M. L. (2005). Multimodality computerized diagnosis of breast lesions using mammography and sonography. *Academic Radiology, 12*(8), 970-979.

Eyal, E., & Degani, H. (2007). Model-based and model-free parametric analysis of breast dynamic-contrast-enhanced MRI. *NMR in Biomedicine*.

Fenton, J. J., Taplin, S. H., Carney, P. A., Abraham, L., Sickles, E. A, D'Orsi, C., Berns, E. A., Cutter, G., Hendrick, R. E., Barlow, W. E., & Elmore, J. G. (2007). Influence of computer-aided detection on performance of screening mammography. *The New England Journal of Medicine, 356*(14), 1399-1409.

Gibbs, P., & Turnbull, L. W. (2003). Textural analysis of contrast-enhanced MR images of the breast. *Magnetic Resonance in Medicine, 50*(1), 92-98.

Giger, M. L., Huo, Z., Kupinski, M. A., & Vyborny, C. J. (2000). Computer-aided diagnosis in mammography. In: M. Sonka, J. M. Fitzpatrick. (Eds.) *Handbook of Medical Imaging Vol. 2, Medical Image Processing and Analysis* (pp. 915-1004). Bellingham, Washington, USA, SPIE Press.

Giger, M. L. (2004). Computer aided diagnosis in diagnostic mammography and multimodality breast imaging. *RSNA Categorical Course in Diagnostic Radiology Physics: Advances in Breast Imaging - Physics, Technology and Clinical Applications,* (pp. 205-217).

Gilhuijs, K. G. A., Deurloo, E. E., Muller, S. H., Peterse, J. L., & Schultze-Kool, L. J. (2002). Breast MR imaging in women at increased lifetime risk of breast cancer: Clinical system for computerized assessment of breast lesions - Initial results. *Radiology, 225*(3), 907-916.

Gupta, S., & Markey, M. K. (2005). Correspondence in texture features between two mammographic views. *Medical Physics, 32*(6), 1598-1606.

Haralick, R. M., Shanmugam, K., & Dinstein, I. (1973). Textural features for image classification. *IEEE Transactions on Systems, Man, and Cybernetics, SMC-3*(6), 610-621.

Horsch, K., Giger, M. L., Vyborny, C. J., & Venta, L. A. (2004). Performance of computer aided diagnosis (CAD) in the interpretation of lesions on breast sonography. *Academic Radiology, 11*(3), 272-280.

Horsch, K., Giger, M. L., Vyborny, C. J., Lan, L., Mendelson, E. B., & Hendrick, R. E. (2006). Classification of breast lesions with multimodality computer aided diagnosis: Observer study results on an independent clinical data set. *Radiology, 240*(2), 357-368.

Huo, Z., Giger, M. L., & Vyborny, C. J. (2001). Computerized analysis of multiple-mammographic views: Potential usefulness of special view mammograms in computer-aided diagnosis. *IEEE Transactions on Medical Imaging, 20*(12), 1285-1292.

Issa, B., Buckley, D. L., & Turnbull, L. W. (1999). Heterogeneity analysis of Gd-DTPA uptake: Improvement in breast lesion differentiation. *Journal of Computer Assisted Tomography, 23*(4), 615-621.

Jackson, A., O'Connor, J. P., Parker, G. J., & Jayson, G. C. (2007). Imaging tumor vascular heterogeneity and angiogenesis using dynamic contrast-enhanced magnetic resonance imaging, *Clinical Cancer Research, 13*(12), 3449-3459.

Jesneck, J. L., Nolte, L. W., Baker, J. A., Floyd, C. E., & Lo, J. Y. (2006). Optimized approach to decision fusion of heterogeneous data for breast cancer diagnosis. *Medical Physics, 33*(8), 2945-2954.

Jiang, Y., Metz, C. E., & Nishikawa, R. M. (1996). A receiver operating characteristic partial area index for highly sensitive diagnostic tests. *Radiology, 201*(3), 745-750.

Jiang, Y., Nishikawa, R. M., Schmidt, R. A., Metz, C. E., Giger, M. L., & Doi, K. (1999). Improving breast cancer diagnosis with computer-aided diagnosis. *Academic Radiology, 6*(1), 22-33.

Kallergi, M. (2004). Computed-aided diagnosis of mammographic microcalcification clusters. *Medical Physics, 31*(2), 314-326.

Karahaliou, A., Skiadopoulos, S., Boniatis, I., Sakellaropoulos, P., Likaki, E., Panayiotakis, G., & Costaridou, L. (2007). Texture analysis of tissue surrounding microcalcifications on mammograms for breast cancer diagnosis. *The British Journal of Radiology, 80*(956), 648-656.

Karahaliou, A., Boniatis, I., Skiadopoulos, S., Sakellaropoulos, P., Arikidis, N., Likaki, E., Panayiotakis, G., & Costaridou, L. (2008a). Breast cancer diagnosis: Analyzing texture of tissue surrounding microcalcifications. *IEEE Transactions on Information Technology in Biomedicine, 12*(6), 731-738.

Karahaliou, A., Vassiou, K., Skiadopoulos, S., Kanavou, D., Yiakoumelos, A., & Costaridou, L. (2008b, in press). Quantifying heterogeneity of lesion uptake in Dynamic Contrast Enhanced MRI for breast cancer diagnosis. *Nuclear Instruments and Methods in Physics Research Section A.*

Kinkel, K., Helbich, T. H., Esserman, L. J., Barclay, J., Schwerin, E. H., Sickles, E. A., & Hylton, N. M. (2000). Dynamic high-spatial-resolution MR imaging of suspicious breast lesions: Diagnostic criteria and interobserver variability. *AJR. American Journal of Roentgenology, 175*(1), 35-43.

Kocur, C. M., Rogers, S. K., Myers, L. R., Burns, T., Kabrisky, M., Hoffmeister, J. W., Bauer, K. W., & Steppe, J. M. (1996). Using neural networks to select wavelet features for breast cancer diagnosis. *IEEE Engineering in Medicine and Biology, 15*(3), 95-102.

Kramer, D., & Aghdasi, F. (1999). Texture analysis techniques for the classification of microcalcifications in digitized mammograms. In *Proc. 5th IEEE AFRICON Conf.* (pp. 395-400), Cape Town, Africa.

Kuhl, C. K., Mielcareck, P., Klaschik, S., Leutner, C., Wardelmann, E., Gieseke, J. & Schild, H. H. (1999). Dynamic breast MR imaging: Are signal intensity time course data useful for differential diagnosis of enhancing lesions? *Radiology, 211*(1), 101-110.

Leichter, I., Lederman, R., Buchbinder, S., Bamberger, P., Novak, B., & Fields, S. (2000a). Optimizing parameters for computer-aided diagnosis of microcalcifications at mammography. *Academic Radiology, 7*(6), 406-412.

Leichter, I., Fields, S., Nirel, R., Bamberger, P., Novak, B., Lederman, R., & Buchbinder, S. (2000b). Improved mammographic interpretation of masses using computer-aided diagnosis. *European Radiology 10*(2), 377-383.

Lucht, R., Knopp, M. V., & Brix, G. (2001). Classification of signal-time curves from dynamic MR mammography by neural networks. *Magnetic Resonance Imaging, 19*(1), 51–57.

Meinel, L. A., & Reinhardt, J. M (2006). Breast MRI computer-aided diagnosis systems. In: J. S. Suri, R. M. Rangayyan (Eds.). *Recent Advances in Breast Imaging, Mammography, and Computer-Aided Diagnosis of Breast Cancer* (pp. 791-832). Bellingham, Washington, USA, SPIE Press.

Meinel, L. A., Stolpen, A. H., Berbaum, K. S., Fajardo, L. L., & Reinhardt, J. M. (2007). Breast MRI lesion classification: Improved performance of human readers with a backpropagation neural network computer-aided diagnosis (CAD) system. *Journal of Magnetic Resonance Imaging, 25*(1), 89-95.

Papadopoulos, A., Fotiadis, D. I., & Likas, A. (2005). Characterization of clustered microcalcifications in digitized mammograms using neural networks and support vector machines. *Artificial Intelligence in Medicine, 34*(12), 141-150.

Paquerault, S., Yarusso, L. M., Papaioannou, J., Jiang, Y., & Nishikawa, R. M. (2004). Radial gradient-based segmentation of mammographic microcalcifications: Observer evaluation and effect on CAD performance. *Medical Physics, 31*(9), 2648-2657.

Park, J. M., Franken, E. A. Jr., Garg, M., Fajardo, L. L., & Niklason, L. T. (2007). Breast tomosynthesis: Present considerations and future applications. *Radiographics, 27* (Suppl 1), S231-240.

Pisano, E. D, Gatsonis, C., Hendrick, E., Yaffe, M., Baum, J. K., Acharyya, S., Conant, E. F., Fajardo, L. L., Bassett, L., D'Orsi, C., Jong, R., & Rebner, M. (2005). Diagnostic performance of digital versus film mammography for breast-cancer screening. *The New England Journal of Medicine, 353*(17), 1773-1783.

Sahiner, B., Chan, H-P, Roubidoux, M. A., Hadjiiski, L. M., Helvie, M. A., Paramagul, C., Bailey, J., Nees, A. V., & Blane, C. (2007). Malignant and benign breast masses on 3D US volumetric images: Effect of computer-aided diagnosis on radiologist accuracy. *Radiology, 242*(3), 716-724.

Sampat, P. M., Markey, M. K., & Bovik, A. C. (2005). Computer-aided detection and diagnosis in mammography. In: A. C. Bovik (Ed.), *Handbook of Image and Video Processing 2nd ed.* (pp. 1195-1217). San Diego, Elsevier Academic Press.

Schnall, M. D., & Ikeda, D. (1999). Lesion diagnosis working group report. *Journal of Magnetic Resonance Imaging, 10*(6), 982–990.

Schnall, M. D., Rosten, S., Englander, S., Orel, S. G., & Nunes, L. W. (2001). A combined architectural and kinetic interpretation model for breast MR images. *Academic Radiology, 8*(7), 591-597.

Sklansky, J., Tao, E. Y., Bazargan, M., Ornes, Ch. J., Murchison, R. C., & Teklehaimanot, S. (2000). Computer-aided, case-based diagnosis of mammographic regions of interest containing microcalcifications. *Academic Radiology, 7*(6), 395-405.

Soltanian-Zadeh, H., Rafiee-Rad, F., & Pourabdollah-Nejad, S. D. (2004). Comparison of multiwavelet, wavelet, Haralick, and shape features for microcalcification classification in mammograms. *Pattern Recognition, 37*(10), 1973-1986.

Stoutjesdijk, M. J., Fuetterer, J. F., Boetes C., van Dieand, L. E., Jager, G., & Barentsz, J. O. (2005). Variability in the description of morphologic and contrast enhancement characteristics of breast lesions on magnetic resonance imaging. *Investigative Radiology, 40*(6), 355–362.

Subramanian, K. R., Brockway, J. P., & Carruthers, W. B. (2004). Interactive detection and visualization of breast lesions from dynamic contrast enhanced MRI volumes. *Computerized Medical Imaging and Graphics, 28*(8), 435-444.

Suri, J. S., Chandrasekhar, R., Lanconelli, N., Campanini, R., Roffilli, M., Chang, R.-F., Guo, Y., Sivaramakrishna, R. et al (2006). The current status and likely future of breast imaging CAD. In: J. S. Suri, R. M. Rangayyan (Eds.). *Recent Advances in Breast Imaging, Mammography, and Computer-Aided Diagnosis of Breast Cancer* (pp. 901-961). Bellingham, Washington, USA, SPIE Press.

Thiele, D. L., Kimme-Smith, C., Johnson, T. D., McCombs, M., & Bassett, L. W. (1996). Using tissue texture surrounding calcification clusters to predict benign vs malignant outcomes. *Medical Physics, 23*(4), 549-555.

Timp, S., Varela, C., & Karssemeijer, N. (2007). Temporal change analysis for characterization of mass lesions in mammography. *IEEE Transactions on Medical Imaging, 26*(7), 945-953.

Tourassi, G. D. (2005). Current status of computerized decision support systems in mammography. *Studies in Fuzziness and Soft Computing: Intelligent Paradigms for Healthcare Enterprises 184,* (pp. 173–208). Springer-Verlag Berlin Heidelberg.

Tsujii, O., Freedman, M. T., & Mun, S. K. (1999). Classification of microcalcifications in digital mammograms using trend-oriented radial basis function neural network. *Pattern Recognition, 32*(5), 891-903.

Twellmann, T., Lichte, O., & Nattkemper, T. W. (2005). An adaptive tissue characterisation network for model-free visualisation of dynamic contrast-enhanced magnetic resonance data. *IEEE Transactions on Medical Imaging, 24*(10), 1256-1266.

Veldkamp, W. J. H., & Karssemeijer, N. (1998). Accurate segmentation and contrast measurement of microcalcifications in mammograms: A phantom study. *Medical Physics, 25*(7), 1102-1110.

Veldkamp, W. J. H., Karssemeijer, N., Otten, J. D. M., & Hendriks, J. H. C. L. (2000). Automated classification of clustered microcalcifications into malignant and benign types. *Medical Physics, 27*(11), 2600-2608.

Vomweg, T. W., Buscema, M., Kauczor, H. U., Teifke, A., Intraligi, M., Terzi, S., Heussel, C. P., Achenbach, T., Rieker, O., Mayer, D., & Thelen, M. (2003). Improved artificial neural networks in prediction of malignancy of lesions in contrast-enhanced MR-mammography. *Medical Physics, 30*(9), 2350-2359.

Wiener, J. I., Schilling, K. J., Adami, C., & Obuchowski, N. A. (2005). Assessment of suspected breast cancer by MRI: A prospective clinical trial using a combined kinetic and morphologic analysis. *AJR. American Journal of Roentgenology, 184*(3), 878-886.

Williams, M. B, Yaffe, M. J, Maidment, A. D, Martin, M. C, Seibert, J. A, & Pisano, E. D. (2006). Image quality in digital mammography: Image acquisition. *Journal of the American College of Radiology, 3*(8), 589-608.

Woods, B. J., Clymer, B. D., Kurc, T., Heverhagen, J. T., Stevens, R., Orsdemir, A., Bulan, O., & Knopp, M. V. (2007). Malignant-lesion segmentation using 4D co-occurrence texture analysis applied to dynamic contrast-enhanced magnetic resonance breast image data. *Journal of Magnetic Resonance Imaging, 25*(3), 495-501.

Wu, Q., & Markey, M. K (2006). Computer-aided diagnosis of breast cancer in MR imaging. In: J. S. Suri, R. M. Rangayyan (Eds.). *Recent Advances in Breast Imaging, Mammography, and Computer-Aided Diagnosis of Breast Cancer* (pp. 791-832). Bellingham, Washington, USA, SPIE Press.

KEY TERMS

Classification: Algorithms aimed at partition the data in two or more classes. They are differentiated as unsupervised (data structure is determined from data itself) or supervised (data structure is determined using *a prior* knowledge or information).

Computer-Aided Detection (CADe): CADe systems in breast imaging are fully automated computer vision algorithms developed to improve radiologists' performance in detecting breast lesions, by identifying suspicious regions in a breast image or series of images.

Computer-Aided Diagnosis (CADx): CADx systems in breast imaging are fully automated computer vision algorithms developed to improve radiologists' performance in characterizing breast lesion status (malignant *vs.* benign), by providing probability estimates of lesions' malignancy.

Feature Extraction: Quantification of image content by means of computer algorithms, aiming to capture tissue alterations, due to underlying biological processes reflected either as morphology or as texture variations, mimicking or complementing radiologist interpretation, used in subsequent pattern analysis.

Feature Selection: Strategy to avoid supervised classification overtraining in case of a high feature dimensionality in small training datasets. Depending on feature selection method and criterion used, sets of the most discriminant features are obtained improving classification accuracy.

Lesion Segmentation: The process of delineating the boundary of a lesion from an image or image series either by use of interactive computer tools (manual) or by automated image segmentation algorithms.

Mammography: The most effective imaging modality in detecting breast lesions such as masses, microcalcification clusters and architectural distortions, providing structural tissue properties by means of X-ray attenuation differences.

ENDNOTES

1 GE Senographe 2000D, Fischer Imaging SenoScan, Lorad Digital Breast Imager, Lorad/Hologic Selenia, GE Senographe DS, Siemens Mammomat Novation DR, GE Senographe Essential and Fuji Computed Radiography Mammography Suite.

2 ImageChecker - R2 Technology Inc., MammoReader™ - Intelligent Systems Software Inc., Second Look™ - CADx Medical Systems Inc., Kodak Mammography CAD Engine - Eastman Kodak Co.

3 CADstream™, by Confirma, Inc. (Kirkland,WA); 3TP Software Option, by CAD Sciences, White Plains (NY); CADimas™, by Alan Penn & Associates., Inc. (Rockville, US).

Chapter XI
Assessment of Stroke by Analysing Carotid Plaque Morphology

E. Kyriacou
Frederick University, Cyprus

C. I. Christodoulou
University of Cyprus, Cyprus

C. Loizou
Intercollege, Cyprus

M.S. Pattichis
University of New Mexico, USA

C.S. Pattichis
University of Cyprus, Cyprus

S. Kakkos
University of Patras Medical School, Greece

A. Nicolaides
Imperial College, UK

ABSTRACT

Stroke is the third leading cause of death in the Western world and a major cause of disability in adults. The objective of this work was to investigate morphological feature extraction techniques and the use of automatic classifiers; in order to develop a computer aided system that will facilitate the automated characterization of carotid plaques for the identification of individuals with asymptomatic carotid stenosis at risk of stroke. Through this chapter we summarize the recent advances in ultrasonic plaque characterization and evaluate the efficacy of computer aided diagnosis based on neural and statistical classifiers using as input morphological features. Several classifiers like the K-Nearest Neighbour(KNN) the Probabilistic Neural Network(PNN) and the Support Vector Machine(SVM) were evaluated resulting to a diagnostic accuracy up to 73.7%.

INTRODUCTION

High-resolution ultrasound has made possible the noninvasive visualization of the carotid bifurcation and for that reason it has been extensively used in the study of arterial wall changes; these include measurement of the thickness of the intima media complex (IMT), estimation of the severity of stenosis due to atherosclerotic plaques and plaque characterization(Reilly, 1983; El-Barghouti, 1996; Elatrozy, 1998). Applications of carotid bifurcation ultrasound include: (1) identification and grading of stenosis of extracranial carotid artery disease often responsible for ischemic strokes, transient ischemic attacks (TIAs) or amaurosis fugax (AF); (2) Follow-up after carotid endarterectomy; (3) evaluation of pulsatile neck mass; (4) investigation of asymptomatic neck bruits: severe internal carotid artery stenosis is a predictive factor for future stroke; (5) cardiovascular risk assessment: the presence of carotid bifurcation atherosclerotic plaques is associated with increased cardiovascular mortality(Joakimsen, 2000; Schmidt, 2003); (6) clinical studies on the effect of lipid-lowering and other medications on carotid intima media thickness(IMT)which includes plaque thickness(Salonen, 2003).

During the last decade, the introduction of computer aided methods and image standardization has improved the objective assessment of carotid plaque echogenicity(El-Barghouti, 1996; Elatrozy, 1998) and heterogeneity(El-Barghouti, 1996; Salonen, 2003) and has largely replaced subjective(visual)assessment(Reilly, 1983; Reilly, 1988) that had been criticized for its relatively poor reproducibility(Arnold , 1987). Through this chapter we are trying to introduce the use of morphological image analysis and automatic classifiers for the creation of an automatic ultrasound image classification system for the estimation of the risk of stroke.

BACKGROUND

Visual Classification of Atherosclerotic Plaque in Ultrasound Imaging

High-resolution ultrasound provides information not only on the degree of carotid artery stenosis but also on the characteristics of the arterial wall including the size and consistency of atherosclerotic plaques. Several studies have indicated that "complicated" carotid plaques are often associated with ipsilateral neurological symptoms and share common ultrasonic characteristics, being more echolucent (weak reflection of ultrasound and therefore containing echo-poor structures) and heterogeneous (having both echolucent and echogenic areas). In contrast, "uncomplicated" plaques which are often asymptomatic tend to be of uniform consistency (uniformly hypoechoid or uniformly hyperechoid) without evidence of ulceration(Reilly, 1983; O'Donnell, 1985; Leahy, 1988; Langsfeld, 1989; Geroulakos , 1993).

Different classifications of plaque ultrasonic appearance have been proposed in the literature. Reilly classified (O'Donnell, 1985) carotid plaques as homogenous and heterogeneous, defining as homogeneous plaques those with "uniformly bright echoes" that are now known as uniformly hyperechoic (type 4) (see below). Johnson(1985) classified plaques as dense and soft, Widder(1990), as echolucent and echogenic based on the their overall level of echo patterns, while Gray-Weale(1988) described 4 types: type 1, predominantly echolucent lesions, type 2, echogenic lesions with substantial (>75%) components of echolucency, type 3, predominately echogenic with small area(s) of echolucency occupying less than a quarter of the plaque and type 4, uniformly dense echogenic lesions. Geroulakos(1993) subsequently modified the Gray-Weale classification by using a 50% area cut off point instead of 75% and by adding a fifth type, which as a result of heavy calcification on its surface cannot be correctly classified.

Regarding the clinical significance of carotid plaque heterogeneity, it seems that the heterogeneous plaques described in the three studies published in the 1980's (Table 1), include hypoechoic plaques. Also heterogeneous plaques in all studies listed in Table 1 contain hypoechoic areas (large or small) and appear to be the plaques which are associated with symptoms or if found in asymptomatic individuals they are the plaques that subsequently tend to become symptomatic.

Table 1. Ultrasound carotid plaque heterogeneity and clinical implications

Author	Year	Ultrasound carotid plaque heterogeneity	Clinical implications
O'Donnell Jr	1985	Visual classification; distinguished fine vs rough and random vs regular texture	Histology study
Aldoori	1987	Visual classification	Plaque classification
Leahy	1988	Plaques containing echolucent components. Homogeneous plaques had uniform consistency suggestive of sclerotic plaques	Heterogeneous plaques more frequently symptomatic and associated with ipsilateral infarction on CT scan
Sterpetti	1988	Mixed high-, medium-, and low-level echoes. Homogenous lesions had uniformly high-medium-level echoes	Heterogeneous plaques became symptomatic more frequently during follow-up
Langsfeld	1989	Predominantly echolucent plaques with a thin "egg shell" cap of echogenicity and echogenic plaques with substantial components of echolucency	Heteroneous plaques more frequently symptomatic. Heterogeneous plaques became symptomatic more frequently during follow-up
Widder	1990	Visual estimation, plaques being classified into four categories (homogeneous, slightly or markedly heterogeneous and non visible)	Histology study
Giannoni	1991	Not provided	Heterogeneous plaques progressed and became symptomatic
ECPSG	1995	Mixed composition	Heterogeneous plaques contained more calcification
Kagawa	1996	Plaques composed of a mixture of hyperechoic, isoechoic and hypoechoic plaques. Normal intima-media complex used to define isoechoicity	Heterogeneous lesions consisted of a mixture of atheroma and fibrosis on histology and demonstrated calcification more frequently than the homogeneous ones
Kardoulas	1996	Mixed echo level pattern	Association of plaque heterogeneity with symptoms less consistent in comparison with echolucency
AbuRahma	1998	Plaques composed of a mixture of hyperechoic,isoechoic and hypoechoic plaques. Normal intima-media complex used to define isoechoicity	Heterogeneous plaques more frequently symptomatic

Natural History Studies

Initially Reilly(1983) suggested that patients with asymptomatic carotid artery disease involving echolucent heterogeneous plaques might be at increased risk of future stroke. In the mid 1990s computers were used to obtain measurements of the grey scale of plaques. Although similar results were obtained by different teams (El-Barghouti,1996; Gronholdt, 2001; Biasi, 1998), different cut off points had to be used by different centres. It became obvious that obtaining ultrasonic images is subjective. If ultrasonic scanning is performed in a relatively dark room the ultrasonographer reduces the gain; in a bright room the gain is increased. It was realised that if reproducible measurements of echodensity or texture were to be made some form of image normalization was essential. Our team has introduced the method of image normalization using blood and adventitia as two reference points with linear (Elatrozy,1998). As a result reproducible measurements of overall plaque echogenicity can be made with a high inter and intra-observer accuracy(Sabetai, 2000; Tegos, 2000).

Finally, our group in Christodoulou(2003), Kyriacou(2007) has shown that it is possible to identify patients at risk of stroke based on texture features extracted from high-resolution ultrasound images of the carotid plaques. For this purpose, multiple texture feature sets and modular neural networks were applied. The developed system(Christodoulou,2003) was able to automatically classify carotid plaques into symptomatic or asymptomatic with a success rate of 73%.

ASSESSMENT OF THE RISK OF STROKE BASED ON MORPHOLOGICAL ANALYSIS

Material

A total of 274 carotid plaque ultrasound images(137 asymptomatic plaques and 137 symptomatic plaques associated with retinal or hemispheric symptoms(33 stroke, 60 TIA, and 44 AF). Patients with cardioembolic symptoms or distant symptoms(> 6 months) were excluded from the study. Asymptomatic plaques were truly asymptomatic if they had never been associated with symptoms in the past where as symptomatic if they had been associated with retinal or hemispheric symptoms(Stroke, TIA or AF), i.e. unstable plaques.

Image Acquisition

The ultrasound images were collected in the Irvine Laboratory for Cardiovascular Investigation and Research, Saint Mary's Hospital, UK, using an ATL(model HDI 3000 - Advanced Technology Laboratories, Seattle, USA) duplex scanner with a 5-10 MHz multifrequency probe. Longitudinal scans were performed using duplex scanning and colour flow imaging. Images were captured according to the protocol mentioned in Nicolaides(2003).

Plaque Segmentation

The plaque identification and segmentation tasks are quite difficult and were carried out manually by a physician or vascular ultrasonographers who are experienced in scanning. The main difficulties are due to the fact that the plaque edges cannot be distinguished from blood based on brightness level difference, or using only texture features, or other measures. Also calcification and acoustic shadows make the problem more complex. Thus, acoustic shadows were excluded. The identification of the outline of hypoechoic plaques was facilitated using a color image indicating the blood flow (see Figure 1). Also, a temporary log image transformation facility was used in order to get a better definition of the edges of the plaque. This guaranteed that the plaque was correctly outlined. The procedure for carrying out the segmentation process, was established by a team of experts and was documented in the ACSRS project protocol(Nicolaides, 2003).

Figure 1 illustrates an ultrasound image with the outline of the carotid plaque and the corresponding color blood flow image. The next step includes feature extraction as described in the following section and Figure 2 illustrates a number of examples of symptomatic and asymptomatic plaques as an expert physician segmented these. The examples were chosen at random. These examples demonstrate the difficulty to distinguish visually between asymptomatic and symptomatic plaques.

Morphological Analysis

Morphological features are motivated from the need to study the basic structure of the plaque. We used two morphological analysis methods in order to quantify morphological features of the plaques. The first one was based on a multilevel approach where the image intensity was thresholded at three different levels, while the second one was based on gray scale morphological analysis.

Morphological features of plaques are strongly associated with events. For example black (echolucent) plaques with white big blobs are considered to be very dangerous. We provide a more detailed discussion on the relationship between morphological methods and clinical expectations in section 3.4.1.

We will next provide a mathematical description of the Pattern Spectrum. In developing the mathematical description, our attempt is to provide an intuition into what the Pattern Spectrum is measuring and how the measurements relate to plaque image analysis. Our presentation is closely related to previously published work in (Dougherty, 1992; Maragos, 1989).

Pattern spectra are defined in terms of translations and dilations of a single structural element. For the morphological analysis carried out in this research we consider the cross '+' structural element. The cross structural element exhibits limited directional selectivity. This is desirable since there is no clearly preferred direction for the analysis. We let the set B to represent the '+' structural element, and define it by its five pixel coordinates

$$B = \{(-1,0),(0,0),(1,0),(0,-1),(0,1)\} \quad (1)$$

We define discrete-set translation by points using

$$B + p = \{(m+i, n+j) : (m,n) \in B\}$$

where

$$p = (i, j) \quad (2)$$

In $B + p$, we are centering the structural element over the point $p = (i, j)$. We define binary dilation using

Figure 1. Selection of a plaque: a.The gray scale and the blood flow colour image are loaded b.User has selected a log transform on the gray scale image for better visualization of the plaque c.The final selected plaque is saved in order to start feature extraction.©2005 IOS Press

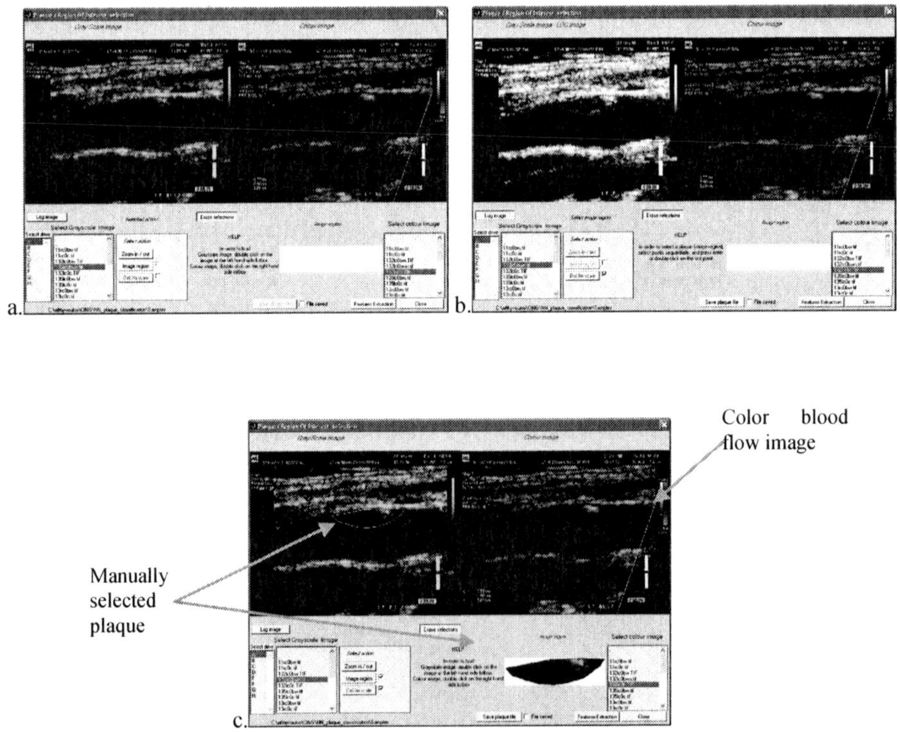

Figure 2. Shows some examples of segmented a) asymptomatic and b) symptomatic plaques. Under each plaque are the type of plaque and several other characteristics.

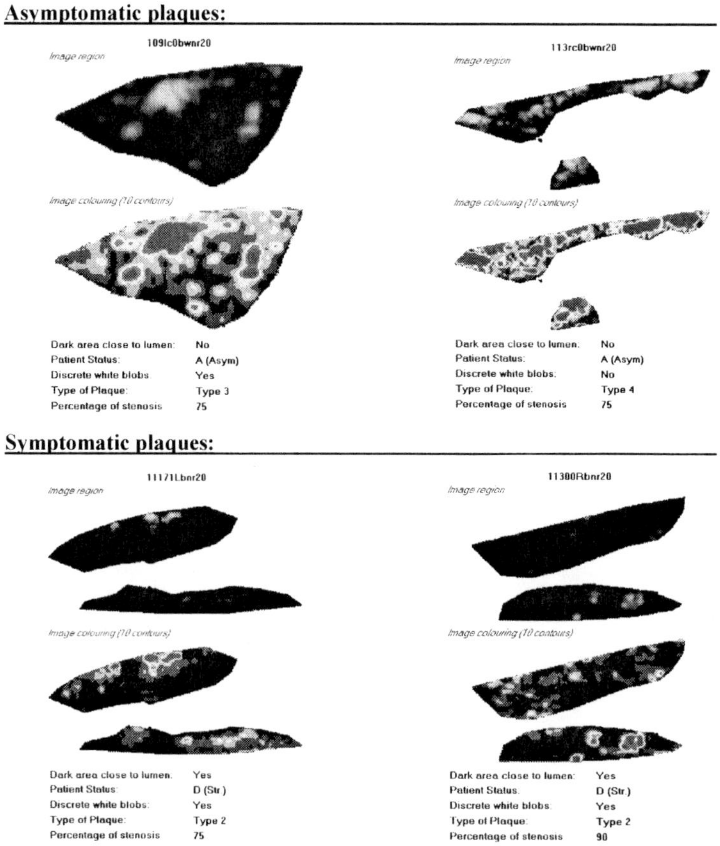

$$X \oplus B = \bigcup_{p \in B} X + p = \{a + b : a \in X \text{ and } b \in B\} \quad (3)$$

The definition leads to the definition of kB that denotes the k-fold expansion of B, and is given by

$$kB = \begin{cases} \{(0,0)\}, & k = 0, \\ \underbrace{B \oplus B \oplus \cdots \oplus B}_{k-1 \text{ dilations}}, & \text{for integer } k > 1. \end{cases} \quad (4)$$

Pattern spectra are defined in terms of openings and closings with kB. We do not have any clear clinical interpretation for the pattern spectra generated by closings with kB. Thus, we will only focus on the pattern spectra generated by openings with kB.

Multilevel Binary Morphological Analysis

In multilevel binary morphological analysis we are interested in extracting different plaque components and investigating their geometric properties. We begin by generating three binary images by thresholding:

$$L = \{(i,j)\text{: such that } f(i,j) < 25\},$$
$$M = \{(i,j)\text{: such that } 25 \le f(i,j) \le 50\},$$
$$H = \{(i,j)\text{: such that } f(i,j) > 50\}. \quad (5)$$

Here, binary image outputs are represented as sets of image coordinates where image intensity meets the threshold criteria. Overall, this multilevel decomposition is closely related to a three-level quantization of the original image intensity. To see this, note that we can simply assign quantization levels to each of the pixels in *L*, *M*, *H* and then use them to provide an approximate reconstruction of the original image.

In *L*, we want to extract dark image regions representing blood, thrombus, lipid or haemorrhage. Similarly, in *H*, we want to extract the collagen and calcified components of the plaque, while in *M*, we want to extract image components that fall between the two. Thus, to decide the threshold levels of (5), we varied the threshold levels so as to extract the desired components from the plaques.

In what follows, we introduce the use of morphological pattern spectra for analyzing the extracted binary images. Our motivation lies in analyzing the structural components of each binary image. We provide a few examples motivated by clinical (visual) observations. Note that if the plaque is captured as a single component in the low intensity image (*L*), or in the high intensity image (*H*), then the plaque is most likely to be stable with little chance for rupture. Also, the plaque will most likely be asymptomatic if the lipid core regions in the low intensity image are made up of small, scattered components. The most dangerous cases occur when image components in the middle image (*M*) appear to be very thin. The risk may be less when image components in the middle image appear relatively thick. We also expect that black (echolucent) plaques with white big blobs to be very dangerous. In this case, we would expect to see large components in both the low image and the high image intensity images (see Figure 3).

We compute normalized pattern spectra for each one of the three binary images *L*, *M*, *H*. Thus, in the following discussion, we will use the symbol *X* to denote any one of the three binary images *L*, *M*, *H*. Binary image erosion is defined using

$$X \odot B = \bigcap_{p \in B} X - p = \{a : B + a \subseteq X\} \quad (6)$$

An opening is then defined in terms of an erosion followed by a dilation:

$$X \circ B = (X \odot B) \oplus B \quad (7)$$

In general, an opening reduces the input image $X \odot B \subseteq X$. However, when the input image can be expressed in terms of translations of the structural element *B*, the opening operation will preserve the input image. We thus write

$$X \circ B = X \quad (8)$$

when

$$X = \bigcup_{p \in S} B + p = B \oplus S = S \oplus B \quad (9)$$

for some set of possible translates *S*. From (8)-(9), we note that an opening will not alter the binary input image provided that the binary image components are "thick and rough enough" to contain all translates of the structural element. On the other hand, any isolated components of *X* that are smaller than *B* will be removed by the opening operation. Here, we define smaller in terms of set operations. We say that a binary image set *A* is smaller than another binary image set *B* if *A* is a proper subset of a translation of *B*. Conversely, any isolated components of *X* that are larger than *B* will not be totally removed from the opening operation (where larger is defined in a similar way).

In general, for any given binary image, an opening outputs an approximation to the input

Figure 3. The three binary level images: (L, M, H) of an asymptomatic and a symptomatic carotid plaque © 2007 Springer(Kyriacou, 2007).

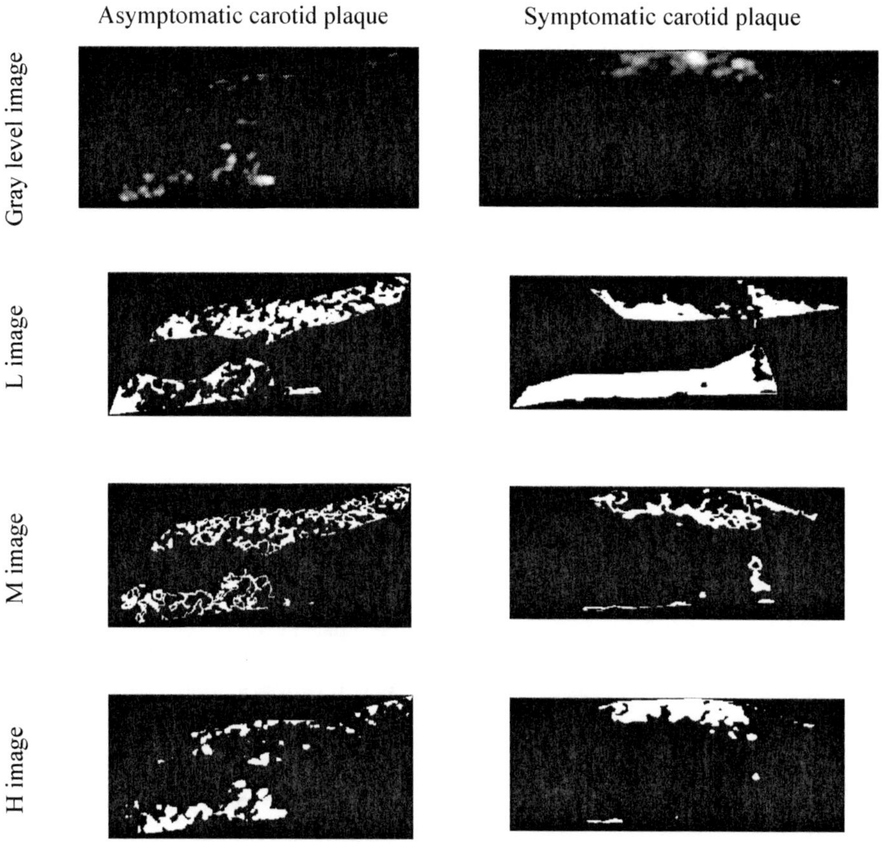

image. This approximation is expressed as a union of translations of the structural element

$$X \circ B = \bigcup_{B+z \subseteq X} B + z \qquad (10)$$

The approximation error image is defined in terms of the set difference $X - X \circ B$. We quantify the approximation error by counting the number of pixels in the difference image. We write $A(S)$ to denote the cardinality of the set S.

For measuring the binary components at different scales, we consider a sequence of openings with the dilated structural element (see (4)):

$$X, X \circ B, X \circ 2B, \ldots, X \circ nB \qquad (11)$$

For our plaque images, we note that the plaques are segmented, and image intensity outside the plaque is assigned to zero (see Figure 1). Thus, for a sufficiently large value of k, kB will outgrow the support of the plaque. When this happens, the opening operation will return the empty-set image. We thus pick n to be the smallest integer for which $X \circ (n+1)B = \varnothing$.

For computing (11), we note that a single opening is needed each time, since the openings can be computed recursively using $X \circ (n+1)B = (X \circ nB) \circ B$. It is also clear from this recursive relationship that the openings generate decreasing images

$$X \circ nB \subseteq \ldots \subseteq X \circ 2B \subseteq X \circ B \subseteq X \quad (12)$$

with decreasing areas

$$A(X \circ nB) \leq \ldots \leq A(X \circ 2B) \leq A(X \circ B) \leq A(X) \quad (13)$$

We form the set difference images using

$$\begin{aligned} d_0(X; B) &= X - X \circ B \\ d_1(X; B) &= X \circ B - X \circ 2B \\ &\vdots \\ d_{n-1}(X; B) &= X \circ (n-1)B - X \circ nB. \end{aligned} \quad (14)$$

The difference images are orthogonal with respect to set intersection

$$d_i(X; B) \cap d_j(X; B) = \varnothing \text{ when } i \neq j \quad (15)$$

We can reconstruct the image using the difference images

$$\begin{aligned} X &= (X \circ nB) \cup \left(\bigcup_{i=0}^{n-1} d_i(X; B)\right) \\ &= \bigcup_{i=0}^{n} d_i(X; B) \end{aligned} \quad (16)$$

We think of the image decomposition given by (16) as a multiscale decomposition where the difference images $d_i(f; B)$ represent information captured at the i-th scale.

The pattern spectrum is also defined in terms of the number of elements in the difference images

$$PS_X(n, B) = A(d_n(X; B)) \quad (17)$$

In (17), we note that the pattern spectra vary with the size of the plaque.

To remove this dependency, we consider a probability density function (*pdf*) measure defined as

$$pdf_X(k, B) = A(d_k(X; B)) / A(X)$$
for $k \geq 0$. (18)

In (18), we note that the normalization is motivated by the reconstruction formula (see (16)). Given the *pdf*-measure, we can also construct the cumulative distribution function (*cdf*) using

$$cdf_f(k, B) = \begin{cases} 0, & k = 0, \\ \sum_{r=0}^{k-1} pdf_f(r, B), & n+1 \geq k > 0. \end{cases} \quad (19)$$

Gray Scale Morphological Analysis

For gray scale morphological analysis, we assume that the input image $f(i, j)$ denotes the (positive) gray scale image intensity at pixel (i, j). At every pixel, for structural element B, we define gray scale dilation by

$$(f \oplus B)(i, j) = \max_{(m,n) \in B+(i,j)} f(m, n) \quad (20)$$

which represents the maximum intensity value over the support of the translated structural element. Similarly, for symmetric structural elements (as is the case for '+'), we define gray scale erosion using the minimum value:

$$(f \odot B)(i, j) = \min_{(m,n) \in B+(i,j)} f(m, n) \quad (21)$$

We then define openings using the new definitions for grey-scale erosions and dilations. Instead of the subset relation, we now have that an opening reduces image intensity in the sense that $f \circ B \leq f$ for every pixel.

Due to the bounds of the extend of the plaque, we are again limited in the maximum number of openings that make sense. Here, instead of the empty set, the limit is the zero-image. The difference images are formed in the same way. For the reconstruction, we use a finite sum instead of a union:

$$\begin{aligned} f &= (f \circ nB) + \left(\sum_{i=0}^{n-1} d_i(f; B)\right) \\ &= \sum_{i=0}^{n} d_i(f; B). \end{aligned} \quad (22)$$

For the gray scale definition of the pattern spectrum we use

$$PS_f(k, B) = \|d_k(f; B)\| \quad (23)$$

where

$$\|f\| = \sum_{(i,j)} f(i,j) \quad (24)$$

We now normalize by the original image intensity

$$pdf_f(k, B) = \|d_k(f; B)\| / \|f\|, \text{ for } k \geq 0 \quad (25)$$

Morphological Analysis Application to Atherosclerotic Carotid Plaques

We begin with a summary. For each plaque we compute the three binary images *L*, *M*, *H* as outlined in (5). For each binary image, we compute the *pdf* and *cdf* distributions as outlined in (18)-(19), for $k = 0,...,70$. Similarly, for gray scale morphological image analysis, we compute the *pdf* and *cdf* distributions based on gray scale erosions and dilations (see (25)). Thus, we compute *pdf* and *cdf* measures on the original gray scale image and the three binary images that are derived from it.

For each one of the four images, the positively-indexed *pdf* and *cdf* measures provide us with normalized size distributions of the white (or brighter) blob-components. These measures are based on binary and gray scale openings. Some examples are shown in Figure 4.

Classification Techniques

The KNN Classifier

The statistical pattern recognition K Nearest Neighbor(KNN) classifier was applied for classifying carotid plaques into two groups(asymptomatic and symptomatic). In the KNN algorithm in order to classify a new pattern, its k nearest neighbors from the training set are identified. The new pattern is classified to the most frequent class among its neighbors based on a similarity measure that is usually the Euclidean distance. In this work the KNN carotid plaque classification system was implemented for values of k = 1, 3, 5, 7 and 9 using for input the eight texture feature sets and morphology features described above(Christodoulou, 2003).

The PNN Classifier

A Probabilistic Neural Network (PNN) classifier was used for developing classification models for the problem under study. The PNN falls within the category of nearest-neighbor classifiers(Candela, 1995). For a given vector **w** to be classified, an activation a_i is computed for each of the two classes of plaques ($i = 1,...,2$). The activation a_i is defined to be the total distance of **w** from each of the M_i prototype feature vectors $\mathbf{x}_j^{(i)}$ that belong to the *i*-th class:

$$a_i = \sum_{j=1}^{M_i} \exp\left[-\beta\left(\mathbf{w} - \mathbf{x}_j^{(i)}\right)^T \left(\mathbf{w} - \mathbf{x}_j^{(i)}\right)\right] \quad (30)$$

where β is a smoothing factor. The normalized activations $\tilde{a}_i = a_i / \sum_{i=1}^{N} a_i$ provide a confidence estimate for the hypothesis that **w** belongs to class *i*. We then classify **w** into the class that yields the highest confidence. An important advantage of the PNN is that it provides confidence estimates for our classification decision. Also, to avoid dependence on the smoothing factor β, the value of β was set to the one that yielded the minimum misclassification error on the training set.

The SVM Classifier

The Support Vector Machine(SVM) was also used for developing classification models for the problem. The method is initially based on nonlinear mapping of initial data set using a function *φ(.)* and then the identification of a hyperplane which is able to achieve the separation of two categories of data. The PNN network performance is compared to an SVM classifier with Gaussian Radial Basis Function(RBF) kernels. Details about the implementation of the SVM algorithm used can be found in(Joachims, 1999).

Feature Selection

A popular way to reduce the dimensionality of a feature vector is Principal Component Analysis (PCA)(Duda,2001). This method can be used in cases when the input features vector is large but the components of this vector are highly correlated. After applying PCA, the data set is represented by a reduced number of uncorrelated features while retaining most of its information content. In this study feature sets were reduced to smaller dimension sets by using only the components which contributed for 98% of the variance in the data set.

Figure 4. Results from a sequence of openings using a '+' structural element on a gray level and a low-intensity image(-image in multi-level binary morphology) of an asymptomatic carotid plaque. The radius of the structural element ranges from 1 to 5 pixels (plotted at 20 pixels/mm). © 2007 Springer (Kyriacou, 2007)

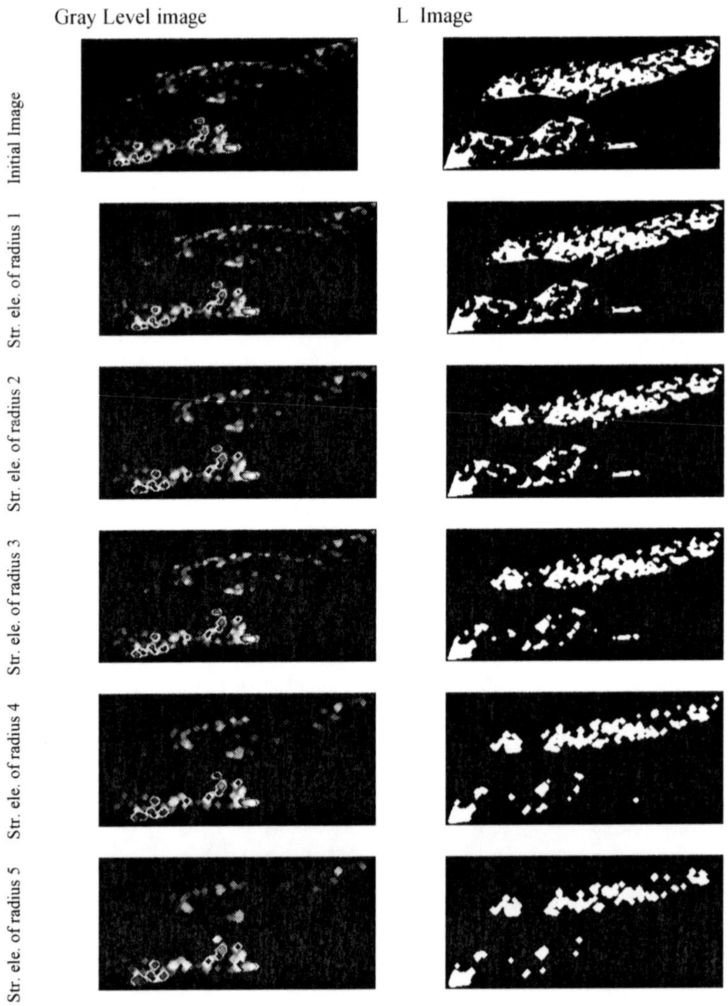

Classification Tests

The leave-one-out estimate was used for validating all the classification models. A total of 274 subsets of size 273 were used for training the classifiers, and the performances of the classifiers were evaluated on the remaining one subset. The performances of the classifier systems were measured using the receiver operating characteristics (ROC) curve parameters . The parameters calculated for ROC curves are the numbers of: (i) true positive (TP), (ii) false positives(FP), (iii) false negatives(FN), and (iv) true negatives(TN). We also compute the Sensitivity(SE) and Specificity(SP. For the overall performance, we provide the correct classification(CC) rate which gives the percentage of correctly classified plaques(Kyriacou, 2007).

RESULTS

The median of the estimated *pdfs* and *cdfs* extracted from the plaques can be seen in Figures 5 and 6. All figures are plotted against the radial size of the structural element. We have divided the results into the two categories of multilevel binary and gray scale morphological analysis.

Results from Multilevel Binary Morphological Analysis

From the results, we observe that the median symptomatic *cdf* is *stochastically* smaller than the median asymptomatic *cdf* for the *L*-images. This means that the median *cdf* for the symptomatic cases assumes equal or smaller values than the asymptomatic *cdf*.

For the *M*-images, the median *cdf* of the asymptomatic cases turned out to be *stochastically* larger to that of TIA&Stroke but smaller to that of Amaurosis Fugax; thus the median *cdfs* of asymptomatic and symptomatic plaques are almost equal. Due to these observations, as expected, the classification results from the *M*-images where relatively lower. Finally, for the *H*-images, the median symptomatic *cdf* turned out to be *stochastically* larger than the asymptomatic *cdf*.

We attempt to relate our measurements to clinical expectations for a known type of dangerous plaques. Consider the case of having a plaque characterized by a dark background with isolated white blobs. This description characterizes dangerous symptomatic plaques. In this case, the uniformity in the dark regions suggests that the symptomatic cdf plot in the *L*-image will be slow to rise, resulting in a cdf that is stochastically smaller than that of the median asymptomatic case. On the other hand, the isolated white blobs will force the cdf of the *H*-image to be stochastically larger than that of the median asymptomatic case. Thus, in this case, both of these observations are in agreement with our measurements. Naturally, we will also need to investigate how to extend these observations for different types of plaques(also see Sterpetti,(1988)).

The *cdfs* and *pdfs* of all plaques were used with the PNN and SVM classifiers. Both classifiers were tested on both the *pdf* and *cdf* feature sets. The first set included features produced for the whole range of scales(1-70) while the second set included the pattern spectra of selected scales(*L*-Images:1,2,3,4,5 , *M*-Images: 3,4,9,11,12, *H*-Images: 2,11,12,15,18, (Panayiotou, 2006) These scales were selected because of their discriminatory power as evaluated using the C4.5 decision trees algorithm(Panayiotou, 2006; Han 2000). The C4.5 was run and the pattern spectra scale with the highest discriminative score was computed. This best scale was then removed and the C4.5 was run again to compute the next best scale. The procedure was repeated 5 times. The dimensionality of the entire pdf/cdf feature vectors from both sets was also reduced using Principal Components Analysis(PCA). For PCA, we selected a small number of components that accounted for 98% of the total variance.

Figure 5. Corresponding median values of the pdfs and cdfs of asymptomatic versus symptomatic plaques for the three different levels(L, M, H images) of multilevel binary morphological analysis. The first line of each sub-plot represents the median cdf and pdf for Asymptomatic vs. Amaurosis Fugax vs.(TIA&Stroke) plaques, while the second line represents the median cdf and pdf for Asymptomatic Vs Symptomatic plaques. In the plot, radius refers to radial spread of the structural element. © 2007 Springer(Kyriacou, 2007)

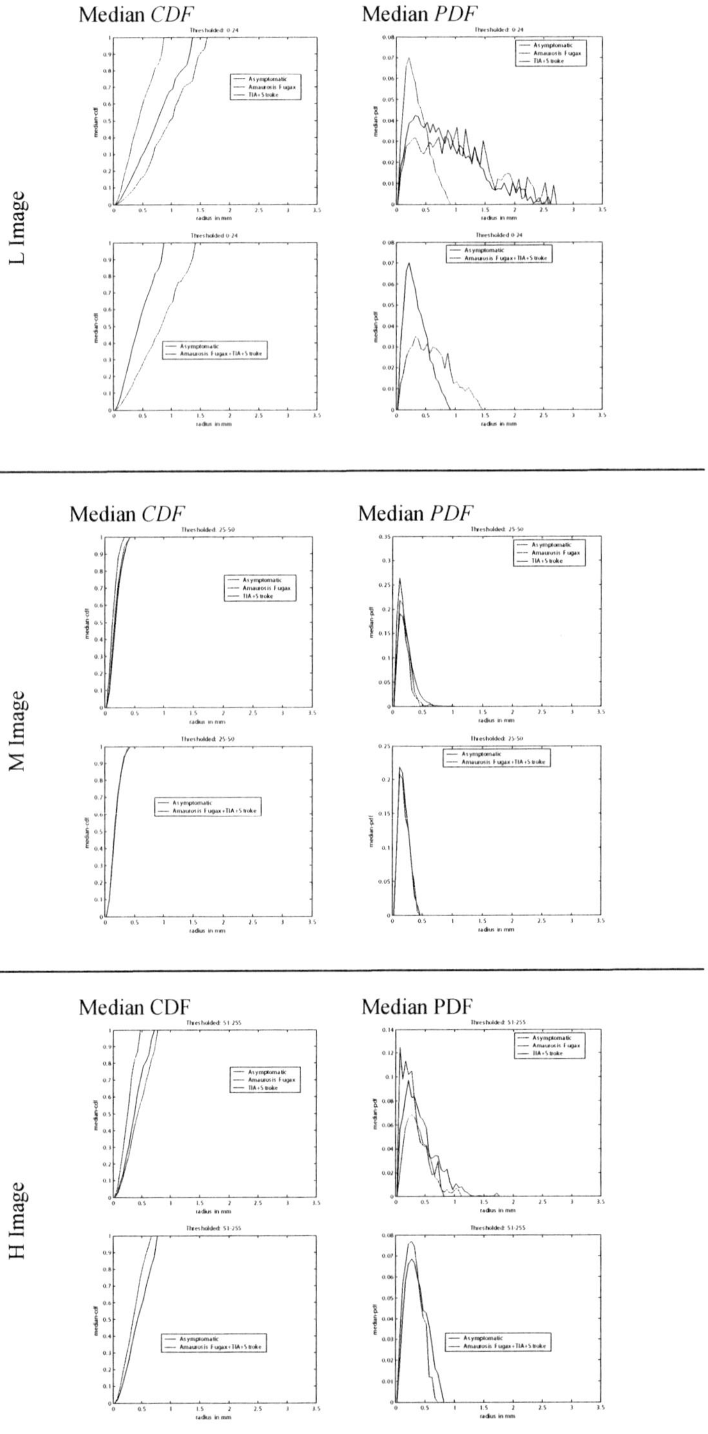

Figure 6. Corresponding median values of the pdfs and cdfs of asymptomatic versus symptomatic plaques for the gray scale morphological analysis. The first row represents the median cdf and pdf for Asymptomatic Vs Amaurosis Fugax Vs(TIA & Stroke) plaques, while the second represents median cdf and pdf for Asymptomatic Vs Symptomatic plaques. © 2007 Springer(Kyriacou, 2007)

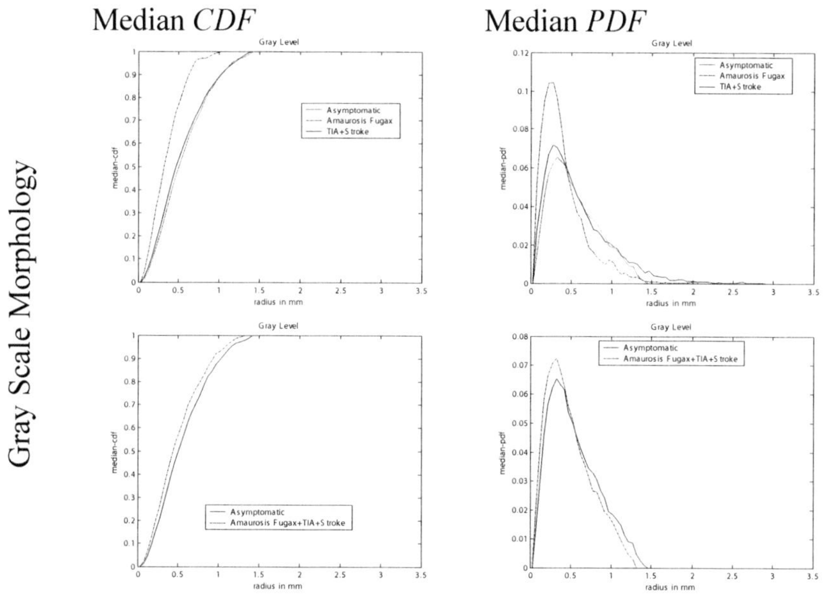

Table 1 presents the results of the ROC analysis for the SVM and PNN classifiers for the different feature sets investigated. Classifiers where tested using features extracted from the *L*, *M* and *H* images and the combination of the three. The highest percentage of correct classifications score was 73.7% and was achieved using the SVM classifier on the features extracted from the *L*-images(*cdf* scales: 1-70 + PCA). For PNN, the highest percentage of correct classifications score achieved was 70.4% for *pdf* scales: 1-70 + PCA. The combination of the three feature sets gave the same highest results as those achieved with the *L*-images feature set.

Results from Gray Scale Morphological Analysis

From the results, we can observe that the median symptomatic *cdf* is *stochastically* larger than the median asymptomatic *cdf*. Recall that this means that the median *cdf* for the symptomatic cases assumes equal or larger values than the asymptomatic *cdf*. The median and box plots of *pdfs* and *cdfs* for gray scale morphological can be seen in Figure 6.

In turn, for the dangerous type of symptomatic plaque discussed in section 4.1, this observation appears to be in agreement with our expectations. Here, the isolated white blobs against a dark background in the symptomatic plaques leads to a larger concentration of the detected components in the lower scales of the pattern spectrum, as compared to the asymptomatic cases. In turn, as for the *H*-images, this cause a rise in the symptomatic *cdf* as compared to the median asymptomatic *cdf* (also see Mavrommatis, 2006).

Again the *cdfs* and *pdfs* of all plaques were used with the PNN and SVM classifiers. Both classifiers were tested on both the *pdf* and *cdf* feature sets.

Table 2. Percentage of correct classifications(%CC), percentage of false positives(%FP), percentage of false negatives(%FN), percentage sensitivity(%SE) and percentage specificity(%SP) of Multi Level morphological features using the SVM and PNN classifiers, for the L, M and H images. Classification models developed for two classes using the leave one out method, with 137 symptomatic and 137 asymptomatic plaques.

	SVM classifier	**%CC**	**%FP**	**%FN**	**%SE**	**%SP**
L Image	SVM rbf spread = 0.4 **PCA** for *pdf* scales 1,2,3,4,5,6	70.80	42.34	16.06	83.94	57.66
	SVM rbf spread = 9.0510 *pdf* scales 1,2,3,4,5,6	69.71	51.09	9.49	90.51	48.91
	SVM rbf spread = 0.1 **PCA** for *cdf* scales 1-70	**73.72**	**36.50**	**16.06**	**83.94**	**63.50**
	SVM rbf spread = 12.8 *cdf* scales 1-70	72.26	37.23	18.25	81.75	62.77
	SVM rbf spread = 1.6 **PCA** for *pdf* scales 1-70	70.07	43.07	16.79	83.21	56.93
	SVM rbf spread = 9.0510 *pdf* scales 1-70	70.80	41.61	16.79	83.21	58.39
	Average Values	71.23	41.97	15.57	84.43	58.03

	PNN classifier	**%CC**	**%FP**	**%FN**	**%SE**	**%SP**
L Image	PNN spread =5 **PCA** for *pdf* scales 1,2,3,4,5,6	66.79	62.77	3.65	96.35	37.23
	PNN spread =5 *pdf* scales 1,2,3,4,5,6	66.79	63.50	2.92	97.08	36.50
	PNN spread =5 **PCA** for *cdf* scales 1-70	**70.07**	**37.96**	**21.90**	**78.10**	**62.04**
	PNN spread =5 *cdf* scales 1-70	**70.07**	**37.96**	**21.90**	**78.10**	**62.04**
	PNN spread =5 **PCA** for *pdf* scales 1-70	**70.44**	**40.88**	**18.25**	**81.75**	**59.12**
	PNN spread =5 *pdf* scales 1-70	69.71	35.77	24.82	75.18	64.23
	Average Values	68.98	46.47	15.57	84.43	53.53

	SVM classifier	**%CC**	**%FP**	**%FN**	**%SE**	**%SP**
M Image	SVM rbf spread = 0.1414 **PCA** for *pdf* scales 3,4,9,11,12	**60.58**	**45.99**	**32.85**	**67.15**	**54.01**
	SVM rbf spread = 0.1 *pdf* scales 3,4,9,11,12	59.49	47.45	33.58	66.42	52.55
	SVM rbf spread = 2.2627 **PCA** for *cdf* scales 1-70	55.47	34.31	54.74	45.26	65.69
	SVM rbf spread = 0.2 *cdf* scales 1-70	59.12	29.93	51.82	48.18	70.07
	SVM rbf spread = 0.4 **PCA** for *pdf* scales 1-70	58.39	37.96	45.26	54.74	62.04
	SVM rbf spread = 0.1 *pdf* scales 1-70	58.39	37.96	45.26	54.74	62.04
	Average Values	58.57	38.93	43.92	56.08	61.07

continued on the following page

Table 2. continued

M Image	PNN classifier	%CC	%FP	%FN	%SE	%SP
	PNN spread =5 **PCA** for *pdf* scales 3,4,9,11,12	48.18	10.95	92.70	7.30	89.05
	PNN spread =5 *pdf* scales 3,4,9,11,12	48.18	10.95	92.70	7.30	89.05
	PNN spread =5 **PCA** for *cdf* scales 1-70	49.27	9.49	91.97	8.03	90.51
	PNN spread =5 *cdf* scales 1-70	48.91	11.68	90.51	9.49	88.32
	PNN spread =5 **PCA** for *pdf* scales 1-70	51.46	9.49	87.59	12.41	90.51
	PNN spread =5 *pdf* scales 1-70	51.09	9.49	88.32	11.68	90.51
	Average Values	49.52	10.34	90.63	9.37	89.66

H Image	SVM classifier	%CC	%FP	%FN	%SE	%SP
	SVM rbf spread = 9.0510 **PCA** for *pdf* scales 2,11,12,15,18,19	58.76	47.45	35.04	64.96	52.55
	SVM rbf spread =12.8 *pdf* scales 2,11,12,15,18,19	58.39	47.45	35.77	64.23	52.55
	SVM rbf spread = 6.4 **PCA** for *cdf* scales 1-70	59.12	42.34	39.42	60.58	57.66
	SVM rbf spread = 0.4 *cdf* scales 1-70	59.12	41.61	40.15	59.85	58.39
	SVM rbf spread = 9.0510 **PCA** for *pdf* scales 1-70	**62.04**	**40.88**	**35.04**	**64.96**	**59.12**
	SVM rbf spread = 0.8 *pdf* scales 1-70	60.22	45.26	34.31	65.69	54.74
	Average Values	59.61	44.17	36.62	63.38	55.84

H Image	PNN classifier	%CC	%FP	%FN	%SE	%SP
	PNN spread =5 **PCA** for *pdf* scales 2,11,12,15,18,19	43.80	24.82	87.59	12.41	75.18
	PNN spread =5 *pdf* scales 2,11,12,15,18,19	43.80	24.82	87.59	12.41	75.18
	PNN spread =5 **PCA** for *cdf* scales 1-70	**59.12**	**48.18**	**33.58**	**66.42**	**51.82**
	PNN spread =5 *cdf* scales 1-70	58.76	48.91	33.58	66.42	51.09
	PNN spread =5 **PCA** for *pdf* scales 1-70	57.66	64.23	20.44	79.56	35.77
	PNN spread =5 *pdf* scales 1-70	55.47	65.69	23.36	76.64	34.31
	Average Values	53.1	46.11	47.69	52.31	53.89

continued on the following page

Table 2. continued

	SVM classifier	%CC	%FP	%FN	%SE	%SP
Combination L M H Images	SVM rbf spread = 6.4 **PCA** for *pdf* scales (Low: 1,2,3,4,5,6) (Med:3,4,9,11,12)(High:19,12,15,11,18,2)	71.90	43.07	13.14	86.86	56.93
	SVM rbf spread =6.4 *pdf*scales(Low:1,2,3,4,5,6) (Med:3,4,9,11,12)(High:19,12,15,11,18,2)	71.90	45.26	10.95	89.05	54.74
	SVM rbf spread = 12.8 **PCA** for *cdf* scales 1-210	69.34	43.80	17.52	82.48	56.20
	SVM rbf spread = 2.2627 *cdf* scales 1-210	71.90	39.42	16.79	83.21	60.58
	SVM rbf spread = 9.0510 **PCA** for *pdf* scales 1-210	70.80	42.34	16.06	83.94	57.66
	SVM rbf spread = 6.4 *pdf* scales 1-210	**73.36**	**39.42**	**13.87**	**86.13**	**60.58**
	Average Values	71.53	42.22	14.72	85.28	57.78

	PNN classifier	%CC	%FP	%FN	%SE	%SP
Combination L M H Images	PNN spread =5 **PCA** for *pdf* scales (Low: 1,2,3,4,5,6) (Med:3,4,9,11,12)(High:19,12,15,11,18,2)	69.34	53.28	8.03	91.97	46.72
	PNN spread =5 *pdf* scales (Low: 1,2,3,4,5,6) (Med:3,4,9,11,12)(High:19,12,15,11,18,2)	69.71	54.01	6.57	93.43	45.99
	PNN spread =5 **PCA** for *cdf* scales 1-210	69.71	37.96	22.63	77.37	62.04
	PNN spread =5 *cdf* scales 1-210	68.61	40.15	22.63	77.37	59.85
	PNN spread =5 **PCA** for *pdf* scales 1-210	**70.44**	**42.34**	**16.79**	**83.21**	**57.66**
	PNN spread =5 *pdf* scales 1-210	**70.07**	**38.69**	**21.17**	**78.83**	**61.31**
	Average Values	69.65	44.41	16.3	83.7	55.6

The first set included features produced for the whole range of scales (1-70) while the second set included the pattern spectra of selected scales(2, 3, 5, 10, 21, and 23) (Panayiotou, 2006), using the C4.5 decision trees algorithm (see section 5.1).

FUTURE TRENDS

What was presented in this chapter is actually an overview of some of the new techniques currently applied for the estimation of the risk of stroke using ultrasound images. Future trends include analysis of plaque video for the estimation of plaque motion; as well as the introduction of several other biochemical measurements or gene analysis models so as to improve the stroke risk estimation models.

CONCLUSION

Concluding, multilevel binary and gray scale morphological analysis features can help us

Table 3. Percentage of correct classifications(%CC), percentage of false positives(%FP), percentage of false negatives(%FN), percentage sensitivity(%SE) and percentage specifity(%SP) of Gray Scale morphological features using the SVM and PNN classifiers. Classification models developed for two classes using the leave one out method, and 137 symptomatic and 137 asymptomatic plaques.

	SVM classifier	%CC	%FP	%FN	%SE	%SP
Gray Scale	SVM rbf spread = 2.2627 **PCA** for *pdf* scales 2,3,5,10,21,23	**66.79**	20.44	45.99	54.01	79.56
	SVM rbf spread = 0.5657 *pdf* scales 2,3,5,10,21,23	65.33	28.47	40.88	59.12	71.53
	SVM rbf spread = 2.2627 **PCA** for *cdf* scales 1-70	63.14	42.34	31.39	68.61	57.66
	SVM rbf spread = 2.2627 *cdf* scales 1-70	62.41	32.12	43.07	56.93	67.88
	SVM rbf spread = 1.1314 **PCA** for *pdf* scales 1-70	60.22	43.80	35.77	64.23	56.20
	SVM rbf spread = 0.5657 *pdf* scales 1-70	**63.14**	**36.50**	**37.23**	**62.77**	**63.50**
	Average Values	63.51	33.95	39.06	60.95	66.06

	PNN classifier	%CC	%FP	%FN	%SE	%SP
Gray Scale	PNNspread =5 **PCA** for *pdf* scales 2,3,5,10,21,23	56.57	22.63	64.23	35.77	77.37
	PNN spread =5 *pdf* scales 2,3,5,10,21,23	56.57	22.63	64.23	35.77	77.37
	PNN spread =5 **PCA** for *cdf* scales 1-70	60.58	36.50	42.34	57.66	63.50
	PNN spread =5 *cdf* scales 1-70	**62.04**	**35.77**	**40.15**	**59.85**	**64.23**
	PNN spread =5 **PCA** for *pdf* scales 1-70	58.76	42.34	40.15	59.85	57.66
	PNN spread =5 *pdf* scales 1-70	60.22	48.91	30.66	69.34	51.09
	Average Values	59.12	34.8	46.96	53.04	65.2

quantify the distribution of blob elements in the atherosclerotic carotid plaques. We have found that there is significant overlap between pattern spectra coming from symptomatic and asymptomatic plaques. Most of the discriminating power was concentrated in the smaller components for lower scales. These results are comparable to results produced using texture analysis algorithms of a similar dataset(Christodoulou, 2003;Kyriacou 2007) as well as results reported by another group(Wilhjelm,1998).

In previous work carried out by our group the highest percentage of correct classifications was 73% using texture features and the self-organising map (SOM) classifier(Christodoulou 2003). Furthermore it was shown in that binary morphological analysis features compare well with the most successful texture feature sets and provide additional information for the identification of individuals at risk of stroke.

REFERENCES

AbuRahma, A. F., Kyer, P. D., Robinson, P. A., et al. (1998). The correlation of ultrasonic carotid plaque morphology and carotid plaque hemorrhage: clinical implications. *Surgery, 124*, 721-8.

Aldoori, M. I., Baird, R. N., Al-Sam, S. Z., et al. (1987). Duplex scanning and plaque histology in cerebral ischaemia. *European Journal of Vascular Surgery, 1*, 159-64.

Arnold, J. A. C., Modaresi, K. B., Thomas, N., et al. (1999) Carotid plaque characterization by duplex scanning. Observer error may undermine current clinical trials. *Stroke, 30*, 61-5.

Biasi, G. M., Mingazzini, P. M., Baronio, L., Piglionica, M. R., Ferrari, S. A., Elatrozy, T. S., Nicolaides, A. N. (1998) Carotid plaque characterization using digital image processing and its potential in future studies of carotid endarterectomy and angioplasty. *Journal of Endovascular Surgery, 5(3)*, 240-6.

Candela, G. T., Grother, P. J., Watson, C. I., Wilkinson, R. A., & Wilson, C. L. (1995). *PCASYS – a pattern-level classification automation system for fingerprints.* Technical report. NISTIR 5647: National Institute of Standards and Technology.

Christodoulou, C. I., Michaelides, S. C., & Pattichis, C. S. (2003). Multi-feature texture analysis for the classification of clouds in satellite imagery. *IEEE Transactions on Geoscience and Remote Sensing, 41(11)*, 2662-2668.

Christodoulou, C. I., Pattichis, C. S., Pantziaris, M., & Nicolaides, A. (2003). Texture Based Classification of Atherosclerotic Carotid Plaques. *IEEE Transactions on Medical Imaging, 22*, 902-912.

Dougherty, E. R. (1992). *An Introduction to Morphological Image Processing*, Belingham. Washington. SPIE Optical Engineering Press.

Dougherty, E. R., Astola, J. (1994). *An Introduction to Nonlinear Image Processing*, Belingham. Washington, SPIE Optical Engineering Press.

Duda, O. R., Hart, E. P., & Stork, D. G. (2001). *Pattern Classification* (pp. 259-265), Willey.

Elatrozy, T., Nicolaides, A., Tegos, T., et al. (1998). The objective characterisation of ultrasonic carotid plaque features. *European Journal of Vascular and Endovascular Surgery, 16*, 223-30.

El-Barghouti, N., Nicolaides, A. N., Tegos, T., et al. (1996). The relative effect of carotid plaque heterogeneity and echogenicity on ipsilateral cerebral infarction and symptoms of cerebrovascular disease. *International Angiology, 15*, 300-6.

European carotid plaque study group (1995). Carotid artery plaque composition - Relationship to clinical presentation and ultrasound B-mode imaging. *European Journal of Vascular and Endovascular Surgery, 10,* 23-30.

Geroulakos, G., Ramaswami, G., Nicolaides, A., et al. (1993). Characterisation of symptomatic and asymptomatic carotid plaques using high-resolution real-time ultrasonography. *British Journal of Surgery, 80,* 1274-7.

Giannoni, M. F., Spezial, F., Faraglia, E., et al. (1991). Minor asymptomatic carotid stenosis contralateral to carotid endarterectomy (CEA). Our experience. *European Journal of Vascular Surgery, 5*, 237-45.

Gray-Weale, A. C., Graham, J. C., Burnett, J. R., et al. (1988). Carotid artery atheroma: comparison of preoperative B-mode ultrasound appearance with carotid endarterectomy specimen pathology. *Journal of Cardiovascular Surgery, 29,* 676-81.

Gronholdt, M. L., Nordestgaard, B. G., Schroeder, T. V., Vostrup, S., & Sillesen, H. (2001). Ultrasonic echolucent carotid plaques predict future strokes. *Circulation, 104,* 68-73.

Han, J. M. Kamber (2000). *Data Mining: Concepts and Techniques*. Morgan Kaufmann.

Joachims, T. (1999). Advances in Kernel Methods - Support Vector Learning In B. Schölkopf, C. Burges, & A. Smola (Eds.), *Making large-Scale SVM Learning Practical.*. MIT Press.

Joakimsen, O., Bønaa, K. H., Mathiesen, E. B., et al. (2000). Prediction of Mortality by Ultrasound Screening of a General Population for Carotid Stenosis: The Tromsø Study. *Stroke*, *31*, 1871-6.

Johnson, J. M., Kennelly, M. M., Decesare, D., et al. (1985). Natural history of asymptomatic carotid plaque. *Archives of Surgery*, *120*, 1010-2.

Kagawa, R., Moritake, K., Shima, T., et al. (1996). Validity of B-mode ultrasonographic findings in patients undergoing carotid endarterectomy in comparison with angiographic and clinicopathologic features. *Stroke*, *27*, 700-5.

Kardoulas, D. G., Katsamouris, A. N., Gallis, P. T. et al. (1996). Ultrasonographic and histologic characteristics of symptom-free and symptomatic carotid plaque. *Cardiovascular Surgery, 4,* 580-90.

Kyriacou, E., Pattichis, M., Pattichis, C. S., Mavrommatis, A., Christodoulou, C. I., Kakkos,S., Nicolaides, A. (2007). Classification of Atherosclerotic Carotid Plaques Using Morphological Analysis on Ultrasound images. *Journal of Applied Intelligence,* Springer. ISSN: 0924-669X (Print) 1573-7497 (Online).

Langsfeld, M., Gray-Weale, A. C., & Lusby, R. J. (1989). The role of plaque morphology and diameter reduction in the development of new symptoms in asymptomatic carotid arteries. *Journal of Vascular Surgery*, *9,* 548-57.

Leahy, A. L., McCollum, P. T., Feeley, T. M., et al. (1988). Duplex ultrasonography and selection of patients for carotid endarterectomy: Plaque morphology or luminal narrowing? *Journal of Vascular Surgery*, *8,* 558-62.

Maragos, P. (1989). Pattern spectrum and multiscale shape representation. *IEEE Transactions on Pattern Analysis and Machine Intelligence*, *11*, 701-715.

Mavrommatis, A. (2006). *Morphology of Carotid US Images*, MSc thesis, Univ. of Cyprus, Nicosia, Cyprus.

Nicolaides, A., Sabetai, M., Kakkos, S.M., Dhanjil, S., Tegos, T., Stevens, J. M., Thomas, D. J., Francis, S., Griffin, M., Geroulakos, G., Ioannidou, E., & Kyriacou, E. (2003). The Asymptomatic, Carotid, Stenosis and Risk of Stroke (ACSRS) study. *International Angiology*, *22(3),* 263-272.

O'Donnell, T. F. Jr., Erdoes, L., Mackey, W. C., et al. (1985). Correlation of B-mode ultrasound imaging and arteriography with pathologic findings at carotid endarterectomy. *Archives of Surgery*, *120*, 443-9.

Panagiotou, S. (2006). *Classification of Plaques Using SVM Class.* MSc thesis, Univ. of Cyprus, Nicosia Cyprus.

Reilly, L. M., Lusby, R. J., Hughes, L., et al. (1983). Carotid plaque histology using real-time ultrasonography. Clinical and therapeutic implications. *American Journal of Surgery, 146*, 188-93.

Sabetai, M. M., Tegos, T. J., Nicolaides, A. N. et. al. (2000). Reproducibility of computer-quantified carotid plaque echogenicity. Can we overcome the subjectivity?. *Stroke*, *39(9),* 2189-2196.

Salonen, R. M., Nyyssonen, K., Kaikkonen, J., et al. (2003). Six-year effect of combined vitamin C and E supplementation on atherosclerotic progression: the Antioxidant Supplementation in Atherosclerosis Prevention (ASAP) Study. *Circulation, 107*, 947-53.

Schmidt, C., Fagerberg, B., Wikstrand, J., et al. (2003). On behalf of the RIS study group. Multiple risk factor intervention reduces cardiovascular risk in hypertensive patients with echolucent plaques in the carotid artery. *Journal of Internal Medicine*, *253*, 430-8.

Sterpetti, A. V., Schultz, R. D., Feldhaus, R. J., et al. (1988). Ultrasonographic features of carotid plaque and the risk of subsequent neurologic deficits. *Surgery, 104,* 652-60.

Tegos, T. J., Sametai, M. M., Nicolaides, A. N. et al. (2000). Comparability of the ultrasonic tissue characteristics of carotid plaques. *Journal of Ultrasound Medicine, 19,* 399-407.

Widder, B., Paulat, K., Hachspacher, J., et al. (1990). Morphological characterization of carotid artery stenoses by ultrasound duplex scanning. *Ultrasound in Medicine and Biology, 16,* 349-54.

Wilhjelm, J. E., Gronholdt, L. M., et al. (1998). Quantitative Analysis of Ultrasound B-Mode Images of Carotid Atherosclerotic Plaque: Correlation with Visual Classification and Histological Examination. *IEEE Transactions on Medical Imaging, 17*(6), 910-922.

KEY TERMS

Stroke: Rapidly developing loss of brain functions due to malfunction in the blood supply to the brain. This can be due to Ischemia(lack of blood supply) or due to haemorrhage.

Gray Scale Ultrasound Carotid Plaque Image: Image produced by using B-Mode ultrasound technique on carotid arteries

Morphology Analysis: Analysis of the morphology of images, describes the structuring elements on an image with no directional sensitivity

Assessment of the Risk of Stroke: Evaluation of the risk that a person has for a stroke event, based on several risk factors and predictors.

Automatic Classifiers: Mathematical functions that can classify events based on several features and previously known cases.

Computer Aided Diagnosis: Diagnosis supported by computer methods, usually by using automatic classifiers in order to get an estimation on the exact diagnosis.

Chapter XII
Quantitative Analysis of Hysteroscopy Imaging in Gynaecological Cancer

Marios Neofytou
University of Cyprus, Cyprus

Marios Pattichis
University of New Mexico, USA

Constantinos Pattichis
University of Cyprus, Cyprus

Eftyvoulos Kyriacou
Frederick University, Cyprus

Vasilios Tanos
Aretaeion Hospital, Nicosia, Cyprus

ABSTRACT

The objective of this chapter is to propose a quantitative hysteroscopy imaging analysis system in gynaecological cancer and to provide the current situation about endoscopy imaging. Recently works, involves endoscopy, gastroendoscopy, and colonoscopy imaging with encouraging results. All the methods are using image processing using texture and classification algorithms supporting the physician diagnosis. But none of the studies were involved with the pre-processing module. Also, the above studies are trying to identify tumours in the organs and no of the are investigates the tissue texture. The system supports a standardized image acquisition protocol that eliminates significant statistical feature differences due to viewing variations. In particular, the authors provide a standardized protocol that provides texture features that are statistically invariant to variations to sensor differences (color correction), angle and distance to the tissue. Also, a Computer Aided Diagnostic (CAD) module that supports the classification of normal vs abnormal tissue of early diagnosis in gynaecological cancer of the endometrium is discussed. The authors investigate texture feature variability for the aforementioned targets encountered in clinical endoscopy before and after color correction. For texture feature analysis, three different features sets were considered: (i) Statistical Features, (ii) Spatial Gray Level Dependence Matrices, and

(iii) Gray Level Difference Statistics. Two classification algorithms, the Probabilistic Neural Network and the Support Vector Machine, were applied for the early diagnosis of gynaecological cancer of the endometrium based on the above texture features. Results indicate that there is no significant difference in texture features between the panoramic and close up views and between different camera angles. The gamma correction provided an acquired image that was a significantly better approximation to the original tissue image color. Based on the texture features, the classification algorithms results show that the correct classification score, %CC=79 was achieved using the SVM algorithm in the YCrCb color system with the combination of the SF and GLDS texture feature sets. This study provides a standardized quantitative image analysis protocol for endoscopy imaging. Also the proposed CAD system gave very satisfactory and promising results. Concluding, the proposed system can assist the physician in the diagnosis of difficult cases of gynaecological cancer, before the histopathological examination.

INTRODUCTION

In the United States, in 2007, it is estimated that over 39,080 new cases will be diagnosed with gynaecological cancer of the endometrium resulting to approximately 7,400 deaths (American Cancer Society). Within the female population, gynaecological cancer accounts for the second highest mortality rate. Early diagnosis and treatment of gynaecological cancer are essential for better quality of life and longer life.

The development of minimally invasive surgery has presented the possibility of new approaches to certain longstanding problems in gynaecology. The initial efforts with hysteroscopy, transabdominal/transvaginal laparoscopy operations have already demonstrated the advantages of endoscopic techniques over traditional open and endovascular approaches. The advantages of laparoscopic/hysteroscopic methods are especially significant in patients with a low risk factor when the operation is usually prophylactic (Cohen et al, 2003).

The objective of this chapter is to provide a standardized protocol for eliminating significant differences in texture feature analysis of endoscopy images that is also used for classifying ROIs into normal and abnormal tissue. For gynaecological cancer, we show that the proposed approach eliminates significant statistical different due to sensor variations (color correction), distance from the tissue (panoramic vs close up) and camera angle. We validate the approach for texture features extracted at difference viewing conditions from: calf endometrium chosen for its resemblance to human tissue, chicken cavities chosen for providing a more realistic laparoscopy/hysteroscopy operation environment, and also verify the findings for human subjects.

The structure of the chapter is as follows. In section II, a brief sections on overview of hysteroscopy/laparoscopy imaging is given. This is followed by methodology, results, discussion, and concluding remarks.

BACKGROUND

In laparoscopic/hysteroscopic imaging, the physician guides the telescope inside the uterine or abdominal cavity investigating the internal anatomy, in search of suspicious, cancerous lesions (Bankman et al, 2000). During the exam, the experience of the physician plays a significant role in identifying suspicious regions of interest (ROIs), where in some cases, important ROIs might be ignored and crucial information neglected (Sierra et al, 2003). The analysis of endoscopic imaging is usually carried out visually and qualitatively (Fayez et al, 1991, based on the subjective expertise of the endoscopist. Therefore, this procedure suffers from interpretational variability, lack of comparative analysis and it is time consuming.

To the best of our knowledge, there are no other studies proposing a standardized quantitative image processing and analysis procedure for the laparoscopic/hysteroscopic imaging for gynaecological cancer. Several endoscopic studies have been reported related to standardisation, that focused on comparing different treatment methods in clinical gynaecological laparoscopy. On the other hand, several CAD systems with most of them based on texture analysis have been reported mainly for colonoscopy with highly promising results (Shi et al, 2006; Bankman et al, 2000; Tjoa et al, 2003; Karkanis et al, 1999; Karkanis et al, 2003), laryngoscopy, (Haralick et al, 1973) and other endosopic imaging modalities. In (Shi et al, 2006), 47 computed tomographic (CT) colonography data sets were obtained in 26 men and 10 women (age range, 42–76 years). Results shown that the use of 3D viewing improves classification accuracy for the three readers and increases significantly the area under the receiver operating characteristic curve. Features maximum polyp width, polyp height, and preparation significantly affected the true positive measure, whereas features like colonic segment, attenuation, surface smoothness, distention, preparation, and true nature of candidate lesions significantly affected the false positive measure. In (Tjoa et al, 2003), A hybrid system was developed for the assessment of colon tissue. It was shown that a slightly higher classification accuracy was achieved when combining texture and color features, versus texture only, or color only features. In (Karkanis et al, 1999) it was shown that the texture spectrum maintains the important structure of different texture classes and also preserves the textural information in the original endoscopic images. In (Karkanis et al, 2003), a CAD system was presented for the detection of tumours in colonoscopic video based on color wavelet covariance (CWC) analysis features. The performance in the detection of abnormal colonic regions corresponding to adenomatous polyps was very high, reaching 97% specificity and 90% sensitivity.

In this chapter, a standardized procedure based on color imaging correction and texture feature extraction, analysis and classification proposed by our group for the analysis of gynaecological tissue is presented (Neophytou et al, 2005; Neophytou et al, 2004; Neophytou et al, 2004; Neophytou et al, 2006; Neophytou et al, 2007). The gamma correction algorithm which is used extensively in many applications for correcting the camera images is applied for correcting the endoscopy images. The usefulness of gamma correction was also demonstrated on endoscopic video processing. In a medical endoscopy video contrast improvement method that provides intelligent automatic adaptive contrast control was presented. The method was based on video data clustering and video data histogram modification, that allowed defining the automatic gamma control range from 0.5 to 2.0. Applying gamma correction on the images, will also limit the variability when analyzing images captured with different cameras, telescopes and endoscopic hardware.

Several textural features were computed in this work based on Statistical Features (SF) (Wu et al, 1992), Spatial Gray Level Dependence Matrices (SGLDM) (Haralick et al, 1973), and Gray level difference statistics (GLDS) (Wenska et al, 1976). Furthermore the diagnostic performance of the texture features was evaluated with two different classifiers: the Probabilistic Neural Network (PNN), and the Support Vector Machine (SVM) (Wenska et al, 1976; Christodoulou et al, 1999; Specht et al, 1990; Joachims et al, 1999; Ebrchart et al, 1990). These classifiers were trained to classify the texture features into normal or abnormal ROIs, with promising success.

METHODOLOGY

We summarize our integrated approach in Figure 1. We break our method into four parts. First, we perform color correction to compensate for sensor variations. Second, we acquire clinical images while carefully controlling the camera angle and distance to the tissue. Third, we perform texture analysis through statistical analysis of the extracted texture features. Fourth, classification analysis is carried out in classifying tissue as normal or abnormal, and comparing the results with the medical expert.

Recording of Endoscopic Video

For image acquisition, we used the medical telescope provided by Wolf (The company Richard WOLF GmbH) (2,8 mm diameter and 30 degrees viewing angle). Endoscopy video was captured using the Circon IP4.1 RGB video camera (The ACMI Corporation). All videos were captured at clinically optimum illumination and focusing. The camera was white balanced using a white surface (white color of the palette) as suggested by the manufacturer. The light source was a 300 Watt Xenon Light Source from ACMI Corporation (The ACMI Corporation). The analog output signal from the camera (PAL 475 horizontal lines) was digitized at 720x576 pixels using 24 bits color and 25 frames per second at two resolutions: (i) approximately 15 pixels/mm for the panoramic view and at (ii) approximately 21 pixels/mm for the close up view. The video was saved in AVI format. Digitization was carried out using the Digital Video Creator 120 frame grabber (The Pinnacle Systems company) that was connected to the PC through the IEEE 1394 port. The capturing conditions were controlled by the physician reflecting the clinical conditions of an operation.

Recording of Testing Targets

The testing targets were obtained from the Edmund Industrial Optics Company (The Edmund Optics company). The general purpose of a test pattern is to correct for variations in the camera sensors. The target contained 24 color squares. Testing images were captured at optimum illumination and focusing based on the experience of the physician, using the camera and the telescope under investigation. Following the above procedure we captured and saved the medical video (AVI format) of the testing palette and then extracted TIFF images of the 24 color squares. The corresponding targets were digitally generated based on the data given by the Edmund Optics Company (The Edmund Optics company) as the ground truth of the experiment.

Color Correction Algorithm

Most of the cameras have a nonlinear relationship between the signal voltage and the light intensity (Haeghen et al, 2000; Jung et al, 2005, Grossberg et al, 2004). We assume that the recorded image intensity is a function of a simple linear model prior to separable non-linear gamma distortion (see general model reported in Fig. 1 of (Grossberg et al, 2004)). We write:

$$\begin{bmatrix} R_p \\ G_p \\ B_p \end{bmatrix} = \begin{bmatrix} a_{11} & a_{12} & a_{13} \\ a_{21} & a_{22} & a_{23} \\ a_{31} & a_{32} & a_{33} \end{bmatrix} \begin{bmatrix} R_{in} \\ G_{in} \\ B_{in} \end{bmatrix} + \begin{bmatrix} k_1 \\ k_2 \\ k_3 \end{bmatrix} \quad (1)$$

where: $[R_{in}\,G_{in}\,B_{in}]^T$ denotes the red (R_{in}), green (G_{in}), and blue (B_{in}) components of the target image intensity and $\begin{bmatrix} R_p & G_p & B_p \end{bmatrix}^T$ denotes the colors of the acquired image. We let **A** denote the transformation matrix and **k** denote the constant offset vector. We then have a gamma model for the non-linear gamma relationship to the recorded image (components: R_{out}, G_{out}, B_{out}):

$$R_{out} = 255\left(\frac{R_p}{255}\right)^{\gamma_R}$$
$$G_{out} = 255\left(\frac{G_p}{255}\right)^{\gamma_G}$$
$$B_{out} = 255\left(\frac{B_p}{255}\right)^{\gamma_B} \qquad (2)$$

To compute all the parameters of the model, we use non-linear least squares (see *lsqnonlin* function in MATLAB (The MathWorks company for software)) by solving equations (1) and (2) for known target images. We estimate matrices **A**, **k** and the gamma values, γ_R, γ_G, γ_B for each color component. To recover the original, target image color components, we invert the color transformations given in equations (1) and (2).

Capturing Video from Experimental Tissue in Panoramic vs. Close Up Views

A total of 40 images (20 panoramic, and 20 close up) were captured from experimental tissue from two calf endometria at distances of 3 and 5 cm for panoramic and close up views respectively (see Figures. 2a and 2b).

A similar experiment was repeated using tissue from a chicken cavity. A total of 200 images (100 panoramic, and 100 close up) were captured from 10 chickens under the same viewing conditions as above.

Capturing Video from Tissue at Two Different Consecutive Angle Views

Similar to the previous experiment, a total of 40 images (20 at angle 1 and 20 at angle 2, with 3 degrees of difference) were captured from two calf endometria (see Figures. 2c and 2d). The same experiments were carried out for the chicken cavity where a total of 200 images from 10 chicken cavities were captured at two different angles.

Capturing Video from the Endometrium

The physician guides the telescope connected to a camera inside the uterus in order to investigate suspicious lesions of cancer. First, he/she investigates the anatomy of the organ and second, in panoramic view, he/she searches for suspicious areas. When a suspicious area is identified the physician switches to close up mode. This procedure is considered to be the standard procedure for identifying ROIs.

A total of 40 videos were recorded from 40 subjects from the endometrium. From these videos, 418 ROIs of 64x64 pixels were cropped and classified into two categories: (i) normal (N=209) and (ii) abnormal (N=209) ROIs based on the opinion of the physician and the histopathological examination.

RGB Transformation to Gray Scale, HSV, YCrCb Systems

All ROIs of 64x64 pixels were extracted from the tissue videos by the physician, for the purpose of clinical endoscopy imaging. The RGB images were transformed to gray scale using

$$Y = (0.299R + 0.587G + 0.114B) \qquad (3)$$

where Y is the intensity image.

For transforming to HSV, we used:

Figure 1. A standardized quantitative image acquisition and analysis protocol in hysteroscopy imaging

Color Correction

1. Calibrate the camera following the guidelines by the manufacturer (i.e. white balance). This provides optimal-viewing calibration that will be environment dependent.
2. Capture the color ROIs using the color palette and their corresponding digitally generated values based on the data given by the manufacturer.
3. Compute the gamma correction parameters.

Image Acquisition

4. Acquire images at an angle that is nearly orthogonal to the object under investigation (only allowing 3 degree deviation) and at distances of 3cm (close-up) to 5cm (panoramic).
5. Manually segment the ROIs under investigation in this examination.
6. Gamma correct the ROI images and visually assess the gamma corrected ROIs. This provides environment-independent calibration.

Texture Analysis

7. Color convert the ROIs from the RGB to the HSV and to the YCrCb systems.
8. Compute texture features (eg: the SF, SGLDM, GLDS feature sets and at different scales) on the gamma corrected ROIs of step 7 each channel of the color systems.
9. Compare texture features extracted from a collection of normal and abnormal cases to determine significant differences. Verify that variations in acquisition angle and distance to object do not yield significant differences.
10. Perform visual expert analysis of the results.

Classification Procedure

11. Train SVM and PNN classification models based on texture features computed at step 8 for differentiating between normal vs abnormal ROIs of the endometrium. This step is applied only for training purposes given that a significant number of cases has been collected and validated based on histopathological examination.
12. Apply texture features on trained SVM and PNN models to derive if ROI is normal or abnormal.
13. Compare (and derive ROC measures) of SVM and PNN models classification of step 12, with experts classification of step 10 classified as normal or abnormal.

Figure 2. ROIs from the calf endometrium under different viewing conditions: (a) panoramic, (b) close up, (c) angle 1 and (d) angle 2.

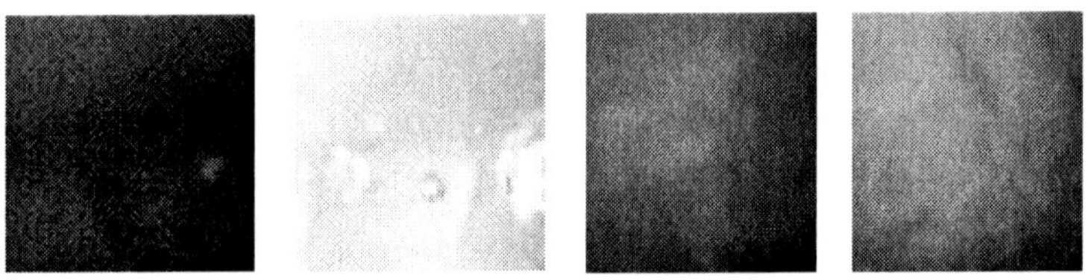

(a) (b) (c) (d)

$$V = \max(R,G,B),$$
$$S = \frac{\max(R,G,B)-\min(R,G,B)}{\max(R,G,B)},$$
$$H = \begin{cases} 3-\dfrac{G-B}{\max(R,G,B)-\min(R,G,B)}, & \text{for } R \geq G,B \\ 1-\dfrac{B-R}{\max(R,G,B)-\min(R,G,B)}, & \text{for } G \geq R,B \\ 5-\dfrac{R-G}{\max(R,G,B)-\min(R,G,B)}, & \text{for } B \geq R,G. \end{cases} \quad (4)$$

For transforming to Y, Cr, Cb, we used:

$$\begin{bmatrix} Y \\ Cr \\ Cb \end{bmatrix} = \begin{bmatrix} 0.299 & 0.587 & 0.114 \\ 0.596 & -0.275 & -0.321 \\ 0.212 & -0.523 & 0.311 \end{bmatrix} \begin{bmatrix} R \\ G \\ B \end{bmatrix} \quad (5)$$

Feature Extraction

Texture features were extracted from the segmented ROI images in order to characterize tissue captured under different viewing conditions, as well as to differentiate between normal and abnormal tissue. A total number of 26 texture features were extracted from endoscopic images (described next). These feature sets were also successfully used in numerous previous works in texture analysis (Petrou et al, 2006). Some of the features used capture complementary textural properties, however, features that were highly dependent or similar with features in other feature sets, were identified through statistical analysis and eliminated. The ROI color images were transformed into gray scale images and the following texture features were computed:

Statistical Features (SF): SF features describe the gray level histogram distribution without considering spatial dependence (Wu et al, 1992).

Spatial Gray Level Dependence Matrices (SGLDM): The spatial gray level dependence matrices as proposed by (Haralick et al, 1973) are based on the estimation of the second-order joint conditional probability density functions that two pixels (*k, l*) and (*m, n*) with distance *d* in direction specified by the angle θ, have intensities of gray level (*i*) and gray level (*j*). Based on the estimated probability density functions, texture measures were extracted, proposed by Haralick et al. (Haralick et al, 1973). For a selected distance *d* (in this work *d=1* was used), and for angles θ = 0°, 45°, 90° and 135° we computed four values for each of the texture measures. The features were calculated for displacements δ=(0,1), (1,1), (1,0), (1,-1), where δ=(Δx, Δy), and their range of values were computed.

Gray level difference statistics (GLDS): The GLDS algorithm (Wenska et al, 1976) is based on the assumption that useful texture information can be extracted using first order statistics of an image. The algorithm is based on the estimation of the probability density p_δ of image pixel pairs at a given distance δ=(Δx, Δy), having a certain absolute gray level difference value. For any given displacement δ=(Δx, Δy), let $f_\delta(x,y)=|f(x,y)-f(x+\Delta_x, y+\Delta_y)|$. Let p_δ be the probability density of $f_\delta(x,y)$. If there are *m* gray levels, this has the form of an *m*-dimensional vector whose *i*th component is the probability that $f_\delta(x,y)$ will have value (*i*). If the picture *f* is discrete, it is easy to compute p_δ by counting the number of times each value of $f_\delta(x,y)$ occurs, where Δx and Δy are integers. Coarse texture images result in low gray level difference values, whereas, fine texture images result in inter-pixel gray level differences with great variances. Features were estimated for the following distances: δ=(d,0), (d,d), (-d,d), (0,d). A good way to analyze texture coarseness is to compute, for various magnitudes of δ, some measure of the spread of values in p_δ away from the origin.

Statistical Analysis

The Wilcoxon rank sum test was applied (Shapiro et al, 1965) to investigate if the texture features exhibited significant statistical difference for different viewing conditions and between texture features extracted before and after gamma correction at $a \leq 0.05$. The Wilcoxon test returns a p-value, which represents the probability of observing the given data by chance if the medians are equal. Small values of p imply that the null hypothesis should be rejected (Gibbons, 1965).

Classification Algorithms

The diagnostic performance of the texture features was evaluated with two different classifiers: the Probabilistic Neural Network (PNN), and the Support Vector Machine (SVM). These classifiers were trained to classify the texture features into two classes: i) normal ROIs or ii) abnormal ROIs. The PNN (Specht, 1990) classifier basically is a kind of Radial Basis Function (RBF) network suitable for classification problems. This classifier was investigated for several spread radius in order to identify the best for the current problem. The SVM network was investigated using Gaussian Radial Basis Function (RBF) kernels; this was decided as the rest of the kernel functions could not achieve so good results. The SVM with RBF kernel was investigated using 10-fold cross validation in order to identify the best parameters such as spread of the RBF kernels (Joachims, 1999). The leave-one-out method was used for validating all the classification models. A total of 418 runs were carried out for training the classifiers, and the performance of the classifiers was evaluated on the remaining one subset (Ebrchart et al, 1990).

The performance of the classifier systems were measured using the parameters of the receiver operating characteristic (ROC) curves: true positives (TP), false positives (FP), false negatives (FN), true negatives (TN), sensitivity (SE), specificity (SP), and precision (PR). We also computed the percentage of correct classifications ratio (%CC) based on the correctly and incorrectly classified cases.

RESULTS

Color Correction Algorithm

The Circon IP4.1 endoscopy camera was used for capturing video from both the testing targets and tissues. In these experiments, the color correction algorithm was run using the recorded test targets and the ground truth images as supplied by Edmund Optics Company. The computed color correction parameters were then used for correcting the images.

Table 1 tabulates the **A, k** and γ values of the R, G, B channels for three different experiments as well as their median values. It is clearly shown that a variability exists between the **A, k**, and γ values for these experiments. The variability documented in Table 1 motivated us to investigate it further.

A database of 209 normal and 209 abnormal ROIs of the endometrium recorded from 40 women was analysed. Images were corrected, using different combinations of the **A, k,** and γ values and their corresponding texture features were computed. Neural network models were trained to classify 100 normal and 100 abnormal endometrium images. The rest of the cases were used for evaluating the performance of the models. The percentage of correct classifications score was computed for the evaluation set. It was found that the texture features computed with the median values of **A**, **k** and γ for the three experiments gave the highest score. The results of these experiments are reported in detail in another study (Neofytou et al, 2007). It was thus decided to use, the median values of **A**, **k** and γ in this study as well. The median gamma values for the three channels $(\gamma_R = 1{,}078,\ \gamma_G = 1{,}046,\ \gamma_B = 1{,}040)$ were very close to unit values.

Table 1. Gamma correction parameters A, k and γ for three different experiments and their median values. (Copyright BioMedical Engineering OnLine, 2007, (Neofytou et al, 2007))

A matrix	No Correction	Exp 1	Exp 2	Exp 3	Median values for Exps 1, 2, 3
a_{11}	1	0.827	0.927	0.975	0.927
a_{12}	0	0.065	0.011	0.105	0.065
a_{13}	0	0.042	0.004	0.104	0.042
a_{21}	0	0.065	0.011	0.105	0.065
a_{22}	1	0.780	0.935	0.895	0.895
a_{23}	0	0.071	0.062	0.134	0.071
a_{31}	0	0.042	0.004	0.104	0.042
a_{32}	0	0.044	0.032	0.023	0.032
a_{33}	1	0.868	1.011	1.044	1.011
k matrix					
k_{11}	0	7.693	1.101	-1.673	1.101
k_{21}	0	10.083	2.090	0.528	2.090
k_{31}	0	-8.161	1.598	-5.689	-5.689
γ matrix					
γ_R	1	1.285	1.078	1.038	1.078
γ_G	1	1.220	1.046	0.999	1.046
γ_B	1	1.180	0.971	1.040	1.040

Capturing Video from Experimental Tissue in Close Up vs. Panoramic Views

The results of the statistical analysis in the close up vs the panoramic view (using experimental tissues) indicates the variability due to the use of different viewing conditions. For this experiment, we use calf endometria, in an environment that is similar to actual operating conditions. Prior to gamma correction, we have found that there was no significance difference between features computed from the panoramic and close-up views (Neofytou et al, 2007). We also repeated these experiments using the chicken cavities, under the same viewing conditions and the same medical equipment. The results were very similar as for the calf endometria (Neofytou et al, 2004).

Capturing Video from Experimental Tissue in Two Different Consecutive Angle Views

We now present statistical analysis results for texture feature values extracted from different angles. Here, we note that gamma correction did not seem to affect the results. There was no significant difference between the texture features values. It is clear that there are no significant differences between texture feature values from different angles, whether we apply gamma correction or not (Neofytou et al, 2004). As before, we also repeated these experiments using the chicken cavities, under the same viewing conditions and the same medical equipment, and the results were similar.

Analysis of Images of Human Endometria

In this subsection we present results from the statistical analysis of ROIs extracted from human endometria. The results are summarized in Table 2. The non-parametric Wilcoxon rank sum test was used to decide if there is a significant difference between normal and abnormal ROIs at a≤0.05. The results indicate that there is a significant difference. Furthermore, as we can see in Table 2, after gamma correction, the entropy values are preserved. From the table, it is clear that the median SGLDM contrast for abnormal cases is dramatically larger than the corresponding median value for the normal ROIs.

Classification Results

Table 3 presents the performance of the different PNN and SVM classification models investigated using the texture features. It is clearly shown that the SVM classifier performed better than the PNN classifier. For the SVM classifier, the best performance was achieved with the SF+SGLDS followed by the SGLDM+GLDS, and SF+SGLDS+GLDS with a percentage of correct classifications (%CC) of 79%, 76%, and 77%, respectively. Similar classification performance to the corrected ROIs was also obtained for all models for the uncorrected ROIs. Moreover, similar performance for all models as given in Table 3 was obtained when the feature sets were transformed using PCA without increasing the %CC.

Table 2. Percentile values of the texture features and statistical analysis for normal (N=209) vs abnormal (N=209) ROIs of the endometrium extracted from 40 subjects. Statistical analysis was carried out after gamma correction but also between the normal/abnormal ROIs before and after gamma correction at a≤0.05. (Copyright BioMedical Engineering OnLine, 2007, (Neofytou et al, 2007))

	Normal ROIs					Abnormal ROIs					Normal vs Abnormal ROIs	Original vs Corrected Images For Normal ROIs	Original vs Corrected Images For Abnormal ROIs
	P5%	P25%	P50%	P75%	P95%	P5%	P25%	P50%	P75%	P95%	H	H	H
SF													
Mean	110,11	138,44	156,06	173,91	204,36	98,48	129,37	144,65	170,48	206,06	1	1	1
Variance	13,23	29,44	54,63	127,94	286,63	31,33	66,9	124,39	223,33	492,3	1	1	1
Median	110,18	138,83	156,44	174,42	203,53	98,2	127,92	143,75	171,43	207,7	1	1	1
Mode	109,95	135,75	156	175	201,05	98	124	146,5	176	211,4	1	1	1
Skewness	-1,01	-0,46	-0,14	0,12	0,56	-1,14	-0,47	-0,14	0,18	0,62	0	0	0
Kurtosis	1,94	2,26	2,64	3,09	4,39	1,82	2,24	2,62	3,16	4,85	0	0	0
Energy	0,02	0,03	0,04	0,06	0,09	0,02	0,02	0,03	0,04	0,06	1	1	1
Entropy	2,66	3,02	3,34	3,68	4,09	3,11	3,44	3,74	3,99	4,32	1	1	1
SGLDM													
Contrast	2,54	3,1	3,82	4,87	12,27	2,55	4,82	7,04	10,99	21,94	1	1	1
Correlation	0,85	0,93	0,96	0,98	0,99	0,91	0,95	0,97	0,98	0,99	1	1	0
Variance	13,02	28,83	53,97	126,41	284,3	30,89	65,53	120,85	221,38	488,55	1	1	1
Homogeneity	0,37	0,45	0,48	0,5	0,53	0,31	0,38	0,42	0,46	0,53	1	1	1
Entropy	4,47	4,93	5,31	5,78	6,28	5,01	5,49	5,93	6,28	6,65	1	1	1
GLDS													
Homogeneity	0,37	0,45	0,48	0,5	0,53	0,31	0,38	0,42	0,46	0,53	1	1	1
Contrast	2,54	3,09	3,81	4,86	12,24	2,55	4,81	7,03	10,97	21,89	1	1	1
Energy	0,17	0,24	0,25	0,27	0,3	0,14	0,18	0,21	0,24	0,3	1	1	1
Entropy	1,37	1,45	1,54	1,64	2	1,37	1,63	1,77	1,96	2,24	1	1	1
Mean	1,18	1,33	1,44	1,63	2,45	1,19	1,62	1,89	2,31	3,16	1	1	1

Table 3. Classification performance of the SVM (PNN) models for the classification of normal and abnormal ROIs of the endometrium based on texture features for the RGB, HSV and YCRCB systems.

SVM (PNN) classifier	%CC	%FP	%FN	%SE	%SP	%PR
			RGB			
SF	75 (66)	21 (18)	28 (49)	71 (50)	78 (81)	77 (72)
SGLDM	72 (67)	23 (25)	31 (40)	68 (59)	76 (74)	74 (70)
GLDS	69 (63)	3 (18)	27 (55)	72 (44)	66 (81)	68 (70)
SF+SGLDM	70 (67)	34 (24)	25 (40)	75 (59)	65 (75)	68 (71)
SF+GLDS	73 (68)	30 (14)	22 (49)	77 (50)	69 (85)	71 (77)
SGLDM+GLDS	74 (67)	22 (21)	29 (43)	70 (56)	77 (78)	76 (72)
SF+SGLDM+GLDS	73 (68)	22 (19)	31 (43)	68 (56)	77 (80)	75 (74)
			HSV			
SF	72 (70)	30 (22)	25 (37)	75 (62)	69 (77)	71 (73)
SGLDM	74 (70)	27 (21)	23 (37)	76 (62)	72 (78)	73 (74)
GLDS	69 (67)	24 (26)	37 (39)	62 (60)	75 (73)	72 (69)
SF+SGLDM	74 (70)	36(21)	15 (37)	84 (62)	63 (78)	69 (74)
SF+GLDS	76 (70)	20 (17)	26 (42)	73 (57)	79 (82)	77 (76)
SGLDM+GLDS	72 (71)	31 (20)	24 (37)	75 (62)	68 (79)	70 (75)
SF+SGLDM+GLDS	75 (69)	30 (21)	19 (39)	80 (60)	69 (78)	72 (73)
			YCrCb			
SF	73 (68)	21 (11)	31 (51)	68 (48)	78 (88)	76 (81)
SGLDM	74 (69)	28 (14)	23 (47)	76 (52)	71 (85)	72 (78)
GLDS	75 (68)	24 (13)	25 (50)	75 (49)	75 (86)	75 (78)
SF+SGLDM	76 (70)	25 (13)	22 (46)	77 (53)	75 (86)	75 (79)
SF+GLDS	**79** (69)	25 (12)	16 (48)	83 (51)	74 (87)	76 (81)
SGLDM+GLDS	**76** (69)	25 (15)	23 (46)	76 (53)	75 (84)	75 (77)
SF+SGLDM+GLDS	**77** (70)	25 (15)	20 (44)	79 (55)	74 (84)	75 (78)

DISCUSSION OF THE RESULTS

For better and consistent classification performance, we limited our study to a distance of 3 cm for close up examinations and a distance of 5 cm for panoramic examinations. We also limited our camera angle variations to remain within 3 degrees. Furthermore, we recommend that the camera should be color corrected. When the proposed standardized protocol is followed, we show that there are no significant differences between texture features extracted from the same type of tissue (normal or abnormal), but under different viewing conditions. On the other hand, even for the same type of tissue, significant differences arise from large variations in the viewing conditions that do not conform to the protocol (as shown in (Neofytou et al, 2007)).

More importantly, after applying the proposed protocol, a large number of texture features show significant differences between ROIs extracted from normal versus abnormal tissues. Findings of this work were published in (Neofytou et al, 2005; Neofytou et al, 2004; Neofytou et al, 2004; Neofytou et al, 2007). To the best of our knowledge, although there are guidelines for performing the endoscopy examination, there are no guidelines for the quantitatively interpretation of the results (American Society for Gastrointestinal Endoscopy), (European Society for Gynaecological Endoscopy). Standardization efforts for reporting endoscopy examinations have been proposed (Yokoi et al, 2006).

Recording of Endoscopic Video

Recent efforts are focused on producing guidelines for gynaecological endoscopy such as gynaecological endoscopy and hysteroscopy (European Society for Gynaecological Endoscopy). These efforts will help the gynaecologist in standardizing the procedure for capturing endoscopic video and will enable the quantitative analysis of tissue pathology. Similar efforts exist in other endoscopic procedures such as gastrointestinal endoscopy and colonoscopy (American Society for Gastrointestinal Endoscopy). Quantitative analysis in these areas is still under investigation. In this study, a complete framework for capturing and analyzing gynaecological endoscopic video was proposed (Scarcanski et al, 2006).

Color Correction Algorithm

Although the importance of the gamma color correction algorithm is widely recommended in the literature, it is rarely used (relevant exceptions are (Neofytou et al, 2007) and (Cohen et al, 2003). We recommend that the gamma color correction algorithm should be used routinely for endoscopic images. This will facilitate the standardised analysis of endoscopic images.

Image Analysis from Experimental Tissue for Different Viewing Conditions

It is shown that there was no significant difference in the texture features for panoramic vs close up views and for small consecutive angles in normal, experimental tissue. Gray scale median, variance and entropy were higher in the close up view compared to the panoramic view, whereas contrast and homogeneity were essentially the same in both views. When comparing two consecutive angles, variance was higher in the smaller angle, whereas median, entropy, contrast and homogeneity were in the same range.

In this study, the close up and panoramic view distances were 3 cm and 5 cm respectively. Another study was carried out by our group where the conditions similar to laparoscopy examination were investigated. In that study the close up and panoramic view distances were 4 cm and 7 cm respectively and similar results to this study were obtained (Neophytou et al, 2004). Similar results were also obtained for texture features obtained from different angles (with a difference of 2 degrees).

However, when the distance between the close up vs panoramic views was higher than 6 cm, significant differences in some texture features were obtained. We have also found that some texture feature values exhibited significant differences when the angle differences were more than 5 degrees.

Human Images from the Endometrium

We have found that a standardized protocol is necessary in order to eliminate any significant differences that may arise due to the lack of color correction. When the proposed standardized protocol is applied, significant differences in texture features are only due to the desired difference between normal versus abnormal tissue. The standardized protocol is essential for subsequent use of texture features in a CAD system in gynaecological cancer. The protocol is also expected to contribute to increased accuracy in difficult cases of gynaecological cancer.

We hope that the proposed standardized protocol will serve as a starting point for allowing

Table 4. Texture characteristics of normal vs abnormal ROIs of the endometrium as these were obtained by interpretation of the texture features values given in Table 2.

	Normal	Abnormal
Gray level	High	Slighthly darker
Variance	Low	Very High
Contrast	Low	High
Homogeneity	Normal range	Slighthly lower
Entropy	Normal range	Slighthly higher

comparisons between different medical centers and images acquired using different medical equipment.

Table 4 tabulates the texture characteristics of normal vs abnormal ROIs as these were obtained by interpretation of the texture features values given in Table 2.

Classification Performance

There was a significant difference in the SF, SGLDM, and GLDS features investigated between the normal and abnormal ROIs as documented in previous sections. Based on the CAD system developed, the highest percentage of correct classifications score was 79% and was achieved for the SVM classifier for the SF+GLDS feature sets. These results support the application of texture analysis for the assessment of difficult cases of normal and abnormal ROIs for gynaecological cancer. The proposed CAD system can be proved to be a useful tool for the gynaecologist during the operation so as to identify suspicious ROIs that should be investigated with histopathological examination.

FUTURE TRENDS

Future work will focus on investigating the usefulness of the proposed methodology in other gynaecological organs, i.e. cervix, and ovary. Moreover, the standardized protocol will be used for investigating if there is variability in the computed texture feature sets between different clinics, as well as in collecting and analyzing more cases. The protocol could also be applied for the provision of telediagnosis or teleconsultation services to rural health centers by experienced clinics during a regular laparoscopy/hysteroscopy examination.

More work is needed towards automating the pre-processing component of the protocol, and more specifically in the automated segmentation of normal and abnormal tissue, not only in freezed laparoscopy/hysteroscopy images, but also in video. It is noted that this is a very difficult task. Multi scale texture analysis, and multi classifier classification should also further be investigated towards differentiating between normal and abnormal tissue. will be explored in the cases of endometrium and ovary cancer increasing the physician diagnosis in difficult cases of gynaecological cancer.

It is hoped that the above mentioned technologies, will help the physician in detecting the disease at its onset, thus offering a better service to the citizen, via the CAD standardized and quantitative analysis. These will facilitate increased prevention, and better monitoring and management of the patient.

CONCLUSION

The use of a standardised protocol for capturing and analyzing endoscopic video will facilitate the wide spread use of quantitative analysis as well as the use of CAD systems in gynaecological endoscopy. The proposed standardized protocol suggests the use of color correction and the use of specific viewing conditions so that there will be no significant differences in texture feature values extracted from the same type of tissue (normal or abnormal). On the other hand, when either color correction is not applied or the standardized viewing conditions are not used, significant differences in texture features can arise, even when they come from the same type of tissue. This implies that the proposed standardized protocol cannot be further simplified by reducing any of its requirements.

When the proposed protocol is applied, we have found that several texture features can be used to discriminate between normal and abnormal tissue since they exhibit significant differences for the two types of tissue investigated. Furthermore, a CAD system was developed based on texture features and classification models for classifying between normal and abnormal endometria with very satisfactory and promising results. Future work will focus on investigating the usefulness of the proposed methodology in other gynaecological organs and clinics, as well as in comparing the findings between the different clinics. Finally, we hope that the proposed system can also be applied to other endoscopic modalities such as colonoscopy and gastroscopy.

ACKNOWLEDGMENT

This study is funded through the Research Promotion Foundation, Cyprus, PENEK 2005, Program for the Financial Support of New Researchers, through the project entitled: Intra-operative Computer Assisted Tissue Image Analysis (CATIA), April 2006 - April 2008. Furthermore this study is partially funded by the program for High Tech Companies of the Ministry of Commerce, Industry and Tourism, Cyprus, through the project Computer Aided Diagnosis system in Gynaecological Endoscopy (CAD_Gen), July 2008 - July 2010.

REFERENCES

American Cancer Society [http://www.cancer.org]

American Society for Gastrointestinal Endoscopy [www.asge.org]

Bankman, I. N., Spisz, T. S., & Pavlopoulos, S. (2000). Two-Dimensional Shape and Texture Quantification, Handbook of medical imaging. Academic Press, Inc.

Christodoulou, C. I., Pattichis, C. S., Pantziaris, M., Tegos, T., Nicolaides, A., Elatrozy, T., Sabetai, M., & Dhanjil, S. (1999). *Multi-feature texture analysis for the classification of carotid plaques.* Presented at the Int. Joint Conf. Neural Networks IJCNN '99, Washington DC.

Cohen, R. V., Schiavon, C. A., Pinheiro, F. J. C., & Correa, J. L. (2003). Laparoscopic Bariatric Surgery: New Technologies, Trends and Perspectives. *Rev Hosp Clin Fac Med Sao Paulo, 58*(5), I-VIII.

Ebrchart, R. C, & Dobbins, R. W. (1990). *Neural Networks PC Tools A Practical Guide.* (Academic Pr., 1990).

European Society for Gynaecological Endoscopy [http://www.esge.org/]

Fayez, J. A., & Vogel, M. F. (1991). Comparison of Different Treatment Methods of Endometriomas by Laparoscopy. *Obstet. Gynecol., 78*, 660-665.

Gibbons, J. D. (1985). *Nonparametric Statistical Inference*. 2nd Ed., M. Dekker.

Grossberg, M. D., & Nayar, S. K. (2004). Modelling the Space of Camera Response Functions. *IEEE Transactions on Pattern Analysis and Machine Intelligence, 26*(10).

Haralick R.M., Shanmugam K., & Dinstein I. (1973). Texture Features for Image Classification. *IEEE Trans. Nov., SMC-3,* 610-621.

Ilgner J., Palm C., Schutz A., Spitzer K., Westhofen M., & Lehmann T. (2003). Colour Texture Analysis for Quantitative Laryngoscopy. *Acta Otolaryngol, 123,* 730-734.

Joachims, T. (1999). Making large-Scale SVM Learning Practical. B. Schölkopf, C. Burges, & A. Smola (Eds.), *Advances in Kernel Methods - Support Vector Learning.* MIT Press.

Jung, Y. H., Kim, J. S., Hur, B. S., & Kang, M. G. (2005). Design of Real-Time Image Enhancement Preprocessor for Cmos Image Sensor. *IEEE Transactions on Consumer Electronics, 46*(1).

Karkanis, S. A., Galousi, K., & Maroulis, D. (1999). Classification of Endoscopic Images Based on Texture Spectrum. ACAI99. *Workshop on Machine Learning in Medical Applications,* Chania, Greece, (pp. 63-69).

Karkanis, S. A., Iakovidis, D. K., Maroulis, D. E., Karras, A. D., & Tzivras, M. (2003). Computer-Aided Tumor Detection in Endoscopic Video using Color Wavelet features. *IEEE Transactions on Information Technology in Biomedicine, 7*(3), 141-152.

Neofytou, M. S., Pattichis, C. S., Pattichis, M. S., Tanos, V., Kyriacou, E. C., & Koutsouris, D. (2007). A Standardised Protocol for Texture Feature Analysis of Endoscopic Images in Gynaecological Cancer. *BioMedical Engineering OnLine, 6*(44). http://www.biomedical-engineering-online.com/content/6/1/44.

Neophytou, M. S., Pattichis, C. S., Pattichis, M. S., Tanos, V., Kyriacou, E., & Koutsouris, D. (2005). The Effect of Color Correction of Endoscopy Images for Quantitative Analysis in Endometrium. *27th Annual International conference of the IEEE Engineering in Medicine and Biology Society,* 1-4 September, Shanghai, China, (pp. 3336- 3339).

Neophytou, M. S., Pattichis, C. S., Pattichis, M. S., Tanos, V., Kyriacou, E., & Koutsouris, D. (2004). Multiscale Texture Feature Variability Analysis in Endoscopy Imaging Under Different Viewing Positions. *CD-ROM Proceedings of the II EFOMP Mediterranean Conference on Medical Physics,* 28-30 April, Limassol, Cyprus.

Neophytou, M. S., Pattichis, C. S., Pattichis, M. S., Tanos, V., Kyriacou, E., Pavlopoulos, S., & Koutsouris, D. (2004). Texture Analysis of the Endometrium During Hysteroscopy: Preliminary Results. *26th Annual International conference of the IEEE Engineering in Medicine and Biology Society,, 2,* 1483-1486. 1-5 September, San Francisco, California, USA.

Neophytou, M. S., Pattichis, C. S., Pattichis, M. S., Tanos, V., Kyriacou, E., & Koutsouris, D. (2006). Texture-Based Classification of Hysteroscopy Images of the Endometrium. *28th Annual International conference of the IEEE Engineering in Medicine and Biology Society,* 30-3 September, New York, USA, (pp. 3005-3008).

Petrou, M., & Sevilla, G. P. (2006). *Image Processing, Dealing with Texture.* John Wiley and Sons.

Plataniotis, K. N., & Venetsanopoulos, A. N. (2000). *Color Image Processing and Applications.* Springer Verlag. Berlin.

Scarcanski, J., Gavião, W., Cunha, S., & João, F. (2005). Diagnostic Hysteroscopy Video Summarization and Browsing. *27th Annual International conference of the IEEE engineering in Medicine and Biology Society,* Shanghai, China, (pp. 5680-5683).

Shapiro, S. S., & Wilk, M. B. (1965). An Analysis of Variance Test for Normality (complete samples). *Biometrika, 52, 3, & 4,* 591-611.

Sheraizin, S., & Sheraizin, V. (2005). Endoscopy Imaging Intelligent Contrast Improvement. *27th Annual International conference of the IEEE engineering in Medicine and Biology Society*, 1-4 September, Shanghai, China, (pp. 6551-6554).

Shi, et al. (2006). CT Colonography: Influence of 3D Viewing & polyp Candidate Features on Interpretation with Computer-Aided Detection. Radiology, 239,768-776.

Sierra, R., Bajka, M., & Szekely, G. (2003). Evaluation of Different Pathology Generation Strategies for Surgical Training Simulators. *Computer Assisted Radiology and Surgery: Proceedings of the 17th International Congress and Exhibition* (pp. 376-381).

Specht, D. F. (1990). Probabilistic Neural Networks. *INNS Neural Networks 3*(1), 109-118.

The ACMI Corporation [www.acmicorp.com]

The company Richard WOLF GmbH [http://www.richard-wolf.com/default.aspx]

The Edmund Optics company [www.edmundoptics.com]

The MathWorks company for software [www.mathworks.com]

The Pinnacle Systems company [www.pinnaclesys.com]

Tjoa, P. M., & Krishnan, M. S. (2003). Feature Extraction for the Analysis of Colon Status from the Endoscopic Images. *BioMedical Engineering OnLine*. [http://www.biomedical-engineering-online.com/content/2/1/9].

Haeghen, V. Y., Naeyaert, J., Lemahieu, I., & Philips, W. (2000). An Imaging System with Calibrated Color Image Acquisition for Use in Dermatology. *IEEE Transactions on Medical Imaging, 19*(7).

Wenska, J. S., Dryer, C. R., & Rosenfeld, A. (1976). A Comparative Study of Texture Measures for Terrain Classification. *IEEE Trans. Syst., Man, Cyber., SMC-6,* 269-285.

Wenzl, R., Lehner, R., Vry, U., Pateisky, N., Sevelda, P., & Husslein, P. (1994). Three-Dimensional Video-endoscopy: Clinical use in Gynaecological Laparoscopy. *Lancet, 344,* 1621–1622.

Wu, C. M., Chen, Y. C., & Hsieh, K. S. (1992). Texture Features for Classification of Ultrasonic liver Images. *IEEE Trans. Med. Imaging, 11,* 141-152.

Yokoi, H., & Fujino, M. A. (2006). Activities for Endoscopy Information Systems Standardization in Japan. *28th Annual International conference of the IEEE engineering in Medicine and Biology Society*, New York, USA, (pp. 5667-5670).

KEY TERMS

Automatic Classifiers: Mathematical functions that can classify events based on several features and previously known cases.

Computer Aided Diagnosis: Diagnosis supported by computer methods, usually by using automatic classifiers in order to get an estimation on the exact diagnosis.

Hysteroscopy Examination: The physician guides the telescope connected to a camera inside the endometrium in order to investigate the cavity.

Chapter XIII
Combining Geometry and Image in Biomedical Systems:
The RT TPS Case

Thomas V. Kilindris
University of Thessaly, Greece

Kiki Theodorou
University of Thessaly, Greece

ABSTRACT

Patient anatomy, biochemical response, as well functional evaluation at organ level, are key fields that produce a significant amount of multi modal information during medical diagnosis. Visualization, processing, and storage of the acquired data sets are essential tasks in everyday medical practice. In order to perform complex processing that involves or rely on image data a robust as well versatile data structure was used as extension of the Visualization Toolkit (VTK). The proposed structure serves as a universal registration container for acquired information and post processed resulted data. The structure is a dynamic multidimensional data holder to host several modalities and/or Meta data like fused image sets, extracted features (volumetric, surfaces, edges) providing a universal coordinate system used for calculations and geometric processes. A case study of Treatment Planning System (TPS) in the stereotactic radiotherapy (RT) based on the proposed structure is discussed as an efficient medical application.

INTRODUCTION

Computer aided medical applications for diagnosis, therapy, simulation or training proliferate gradually in everyday practice heavily relying on image data (Dawson and Kaufmann, 1998; Spitzer & Whitlock, 1998). Radio therapy planning, surgery as well medical simulation requires anatomic and physical modeling of the whole or part of the human body. Further on *in silico* functional study of the human body physiology requires the interoperation of several models to approximate an as real as possible behavior (Noble, 2002; Gavaghan, Garny, Maini, & Kohl, 2006; Seemann, Hoeper, Doessel, Holden, & Zhang, 2006). Major sources of real world data related to anatomical details are tomographic image sets. Tomographic image sets of 3D solid objects are in general stacked 2D cross-sectional images of the inspected object that contain geometric information mixed with material properties of the solid in terms of radiation absorbance.

The modality used to obtain the tomographic set determines the geometric accuracy of anatomical regions, the resolution of material properties as well functional characteristics. The almost annual doubling in computer power permits today real time manipulation of simultaneous multimodal datasets representation also know as image fusion and 3D image registration. Sometimes modalities act complementary in cases of sparse acquired datasets (Shim, Pitto, Streicher, Hunter P. J. & Anderson I. A. 2007). In order to study physiological function of internal organs several models have been proposed ranging from simple calculation diagrams to complex animated 3D solid models (France et al. 2005; Noble 2002; Seemann, 2007; Selberg & Vanderploeg, 1994; Spirka & Damasa, 2007). Almost all models involve dynamics and geometry. Physiological functions rule dynamics, dynamics produce data and data become finally visualized (Freudenberg, Schiemann, Tiede, & Hoehne, 2000). Soft tissue simulation used extensively in computer assisted surgery planning or training is an example. Tissue is modeled as a deformable object while collision detection between the virtual surgery instruments or even neighbor organs is used. Deformation is modeled according to physiological data while collision detection queries the geometric models to undertake the desired action for example simulated tissue ablation, rapture (Nealen et al. 2005; Teschner et al., 2005).

The Visible Human Project is another reference project that serves educational as well research (Ackerman 1998; Robb & Hanson 2006). Using the multimodal sets of the project (CT, MRI, CRYO) volume reconstruction of the human body both female and male is possible. Especially today where computational power and special graphics hardware is widely available at the cost of regular home personal computer the realization of a virtual dissection is feasible (Spitzer et al. 2004). One successful example is the Voxel-Man navigator (Schiemann, Tiede & Hoehne, 1997). Image guided techniques can assist both surgery and diagnosis. Virtual Endoscopy is an example of simulated endoscopic examination for diagnostic purposes (Robb, 1999). Reconstruction of the anatomy is done using tomographic imagesets and a fly through visualization is adopted to provide the analogous of real endoscopy. Once again improvements in the medical scanning systems combined with progress in computer systems lead to a novel approach of diagnostic medical imaging. Finally therapy planning systems in medicine make extensive use of imageset. Either directly or indirectly used to extract volumetric – geometric characteristics and 3D models those systems become essential in calculating complex therapeutic schemes like stereotactic radiotherapy, IMRT, neurosurgery, liver surgery orthopedics surgery etc (Mock et al. 2004; Shim et al. 2007).

All these systems are relative new and are undergoing an evaluation period where knew concepts from already established knowledge areas are reused. An example mentioned above is collision detection. Collision detection concept serves gaming from the very first day when primitive bouncing ball games debuted to the virtual reality implementation of industrial standard simulators. Data structures are continuously tested in the complex field of computer visualization.

Finally the most critical part is the man machine interface. But poor human interaction with application's functional dynamics can render useless even a state of the art system. Thus a lot of new techniques, input devices, displays, and controllers exist to fulfill the principal need for as possible high reality representation of the real world.

BACKGROUND

The primary task in spatial modelling of the human body is to regain real world patient's geometry from the available image data. Since the introduction of CT and MRI image datasets in medical diagnosis this task is mentally performed by the physician. Tilling cross-sectional images across a light box can reduce the size of area in interest as well the ability of the physician to traverse in space along planar data. Computer aided reconstruction was introduced (Robb et al, 1974; Herman & Liou, 1977) known as 3D reconstruction. On the 2D interactive visual display systems (computer monitors) this is done successful using different techniques like ray tracing, volume rendering [etc.] The amount as well the nature of data are more photometric than geometric thus it is extremely difficult to perform several morphometric measurement or even distance calculation between points in those data sets. A polygonal approximation of the external surface of the ventricle can be easily used to calculate any metrics like volume or surface distance. Applying a flow approximation model that involves finite element methods on the polygonal surface modelled vena cava is more efficient and feasible than to apply the simplest flow law in a point cloud that represents spatially the amount of absorbed energy. The results of the 3D reconstruction are geometric constructs with defined spatial boundaries composed by planar polygons also called polygonal approximations. (Fig. 1)

Polygonal approximations may vary in resolution as well in the type of primitive planar polygons used. The simplest planar polygon to manipulate mathematically and handle unambiguously by graphics rendering hardware is the triangle therefore the approximation tends more to triangulation. It is shown that any polygon can be divided in triangles. As already explained for practical reasons triangles were the first and are still used as the most favoured primitive polygon type to approximate surfaces. Polygonal surface approximations can be viewed in general as a fitting problem, a point set in R^3 space has to be fitted in one ore more possible surface approximations embedded in R^3 space. In most cases the point set is derived from a tomographic image set where the sliced nature ensures that points are rather layered than arbitrarily distributed in a cloud manner like the points acquired using a 3D digitizer.

The procedure to extract an anatomical meaningful region enclosed by a planar curve, the boundary of the anatomical unit, is called contouring or contour extraction. Contour extraction plays a key role in anatomical surface reconstruction. Algorithms that directly extract a surface (also called an isosurface) from a 3D point data set are well known and are extensively optimised. The famous Marching Cubes (MC) algorithm (Lorensen & Cline, 1987) or later improvements of it (Brodlie & Wood, 2001; Lopes & Brodlie, 2003) in surface extraction speed, resolution as well accuracy are widely used to extract surface on relatively large well defined anatomical units like bones. Application of the algorithm to smaller soft tissue areas does not always supply acceptable results even if fed by MRI image datasets. Using extracted planar contours the previous mentioned problem becomes a problem to combine points of adjacent slices that are not evenly spaced along adjacent contours. Although introduced in the early day of graphical computing (Kepel 1975, Fuchs, Kedem & Uselton, 1977) it is still an active research topic (Jones & Chen, 1994; Berzin 2002). Contouring algorithms often produce high detail contours. In order to reduce the level of detail, unnecessary or redundant vertices have to be removed using Vertex reduction filters applied to each contour line. These filters operate at each point that forms the polygonal contour line. A very simple one is the n-th point where the every n-th point is part of the output contour line but has the disadvantage that it is sensitive to the start point as well essential characteristics of the contour line might be lost arbitrarily. More complex algo-

Figure 1. Demonstrating part of the external surface of the head triangulated and embedded into a CT slice

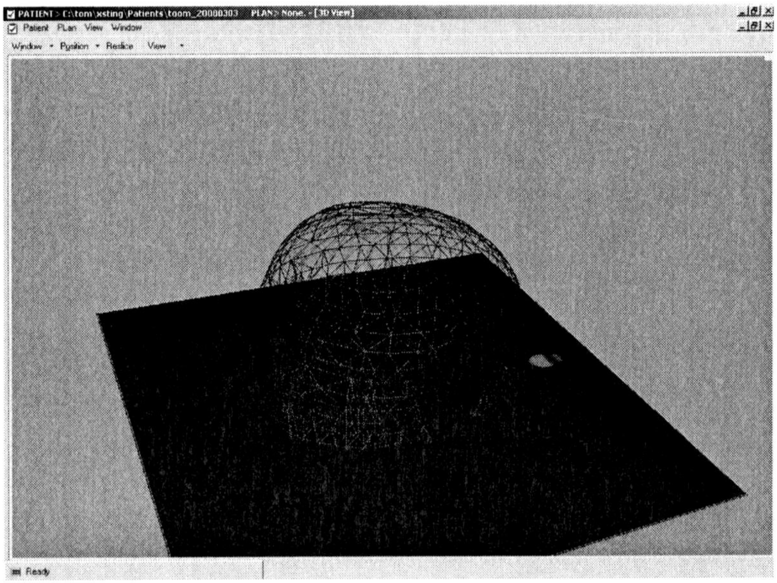

rithms preserve local geometrical characteristics (ie curvature) according to predefined tolerance metrics (distance, energy functions etc) without sacrificing global geometry of the processed line (Douglas and Peuckert 1973; Reuman and Witkam 1974). The reduction can be also done at a later stage on higher dimension by merging/eliminating triangular elements based on spatial smoothing criteria or other restrictions or requirements. Sometimes regeneration of the triangular mesh is needed. A collection of some classical algorithms to achieve polygonal mesh manipulation can be found in several survey and reviews (Heckbert & Garland 1997; Luebke, 2001).

Unlike geometric surfaces that can be described using equation sets in general point reconstructed surfaces do not have straight forward analytical expressions that can participate in transformations, actual processing is performed on their corresponding surface points. A set of powerful and well explored surface categories are the implicit surfaces. These surfaces can be expressed as the zero level set of a function $f(x,y,z)$. Implicit surfaces have some useful properties that are exploited in computer graphics as implicit surface modelling, especially in solids modelling, animation and simulation. One of their property extensively used is the intrinsic space division they provide. Consider the equation of a sphere of radius r in 3D space placed at the origin

$$x^2 + y^2 + z^2 = r^2 \qquad (1)$$

Rewriting the equation as the zero level set we can classify every point in $\mathfrak{R}^3$ according to the spheres surface as "inside"/ "outside" or at surface by checking the sign of $f(x,y,z)$. Thus an implicit surface divides the 3D space in a known way. It is also easy to combine implicit surfaces and form more complex surfaces or solid shapes by setting a tree like structure where the leaves are surfaces and the branches are operators in this case the root will represent the resulted final stage of construction. This method is know as Construc-

Figure 2. Visualizing the «inside/outside» property of the universal matrix voxels. Grey voxels are inside black voxels are outside. The implicit surface (patch) used to classify the voxels is also visible. Voxels have been intentionally shrinked for better visual perception

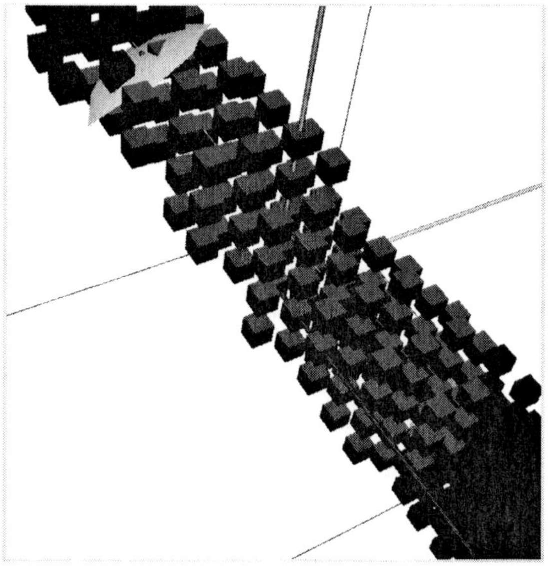

tive Solid Geometry (CSG). The resulted construct has the same property regarding classification of points in space therefore it is easy to built complex constructs approximating real world constructs and interact , manipulate or perform collision detection. We have successfully expanded this property to polygonal reconstructed shapes by imitating the classification behavior of implicit surfaces permitting the participation of these functions to CSG driven simulation applications. Fig. 2 and Fig. 3

REGISTRATION AND FUSION OF MODALITIES AND GRAPHICS IN STEREOTACTIC RADIOTHERAPY

Stereotactic Radiotherapy as well Radiosurgery make intensive use of image extracted features. Main concerns in therapy planning and irradiation procedure are proper localisation of the lesion in terms of diagnosis and definition in real world coordinate system as well calculation of the spatial distribution of deposited energy, called dose, on the lesion and healthy tissue. Further on possible successive sessions required need also follow up evaluation and verification based on new datasets and physical examinations acquired. Special systems are developed to assist this procedure called Treatment Planning Systems (TPS). Those systems simulate the irradiation room world by modelling precisely all devices involved in the plan like the linear accelerator (LINAC) the patient table and the patient itself to perform geometric verification in 3D space of patient placement, lesion targeting, functional feasibility and finally accepted volume dose distribution. The data input to the system are single or multimodal tomographic image sets representing the desired body anatomy where the lesion is located. Stereotactic radiotherapy is widely known for successful treatment of malignances into the head. Its almost spherical geometry that

Figure 3. A closer look at the implicit surface patch

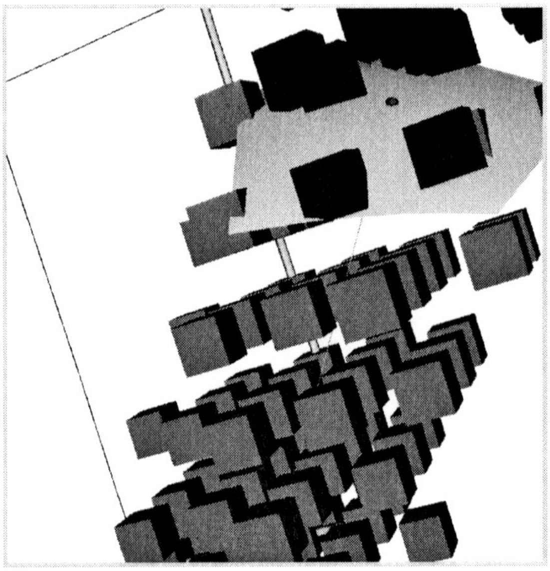

is easily accessed by the rotational LINAC as well the homogeneity of the brain tissue that allows fast dose calculation made it an excellent field of therapeutic application. Stereotactic radiotherapy can be also applied to treat almost any part the human body (Stereotactic Body Radiotherapy). Specific areas with high spatial density of different anatomical structures (spinal cord, blood vessels, trachea, lymphatic network etc) like the neck require sophisticated calculating power demanding TPS to achieve feasibility of irradiation within the required therapeutic, safety and geometrical constraints. A novel mounting approach of the LINAC on a robotic arm combined with a six freedom degree patient table and a patient movement synchronisation system is the state of the art in radiotherapy. The CyberKnife as it is called has been applied to lung (Brown et al. 2007; Cessaretti et al. 2008), pancreas, prostate (Fuller et al. 2008), neck, and spinal cord (Sahgal, Larson, & Chang, 2008) cancer treatment promising higher dose accuracy and almost total body access.

The patient images used for the simulated reconstruction presented were axial scans of the head. The image size was 256 x 256 or 512 x 512 pixels. Two types of slices are used fine and normal slices with 1.0 and 5.0 mm thickness respectively. The total size of the stack is 40 to 80 slices. Normal slices are used to define the exterior of the head and provide also landmarks for proper localisation of the imageset regarding the real world coordinate system. Fine slices include the lesion which is usual soft tissue. After successful localisation contour extraction (also know as delineation) of all organs or anatomic areas has to be performed in order to reconstruct their models in 3D space. Contour extraction can be done manually, semi automatically and automatically. In case of manual contour extraction the physician marks every point that belongs to the contour trying to follow it based on visual distinction of the boundaries. Proper contrast level is applied using window and slope settings in order to locate anatomic areas. All the points are linearly connected and form a closed contour.

The semi automatic way works also in planar mode but for every contour on a particular slice a physician indicates the point that is part of the external surface of desired organ or anatomical area. The selected Hounsfield Unit (HU) selected is used by a contour extraction algorithm as the isoline value and the points that belong to the corresponding isoline are generated. It is possible that more than one closed isoline exist, in this case manual intervention determines the correct one although automatic detection and correction can be implemented by advising already delineated contours or anatomic atlas retrieved prototypes. (Falcao & Udupa 2000; Faerber, Ehrhardt, & Handels 2007). The last method can be also used for automatic contour extraction. Pateint slices are registered with an anatomic atlas and necessary seed points are automatically transferred to initiate contouring algorithms. (Faerber, Ehrhardt, & Handels 2005) Physicians have to review the generated contours and accept or modify them to the anatomical detail desired.

Intermediate slice imaging data can be artificially generated using several classical interpolation methods (Lehmann, Goenner, & Spitzer 1999) or image registration techniques (Penney et al. 2004; Frakes et al 2008). Once delineation process is complete the image stack contains overlaid planar curves or to be more accurate a point set that is line connected to form a linear approximation of a set of contour curves. There are no interslice connections yet established. All these contour curves will be used to form a closed, watertight hull that encloses the area of interest in 3D space. The hull surface is composed by triangular elements that interconnect points of adjacent slices. A lot of hull generation algorithms exist. Some of them can directly operate on point clouds (points distributed in 3D space) were other require a planar layout of points. The connection element between points is still a linear segment and the representation is a connectivity list that indicates a traversal direction from one point to the next. While constructing contours and hulls the problem of direction is important because a lot of other issues like normals direction on planar elements are directly related. In order to ensure that the reconstructed hulls normals direction is consistent all contour lines extracted are filtered to maintain clockwise or counter clockwise connection. Once the global direction is set the connection of the points of the individual triangles has to be the same to ensure that each normal vector on every triangle will point outside the hull. This convention is stressed because the characterization algorithm used to determine and construct the models inside/outside map requires consistent normals direction. Also the light and transform algorithm of the render engine will produce a messy image (obscured and darkened areas) making 3D image perception difficult (Borodin, Zachmann & Klein, 2004).

The user saved structures that model organs and anatomic units are automatically saved as implicit surface constructs. These constructs consist of the polygonal data that is needed to represent the surface; the point set an octtree and normals cache. The octtree is a treelike data structure for space subdivision like the quad trees in planar subdivision. The use of octtrees speeds up point, elementary triangle retrieval of the polygonal surface. The normals cache is actually an array holding the normal vectors for every individual triangular element. Generation of the normals cache and the octtree is done upon creation of the implicit surface. Both of them are needed to speedup the point classification algorithm. As already mentioned any given point in 3D space can be characterized relative to an implicit surface. The implicit surface construct using its own classification algorithm replies to the call surfA->InOut() returning only three values 1, -1 and 0 representing outside, inside and "at surface" respectively.

All structures are embedded into a particular 3D data structure that acts as the universal container for the modeling environment. The structure has rectilinear grid for space subdivision. The cells composing this grid are called voxels. Depending on the implemented simulation, the size of the hexahedral voxels may be non equal for every side of the cell allowing a more dense resolution in areas required. Once an implicit surface construct is embedded into the universal container a new attribute is generated and added to the voxels that is used to label all voxels of the container as inside/outside the embedded surface or to be more concrete if the implicit surface represents the patient left eye "belongs to LE". Subsequent embedding of implicit surface structures causes a universal voxel to be multiple labeled. Specific volume data can be easily queried out of the universal data structure by counting the voxel labeled to the organ of interest. The particular developed TPS for radiotherapy uses a complex hexahedral grid based on the acquired patient image spatial resolution. The hexahedral cells have quadratic section matched to image resolution while the height of each cell depends whether the cells have normal or fine slice embedded into them. It is also possible to work entirely on the fine resolution by interpolating missing slices between normal slices but the result does not justify the computation overhead. In stereotactic radiotherapy the therapeutic dose is delivered partially to the patient using more irradiation beams that form fans rather than single beams. The benefit of this concept is that all irradiation beams are positioned to converge to a common area accumulating maximum energy as close as possible at the lesion. The placement of the beams as well the arcs traversed by individual beams is a problem that does not have a single solution. Restrictions apply to the path of every beam regarding sensitive or even forbidden anatomic units. These have to be either totally omitted or the dose should be kept below an upper limit. As already mentioned irradiation beams are generated by LINACs that are machines with a rotating gantry around a center called the isocenter. The gantry can rotate either clockwise or counterclockwise up to 180 degrees. The patient table rotates as well around the same the isocenter but the semi circle drawn is always on a plane perpendicular to the rotation plane of the gantry. It is obvious that while the gantry rotates to irradiate it should not in any way collide with the patient. Thus operational restrictions and machine limitations have to be taken in account during therapy planning. Using a simulated view of the beam also called "beams eye view" (BEV) the physician can see how the beam will interact with anatomic structures. Visual guidance ensures that the beams avoid them and a proper set of starting and ending angle are chosen for the rotating gantry position.

Isocenter placement is also a critical planning stage. Sometimes more than one isocenter are needed to cover adequately the whole volume of the lesion. Every isocenter has its own set of beams and has to be verified as already mentioned.

Once all preconditions are set the simulation starts firing beams passing through the isocenter across our geometric constructs registering energy deposition on the respectively cells contained into the beam's path. The calculation of the dose $D(v)$ on a given voxel v is given by the following simplified formula:

$$D(v) = TPR(d(v)) \cdot OAR(d(v), offset(v)) \cdot C \quad (2)$$

Function $d(v)$ is the depth of voxel(cell) v referred to the beams entry point in patients external surface (skin). The function $offset(v)$ is the distance of voxel v to the beams centerline. $TPR(d)$ is the Tissue Phantom Ratio at phantom depth d while $OAR(d, off)$ is the off-axis ratio at depth d and distance off from the beam's centerline entering the phantom. C is a collimator specific precalculated correction constant that justifies the circular field of the beams to a predefined square sectioned radiation field at a standard source detector distance.

The dose contents of the the voxels involved are added up and stored as new attribute to the voxel representing the total dose. Quality evaluation of the treatment plan requires visualization of the total dose as well computation some metrics. The total dose data is a volumetric dataset like the initial imageset. Visualization of dose data can be done either in 2D or 3D after normalization against a special user selected point (max. dose, dose at isocenter, specific point in patients body) Both of them require overlay with acquired patient images as well any delineated organs to percept the actual effect. In 2D visualization the dose is usually color coded in contrast to the gray scaled CT/MRI images. Radiotherapists prefer to view isodose curves instead of colored areas overlaid on grey scaled images. At this point automatic multiple contour extraction algorithms give a set of isodose lines. Every isodose line is carefully examined traversing through CT/MRI slices for the anatomic structures enclosed.

In 3D the only meaningful visualization of the total dose data is the extracted isosurfaces (Fig. 4). These isosurfaces show the volume of lesion enclosed that receives the specific dose. Only one surface at a time is meaningful to be displayed. Control on the isosurface opacity can highly contribute to spatial perception of the relative volume covered. Usually more than one treatment plans are generated as a result of optimization. Dose profiles are compared and the best plan is set for implementation.

Stereotactic Radiotherapy is in its nature an extended registration and fusion process. (Pellizari 1998). Multimodality coordinates (CT, MRI, PET, MR-Spectroscopy etc), machine – room coordinates (LINAC, table), patient body coordinates (lesion) as well the therapeutic plan (expected dose) have to be co-registered on the physical patient. Therefore spatial precision is essential in stereotactic radiotherapy. Proper positioning of the patient has to be ensured by any means. Any movement of the patient during dose delivery should be avoided. Specially designed frames have been developed and applied to patients to achieve this goal as well to provide a physical reference coordinates frame that is also used for fast registration of patient multimodal images. It is known that CT scans provide accurate anatomical information with high spatial resolution while MRI, has excellent soft tissue contrast and PET, MR-Spectroscopy etc reveal functional disorders sometimes down to metabolic level. This mutual information derived from the multimodality can be combined to precisely locate the lesion using the delineation process described above. (Maintz and Viergever 1998;. Pluim, Maintz, & Viergever, 2003);

Advanced image registration techniques promise frameless treatment (Eggers, Muehling, & Marmulla, 2006) while real time registration might compensate respiration movement that elastically deforms the torso geometry affecting internal organs boundaries. (Rietzel, Chen, Choi, & Willet, 2005; Lu et al 2006; McClelland et al. 2006).

The whole simulation environment of the TPS was coded in C++. Imageset and dataset processing, environment modeling and graphics realization was done using kitware's Visualization Toolkit (VTK). (Schroeder, Martin, & Lorensen, 1998). The proposed structures were designed according to VTK's interface model ensuring seamless integration and easy usage to already experienced developers.

FUTURE TRENDS

Geometric concepts in biomedical systems are intrinsically related to biomedical images. In most cases images are the starting point to lead to representation of world's real models. In prototyping the order is reversed but the common point is still high fidelity representation. Following the chain from the acquired image sets to 3D representation and user interaction almost all points need constant improvement. Multi slice medical scanners may increase spatial resolution and scanning speed producing more data to be processed at later processing stage. Consider

Figure 4. Demonstrating 3D dose representation. The object in red is the target volume while the olive colored surface embedded in it is the isosurface of a specific user selected dose level. The arcs are the 4 beam used to deliver dose to the target. The external surface of the head is colored orange.

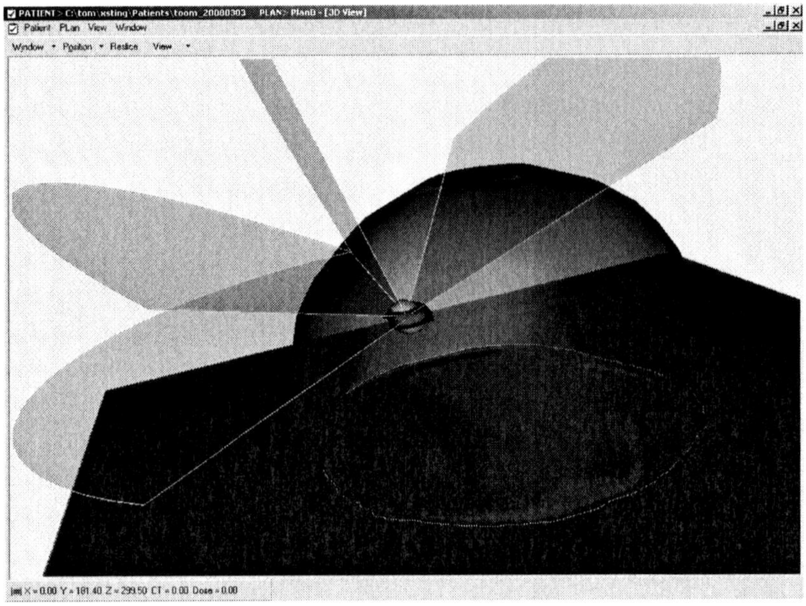

dynamic, real time processing of the imageset generated and existing graphic hardware reaches its limits. This data flooding overwhelms today's multicore general purpose CPU as well volatile memory bandwidth and size. Also processing software should encourage the development and use of well defined, high quality libraries, toolkits, classes even total development platforms stressing constant optimization and reusability of code. Dynamics in models might be handled by specialized hardware. Recall in early 90's the term GPU was more fiction than fact while the first SuperVGA adapters proudly displayed true color images to CRT monitors. Today's dedicated graphics processors pose units that perform higher than general purpose CPU raising the interest for general purpose GPU.

Constructional limits posed by solid state physics have been always the nightmare of microelectronics to disturb/cancel Moore's law. Core redesign of CPUs entering parallelism using multiple identical cores and promising novel nanomaterials might keep the Moore's law valid for the near future. Specialized processors might strongly support some highly repeatable tasks. Today PhysX, a dedicated physics processor unit (PPU) starts offering physics calculation offering universal collision detection, rigid-body dynamics, soft-body dynamics and deformation, fluid dynamics, and smart particle systems in gaming industry. But hardware is not a sole contributor, software needs also redesign and refactoring to exploit as more as possible the available or future GPU hardware platform. Thus the co-evolution algorithms-architecture leads to a Chicken/Egg problem.

Although fundamental limits of image registration are continuously studied (Robinson & Milanfar, 2004; Yetik & Nehorai 2006) the topic is still an open research and application field

(Orchard 2008). New and old hardware platforms (GPU, VLSI) are investigated promising high performance for sophisticated registration algorithms (Gupta & Gupta 2007; Samant, Xia, Muyan-Oezcelik & Owens, 2008). New optimization techniques and parallel implementation of the registration process (Wachowiak & Peters, 2006) show significant speed up maintaining robustness and accuracy.

The final part of the chain is human visual perception and interaction. Beside tremendous improvement in imaging and processing hardware the terminal visualization display remains 2-dimensional. The demand for real 3D display system is an old but still active research field for wide area of applications. There exist some implementations with acceptable spatial perception of the objects displayed. A commercially available system using dome shaped display unit offers color 3D projection for RT planning (Napoli et al., 2008). Some recent research has announced the development of an updatable flat monochrome holographic display (Tay et al. 2008).

Finally virtual reality environments offer a new perception in medical training and treatment planning. In some surgical operations instead of looking to an image guiding display system information is directly projected in front of the surgeons view field (Lorensen et al. 1993). Wearing a special head mounted display (HMD) visual system graphical information is overlayed to the surgeons view field (Grimson et al 1996). The information may be a CT/MRI image or synthetic graphical simulated information. This is a typical application of augmented reality. In general augmented reality is actually an image registration problem in real time. A visual system (camera) is used to provide the real world image while a computer is synthesizing the composed – overlaid image to be projected. The problems to be solved in real time are real scene light matching, real world – object coordinate systems transformation and matching (Uenohora & Kanade, 1995). The benefits of augmented reality eliminate the use of stereotactic frames because solving the coordinate transformation a virtual universal real time coordinate system accompanies the patient thus any externally attached positioning devices can be omitted (Grimson et al, 1996). Total immersion virtual reality is also promising a new dimension in medical training and education. Simulating a complete environment (i.e. operation room) by synthesizing the scene with graphically modeled 3D objects enhances spatial reality perception. A radiotherapy room has been simulated (Philips, Ward & Beavis, 2005) using this type of virtual reality for training. The linac movement was controlled by a real handheld device. Although VR systems progress in the visual part of reality the lack of proper human interaction. User interaction is mainly done using keyboard and pointing device. In some cases joysticks are used to move or traveling through 3D scenes. In surgical and laparoscopy simulators the sense of touch is essential. Special controls that imitate force feedback using haptics technology are explored (Westerbring-van der Putten, Goossens, Jakimowicz, & Dankelman, 2008).

CONCLUSION

Visualization of geometric features embedded in biomedical images is essential for medical spatial perception. We have presented an application framework for image and geometry coregistration by extending functionality of an already existing, reliable and widely used visualization toolkit. High speed computing at medium cost permits to switch from the classic 2 dimensional patient images to 3 dimensional patient anatomy reconstruction. Establishing a universal matrix where all geometrical structures and image reside, interact and register topological and functional data might serve as basic framework to build simulation application. A real application in stereotactic radiotherapy treatment planning that is based on the particular framework was presented in detail. There are functional topics in the application that can be optimized to increase performance in repeated treatment planning. To enhance the framework the parameter of time to support motion could be a possible extension serving real time dynamics where needed. On the other hand evolving hardware like virtual reality supporting devices could give another perspective of design and simulation in biomedical systems.

REFERENCES

Ackerman, M. (1998). The visible human project. *Proceedings of the IEEE, 86*(3), 504–511.

Berzin, D., & Hagiwara, I. (2002). Minimal area for surface reconstruction from crosssections, *The Visual Computer, 18*, 437–444.

Borodin, P., Zachmann, G., & Klein, R. (2004). Consistent Normal Orientation for Polygonal Meshes. *Computer Graphics International 2004* (CGI), June 16–19, Crete, Greece. IEEE Computer Society Press.

Brodlie, K., & Wood, J. (2001). Recent Advantages in Volume Visualization. *Computer Graphics Forum, 20*(2), 125-148.

Brown, W. T., Wu, X., Amendola, B., Perman, M., Han, H., Fayad, F., Garcia, S., Lewin, A., Abitbol, A., de la Zerda, A., & Schwade, J. G. (2007). Treatment of early non-small cell lung cancer, stage IA, by image-guided robotic stereotactic radioablation--CyberKnife. *The Cancer Journal, 13*(2), 75-7.

Cesaretti, J., Pennathur, A., Rosenstein, B. S., Swanson, S. J., & Fernando, H. (2008). Stereotactic Radiosurgery for Thoracic Malignancies. *The Annals of Thoracic Surgery, 85*(2), 785–791.

Dawson, S. L., & Kaufman, J. A. (1998). The imperative for medical simulation. *Proceedings of the IEEE 8*(3), 479–483.

Douglas, D. H., & Peucker, T. K. (1973). Algorithms for the Reduction of the Number of Points Required to Represent a Line or its Character. *The American Cartographer, 10*(2), 112-123.

Eggers, G., Mühling, J., & Marmulla, R. (2006). Image-to-patient registration techniques in head surgery. *International Journal of Oral and Maxillofacial Surgery, 35*(12), 1081-95.

Faerber, M., Ehrhardt, J., & Handels, H. (2005). Automatic atlas-based contour extraction of anatomical structures in medical images. *International Congress Series, 1281*, 272–277.

Faerber, M., Ehrhardt, J., & Handels, H. (2007). Live-wire-based segmentation using similarities between corresponding image structures. *Computerized Medical Imaging and Graphics, 31*, 549–560.

Falcao, A., & Udupa, J. (2000). A 3D generalization of user-steered live-wire segmentation. *Medical. Image Analysis, 4*(4) 89–402.

Frakes, D. H., Dasi, L. P., Pekkan, K., Kitajima, H. D., Sundareswaran, K., Yoganathan, A. P., & Smith, M. J. T. (2008). A New Method for Registration-Based Medical Image Interpolation. *IEEE Transactions on Medical Imaging, 27*(3), 370-377.

France, L., Lenoir, J., Angelidis, A., Meseure, P., Cani, M.-P., Faure, F., & Chaillou, C. (2005). A layered model of a virtual human intestine for surgery simulation. *Medical Image Analysis,* (9).

Freudenberg, J., Schiemann, T., Tiede, U., & Hoehne, K. H. (2000). Simulation of cardiac excitation patterns in a three-dimensional anatomical heart atlas. *Computers in Biology and Medicine, 30*, 191-205.

Fuchs, H., Kedem, Z. M., & Uselton, S. P. (1977). Optimal surface reconstruction from planar contours. *Commun ACM, 20*, 693–702.

Fuller, D. B., Naitoh, J., Lee, Ch., Hardy, S., & Jin, H. (2008). Virtual HDR CyberKnife Treatment for Localized Prostatic Carcinoma: Dosimetry Comparison With HDR Brachytherapy and Preliminary Clinical Observations. *International Journal of Radiation Oncology, Biology, Physics, 70*(5), 1588-1597.

Gavaghan, D., Garny, A., Maini, P. K., & Kohl, P. (2006). Mathematical models in physiology. *Phil. Trans. R. Soc. A 364*, 1099–1106.

Grimson, W. E. L., Ettinger, G. J., White, S. J., Lozano-Perez, T., Wells, W. M., III., & Kikinis, R. (1996, April). An Automated Registration Methods for Frameless Stereotaxy, Image Guided Surgery, and Enhanced Reality Visulatization. *Medical Imaging, IEEE Transactions, 15*(2), 129-140.

Gupta, N., & Gupta, N. (2007). A VLSI Architecture for Image Registration in Real Time. *IEEE Transactions on VLSI, 15*(9), 981-989.

Heckbert, P., & Garland, M. (1997). Survey of Polygonal Surface Simplification Algorithms. *Siggraph 97 Course Notes, 25*. ACM Press.

Herman, G. T., & Liu, H. K. (1977). Display of three dimensional information in computed tomography. *J Comput Assist Tomogr, 1*, 155–160.

Jones, M. W., & Chen, M. (1994). A new approach to the construction of surfaces from contour data. *Comput Graph Forum, 13*, 75–84.

Keppel, E. (1975). Approximating complex surfaces by triangulation of contour lines. *IBM J Res Dev 19*(1), 2–11.

Lu, W., Olivera, G. H., Chen, Q., Chen M-L., & Ruchala, K. J. (2006). Automatic re-contouring in 4D radiotherapy. *Physics in Medicine and Biology, 51*, 1077–1099.

Lehmann, T. Goenner, C., & Spitzer K. (1999). Survey: Interpolation Methods in Medical Image Processing. *IEEE Transactions on Medical Imaging,18*(11), 1049-1075.

Lopes, A., & Brodlie, K.(2003). Improving the robustness and accuracy of the marching cubes algorithm for isosurfacing. *IEEE Transactions on Visualization and ComputerGraphics, 9*, 16–29.

Lorensen, W. E., & Cline, H. E. (1987). Marching cubes: A high resolution 3D surface construction algorithm. *In Proceedings of the 14th annual conference on Computer graphics and interactive techniques*. (pp. 163–169). ACM Press.

Lorensen, W., Cline, H., Nafis, C., Kikinis, R., Altobelli, D., & Gleason, L. (1993). Enhancing Reality in the Operating Room. *Proceedings of the 1993 IEEE Visualization Conference* (pp. 410-415).

Luebke, D. (2001). A Developer's Survey of Polygonal Simplification Algorithms. *IEEE Computer Graphics &Applications,* (pp. 24-35).

McClelland, J. R., Blackall, J. M., Tarte, S., Chandler, A. C., Hughes, S., Ahmad, S., Landau, D. B., &Hawkes, D. J. (2006). A continuous 4D motion model from multiple respiratory cycles for use in lung radiotherapy. *Medical Physics, 33*, 3348–3358.

Mock, U., Georg, D., Bogner, J., Auberger, T., & Potter, R. (2004). Treatment planning comparison of conventional, 3D conformal, and intensity-modulated photon (IMRT) and proton therapy for paranasal sinuscarcinoma. *Int J Radiat Oncol Biol Phys, 58*(1), 147–154. [3D reduces dose delivered].

Maintz, J. B. A., & Viergever, M. A. (1998). *A Survey of Medical Image Registration Medical Image Analysis, 2*(1), 1–37.

Napoli, J., Stutsman, S., Chu, J. C. H., Gong, X., Rivard, M. J., Cardarelli, G., Ryan, T. P., & Favalora, G. E. (2008). Radiation therapy planning using a volumetric 3-D display: PerspectaRAD. *Proceedings of SPIE-IS&T Electronic Imaging, SPIE, 6803.*

Nealen, A., Muller, M., Keiser, R., Boxerman, E., & Carlson, M. (2005). Physically based deformable models in computer graphics. In *Eurographics 2005, State of the Art Report* 2005.

Noble, D. (2002). Modeling the Heart from Genes to Cells to the Whole Organ. Science, *295*(5560), 1678-1682.

Pelizzari, C. A. (1998). Image Processing in Stereotactic Planning: Volume Visualization and Image Registration. *Medical Dosimetry, 23*(3), 137–145.

Penney, G. P., Schnabel, J. A., Rueckert, D., Viergever, M. A., & Niessen, W. J. (2004). Registration-Based Interpolation. *IEEE Transactions on Medical Imaging, 23*(7), 922-926.

Phillips, R., Ward, R., & Beavis, A. (2005). Immersive visualization training of radiotherapy treatment. In *Medicine Meets Virtual Reality Conference (MMVR 13)* (pp. 390–396) (Long-Beach, California), IOS Press.

Pluim, J. P. W., Maintz, J. B. A., & Viergever, M. A. (2003). Mutual-Information-Based Registration of Medical Images: A Survey. *IEEE Transactions on Medical Imaging, 22*(8), 986-1004.

Reumann, K., & Witkam, A. P. M. (1974). Optimizing Curve Segmentation in Computer Graphics. I*nternational Computing Symposium. Amsterdam, North Holland*, (pp. 467- 472).

Rietzel, E., Chen, G. T., Choi, N. C., & Willet, C. G. (2005). Four-dimensional image-based treatment planning: Target volume segmentation and dose calculation in the presence of respiratory motion. *International Journal of Radiation Oncology Biology and Physics, 61*, 1535–1550.

Robb, R. A., Greenleaf, J. F., Ritman, E. L., Johnson, S. A., Sjostrand, J. D., Herman, G. T., & Wood, E. H. (1974). Three-dimensional visualization of the intact thorax and contents: a technique for cross-sectional reconstruction from multiplanar x-ray views. *Comput Biomed Res, 7*, 395–419.

Robb, R. A. (1999). Virtual endoscopy: development and evaluation using the Visible Human Datasets, *Computerized Medical Imaging and Graphics*, (24), 133–151.

Robb, R. A., & Hanson, D. P. (2006). Biomedical Image Visualization Research Using the Visible Human Datasets. *Clinical Anatomy, 19*, 240–253.

Robinson, D., & Milanfar, P. (2004). Fundamental Performance Limits in Image Registration. *IEEE Transactions on Image Processing,13*(9), 1185-1199.

Sahgal, A., Larson, D. A., & Chang, E. L. (2008). Stereotactic body radiosurgery for spinal metastases: a critical review. *International Journal of Radiation Oncology, Biology, Physics., 71*(3), 652-65.

Samant, S. S., Xia, J., Muyan-Özçelik, P., & Owens, J. D. (2008). High performance computing for deformable image registration: Towards a new paradigm in adaptive radiotherapy. *Medical. Physics., 35*(8), 3546-3553.

Seemann, G., Hoeper, Ch., Doessel, O., Holden, A. V., & Zhang, H. (2006). Heterogeneous three-dimensional anatomical and electrophysiological model of human atria. *Phil. Trans. R. Soc., A 364*, 1465–1481.

Sellberg, M. S., & Vanderploeg, M. J. (1994). Virtual human: A computer graphics model for biomechanical simulations and computer-aided instruction. *Proceedings of the 16th Annual International Conference of the IEEE Engineering in Medicine and Biology Society, Engineering Advances: New Opportunities for Biomedical Engineers, IEEE*, New York, NY, (pp. 329–330).

Schroeder, W., Martin, K., & Lorensen, W. (1998). *The Visualization Toolkit: An Object-Oriented Approach to 3D Graphics*. Prentice Hall.

Schiemann, T., Tiede, U., & Höhne, K. H. (1997). Segmentation of the visible human for high-quality volume-based visualization. *Medical Image Analysis, 1*(4), 263-70.

Shim, V. B., Pitto, R. P., Streicher, R. M., Hunter, P. J., & Anderson, I. A. (2007). The use of sparse CT datasets for auto-generating accurate FE models of the femur and pelvis. *Journal of Biomechanics, 40*, 26–35.

Spirka, T. A., & Damaser, M. S. (2007). Modeling physiology of the urinary tract. *Journal of Endourology, 21*(3), 294-299.

Spitzer, V. M., & Whitlock, D. G. (1998). The visible human data set: the anatomical platform for human simulation. *Anat. Rec. (New Anat.,) 253*, 49–57.

Spitzer, V., Spitzer, G., Lee, C., Reinig, K., Granas, L., Graus, K., & Smyth, P. (2004). VH Dissector: A platform for curriculum development and presentation for the anatomical arts and sciences. In *Medicine Meets Vitual Reality 12* (Newport Beach, California), IOS Press, (pp. 127–129).

Tay, S., Blanche, P.-A., Voorakaranam, R. A., Tunc, V., Lin, W., Rokutanda, S., Gu, T., Flores, D., Wang, P., Li, G., St Hilaire, P., Thomas, J., Norwood, R. A., Yamamoto, M., & Peyghambarian, N. (2008). An updatable holographic three-dimensional display. *Nature Letters, 451*, 694-698.

Teschner, M., Kimmerle, S., Heidelberger, B., Zachmann, G., Raghupathi, L., Fuhrmann, A., Cani, P. M., Faure, F., Magenat-Thalmann, N., Strasser, W., & Volino, P. (2005). Collision detection for deformable objects. *Computer Graphics Forum, 24*(1), 61–81.

Uenohara, M., & Kanade, T. (1995). Vision-Based Object Registration for Real-Time Image Overlay. In N. Ayache (Ed.), *Computer Vision, Virtual Reality and Robotics in Medicine: CVRMed '95* (pp. 14-22). Berlin: Springer-Verlag.

Wachowiak, M. P., & Peters, T. M. (2006). High-Performance Medical Image Registration Using New Optimization Techniques. *IEEE Transactions on Information Technology in Biomedicine, 10*(2), 344-353.

Westerbring-van der Putten, E. P., Goossens, R. H. M., Jakimowicz, J. J., & Dankelman, J. (2008). Haptics in minimally invasive surgery – a review. *Minimally Invasive Therapy, 17*(1), 3–16.

Yetik, I. S., & Nehorai, A. (2006). Performance Bounds on Image Registration. *IEEE Transactions on Signal Processing, 54*(5), 1737-1749.

KEY TERMS

Contouring: A subdivision process where a set of points logically connected forms a construct that represents a common characteristic feature in general. On a 2D space contouring generates lines while on a 3D space beside lines and surfaces.

Dose Calculation/Optimization: The procedure to determine the body absorbed energy in both the lesion and healthy tissue. The optimization of the process is inherent due to steep dose delivery around the target.

Image Fusion: Simultaneous presentation of multimodal registered images on a visual media.

Image Registration: Registration of images in a common known reference coordinate system.

Implicit Surface Modeling: Specific modeling process that approximates every geometrical model using implicit mathematical functions as analytical surface representation constructing complex geometric representations maintaining mathematical functionality of the final model.

Multimodal Imaging (Multispectral): Images of the same object using different physical acquisition technology the term is widely used for medical imaging while multispectral refers to satellite imaging and survey.

Octtrees: 3D space divison data structures analogous to 2D quad trees. Used for storage, compression, collision detection, point search etc.of 3D models.

Stereotactic Radiotherapy: A Radiation therapy procedure that requires precise localization of the target area to deliver fractioned prescribed dose by means of convergent or not beams.

Surface Reconstruction: The reconstrunction of geometrical surface The surface might by a point cloud, know contours of the recoctructed surface, known gradients.

Treatment Planning System (TPS): A computer based system used to simulate, calculate and optimize the radiotherapy treatment of patients. The main tasks are lesion localization, radiation plan generation according to safety and health constaints and geometric feasibility plan optimization.

Visualization Toolkit (VTK): An open source graphical toolkit widely used as a common extendable customizable platform for scientific visualization.

Chapter XIV
Internal Radionuclide Dosimetry using Quantitative 3-D Nuclear Medical Imaging

Ioannis Tsougos
University of Thessaly, Greece

George Loudos
Technological Educational Institute of Athens, Greece

Panagiotis Georgoulias
University of Thessaly, Greece

Konstantina S. Nikita
National Technical University of Athens, Greece

Kiki Theodorou
University of Thessaly, Greece

ABSTRACT

Quantitative three-dimensional nuclear medical imaging plays a continuously increasing role in radionuclide dosimetry, allowing the development of patient – specific treatment planning systems. The established method for dosimetry is based on the measurement of the biokinetics by serial gamma camera scans, followed by calculations of the administered activity and the residence times, resulting in the radiation absorbed doses of critical organs. However, the quantification of the activity in different organs from planar data is hampered by inaccurate attenuation and scatter correction as well as due to background and organ overlay (Glatting 2006). Alternatively, dosimetry based on quantitative three-dimensional data is more accurate and allows a more individualized approach, provided that all effects that degrade the quantitative content of the images have been corrected for. In addition inhomogeneous organ accumulation of the radionuclide can be detected and possibly taken into account (De Jong 2004). This chapter provides adequate information on internal emitter dosimetry and a state of the art review of the current methodology.

INTRODUCTION

In order to estimate the absorbed dose for all significant tissues in nuclear medicine, one must determine for each tissue the quantity of energy absorbed per unit mass. This yields the quantity absorbed dose, and can be extended to the calculation of dose equivalent if desired. This response and the prediction of toxicity is essential to rational the implementation of cancer therapy.

Nevertheless, to state that the absorbed dose alone would predict the radiobiologic response of tissue is an oversimplification that would certainly lead to hypo- or hyper- estimation of the radiation induced effects. It has already been recognized in radiotherapy that the response is affected by a number of parameters such as: the type of radiation (LET), the rate at which absorbed dose is delivered, the radiobiologic characteristics of the tumor or normal tissue etc. Moreover the anatomical characteristic of the patients have to be taken into account, since the presence of different structures affects the distribution of radiation dose.

Presently, nuclear medicine dosimetry is based on the measurement of the biokinetics of the radionuclide by serial gamma camera scans, followed by calculations comprising three steps. First the percentage of administered activity of the radiopharmaceutical must be determined for the accumulating organs for several scan times. Second these biokinetic data must be integrated to obtain the percentage of the number of decays in the source organs, i.e the residence times and third, the radiation absorbed doses of critical organs must be determined.

However, using planar data to quantify the activity in different organs may be severely affected by several factors, such as the inaccurate attenuation and scatter correction as well as the background and organ overlay.

Dosimetry that takes into account quantitative 3-dimensional data is more accurate and obviously allows the so called 'tailor made' approach, in terms of the individualization of therapy on each specific patient. Nevertheless there are factors that can potentially degrade the quantitative content of the images, or insert erroneous data, such as the inhomogeneous organ accumulation of the radionuclide, which have to be detected and taken into account.

The research on dosimetry is focused on the development of software tools, which allow the use of tomographic functional data (PET-SPECT) in conjunction with anatomical information from CT or MRI, providing a more accurate and detailed description of the individual patient situation. Firstly anatomical and functional data need to be registered and fused and then manual or automated Regions Of Interest (ROIs) are drawn. Hence dose calculation is based on dose kernel convolution methods, reliant on convolving the radioactivity distribution with a medium specific radionuclide dose-kernel, defined as the adsorbed dose per decay at a point away from the source. The innovation consists in the application of the CT information, which allows the use of different dose kernels depending on the different evaluated structures.

BACKGROUND

Absorbed Dose Definitions and Calculations

The biologic responses of radionuclide therapy are mediated by a well defined physical quantity, the absorbed dose, defined as the energy absorbed per unit mass of tissue. Absorbed dose is a non-stochastic quantity applicable to both indirectly and directly ionizing radiations. For indirectly ionizing radiations, energy is imparted to matter in a two step process. In the first step (resulting in kerma) the indirectly ionizing radiation transfers energy as kinetic energy to secondary charged particles. In the second step these charged particles transfer some of their kinetic energy to the medium (resulting in absorbed dose) and lose some of their energy in the form of bremsstrahlung (electromagnetic radiation produced by the deceleration of a charged particle, such as an electron, when deflected by another charged particle, such as an atomic nucleus) losses.

- The absorbed dose is related to the stochastic quantity energy imparted. The absorbed dose is defined as the mean energy ε imparted by ionizing radiation to matter of mass m in a finite volume V by:

$$D = \frac{d\bar{\varepsilon}}{dm} \qquad (1)$$

- The energy imparted ε is the sum of all energy entering the volume of interest minus all energy leaving the volume, taking into account any mass-energy conversion within the volume.

The unit of absorbed dose is joule per kilogram ($J \cdot kg^{-1}$). The special name for the unit of absorbed dose is the gray (Gy).

Specifically for radionuclide therapy the energy absorbed in a particular mass of tissue is defined as:

E = number of radionuclide disintegrations in a particular volume x energy emitted per disintegration of the radionuclide x fraction of emitted energy that is absorbed by a particular (target) mass. (Sgouros 2005)

Depending on the identity of the radionuclide, particles or rays of characteristic energy and abundance will be given off at a rate dependent on the amount of activity present.

Most of the quantities needed for a calculation of dose are now defined: the energy per decay (and number per decay), activity and mass of the target region. One other factor needed is the *fraction of emitted energy* that is absorbed within the target. This quantity is most often called the absorbed fraction and is represented by the symbol φ. For photons (gamma rays and x rays) some of the emitted energy will escape objects of the size and composition of interest to internal dosimetry (mostly soft tissue organs with diameters of the order of centimetres). For electrons and beta particles, most energy is usually considered to be absorbed, so we usually set the absorbed fraction to 1.0. Electrons, beta particles and the like are usually grouped into a class of radiations referred to as 'nonpenetrating' emissions, while x and gamma rays are called 'penetrating' radiations. Subsequently a generic equation for the absorbed dose rate in our object as:

$$\dot{D} = \frac{kA\Sigma_i n_i E_i \phi_i}{m} \qquad (2)$$

where $\dot{D}$ is the absorbed dose rate (rad h^{-1} or Gy s^{-1}), A is the activity (μCi or MBq), n is the number of radiations with energy E emitted per nuclear transition, E is the energy per radiation (MeV), φ is the fraction of energy emitted that is absorbed in the target, m is the mass of target region (g or kg) and k is the proportionality constant (rad g μCi^{-1} h^{-1} MeV^{-1} or Gy kg MBq^{-1} s^{-1} MeV^{-1}).

The equation of the cumulative dose would be shown as:

$$D = \frac{k\tilde{A}\Sigma_i n_i E_i \phi_i}{m} \qquad (3)$$

where D is the absorbed dose (rad or Gy) and $\tilde{A}$ is the cumulated activity (μCi h or MBq s). (Stabin 2005)

The term ϕ accounts for the emission type, energy, and also the geometry and characteristics of the source or target tissue, to provide a net factor that converts the total energy emitted in a particular source region to that absorbed in the region or in other regions. The absorbed fraction factor ϕ is generally determined by Monte Carlo calculations (Sgouros 2005, Loevinger 1988, Snyder 1978).

Dosimetry Systems

Medical Internal Radiation Dose (MIRD) System

The system that defined medical internal dosimetry for many years, is the system developed in 1988 by the Medical Internal Radiation Dose (MIRD) Committee of the Society of Nuclear Medicine (Loevinger 1988). The equation for absorbed dose in the MIRD system is as follows:

$$D_{r_k} = \sum_h \tilde{A}_h\, S(r_k \leftarrow r_h) \qquad (4)$$

In this equation, r_k represents a target region and r_h represents a source region. The cumulated activity is given in the term $\tilde{A}$.

Hence all other terms of the basic equation are lumped in the *S* factor, that is:

$$S(r_k \leftarrow r_h) = \frac{k\sum_i n_i E_i \varphi_i (r_k \leftarrow r_h)}{m_{r_k}} \qquad (5)$$

The use of the '*S* factor' approach greatly facilitated dose calculations. This was accomplished by isolating and tabulating values for those factors of the absorbed dose calculation that could be generalized.

The S values were initially calculated based on idealized models of human anatomy defined as a collection of appropriately placed distinct organ volumes with mass and composition that were selected to reflect a typical or standard human anatomy.

The absorbed fractions required for the determination of the S values were calculated for each radionuclide by taking into account a certain number of decays uniformly distributed throughout each idealized organ volume, while the absorbed fraction from each source–target organ pair was calculated by Monte Carlo simulations (Snyder 1978).

Of course these calculations were performed with very limited computational power, resulting in several simplifying assumptions. Therefore the application of these values to real patient anatomies that deviate from the idealized model would certainly lead to errors.

These potential errors led several groups to develop better generations of anthropomorphic phantoms after the development of the Snyder phantom (Snyder 1969). For example the development of the series of phantoms by Cristy and Eckerman (1987) allowed dose calculations for different size and age, by including six phantoms representing children and adults of both genders. According to Stabin (2006) "absorbed fractions for photons at discrete energies were published for these phantoms, which contained approximately 25 source and target regions. Tables of *S* values were never published, but ultimately were made available in the MIRDOSE computer software (Stabin 1996)."

Moreover Stabin *(*1995) modelled the changes to the uterus, intestines, bladder and other organs that occur during pregnancy and included specific models for the foetus, foetal soft tissue, foetal skeleton and placenta, in an adult female model. The *S* values for these phantoms were also made available through the MIRDOSE software.

Other structures or particular organs have also been described by detailed models, such as the eye (Eckerman *1981*, Holman *1983*), brain (Eckerman *1981*, Bouchet *1999*), peritoneal cavity (Watson *1989*), prostate gland (Stabin 1994), bone (Eckerman and Stabin 2000, Bouchet *1999*), and rectum (Mardirossian *1999*, Cross 1992).

Moreover in order to represent tumours small unit density spheres have also been introduced (Stabin and Konijnenberg 2000).

The evolution of such phantoms from the early beginning with the MIRD 5 Phantom, to the latest NURBS adult model is suggestively illustrated in the following figure (based on Stabin (2006)).

Figure 1. The evolution of the idealized models of human anatomy, utilized to aid the internal nuclear dosimetry.

MIRD 5 Phantom (Snyder *et al* 1978)	VIP Man Phantom (Xu *et al* 2000)	NURBS-based adult male model (Segars 2001)
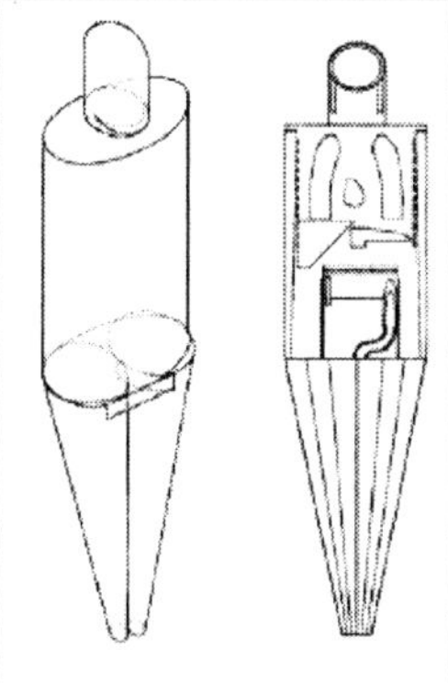	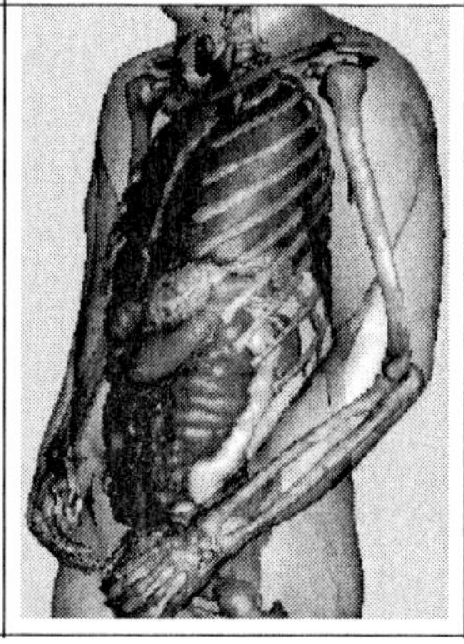	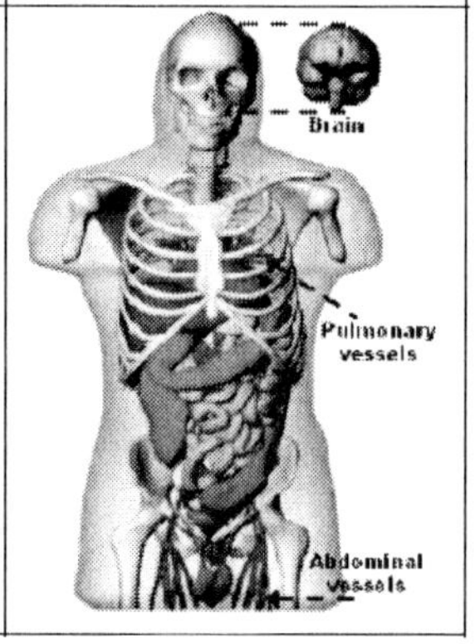

Phantom Based Dosimetry Software

Several groups have utilized the MIRD methodology by developing software where the S factors are implemented. MABDOSE (Johnson 1999) allows the user to place spherically shaped tumors within the simplified anatomic model originally described by the MIRD Committee. The most widely used, was the MIRDOSE software with versions 1, 2, 3 and 3.1 (Stabin 1996). The code automated the calculation of internal dose for a large number (>200) of radiopharmaceuticals in 10 different anthropomorphic models with great success, until it was replaced by a newer code called OLINDA/EXM (Organ Level INternal Dose Assessment with EXponential Modelling) (Stabin *2005*). This software includes data for more than 800 radionuclides resulting in S values specific to 10 phantoms and 5 organ models. The program also includes α-particle emitters and a pharmacokinetic module that may be used to determine organ cumulated activities, as well as the ability to perform minor patient-specific adjustments to doses reported for the standard phantoms.

Image Based Dosimetry Software

The use of 3D imaging modalities, such as PET/CT and SPECT/CT allowed the use of tomographic functional data and anatomical data to be implemented towards the development of patient-specific nuclear medicine dosimetrical systems. This was made possible by the increase in computer processing power and the implementation of point-kernel or Monte Carlo calculation methodologies for the estimation of absorbed fractions.

In order to accomplish 3D image based dosimetry, one would need two requisites. The first requisite is a 3D anatomic imaging study, in order to define the anatomy and provide tissue density information (e.g CT or MRI), in conjunction with a 3D imaging of the radioactivity distribution (e.g. PET or SPECT). The second requisite would be an expedient software that implements the absorbed fraction calculation (point kernel or Monte Carlo) in order to estimate the spatial distribution of the absorbed dose.

Based on the aforementioned idea several groups sought to contribute to the development of such software, including the following efforts: the 3D-Internal Dosimetry (3D-ID) code (Kolbert

1997), the RTDS code (Liu 1999) the DOSE3D code (Clairand 1999) and the SIMDOS code (Dewaraja 2005).

The most fully developed and widely used software package until now is the 3D-ID, which is able to perform both Monte Carlo and point-kernel based calculations. The 3D-ID software package accomplished the two requisites mention above. It takes the distribution of radiolabeled antibody for a given patient (from SPECT or PET) and combines it with anatomic information (from CT or MRI) to yield absorbed dose estimates that are specific to a particular patient's biodistribution and anatomy (Sgouros 1990, Sgouros 1993, Kolbert 1997, Sgouros 2003-2004).

This work introduced the concept of dose volume histograms for internally administered radionuclides in a clinical trial of ^{131}I-labeled anti-B1 antibody. Nevertheless the analysis did not reveal a statistically significant dose–response relationship (Sgouros 2003), but Koral (2002) were able to demonstrate a dose–response relationship, using a more robust and validated SPECT quantitation methodology in a selected subset of 15 patients with pelvic or abdominal tumors.

Internal Dosimetry using Quantitative 3-D Nuclear Medical Imaging

The Difference Compared to External Beam Therapy

In order to understand the limitations, problems, challenges and research directions of Targeted Radiotherapy (TRT) dosimetry, it is useful to consider its standard clinical practice and compare it with external beam therapy. Currently, in almost all TRT treatments the administered activity is fixed; the clinician empirically modifies them according to patient characteristics including age, size and clinical findings (Flux 2006). However, clinical studies have shown that this approach leads to errors in the order to 30%-100% or even higher. The main reason for such errors is that the absorbed dose is not only a function of the administered dose, but is highly correlated to a number of other factors that are patient specific, including both anatomical and functional variations. It is obvious that no radiation oncologist or medical physicist would suggest the same protocol in all patients with a certain type o cancer (Siegel 2002); Variations in beam type, energy, beam exposure time, geometry, etc are decided for different patients.

The Importance

The importance of the need of personalized dosimetry in TRT is stated in the EU council directive 97/43/EURATOM (Nuis A 1997) in which it is stated that "For all medical exposure of individuals for radiotherapeutic purposes exposures of target volumes shall be individually planned; taking into account that doses of non-target volumes and tissues shall be as low as reasonably achievable and consistent with the intended radiotherapeutic purpose of the exposure." However, the physical principles of TRT make it a very complicated problem as compared to external beam therapy. For as accurate as possible absorbed dose estimation and personalization, information about radioisotope type, radiopharmaceutical kinetics, patient anatomy and disease characteristics is needed; this information can be known, measured or estimated.

The Components in TRT

Radioisotope type defines the particles emitted by the used radionuclide. They can be alpha, beta particles, gamma rays or a combination. The type of the emitted particles and their energy is known. However, the interaction between particles and tissue is a statistical process and accurate calculations are not straight forward. Radiopharmaceutical kinetics gives information about a) where the radionuclide is concentrated,

b) in what percentage (at least theoretically), c) how fast it accumulates in target organs (both tumors and normal organs) and d) for how long it remains in these areas (Stabin and Flux 2007). Patient anatomy provides accurate information about tumor(s) and organs size, as well as possible non homogeneous areas. Finally, the disease type plays a critical role in the selection of radiopharmaceuticals and can affect their kinetic properties. TRT dosimetry aims to personalize the abovementioned parameters and overcome the limitations of the standard procedures (Cremonesi 2006). An accurate dose calculation model must address all those issues.

Imaging

Imaging plays a critical role since image provides the personalized anatomical as well as functional information (Bardies 2006). The most evident information that (tomographic) imaging provides is the location, the size and the volume of the organs and the tumor. This is a standard procedure in all therapeutic schemes and CT or MRI imaging are suitable modalities. It is important to mention that in a kidney dosimetry study (Pauwels 2005), the inclusion of the actual kidney masses (derived from CT) lead to a significant rescale in absorbed doses. The new values differed up to 100% and explained the unexpected renal toxicity in patients with small kidney.

While anatomical imaging has obvious importance, the functional imaging techniques SPECT and PET provide complementary information about tracers kinetics and tumors functionality. First of all, it must be emphasized that in most cases the imaging tracer is different from the therapeutic one. Thus, it is necessary to correlate the behavior of the imaging and the therapeutic radiopharmaceutical (Siegel 1999). However, there are significant research efforts towards the use of radiolabeled peptides (Cremonesi 2006), especially on those that emit gamma rays, which permit 3D imaging of the therapeutic radionuclides distribution.

When using a proper imaging tracer, variations in accumulation in tumors can be depicted. Planar scintigraphic imaging provides functional information but is limited to one projection plane. Image quantification is not possible due to organs overlapping, low resolution, attenuation, scattering, collimator penetration and system dead time. Although such problems appear in conventional diagnostic planar imaging, the use of higher energy isotopes makes those effects more severe. Tomographic SPECT imaging overcomes the problem of organs overlapping. In addition more advanced iterative reconstruction algorithms allow system and acquisition parameters to be included in reconstruction process and partially compensated. PET is currently the most robust technique for the acquisition of quantified functional images. Compared with SPECT it offers ~100 times higher sensitivity, which significantly improves SNR, thus quantification. Moreover, attenuation and scatter correction have been well studied in PET, while the lack of collimator minimizes penetration errors. Finally PET/CT, which has practically replaced PET, combines both functional and anatomical information and is continuously gaining acceptance in dosimetry.

Monte Carlo

The role of Monte Carlo (MC) simulations in dosimetry could be divided into four major categories: (a) use of MC for the simulation of particles-matter interaction, (b) modeling of physical phenomena through image acquisition process, (c) optimization of imaging system design and acquisition protocols, (d) use of MC for dose calculation. Although, the latter in principle fully addresses the problem of personalized absorbed dose calculation, there are practical computational limitations, which cannot permit the clinical application of MC.

A number of Monte Carlo packages have been developed and validated for a number of applications including dosimetry. On the one hand, there are generic MC code such as EGSnrc (Nelson 1985), Geant4 (Agostinelli 2003), or MCNP (Briesmeister 2000), which have can be used in a variety of nuclear physics applications. Their main advantages are the wide use and validation, as well as continuous support and update. However, there are limitations on specific applications e.g. time management, simulation of low energy photons etc. The later is rather important in the case of dose calculation. On the other hand a number of MC packages have been designed in order to address specific problems such as SPECT and PET imaging, namely SIMIND (Ljungberg 1989), simSET (Harrison 1993) and GATE (Jan 2004). The main advantage of those packages is the relatively simple geometry construction, the fast implementation of simulation code and usually the performance advantages since they are optimized on specific applications. However, there are disadvantages such as limits in the physics description and issues concerning maintenance, support and upgrades.

As a first step, MC can be used in order to accurately model all physical processes related to particles generation and interaction with matter. Usually, patient body is descretized in voxels. Their size is determined by the available modality resolution. In the case of CT submillimeter resolution is possible, while in SPECT and PET voxel size is usually some millimeters. A different material is assigned in each voxel. Thus, MC code can model physical processes by taking into account patients' anatomical map. In order to select the appropriate MC code two requirements are needed: a) accurate and detailed physics simulation, b) possibility to introduce anatomical maps into the simulation. Thus, patient specific emission voxels can be defined (e.g. from SPECT or PET images), as well as absorption voxels (e.g from CT or MRI images).

MC is a widely used tool for the simulation, study and modeling of several processes that limit accuracy of tomographic and planar images. Details about the role of MC in image corrections can be found elsewhere (Zaidi and Hasegawa 2003). In dosimetry the role of MC is to provide additional tools and methods that will improve image quantification, thus increase the accuracy of functional planar, SPECT or PET images. The main steps include scanner and source simulation. Then MC is used e.g to study scatter distributions for a particular scanner and acquisition configuration and include this information in reconstruction probability matrix. In addition, MC is a very useful tool for modeling collimator penetration in scintigraphic and SPECT imaging and improve image resolution. The importance of attenuation correction in PET and SPECT and the use of CT for the calculation of the attenuation map is another challenging problem; MC can be used in order to correlate CT X-rays attenuation coefficients to gamma ray photons attenuation, resulting to improved quantification. While MC is used for modeling those effects one critical parameter is the possibility to introduce advanced phantoms including patient imaging data. This leads to advanced correction techniques optimized for human studies and specific scanners.

MC is also used for scanner and imaging protocols optimization. When scanner geometry is accurately modeled, it is possible to assess the effects of patient size and injected dose on system's count rate e.g. NECR estimation in PET (Watson 2005). The use of anthropomorphic phantoms and MC simulations is increasingly being used for modeling heart and respiration motion. The latter one can severely affect image quantification, especially in the case of CT attenuation correction (Osman 2003). The NCAT phantom that includes respiratory motion pattern, in combination with MC toolkits that can simulate time dependent phenomena are being used for respiratory motion compensation.

Finally, MC can be used in order to directly calculate absorbed dose provided that patient geometry, radionuclide type and concentration locations are known (Kolbert 1997). Initially, MC was used in order to derive dose kernels in water and calculate absorbed dose using convolution methods (Furhang 1996). This method assumed a uniform patient body, although it is possible to use CT values in order to define different regions and use dose kernels for other materials. A purely MC based dosimetry includes a) import of the CT scan, in order to define patient attenuation map; b) import of the SPECT or PET scan (possibly with selected ROIs) in order to define emission map and c) use of MC in order to model dose distribution.

Dose Calculation using NM Information and Dose Kernels

The strategy for dose calculation is summarized in figure 2. It can be divided in four major steps, as it has already been described. Some key points are highlighted.

Dose kernels are defined as the absorbed dose per decay at a point r away from the source. Dose kernels are usually generated using MC simulations. A common strategy is the simulation of a point source in a homogeneous media and the calculation of absorbed dose as a function of distance from the source. MC simulation must take into account transport of initial photons and all resulting particles.

According to Furhang (1996) the dose kernel in cGy/Bq-s is given by the formula:

$$K(r)=\left(\frac{dose(r)}{4\pi r^2}\right)\left(\frac{n_{dec}}{n_{total}}\right)\cdot 1.0602\times 10^{-8} \quad (6)$$

where n_{dec} is the number of photons per decay, n_{total} is the total number of histories per simulation, and $1.602x10^{-18}$ is an MeV/g-cGy conversion factor. Two examples of the dose kernel for I^{125} and Sm^{153} are shown in Figure 3.

In order to calculate absorbed dose a specific dose distribution must be given (usually derived from a functional image). Then it is possible to fit the kernel to an algebraic expression such as:

$$k(r)=\sum_i^{i_{max}}\left(\frac{a_{-2}}{r^2}+\frac{a_{-1}}{r}+a_0+a_1r+a_2r^2\right)_i e^{-m_ir}(cGy/Bq-s) \quad (7)$$

Depending on the isotope i can range between 1 and 3. Dose is determined by convolving those kernels with the activity of the nuclear medicine image in 3D space. To speed up the process it is possible to work in Fourier domain and replace convolution, by multiplication.

The main drawback of the method is the difficulty of incorporating tissue inhomogeneity, eventhough it is known from anatomical images. The dose kernel can only be generated assuming an infinite, homogeneous medium. In addition grid size affects both accuracy of kernel calculation as well as simulation time (Liu 1998). Use of different kernels and functional information is possible, which will increase computational time and algorithmic complexity.

Direct Dose Calculation using Monte Carlo Packages

When MC is used for absorbed dose calculation patient-specific information is used; Patient body is discretized in voxels and each voxel is treated as a unique medium having a uniform p and Z value. A SPECT or PET image is used in order to provide cumulated activity and determine the number of photon emissions at each voxel. A CT or MRI image is used to distinguish between water and bone, to evaluate the equivalent pathlengths, and to discard particles escaping the body. This approach can accurately account for p and Z variations within the human body by simulating particle transport and tallying the energy deposited (Furhang 1996). However, the voxel dimension is an upper limit on the step

Figure 2. A summary of the dose calculation plan

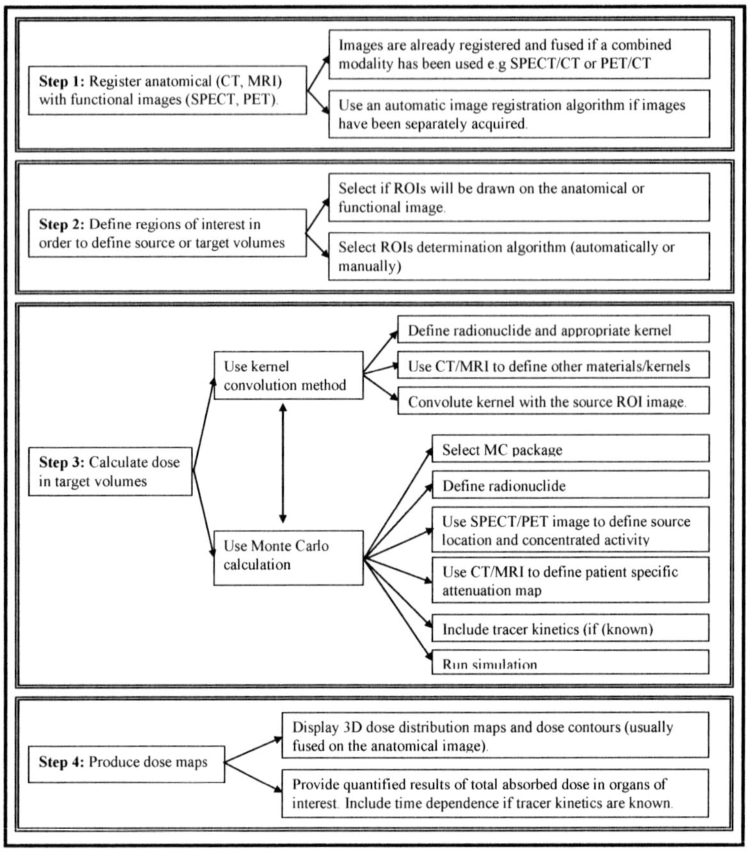

Figure 3. Dose kernels for I125 and Sm153. The plot shows the absorbed dose x r2 (cGy.cm2/Bq.sec) on the Y axis, versus the distance r in cm on the X axis.

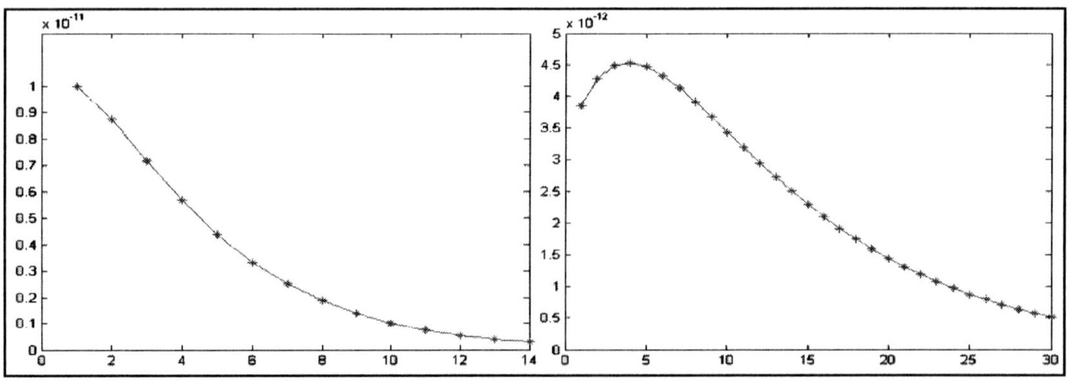

Figure 4. An example of the 3-D dose kernel calculation implemented in the registered anatomical and functional image information.

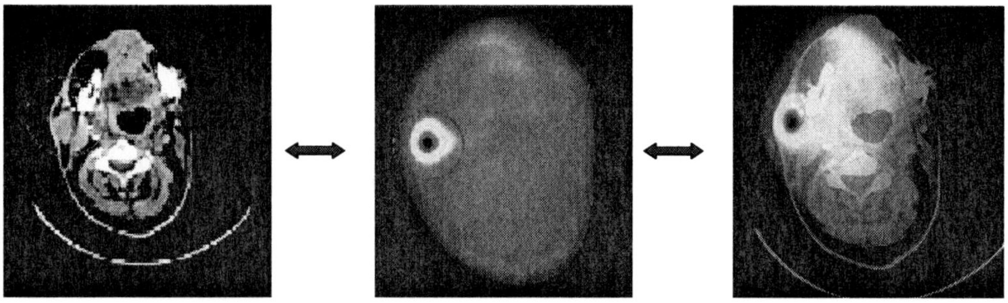

size, and thus requires resampling of interaction parameters at every voxel.

Depending on the estimated activity on the source organ, photons are generated; Initial photon positions can be uniformly sampled within each voxel. Each photon is emitted with a random direction and with energy sampled from the radionuclide emission spectrum (Weber 1989). Media differentiation is determined by setting a water-bone density threshold and Z of each voxel can be determined from a CT image. Given the medium cross sections and the particle energy, the MC code either locally deposits the particle, or provides the direction and the distance, T, to the next interaction in the corresponding infinite homogeneous medium having unit density. The process continues until the particle escapes patient geometry, or particle energy falls below a preselected energy threshold (e.g. 10 keV) and the particle energy is assumed locally absorbed.

Absorbed dose can be given by such an expression

$$Dose(x,y,z) = \frac{E}{V}\left\{\left(\frac{\mu_{ab}}{\rho}(E)\right)_{medium} \cdot T_{x,y,z}, \quad E > 10KeV\right.$$

$$\frac{1}{\rho_{x,y,z}}, \quad E \leq 10KeV$$

where x,y,z are target voxel coordinates, E is the photon energy in MeV, V is the voxel volume in cm^3, $\mu_{ab}(E)/\rho$ is the mass energy absorption coefficient that depends on the voxel medium and is measured in cm^2g^{-1} and $T_{x,y,z}$ is the pathlength across voxel x,y,z in cm.

FUTURE TRENDS

Uncertainties in Absorbed Dose Calculations

The quality and accuracy of the input data implemented in dosimetry software, determines the validity of the overall internal dose assessment. Efforts to measure attenuation correction, scatter correction, overlapping and irregularly shaped organs, and the measurement of patient thickness and background correction factors, are always subject to analytical errors. (Fischer 2003).

According to the ICRP (1988), the likely error associated with the aforementioned measurements and the direct measurement of activity in a patient's organ can reach up to a factor of 2, or about ± 100%, while the error associated with the use of a mathematical construct such as the MIRD phantom to represent the actual size and mass of a patient and internal organ is about ± 20 to 60%. The optimization of the measurement techniques by the implementation of 3D data and the customization of the actual patient size and organ weight can reduce the overall uncertainty of an organ dose estimate to about ± 30%. (Fischer 2000)

The use of phantoms and standard models in the dosimetry of internal emitters never included the tabulation of S values for tumors, correctly so, because obviously tumors do not have definite absorption or standard dimensions or certain positions in the human body. Although this has not been a concern in diagnostic nuclear medicine, in therapeutic nuclear medicine the absorbed dose to tumors is of outmost importance in order to evaluate the treatment efficacy.

The expectation that radionuclide dosimetry could be used to plan radionuclide therapy in the same way that dosimetry is used to plan external beam radiotherapy has yet to be met. In large part, this unfulfilled expectation is the direct result of the many variables involved in determining the biologic effect of targeted radionuclides.

The objective in cancer radiotherapy is to design treatments that result in minimum normal tissue complication and maximum tumour control probabilities. To accomplish this goal, a quantitative description of the organ response to radiation is of great importance. This can be achieved by determining the relationship between the 3-D dose distribution and organ radiation response (Tsougos 2005). Several "biomathematical" models (radiobiological response models) have been developed to estimate the radiation-induced symptoms. The aim was to quantify the normal tissue response to irradiation thus translating the dose delivered to normal tissue complication probability, NTCP, or the dose delivered to the tumour, calculating the tumour control probability (TCP) (Kutcher 1991, Burman 1991). Towards that direction several groups have derived radiobiological parameters, which are used in empirical models by comparing the predicted response values with the observed incidence of radiation complications. Some of the models have started to be gradually implemented in the clinical practice as a helping tool in external radiotherapy, but there is no such attempt in internal dosimetry yet.

Meredith (2002) summarized the current knowledge in the relationship between results from internal and external sources of radiation, and concluded in three specific problems that still apply.

The first problem is that in internal dosimetry the factors such as the lack of radionuclide homogeneity within the tissues, or the tissue density changes which may have affected the image quantification are not carefully taken into account, resulting in less accurate data comparing to external dose data. The second problem is that tracer studies used to establish the biokinetics (and thus the dosimetry) may have different biokinetic patterns than when the full therapeutic dose is given, as has been documented in several studies. The last problem is the lack of uniformity on the reporting of internal dose results, which depends on the different use of image quantification methods, computer programs, dose conversion factors, etc.

CONCLUSION

Internal radionuclide dosimetry has evolved greatly since the 1970s with the development of the MIRD models and calculational techniques; however it still stands at an early stage of development.

The physics of absorbed dose estimation is improving by the active research in the fields of patient-specific dosimetry supported by the application of 3D imaging. The availability of faster and more efficient computers, improved and accurate Monte Carlo methods and imaging devices that support both anatomy and radioactivity tomography (PET / CT) will push internal dosimetry into a new era of individualized therapy.

Nevertheless, two important prerequisites should be considered when implementing internal dosimetry software. First the image input for dosimetric calculations should be quantitative because the validity of the data input is crucial for the output. Moreover it has to be noted that the correction of the images for all effects that degrade the quantitative content is especially difficult to achieve for SPECT or PET images obtained using non-pure positron emitting nuclides. (Glatting 2006).

Albeit, a treatment planning approach to radionuclide therapy like in external radiotherapy will eventually require incorporation of biologic and radiobiologic considerations in order to predict response in an individual patient, and efforts in this direction are just beginning.

REFERENCES

Agostinelli, S. (2003). Geant4—a simulation toolkit. *Nuclear Instruments and Methods in Physics Research, A 506,* 250–303.

Bardies, M., Flux, G., Lassmann, M., Monsieurs, M., Savolainen, S., Strand, S. E. (2006). Quantitative imaging for clinical dosimetry. *Nuclear Instruments and Methods in Physics Research, A 569,* 467–471.

Briesmeister, J. F. (2000). *Report LA-13709-M.* Los Alamos National Laboratory, NM.

Bouchet, L. G. Jokisch, D. W., & Bolch, W. E. (1999). A three-dimensional transport model for determining absorbed fractions of energy for electrons within trabecular bone. *J. Nucl. Med., 40,* 1947–66.

Burman, C., Kutcher, G. J., & Emami, B. (1991). Fitting of normal tissue tolerance data to an analytical function. *Int. J. Radiat. Biol. Phys., 21,* 123-35.

Clairand, I., Ricard, M., Gouriou, J., Di Paola, M., & Aubert, B. (1999). DOSE3D: EGS4 Monte Carlo code-based software for internal radionuclide dosimetry. *J. Nucl. Med., 40,* 1517–23.

Cremonesi, M., Ferrari, M., Bodei, L., Tosi, G., & Paganelli, G. (2006). Dosimetry in Peptide Radionuclide Receptor Therapy: A Review. *J Nucl Med 2006, 47,* 1467–1475.

Cristy, M., & Eckerman, K. (1987). Specific absorbed fractions of energy at various ages from internal photons sources *ORNL/TM-8381 V1-V7* (Oak Ridge, TN: Oak Ridge National Laboratory).

Dewaraja, Y. K., Wilderman, S. J., Ljungberg, M., Koral, K. F., Kenneth, Z., & Kaminiski, M. S. (2005). Accurate dosimetry in 131I radionuclide therapy using patient-specific, 3-dimensional methods for SPECT reconstruction and absorbed dose calculation. *J. Nucl. Med., 46,* 840–9.

Eckerman, K., & Stabin, M. (2000). Electron absorbed fractions and dose conversion factors for marrow and bone by skeletal regions. *Health Phys., 78,* 199–214.

Eckerman, K. F., Cristy, M., & Warner, G. G. (1981). Dosimetric evaluation of brain scanning agents. In E. E. Watson, A. T. Schlafke-Stelson, J. L. Coffey, & R. J. Cloutier (Eds.), *3rd Int. Radiopharmaceutical Dosimetry Symp.* (Rockville, MD: U.S. Department of Health and Human Services, Food and Drug Administration) (pp. 527–40). *HHS Publication* FDA 81-8166.

Fischer, D. R. (2003). Assessments for high dose radionuclide therapy treatment planning. *Radiation Protection Dosimetry, 105*(1–4), 581–586.

Fisher, D. R. (2000). Internal dosimetry for systemic radiation therapy. *Semin. Radiat. Oncol., 10*(2), 123–132.

Glatting, G., Landmann, M., Wunderlich, A., Kull, T., Mottaghy, F. M., Reske, S. N. (2006). Internal radionuclide therapy: Software for treatment planning using tomographic data. *Nuklearmedizin, 45*(6), 269-72.

Flux, G., Bardies, M., Monsieurs, M., Savolainen, S., Strand, S. E., & Lassmann, M. (2006). The

Impact of PET and SPECT on Dosimetry for Targeted Radionuclide Therapy. *Z. Med. Phys., 16*, 47–59.

Furhang, E. E., Sgouros, G., & Chui, C. S. (1993). Radionuclide photon dose kernels for internal emitter dosimetry. *Med. Phys., 23*(5), May 1996.

Harrison, R. J. (n. d.). *Nucl. Med., 34,* 60.

Holman, B. L., Zimmerman, R. L., Shapiro, J. R., Kaplan, M. L., Jones, A. G., & Hill, T. C. (1983). Biodistribution and dosimetry of *n*-isoproyl *p*-123I iodoamphetamine in the primate. *J. Nucl. Med., 24*, 922–31.

Johnson, T. K., McClure, D., & McCourt, S. (1999). MABDOSE. I: characterization of a general purpose dose estimation code. *Med Phys.* 1999, *26*, 1389 –1395.

Jan, S. (2004). GATE: a simulation toolkit for PET and SPECT. *Phys. Med. Biol., 49*(2004), 4543–4561.

Johnson, T. K., McClure, D., & McCourt, S. (2000). MABDOSE. II: validation of a general purpose dose estimation code. *Med Phys., 26*, 1396 –1403.

ICRP. (1988). Radiation dose to patients from radiopharmaceuticals. *ICRP Publication, 53. Ann. ICRP 18*(1–4) (Oxford: Pergamon).

Kolbert, K. S., Sgouros, G., Scott, A. M., Bronstein, J. E., Malane, R. A., Zhang, J., Kalaigian, H., McNamara, S., Schwartz, L., & Larson, S. M. (1997). Implementation and evaluation of patient-specific three-dimensional internal dosimetry. *J. Nucl. Med., 38*, 301–8.

Kutcher, G. J., Burman, C., Brewster, L., Goitein, M., & Mohan, R. (1991). Histogram reduction method for calculating complication probabilities for 3-dimensional treatment planning evaluations. *Int. J. Radiat. Oncol. Biol. Phys., 21*, 137-46.

Koral, K. F., Francis, I. R., & Kroll, S. (2002). Volume reduction versus radiation dose for tumors in previously untreated lymphoma patients who received iodine-131 tositumomab therapy. Conjugate views compared with a hybrid method. *Cancer, 94*, 1258–1263.

Liu, A., Williams, L., Lopatin, G., Yamauchi, D., Wong, J., & Raubitschek, A. (1999). A radionuclide therapy treatment planning and dose estimation system. *J. Nucl. Med., 40*, 1151–3.

Loevinger R, Budinger T and Watson E 1988 *MIRD Primer for Absorbed Dose Calculations* (New York: Society of Nuclear Medicine)

Ljungberg M and Strand SE, Comput. Methods Prog. Biomed. 29 1989 257–72.

Nelson WR, Hirayama H, and Rogers DW, "The EGS4 code system," SLAC Report No. 265 (SLAC, Stanford, CA, 1985).

Nuis A,: Health protection of individuals against the dangers of ionising radiation in relation to medical exposure: Council directive 97/43 EURATOM 30-6-1997

International Commission on Radiological Protection (ICRP) 1975 report of the Task Group on Reference Man *ICRP Publication 23* (New York: Pergamon)

Osman MM, Cohade C, Nakamoto Y, Wahl RL, Respiratory motion artifacts on PET emission images obtained using CT attenuation correction on PET-CT, Eur J Nucl Med Mol Imaging (2003) 30:603–606.

Pauwels S, Barone R, Walrand S, . Practical dosimetry of peptide receptor radionuclide therapy with 90Y-labeled somatostatin analogs. J Nucl Med. 2005;46(suppl 1):92S–98S.

Poon E and Verhaegen F, Med Phys 32 (6), 1696 (2005).

Siegel, J.A., Thomas, S.R., Stubbs, J.B., Stabin, M.G., Hays, M.T., Koral, K.F., Robertson, J.S.,

Howell, R.W., Wessels, B.W., Fisher, D.R., Weber, D.A., Brill, A.B.: MIRD pamphlet no. 16: Techniques for quantitative radiopharmaceutical biodistribution data acquisition and analysis for use in human radiation dose estimates. J Nucl Med 40 (1999) 37S–61S

Siegel JA, Stabin MG, Brill AB. The importance of patientspecific radiation dose calculations for the administration of radionuclides in therapy. Cell Mol Biol (Noisy-Le-Grand) 2002; 48(5):451-9.

Snyder WS, Fisher HL, Ford MR, Warner GG. Estimates of absorbed fractions for monoenergetic photon sources uniformly distributed in various organs of a heterogeneous phantom. *J Nucl Med.* 1969;10(suppl):7S–52S.

Snyder WS, Ford MR, Warner GG. *Estimates of Specific Absorbed Fractions for Photon Sources Uniformly Distributed in Various Organs of a Heterogeneous Phantom.* MIRD Pamplet No. 5, rev. New York, NY: Society of Nuclear Medicine; 1978.

Sgouros G, Barest G, Thekkumthala J, . Treatment planning for internal radionuclide therapy: three-dimensional dosimetry for nonuniformly distributed radionuclides. J Nucl Med. 1990; 31:1884 –1891.

Sgouros G, Chiu S, Pentlow KS, . Three-dimensional dosimetry for radioimmunotherapy treatment planning. J Nucl Med. 1993;34:1595–1601.

Sgouros G, Squeri S, Ballangrud AM, . 2003;Patient-specific, 3-dimensional dosimetry in non-Hodgkin's lymphoma patients treated with 131I-anti-B1 antibody: assessment of tumor dose-response. J Nucl Med. 44:260 –268.

Sgouros G, Kolbert KS, Sheikh A, . 2004;Patient-specific dosimetry for 131I thyroid cancer therapy using 124I PET and 3-dimensional-internal dosimetry (3D-ID) software. J Nucl Med. 45:1366 –1372.

Sgouros G. 2005 Dosimetry of internal emitters. J Nucl Med. Jan;46 Suppl 1:18S-27S.

Stabin MG. 1996 MIRDOSE: personal computer software for internal dose assessment in nuclear medicine. *J Nucl Med.*; 37:538 –546.

Stabin M G, Sparks R B and Crowe E 2005 OLINDA/EXM: the second-generation personal computer software for internal dose assessment in nuclear medicine *J. Nucl. Med.* 46 1023–7

Stabin M G 1994 A model of the prostate gland for use in internal dosimetry *J. Nucl. Med.* 35 516–20

Stabin M 1996 MIRDOSE—the personal computer software for use in internal dose assessment in nuclear medicine *J. Nucl. Med.* 37 538–46

Stabin MG and Konijnenberg M 2000 Re-evaluation of absorbed fractions for photons and electrons in small spheres *J. Nucl. Med.* 41 149–60

Stabin M G, Konijnenberg M, Knapp F F Jr and Spencer R H 2000 Monte Carlo modeling of radiation dose distributions in intravascular radiation therapy *Med. Phys.* 27 1086–92

Stabin M G, Sparks R B and Crowe E 2005 OLINDA/EXM: the second-generation personal computer software for internal dose assessment in nuclear medicine *J. Nucl. Med.* 46 1023–7

Stabin MG, Flux GD, Internal dosimetry as a tool for radiation protection of the patient in nuclear medicine, Biomed Imaging Interv J 2007; 3(2): e28.

Tsougos I, Mavroidis P Rajala J, Theodorou K, Jarvenpaa R, Pitkanen MA, Holli K, Ojala AT, Lind BK, Hyodynmaa S, Kappas C. 2005 Evaluation of dose-response models and parameters predicting radiation induced pneumonitis using clinical data from breast cancer radiotherapy *Phys. Med. Biol.* 50 3535-54

Watson E W and Stabin M G 1984 BASIC alternative software package for internal dose calculations Computer Applications in Health Physics: Proc. 17th Midyear Topical Symposium of the Health Physics Society (Pasco, WA, 5–9 February 1984) pp 7.79–7.86

Watson E E, Stabin M G, Davis J L and Eckerman K F 1989 A model of the peritoneal cavity for use in internal dosimetry J. Nucl. Med. 30 2002–11

Watson CC, Casey ME, Bendriem B, Carney JP, Townsend DW, Eberl S, Meikle S, DiFilippo FP, Optimizing Injected Dose in Clinical PET by Accurately Modeling the Counting-Rate Response Functions Specific to Individual Patient Scans, J Nucl Med 2005; 46:1825–1834.

Xu XG,Chao T Cand Bozkurt A 2000 VIP-man: an image-based whole-body adult male model constructed from colour photographs of the visible human project for multi-particle Monte Carlo calculations *Health Phys.* 78 476–86

Zaidi H, Labbe C and Morel C, Parallel Comput. 24 (1998) 1523–36.

KEY TERMS

Absorbed Dose: A general term denoting the quantity of radiation or energy absorbed. For special purposes it must be appropriately qualified. It is defined as absorbed dose per unit mass.

Dosimetry: The accurate measurement of the absorbed dose.

Monte Carlo: An analytical technique in which a large number of simulations are run using random quantities for uncertain variables and looking at the distribution of results to infer which values are most likely.

Nuclear Medicine: The branch of medicine concerned with the use of radioisotopes in the diagnosis, management, and treatment of disease. Nuclear medicine uses small amounts of radioactive materials or radiopharmaceuticals, substances that are attracted to specific organs, bones, or tissues.

Radionuclide Therapy: A form of cancer therapy, by the use of radionuclides that localise to certain organs (e.g., radioactive iodine or gallium), and deliver cytotoxic radiation doses to tumours.

Tomographic Data: Data acquired by radiologic / nuclear medicine imaging techniques for making detailed three-dimensional images of a plane section of a solid object.

Treatment Planning: A system that calculates the dose that will be absorbed by a radionuclide therapy.

Chapter XV
Diffusion Tensor Imaging and Fiber Tractography

Evanthia E. Tripoliti
University of Ioannina, Greece

Dimitrios I. Fotiadis
University of Ioannina, Greece

Konstantia Veliou
Magnetic Tomography of Epirus, Greece

Charalambos Bougias
University Hospital of Ioannina, Greece

ABSTRACT

Diffusion Tensor Imaging (DTI) is a magnetic resonance imaging (MRI) modality which can significantly improve our understanding of the brain structures and neural connectivity. DTI measures are thought to be representative of brain tissue microstructure and are particularly useful for examining organized brain regions, such as white matter tract areas. DTI measures the water diffusion tensor using diffusion weighted pulse sequences which are sensitive to microscopic random water motion. The resulting diffusion weighted images (DWI) display and allow quantification of how water diffuses along axes or diffusion encoding directions. This can help to measure and quantify the tissue's orientation and structure, making it an ideal tool for examining cerebral white matter and neural fiber tracts. In this chapter the authors discuss the theoretical aspects of DTI, the information that can be extracted from DTI data, and the use of the extracted information for the reconstruction of fiber tracts and the diagnosis of a disease. In addition, a review of known fiber tracking algorithms is presented.

INTRODUCTION

A major challenge for neuroscience is to understand brain function in terms of connectional anatomy and the dynamic flow of information across neuron networks. In the last 10-15 years, MR imaging techniques have been increasingly applied to the study of molecular displacement (diffusion) in biological tissues. The MR measurement of an effective diffusion tensor of water in tissues can provide unique biological and clinical information that is not available by other imaging modalities. For this purpose Diffusion Tensor Imaging is applied. DTI is an MRI modality which emerged as a powerful method for investigating white matter architecture. Diffusion is the random translational or Brownian motion of molecules and can be either isotropic or anisotropic depending on the characteristics of the tissue. The diffusion anisotropy can be fully characterized, providing more details on tissue microstructure. Fiber tracking in the brain is the most advanced application, which in combination with fMRI might open a window on brain connectivity and the understanding of brain function. In this chapter we describe the tensor theory used to characterize molecular diffusion in white matter, and the information that can be extracted from DTI data. We review techniques for acquiring relatively high resolution diffusion-sensitive MR images and computer-based algorithms that allow the generation of white matter fiber tract maps from the tensor data. We discuss the role of these white matter maps in the assessment or diagnosis of white matter diseases and the way that can be combined with fMRI data to produce a clear view of brain function and connectivity (Bihan, 2001; Melhem, 2002; Nucifora 2007).

BACKGROUND

Diffusion is the random translation or Brownian motion of molecules which is driven by internal thermal energy. The mobility of molecules can be characterized by a physical constant, the diffusion coefficient D. The random motion of molecules, in the presence of a strong magnetic gradient results in MR signal loss as a consequence of the dephasing of spin coherence. The signal attenuation depends on D and on the *b*-factor and is given by (Basser, 1994; Basser, 1998; Bihan, 2001; Le Bihan, 1991; Mattiello, 1994; Mattiello, 1997; Melherm 2002):

$$A = exp(-b^{*}\mathrm{D}) \tag{1}$$

The *b*-value expresses the degree of diffusion weighting and it is determined by the type of the sensitizing gradient scheme implemented in the MR experiment. It is given by:

$$b = \gamma^2 G^2 \delta^2 (\Delta - \delta/3) \tag{2}$$

where γ is the gyromagnetic ration, G is the strength of gradients, $\triangle$ is the duration of gradients and δ is the time between gradients.

Adding two diffusion-sensitizing gradients before and after the refocusing pulse of a spin-echo sequence constitutes the basis of the diffusion-weighted MR imaging. The signal intensity S in each voxel of a DWI is affected by the choice of b value, the pulse sequence time echo and by two parameters: a) the apparent diffusion coefficient (*ADC*) and b) the spin-spin relaxation time (T2). Apparent diffusion coefficient reflects molecular diffusivity in the presence of restrictions. The following equation describes the relationship between signal intensity and those parameters (Basser, 1994; Basser, 1998; Bihan, 2001; Le Bihan, 1991; Mattiello, 1994; Mattiello 1997):

$$S = S_0 e^{-b(ADC)} \tag{3}$$

where *ADC* is given as:

$$ADC = -\frac{1}{b}\ln\left(\frac{S}{S_0}\right) \quad (4)$$

and S_0 is the signal intensity for b=0.

If the diffusion is the same in all directions is called isotropic. In small structures, as axons, the diffusion is restricted to some directions more than others. In that case the diffusion is called anisotropic. Diffusion anisotropy can no longer be characterized by the constant D, but requires a tensor D. A tensor is a mathematical quantity which describes the properties of an ellipsoid in the three dimensional space:

$$D = \begin{bmatrix} D_{xx} & D_{xy} & D_{xz} \\ D_{yx} & D_{yy} & D_{yz} \\ D_{zx} & D_{zy} & D_{zz} \end{bmatrix} \quad (5)$$

The diagonal elements of D represent the apparent diffusion coefficient along the x, y, z direction, while the off diagonal elements represent the correlation between the diffusion in perpendicular directions. The tensor D is symmetric ($D_{ij} = D_{ji}$, $i,j = x,y,z$ $i \neq j$) and positive definite. The determination of tensor D can be achieved by applying diffusion sensitizing gradients in at least six directions in addition to a non-diffusion weighted image(b = 0). An important property of the tensor is that it be diagonalized. The diagonalization of the tensor D is necessary in order to determine the basic diffusion directions. The diagonalization leaves only three non zero elements along the main diagonal of the tensor (Basser, 1994; Basser, 1998; Bihan, 2001; Le Bihan, 1991; Mattiello, 1994; Mattiello, 1997; Melhem, 2002):

$$\hat{D} = \begin{bmatrix} \lambda_1 & 0 & 0 \\ 0 & \lambda_2 & 0 \\ 0 & 0 & \lambda_3 \end{bmatrix}. \quad (6)$$

The diagonal elements, which are called eigenvalues, reflect the shape of the ellipsoid and their sum reflects the size of the ellipsoid. An eigenvector v corresponds to each eigenvalue and determines the main direction of the diffusion. The eigenvector of the largest eigenvalue corresponds to the direction of the main diffusion direction (Figure 1) (Basser, 1994; Basser, 1998; Bihan, 2001; Le Bihan, 1991; Mattiello, 1994; Mattiello, 1997; Melhem, 2002).

Figure 1. Eigenvalues and eigenvectors

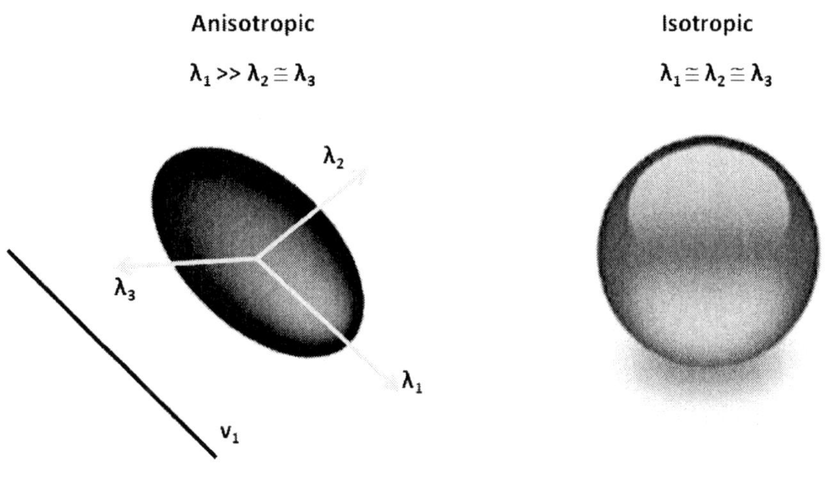

EXTRACTED INFORMATION FROM DTI DATA

The DTI data can be analyzed in two ways to provide information on the microstructure and the architecture for each voxel (Conturo, 1996; Hsu, 1995). Those are the mean diffusivity and the degree of anisotropy. The mean diffusivity $\hat{\lambda}$ characterizes the overall mean-squared displacement of molecules and the presence of obstacles to diffusion (Figure 2a):

$$\hat{\lambda} = \frac{\lambda_1 + \lambda_2 + \lambda_3}{3} \qquad (7)$$

The degree of anisotropy describes the variation of molecular displacements in the space and it is related to the presence of oriented structures. The most commonly used invariant measures are:

- **Relative Anisotropy (RA):** it represents the ratio of the anisotropic part of D to its isotropic part and is given as (Figure 2b):

$$RA = \sqrt{\frac{1}{3}}\sqrt{\frac{(\lambda_1 - \hat{\lambda})^2 + (\lambda_2 - \hat{\lambda})^2 + (\lambda_3 - \hat{\lambda})^2}{\hat{\lambda}^2}} \qquad (8)$$

- **Fractional Anisotropy (FA):** it measures the fraction of the magnitude of D that can be ascribed to anisotropic diffusion and is given as (Figure 2c):

$$FA = \sqrt{\frac{2}{3}}\sqrt{\frac{(\lambda_1 - \hat{\lambda})^2 + (\lambda_2 - \hat{\lambda})^2 + (\lambda_3 - \hat{\lambda})^2}{\lambda_1^2 + \lambda_2^2 + \lambda_3^2}} \qquad (9)$$

- **Volume Ratio (VR):** it represents the ratio of the volume of the ellipsoid to the volume of a sphere of radius $\hat{\lambda}$ and is given as (Figure 2d):

$$VR = \frac{\lambda_1 * \lambda_2 * \lambda_3}{\hat{\lambda}^3} \qquad (10)$$

The main direction of the diffusivities is linked to the orientation of the structures.

Anisotropy maps are often color encoded (color maps) and represent directional information of the principal eigenvector (Pierpaoli, 2002; Pierpaoli, 1996; Sorensen, 1999). White matter color maps are created on the basis of the three vector elements of the principal eigenvector for each voxel. The absolute values of the vector elements are assigned to red (v_x element), green (v_y element) and blue (v_z element). If the principal eigenvector is 45° between the *x*- and *y*-axes, yellow (red plus green) is assigned to the voxel. The intensity of the color of each voxel is determined by the degree of the fractional anisotropy (Figure 2d).

DATA ACQUISITION

To extract all necessary information from DTI data, the full tensor must be determined. This is accomplished by collecting a b_0 image and diffusion weighted images along six gradient directions, using diffusion-sensitized MRI pulse sequences. The process of data acquisition in DTI consists of two steps: a) diffusion sensitization and b) spatial encoding. DTI is influenced by the strength, the number and the orientation of the gradients. Although, the increase of the number of sensitizing gradient directions improves the accuracy of diffusion tensor estimates and fiber tracking applications, the optimal number of gradients and their orientation is widely discussed (Bihan, 2001; Melhem, 2002; Nucifora, 2007).

A variety of spatial encoding schemes has been proposed for diffusion tensor MR imaging. The most commonly schemes used in practice are based on echo-planar readout and include single-shot and multi-shot techniques. Multi-shot techniques provide higher spatial resolution, higher signal to noise ratio, low susceptibility-related distortion but longer data acquisition time which makes them more susceptible to artefacts related to respiration, cerebrovascular and cere-

Figure 2. DTI data: (a) Mean Diffusivity, (b) Relative Anisotropy, (c) Fractional Anisotropy, (d) Volume Ratio and (e) Color Map.

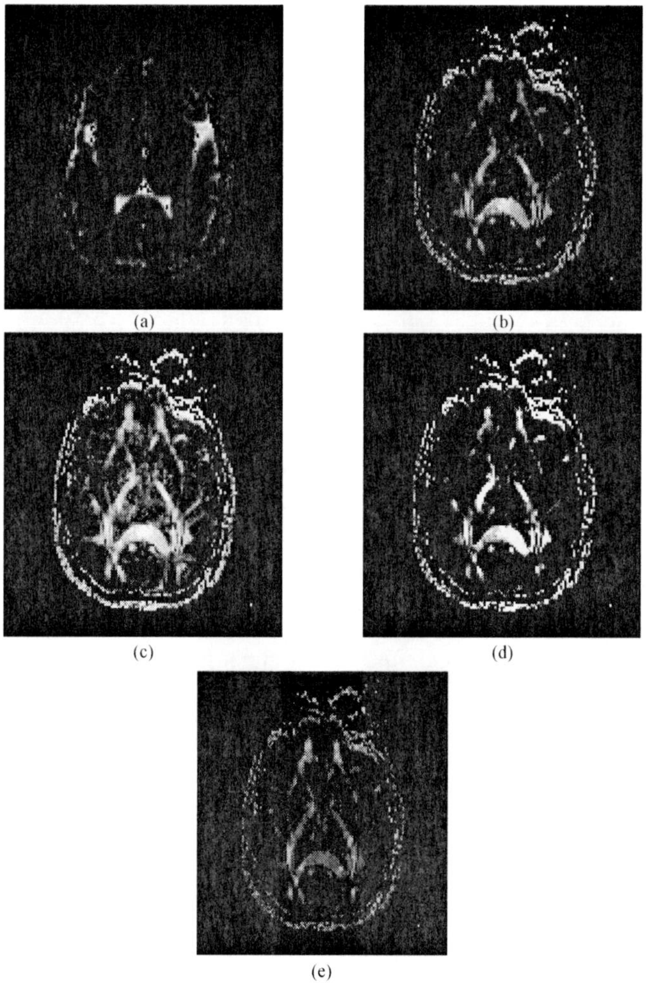

brospinal fluid flow, eye motion and involuntary head motion.

The presence of such artefacts during data acquisition may lead to signal tissue misinterpretation. Therefore, scan times are kept short, by using large voxel sizes and fast acquisition techniques such as echo-planar imaging. Artefacts such as eddy currents are removed during preprocessing and can be further reduced with a modified acquisition, such as gradient and spin echo (GRASE), fast spin-echo and line scanning techniques (Alexander, 1997; Alexander, 2005; Anderson, 2002; Armitage, 2001; Chang, 2005; Hasan, 2001; Haselgrove, 1996; Jones, 1999; Jones, 2004; Kingsley, 2004; Nucifora, 2007; Rohde, 2004; Rohde, 2005; Turner, 1991; Xing, 1997).

Line scanning is occasionally used in imaging children due to its inherent insensitivity to variations in the phase of the MR signal induced by physiologic motion. Alternatively navigator information can be acquired during a multi-shot sequence to account for motion during reconstruction. One such approach is periodically rotated overlapping parallel lines with enhanced reconstruction, or PROPELLER, DT imaging, which acquires data in a rotating blade of k-space. Similarly, self-navigated interleaved spiral, or SNAILS, DT imaging acquires data through a spiral in k-space. In both cases, the oversampled center of k-space provides the navigator data (Finsterbusch, 2000; Forbes, 2002; Gudbjartsson, 1996; Pipe, 2006; Pipe, 2002).

Pulsation of cerebrospinal fluid and cardiac pulsation can be corrected by decreasing voxel size or using fluid-attenuated inversion-recovery diffusion weighted imaging and cardiac gating, respectively. Susceptibility artefacts are addressed by applying a single-shot stimulated echo acquisition or multi-shot diffusion protocol which does not introduce phase errors due to subject motion. Finally, parallel imaging has been proven useful in reducing susceptibility artefacts both in single-shot and multi-shot acquisitions. Parallel imaging strategies combine the signal intensity from individual coil elements of an RF coil array to accelerate MR imaging data acquisition without interfering with the contrast mechanisms. This reduces the distortions seen in echo planar imaging (EPI), but has the disadvantage that the signal to noise ratio (SNR) is lower. Because the intrinsic SNR of an MR imaging scanner is roughly proportional to the field strength, the combination of multicoil receiver arrays with parallel imaging techniques on high field magnets has produced good quality DT MR imaging data (Bammer, 2003; Bhagat, 2004; Falconer, 1997; Hirsch, 1999; Kwong, 1991; Pagani, 2007; Papadakis, 2002; Riesebeg, 2005; Skare, 2001).

Although tensor model can represent most white matter regions, it does not adequately describe voxels with crossing diverging or converging white matter tracts. These fiber tracts theoretically could be resolved using improved voxel resolution. However, multiple directions of diffusion within a single voxel are modeled using higher order vectors. These methods generally involve the examination of q-space, which contains the Fourier transform of diffusion properties. Depiction of most fiber tracts was improved using 3T DT tractography compared with depiction using 1.5T tractography. More specifically DT tractography at 3T enables improved visualization of the corticospinal tract compared to DT tractography at 1.5T. 3T tractography of the superior longitudinal fasciculus, corpus callosum, and fornix has some advantages over 1.5T tractography. Further refinement of efficient MR sequences are needed to improve the image quality and reliability of 3T DT tractography (Basser, 1994; Lazar, 2003; Okada, 2006; Ozarslan, 2003; Pierpaoli, 196; Tuch, 2002).

FIBER TRACKING ALGORITHMS

A variety of methods for the reconstruction of fiber tracts within white matter using DTI data has recently been suggested. Those methods are deterministic and probabilistic. Deterministic methods are based on line propagation algorithms which use local tensor information for each step of the propagation. Techniques differ in the way that information from neighboring pixels is incorporated to define smooth trajectories or to minimize noise contributions. More specifically, simple line propagation techniques which connect voxels using local tensor information (local principal eigenvector orientation), are incapable of providing accurate representation of white matter tracts. To overcome this problem line propagation using continuous, rather than discrete, number fields are employed to provide connections which follow the actual white matter tract. Furthermore, line propagation techniques can be further improved to create a smooth (curved) path by interpolating the vector of the principal axis or the whole diffusion tensor for each coordinate as a line is propagated. The probabilistic methods are based on global energy minimization to find the energetically most favorable path between two predetermined voxels (Bahrens, 2003; Basser, 2000; Conturo, 1996; Jackowski, 2005; Lazar,

2003; Masutani, 2003; Mori, 1999; Mori, 2002; Parker, 2003; Parker, 2002; Westin, 2002).

Line Propagation Techniques

Assuming that the orientation of the dominant component of the diagonalized diffusion tensor represents the orientation of dominant axonal tracts, DTI can provide a 3D vector field, in which each vector represents the fiber orientation. A simple way to reconstruct a 3D trajectory from a 3D vector field is to propagate a line from a seed point following the local vector orientation. This starts from a seed point and follows the principal eigenvector of the current voxel. This voxel is connected to the adjacent one toward which the fiber direction is pointing. However, if a line is propagated simply by connecting pixels, which are discrete entities, the vector information contained at each pixel may not be fully reflected in the propagation and the real tract cannot be represented. To overcome these problems line propagation with continuous vector field can be used. Tracking is launched from a seed voxel from which a line is propagated in the direction of eigenvector which is associated with the largest eigenvalue. At the point where the line leaves the voxel and enters the next the direction is changed to that of the principal eigenvector of the neighboring voxel. In order to create a smooth path, which is more accurate when the curvature of a reconstructed line is steep with respect to the imaging resolution, an interpolation method is used. When propagation moves to a new voxel a distance-weighted averaged of nearby vectors orientation is computed or the diffusion tensors are interpolated as a line propagates (Figure 3). The choice between the two approaches (continuous propagation and interpolation) depends on the degree of curvature of the tract of interest with respect to the imaging resolution. In other words if the resolution is low and bending in the reconstructed path are evident, interpolation provides an advantage in terms of accuracy. On the other hand, if the resolution is sufficiently high the simple continuous line propagation is faster.

Line propagation is terminated when one of the following criteria holds: (a) a fractional anisotropy threshold equals to 0.2. This termination criterion helps to exclude gray matter and to segment white matter tracts which are separated by gray matter, (b) the change between pixels angle ranges from 35° to 45°. In general, it is preferable to set a threshold which prohibits a sharp turn during line propagation. In the cases when two white matter tracts are close the angle becomes an important criterion for adequate segmentation. The significance of this terminating criterion depends on the particular trajectories of tracts of interest and the image resolution (Basser, 2000; Conturo, 1999; Lazar, 2001; Lori, 1999; Mori, 1998; Mori, 1999; Mori, 2002; Stieltjes, 2001; Xue, 1999).

Figure 3. Line propagation: (a) Discrete vector field, (b) continuous vector field, (c) interpolation method

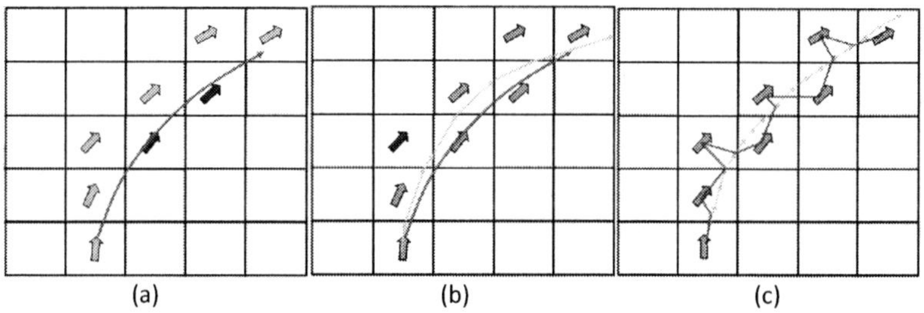

Figure 4. White matter fiber tracking from different regions of the brain

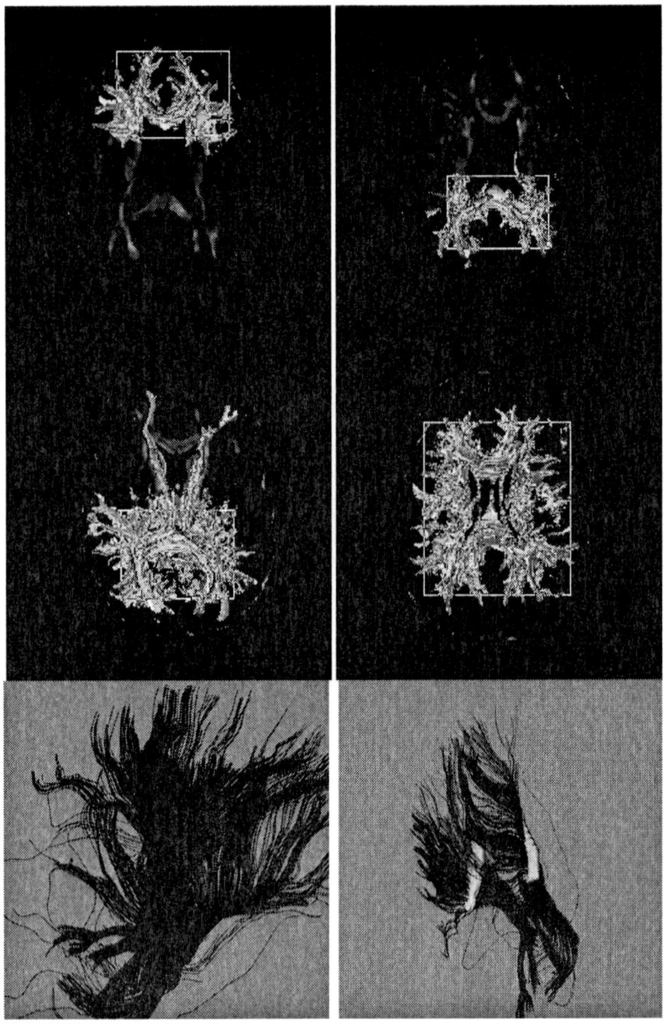

Results of fiber tracking algorithms using line propagation techniques are shown in Figure 4.

Energy Minimization Techniques

Fast marching and simulated annealing methods belong to this category (Parker, 2000; Tuch, 2001). In the stationary formulation of the level set theory, the evolution of a front allows a time of arrival, T, from a starting point to any point in the image to be determined. The rate, F, at which the front evolves, is related to T by:

$$|\nabla T| F = 1 \tag{11}$$

F is defined in the direction normal to the front. Usually the propagation of the front is governed by the image intensity and other constraints, such as the curvature of the front. F can be calculated as:

$$F(r) = A|\varepsilon_1(r) * n(r)| \tag{12}$$

where r is the front; n is the unit normal to the front; ε_1 is the principal eigenvector of diffusion; and

A is the value of fractional anisotropy. The front propagates at the point of smallest T (highest F); at the point where the principal eigenvector direction is most similar to the normal to the front. As the front propagation proceeds from one or more seed points, each voxel is assigned an arrival time. Once the front propagation has finished, a map of arrival times from the seed point(s) to the rest of the brain is obtained. This may be interpreted as a likelihood of a connection map. Points that are well connected to the seed region(s) have short arrival times; those far away or poorly connected have larger arrival times. To determine the most likely path between any point within the arrival time map and the seed point(s), a set of link points is defined. From each one of these, the gradient of steepest descent in T is found, giving the most likely path back to the seed point(s). Hence, a trace of the best connection(s) between the seed point(s) and the link point(s) is created.

If two arbitrary points are chosen in a 2D vector field, the most favorable way to connect them is through simulated annealing, a technique which minimizes the effect of noise in a global fashion. Two initial ROIs are selected initially based on knowledge of the anatomy of the brain. Alternatively, the amount of the lowest energy can be used to estimate the "likeliness" of the connection. For example, if two selected ROIs are not connected by the real tract, the energy to force a connection between them must be large even for the energy minimized path. This approach can be extended to create the "connectivity map".

The techniques discussed above are all based on the principle that a clear principal axis can be defined inside an MRI voxel, which means that the voxel occupies a single tissue and that the vector can be connected to a neighboring voxel. In some situations these assumptions are violated, so some approaches, that were recently suggested to address them, are discussed below.

The assumption that the direction of the largest principal eigenvector (principal axis) aligns with a single local fiber orientation is not always true. Until recently, this problem requires termination of tracking. To better quantify this judgment, indices for the cigar (C_c) and planar (C_p) shaped ellipsoids have been defined and new computer-based tracking approaches have been presented. These techniques are:

1. **Tensor line** (Lazar, 2000; Weinstein, 1999): It uses not only the principal eigenvector ε_1, but the entire diffusion tensor, D, to determine the propagation direction. The diffusion tensor defines a deflected direction, $v_{out} = D^*v_{in}$, where v_{in} is the initial direction. The propagation direction is given as: $v_{prop} = (1-a)^*v_{in} + a^*\, v_{out}$ where a is a user defined weighting factor. Studies have demonstrated that this approach can successfully reconstruct major fiber bundles and the results are more robust and reproducible under conditions of high noise.
2. **Surface line** (Zhang, 2001): The algorithm begins by generating many streamtubes (which represent linear anisotropy) and streamsurfaces (which represent planar anisotropy) and then selects some of them in order to create a representative subset. Initially, each voxel with a linear or planar anisotropy value greater than some threshold has a representative streamtube or a streamsurface. The criteria for selecting the subset include the size of the structure, the average anisotropy in the region containing the structure, and the similarity of the structures. Structures with low scores on these criteria are not included.
3. **Diffusion spectrum** (Frank, 2001; Wedeen, 2000): This technique images a distribution of fiber orientations within each voxel, mapping within each MRI voxel the 3D probability density function (PDF) of proton diffusion using q space diffusion MRI and Fourier transform (FT) encoding and reconstruction. Similarly, it was demonstrated that the degree of anisotropy can be directly

estimated from the high angular resolution acquisition (43 orientations) without using any tensor calculation.

When there are multiple populations of tracts within a pixel, the above techniques can improve tractography results by detecting and visualizing such pixels (stream surface technique), providing more robust tracking (tensor line technique) and better describing tract architecture within a pixel through an increased number of measurements (diffusion spectrum technique). However, simple unconstrained DTI tract tracing cannot distinguish whether two tracts are crossing or kissing within a pixel. In this case there are three options: a) terminate tracking when a pixel with non-cigar-shape anisotropy is met, b) use anatomical knowledge so that the tracking can penetrate the ambiguous regions by finding a path with minimum energy and c) take into account the existence of consistent artefacts in the tracking results that go through particular anatomical regions. These artefacts may include missing branches and/or systematic mislabeling of adjacent tracts.

Even though there is no error in the DTI measurement process, noise and partial volume effect (PVE) make fiber tracking a complicated process. The first factor is largest for the linear line propagation models and smaller for the other techniques which use fitting, regularization and/or energy minimization processes. Partial volume effect is directly related to the noise since image resolution must be increased to reduce PVE, leading to lower SNR. The enhancement of SNR, as a postprocessing step, results in the reduction of resolution and, hence, increases PVE. The minimization of the errors can be achieved by the following two approaches:

1. **Knowledge-based multiple-ROI approach** (Mori, 2002; Stieltjes, 2001; Xing, 1997): A drawback of this approach is that it can, in many cases, be applied only to anatomically well-documented tracts, imposing limitations on the discovery of new tracts. However, it has a significant advantage since the location of many tracts can be identified in living humans non-invasively.
2. **Probabilistic approach** (Mori, 2002): Assuming that errors due to noise and PVE are random, they are expected to have low reproducibility if the same subject is repeatedly scanned and the results are superimposed. Poor brain normalization quality may lead to obscure definition of smaller tracts of interest, and thus decreasing detection of abnormalities. These limitations become especially apparent for the smaller fiber structures near the cortical areas of the brain.

ANALYSIS OF DTI

In section 3 the features which can be extracted from DTI data are reported. Those are scalars or tensors and permit the use of a variety of statistical techniques for group analysis. Scalar DTI measures such as anisotropy, diffusivity and probability maps are compared using histogram, ROI or voxel-based analysis techniques (Anbeek, 2004; Biligili, 2004; Cerignani, 2003; Ciccarelli, 2003; Davatzikos, 2004; Jones, 2005; Lin, 2005; Mascalchi, 2002; Nyul, 1999; Steens, 2004; Tzouio-Mazoyer, 2002).

Histogram analysis does not require any presuppositions related to anatomy or pathologic features, making it suitable for widespread diseases such as multiple sclerosis or small vessel ischemic disease. On the other hand only global conclusions can be drawn on the composition of white gray matter. This may be a disadvantage when considering lesions in the brain since their effects often depend on their location.

ROI analysis is used to test hypothesis for specific regions where the disease is suspected. Any significant differences that are detected can be ascribed to the ROI, thus, offering a possible correlation between structure and function. ROIs drawn on DTI may suffer from artefacts and decreased resolution, whereas those drawn on higher resolution images must be accurately registered to the DT images. In this case registration must be performed carefully.

Voxel-by-voxel analysis depends usually less on the operator and can be more easily automated than ROI analysis, but it can only be performed after intersubject registration.

APPLICATIONS

Analysis of DTI aims to demonstrate the relationship between the white matter structure and the function of the anatomical region that is depicted. In this section application of DWI and DTI in disorders of the central nervous system are reviewed. We emphasize diseases mainly affecting the white matter such as dementia, neoplasm, epilepsy, ischemic, psychiatric and demyelinating diseases (Horsfield, 2002; Nucifora, 2007).

In premature newborns, increased anisotropy is found in developing cortical gray matter rather than in unmyelinated white matter, and cortical anisotropy steadily decreases during the first few months of life. This reflects the radial anisotropy of the glial scaffolding that guides the migration of neurons to the cortex.

Although mild decreases in anisotropy are a normal result of aging, DT imaging has shown additional abnormalities in patients with several types of dementia and neurodegenerative diseases. A study of patients with early Parkinson disease demonstrated decreased anisotropy in the substantia nigra but normal anisotropy in the putamen and caudate nucleus. Increased diffusivity and decreased anisotropy were found in the corpus callosum and the frontal temporal and parietal white matter in both patients with Alzheimer Disease (AD) and those with lewy body dementia.

Since schizophrenia may involve disordered brain connectivity, many investigators have used DTI to demonstrate a variety of white matter abnormalities, often correlated with performance on neuropsychiatric tests. Decreased anisotropy in the white matter subserving language centers has been correlated with the presence of auditory hallucinations and also decreased anisotropy has been ascribed in the arcuate fasciculus of children with behavioral disorders, in the prefrontal white matter of the patients with bipolar disorder, and in the right superior frontal gyrus of elderly patients with depression.

The specificity of DTI measures for white matter abnormalities has spurred its use in demyelinating diseases, particularly multiple sclerosis. Several studies have demonstrated increased diffusivity and decreased anisotropy which vary with the degree and type of contrast enhancement. However, DTI has also demonstrated abnormalities in normal appearing white matter and gray matter.

The use of DTI in ischemic diseases is expanding well beyond its proven role in the detection of early acute ischemia into the domain of prognosis and long-term management of ischemic sequelae. Patients with cerebral autosomal dominant arteriotherapy with subcortical infarcts and leukoencephalopathy, or CADASIL, syndrome demonstrated decreased anisotropy and increased diffusivity in normal appearing white matter representing early ischemia. DTI abnormalities in the frontal lobes and cingulated fasciculus have been associated with specific types of cognitive impairment in this disease.

The changes in diffusivity may have important implications in the delineation of tumor margins beyond what is currently demonstrated with conventional imaging. Also, they may be used to predict tumor response to chemotherapy and radiation. Furthermore, the neurosurgical uses for tractography are not limited to oncology. There are multiple examples of the use of tractography in surgical planning for epilepsy. Intra-operative maps of language centers in epilepsy have been analyzed with tractography to suggest locations of eloquent white matter. Tractography has also been used to determine whether seizure foci involved the visual radiations, and findings were in concordance with cortical visual evoked potentials.

FUTURE TRENDS

The full potential of DTI will probably not be realized until it is integrated with other image modalities to obtain rich characterization of white matter. The most intriguing application is the integration of tractography with functional imaging. Activation maps are the natural complement of tractography. A temporal relationship between activated foci implies the existence of subservient fiber tracts, whereas anatomic connectivity between two regions of the brain suggests a functional relationship. The excellent correlation of BOLD functional MR data with tractography findings in motor and visual cortex may illustrate the future of structure function investigations in the brain, ultimately to culminate in a comprehensive description of the "human connectome".

CONCLUSION

Diffusion magnetic resonance imaging is an evolving tool in the examination of central nervous system. Techniques such as diffusion tensor imaging offer a glimpse into brain microstructure at a scale which is not easily accessible with other modalities, in some cases improving the detection and characterization of white matter abnormalities. DTI is the only non-invasive approach available to track white matter fibers and therefore has a tremendous impact on the brain function studies. With DTI, diffusion anisotropy effects can be fully extracted, characterized and exploited providing even more exquisite details on tissue microstructure. The DTI demonstrates subtle abnormalities in a variety of diseases, thus, can have a broad range of possible applications. The most advanced application is tractography. Fiber tracking techniques offer an overall view of brain anatomy, including the degree of connectivity between different regions of brain. Optimal utilization of the wide range of data provided with DTI requires attention during acquisition and analysis. Although, first results of incorporation of DTI in clinical practice, especially in the assessment of brain tumors, diffuse axonal injury, pediatric brain development and cerebral infarcts, are promising, DTI is not fully utilized. The full potential of DTI will be realized when it will be integrated with other image modalities such as functional MRI. Activation maps are the natural complement of tractography. This combination of fMRI and DTI will open a window on the brain connectivity issues.

REFERENCES

Alexander, A. L., Tsuruda, J. S., & Parker, D. L. (1997). Estimation of eddy current artifacts in diffusion-weighted echo-planar images: the use of bipolar gradients. *Magnetic Resonance in Medicine, 38,* 1016-1021.

Alexander, D. C., & Barker, G. J. (2005). Optimal imaging parameters for fiber-orientation estimation in diffusion MRI. *NeuroImage, 27,* 357-367.

Anbeek, P., Vincken, K. L., van Osch, M. J., Bisschops, R. H., & van der Grond, J. (2004). Probabilistic segmentation of white matter lesions in MR imaging. *Neuroimage, 21,* 1037-1044.

Anderson, J. L., & Skare, S. (2002). A model-based method for retrospective correction of geometric distortions in diffusion-weighted EPI. *NeuroImage, 16,* 177-199.

Armitage, P. A., & Bastin, M. E. (2001). Utilizing the diffusion-to-noise ratio to optimize magnetic resonance diffusion tensor acquisition strategies for improving measurements of diffusion anisotropy. *Magnetic Resonance in Medicine, 45,* 1056-1065.

Bahrens, T. E., Johansen-Berg, H., & Woolrich, M. W. (2003). Non-invasive mapping of connection between human thalamus and cortex using diffusion imaging. *Nature Neuroscience, 6,* 750-757.

Bammer, R. (2003). Basic principles of diffusion-weighted imaging. *European Journal of Radiology, 45,* 169-184.

Basser, P. J., Mattiello, J., & Bihan, D. L. (1994). Estimation of the effective self-diffusion tensor from the NMR spin echo. *Journal of Magnetic Resonance, 103,* 247-254.

Basser, P. J., Pajevic, S., Pierpaoli, C., Duda, J., & Aldroubi, A. (2000). In vitro fiber tractography using DT-MRI data. *Magnetic Resonance in Medicine, 44,* 625-632.

Basser, P. J., & Pierpaoli, C. (1998). A simplified method to measure the diffusion tensor from seven MR images. *Magnetic Resonance in Medicine, 39,* 928-934.

Bhagat, Y. A., & Beaulieu, C. (2004). Diffusion anisotropy in subcortical white matter and cortical gray matter: changes with aging and the role of CSF-suppression. *Journal of Magnetic Resonance Imaging, 20,* 216-227.

Bihan, D. L., Mangin, J., Poupon, C., Clark, C. A., Pappata, S., Molko, N., & Chabriat, H. (2001). Diffusion Tensor Imamging: Concepts and Applications. *Journal of Magnetic Resonance Imaging, 13,* 534-546.

Bilgili, Y., & Unal, B. (2004). Effect of region of interest on interobserver variance in apparent diffusion coefficient measures, *American Journal of Neuroradiology, 25,* 108-111.

Cerignani, M., Bammer, R., Sormani, M. P., Fazekas, F., & Filippi, M. (2003). Inter-sequence and inter-imaging unit variability of diffusion tensor MR imaging histogram-derived metrics of the brain in healthy volunteers. *American Journal of Neuroradiology, 24,* 638-643.

Chang, L. C., Jones, D. K., & Pierpaoli, C. (2005). RESTORE: robust estimation of tensors by outlier rejection. *Magnetic Resonance in Medicine, 53,* 1088-1095.

Ciccarelli, O., Toosy, A. T., Parker, G. J., Wheeler-Kingshott, C. A. M., Barker, G. J., Miller, D. H., & Thompson A. J. (2003). Diffusion tractography based group mapping of major white-matter pathways in the human brain. *NeuroImage., 19,* 1545-1555.

Conturo, T. E., Lori, N. F., Cull, T. S., Akbudak, E., Snyder, A. Z., Shimony, J. S., McKinstry, R. C., Burton, H., & Raichle, M. E. (1999). Tracking neuronal fiber pathways in the living human brain, *Proceedings of National Academy of Sciences USA, 96,* 10422-10427.

Conturo, T. E., McKinstry, R. C., Akbudak, E., & Robinson, B. H. (1996). Encoding of anisotropic diffusion with tetrahedral gradients: A general mathematical diffusion formalism and experimental results. *Magnetic Resonance in Medicine, 35,* 399-412.

Davatzikos, C. (2004). Why voxel-based morphometry analysis should be used with great caution when characterizing group differences. *NeuroImage, 23,* 17-20.

Falconer, J. C., & Narayana, P. A. (1997). Cerebrospinal fluid-suppressed high-resolution diffusion imaging of human brain. *Magnetic Resonance in Medicine, 37,* 119-123.

Finsterbusch, J., & Frahm, J. (2000). Diffusion tensor mapping of the human brain using single-shot line scan imaging. *Journal of Magnetic Resonance Imaging, 12,* 388-394.

Forbes, K. P., Pipe, J. G., Karis, J. P., & Heiserman, J. E. (2002). Improved image quality and detection of acute cerebral infarction with PROPELLER diffusion weighted MR imaging. *Radiology, 225,* 551-555.

Frank, L. R. (2001). Anisotropy in high angular resolution diffusion-weighted MRI. *Magnetic Resonance in Medicine, 45,* 935-939.

Gudbjartsson, H., Maier, S. E., Mulkern, R. V., Morocz, I. A., Patz, S., & Jolesz, F. A. (1996). Line scan diffusion imaging. *Magnetic Resonance in Medicine, 36,* 509-519.

Hasan, K. M., Parker, D. L., & Alexander, A. L. (2001). Comparison of gradient encoding schemes for diffusion-tensor MRI. *Journal of Magnetic Resonance Imaging, 13,* 769-780.

Haselgrove, J. C., & Moore, J. R. (1996). Correction for distortion of echo-planar images used to calculate the apparent diffusion coefficient. *Magnetic Resonance in Medicine, 36,* 960-964.

Hirsch, J. G., Bock, M., Essig, M., & Schad, L. R. (1999). Comparison of diffusion anisotropy measurements in combination with the flair –technique. *Magnetic Resonance in Medicine, 17,* 705-716.

Horsfield, M., & Jones, D. (2002). Applications of diffusion-weighted and diffusion tensor MRI to white matter diseases – a review. *NMR in Biomedicine, 15,* 570-57.

Hsu, E. W., & Mori, S. (1995). Analytical expressions for the NMR apparent diffusion coefficients in an anisotropic system and a simplified method for determining fiber orientation. *Magnetic Resonance in Medicine, 34,* 194-200.

Jackowski, M., Kao, C. Y., Qiu, M., Constable, R. T., & Staib, L. H. (2005). White matter tractography by anisotropic waveform evolution and diffusion tensor imaging. *Medical Image Analysis, 9,* 427-440.

Jones, D. K., Horsfield, M. A., & Simmons, A. (1999). Optimal strategies for measuring diffusion in anisotropic systems by magnetic resonance imaging. *Magnetic Resonance in Medicine, 42,* 515-525.

Jones, D. K., Symms, M. R., Cerignani, M., & Howard, R. J. (2005). The effect of filter size on VBM analyses of DT-MRI data. *NeuroImage, 26,* 546-554.

Jones, D. K. (2004). The effect of gradient sampling schemes on measures derived from diffusion tensor MRI: a Monte Carlo study. *Magnetic Resonance in Medicine, 51,* 807-815.

Kingsley, P. B., & Monahan, W. G. (2004). Selection of the optimum b factor for diffusion-weighted magnetic resonance imaging assessment of ischemic stroke. *Magnetic Resonance in Medicine, 51,* 996-1001.

Kwong, K. K., McKinstry, R. C., Chien, D., Crawley, A. P., Pearlman, J. D., & Rosen, B. R. (1991). CSF-suppressed quantitative single-shot diffusion imaging. *Magnetic Resonance in Medicine, 21,* 157-163.

Lazar, M., & Alexander, A. L. (2003). An error analysis of white matter tractography methods: synthetic diffusion tensor field stimulations. *NeuroImage, 20,* 1140-1153.

Lazar, M., & Alexander, A. L. (2001). Error analysis of white matter tracking algorithms (streamlines and tensorlines) for DT-MRI. *Proceedings of International Society of Magnetic Resonance in Medicine*, (pp. 506), Glasgow, UK.

Lazar, M., Weinstein, D., Hasan, K., & Alexander, A. L. (2000). Axon tractography with tensorilines. *Proceedings of International Society of Magnetic Resonance in Medicine,* (pp. 482), Denver, CO.

Lazar, M., Weinstein, D. M., & Tsuruda, J. S. (2003). White matter tractography using diffusion tensor deflection. *Human Brain Mapping, 18,* 306-321.

Le Bihan, D. (1991). Molecular diffusion nuclear magnetic resonance imaging. *Magnetic Resonance in Medicine, 7,* 1-30.

Lin, C. Y., Sun, S. W., Hong, C. Y., & Chang, C. (2005). Unsupervised identification of white matter tracts in a mouse brain using a directional correlation-based region growing (DCRG) algorithm. *NeuroImage, 28,* 380-388.

Lori, N. F., Akbuda, E., Snyder, A. Z., Shimony, J. S., & Conturo, T. E. (1999). Diffusion tensor tracking of human neuronal fiber bundles: Simulation of effects of noise, voxel size and data interpolation. *Proceedings of International Society of Magnetic Resonance in Medicine*, (pp. 775), Denver, CO.

Mascalchi, M., Tessa, C., Moretti, M., Della Nave, R., Boddi, V., Martini, S., Inzitari, D., & Villari, N. (2002). Whole brain apparent diffusion coefficient histogram: a new tool for evaluation of leukoaraiosis. *Journal of Magnetic Resonance Imaging, 15,* 144-148.

Masutani, Y., Aoki, S., Abe, O., Hayashi, N., & Otomo, K. (2003). MR diffusion tensor imaging: recent advance and new techniques for diffusion tensor visualization. *European Journal of Radiology, 46,* 53-56.

Mattiello, L., Basser, P. J., & Bihan, D. L. (1994). Analytical expression for the b matrix in NMR diffusion imaging and Spectroscopy. *Journal of Magnetic Resonance, 108,* 131-141.

Mattiello, L., Basser, P. J., & Bihan, D. L. (1997). The b-matrix in diffusion tensor echo-planar imaging. *Magnetic Resonance in Medicine, 37,* 292-300.

Melhem, E. R., Mori, S., Mukundan, G., Kraut, M. A., Pomper, M. G., & van Zijjl, P. C. M. (2002). Diffusion Tensor MR Imaging of the Brain and White Matter Tractography. *American Journal of Radiology, 178,* 3-16.

Mori, S., Crain, B. J., & van Zijl, P. C. (1998). 3D brain fiber reconstruction from diffusion MRI. *Proceedings of International Conference on Functional Mapping of the Human Brain*, Montreal.

Mori, S., Fredericksen, K., van Zijil, P. C. M., Stieltjes, B., Kraut, A. K., Solaiyappan, M., & Pomper, M. D. (2002). Brain white matter anatomy of tumor patients using diffusion tensor imaging. *Annals of Neurology, 51,* 377-380.

Mori, S., Grain, B. J., Chacki, V. P., & van Zijl, P. C. (1999). Three-dimensional tracking of axonal projections in the brain by magnetic resonance imaging. *Annals of Neurology, 45,* 26-269.

Mori, S., Kaufmann, W. E., Davatzikos, C., Stieltjes, B., Amodei, L., Fredericksen, K., Pearlson, G. D., Malhem, E. R., Solaiyappan, M., Raymond, G. V., Moser, H. W., & van Zijil, P. C. M. (2002). Imaging cortical association tracts in human brain. *Magnetic Resonance Imaging, 47,* 215-223.

Mori, S., & van Zijil, P. C. M. (2002). Fiber tracking: principles and strategies – a technical review. *NMR in Biomedicine, 15,* 468-480.

Nucifora, P. G. P., Verma, R., Lee, S., & Melherm, E. R. (2007). Diffusion-Tensor MR Imaging and Tractography: Exploring Brain Microstructure and Connectivity. *Radiology, 245,* 367-384.

Nyul, L. G., & Uduppa, J. K. (1999). On standardizing the MR image intensity scale. *Magnetic Resonance in Medicine, 42,* 1072-1081.

Okada, T., Miki, Y., Fushimi, Y., Hanakawa, T., Kanagaki, M., Yamamoto, A., Urayama, S., Fukyama, H., Hiraoka, M., & Togashi, K. (2006). Diffusion-Tensor Fiber Tractography: Intaindividual Comparison of 3.0-T and 1.5-T MR imaging. *Radiology, 238,* 668-678.

Ozarslan, E., & Mareci, T. H. (2003). Generalized diffusion tensor imaging and analytical relationships between diffusion tensor imaging and high angular resolution diffusion imaging. *Magnetic Resonance in Medicine, 50,* 955-965.

Pagani, E., Bammer, R., Horsfield, M. A., Rovaris, M., Gass, A., Ciccarelli, O., & Filippi, M. (2007). Diffusion MR Imaging in Multiple Sclerosis: Technical Aspects and Challenges. *American Journal of Neuroradiology, 28,* 411-420.

Papadakis, N. G., Martin, K. M., Mustafa, M. H., Wilkinson, I. D., Griffiths, P. D., Huang, C. L. H., & Woodruff, P. W. R. (2002). Study of the effect of CSF suppression on white matter diffusion anisotropy mapping of healthy human brain. *Magnetic Resonance in Medicine, 48,* 394-398.

Parker, G. J., Haroon, H. A., & Wheeler-Kingshott, C. A. (2003). A framework for a streamline-based probabilistic index of connectivity (PICo) using a structural interpretation of MRI diffusion measurements. *Journal of Magnetic Resonance Imaging, 18,* 242-254.

Parker, G. J., Stephan, K. E., & Barker, G. J. (2002). Initial demonstration of in vivo tracing of axonal projections with the human brain using diffusion tensor imaging and fast marching tractography. *NeuroImage, 15,* 797-809.

Parker, G. J. (2000). Tracing fiber tracts using fast marching. *Proceedings of International Society of Magnetic Resonance*, (pp. 85), Denver, CO.

Pierpaoli, C. (2002). Inferring structural and architectural features of brain tissue from DT-MRI measurements. *CNS Spectrums , 7,* 10-515.

Pierpaoli, C., Jezzard, P., Basser, P. J., Barnett, A., & Di, C. G. (1996). Diffusion tensor MR imaging of the human brain. *Radiology, 201,* 637-648.

Pipe, J. G., & Zwart, N. (2006). Turboprop: improved PROPELLER imaging. *Magnetic Resonance in Medicine, 55,* 380-385.

Pipe, J. G., Farthing, V. G., & Forbes, K. P. (2002). Multi-shot diffusion-weighted FSE using PROPELLER MRI. *Magnetic Resonance in Medicine, 47,* 42-52.

Rieseberg, S., Merboldt, K. D., Kuntzel, M., & Frahm, J. (2005). Diffusion tensor imaging using partial Fourier STEAM MRI with projection onto convex subsets reconstruction. *Magnetic Resonance in Medicine, 54,* 486-490.

Rohde, G. K., Barnet, A. S., Basser, P. J., Marenco, S., & Pierpaoli, C. (2004). Comprehensive approach for correction of motion and distortion in diffusion-weighted MRI. *Magnetic Resonance in Medicine, 51,* 103-114.

Rohde, G. K., Barnett, A. S., Basser, P. J., & Pierpaoli, C. (2005). Estimating intensity variance due to noise in registered images: applications to diffusion tensor MRI. *NeuroImage, 26,* 673-684.

Skare, S., & Andersson, J. L. (2001). On the effects of gating in diffusion imaging of the brain using single shot EPI. *Magnetic Resonance in Medicine, 19,* 1125-1128.

Sorensen, A. G., Wu, O., Copen, W. A., Davis, T. L., Gonzalez, R. G., & Koroshetz, W. J. (1999). Human acute cerebral ischemia: Detection of changes in water diffusion anisotropy by using MR imaging. *Radiology, 212,* 785-792.

Steens, S. C., Admiraal-Behloul, F., Schaap, J. A., Hoogenraad, F. G. C, Wheeler-Kingshott, C. A. M., le Cessie, S., Tofts, P. S., & van Buchem, M. A. (2004). Reproducibility of brain ADC histograms. *European Radiology, 14,* 425-430.

Stieltjes, B., Kaufmann, W. E., van Zijil, P. C. M., Fredericksen, K., Pearlson, G. D., & Mori, S. (2001). Diffusion tensor imaging and axonal tracking in the human brainstem, *NeuroImage, 14,* 723-735.

Tuch, D. S., Reese, T. G., Wiegell, M. R., Makris, N., Belliveau, J. W., & Wedeen, V. J. (2002). High angular resolution diffusion imaging reveals intravoxel white matter fiber tractography. *Magnetic Resonance in Medicine, 48,* 577-582.

Tuch, D. S., Wiegell, M. R., Reese, T. G., Belliveau, J. W., & Wedeen, V. (2001). Measuring cortico-cortical connectivity matrices with diffusion spectrum imaging. *Proceedings of International Society of Magnetic Resonance in Medicine*, (pp. 502), Glasgow, UK.

Turner, R., Le Bihan, D. J., & Chesnick, A. S. (1991). Echo-planar imaging of diffusion and perfusion. *Magnetic Resonance in Medicine, 19,* 247-253.

Tzouio-Mazoyer, N., Landeau, B., Papathanasiou, D., Crivello, F., Etard, O., Delcroix, N., Mazoyer, B., & Joliot, M. (2002). Automated anatomical labeling of activations in SPM using a macroscopic anatomical parcellation of the MNI MRI single-subject brain. *NeuroImage, 15,* 273-289.

Wedeen, V., Reese, T. G., Tuch, D. S., Weigel, M. R., Dou, J. G., Weiskoff, R. M., & Chessler, D. (2000). Mapping fiber orientation xpectra in cerebral white matter with fourier-transform diffusion MRI. *Proceedings of International Society of Magnetic Resonance in Medicine*, (pp. 82), Denver, CO.

Weinstein, D., Kindlmann, G., & Lundberg, E.C. (1999). Tensorline: advection diffusion based propagation through diffusion tensor fields. *Proceedings IEEE Visualization*, (pp. 249-253), San Francisco, CA.

Werring, D. J., Toosy, A. T., Clark, C. A., Parker, G. J., Barker, G. J., Miller, D. H., & Thompson, A. J. (2000). Diffusion tensor imaging can detect and quantify corticospinal tract degeneration after stroke. *Journal of Neurology, Neurosurgery, and Psychiatry, 69,* 269-272.

Westin, C. F., Maier, S. E., Mamata, H., Nabavi, A., Jolesz, F. A., & Kikinis, R. (2002). Processing and visualization for diffusion tensor MRI. *Medical Image Analysis, 6,* 93-108.

Xing, D., Papadakis, N. G., Huang, C. L., Lee, V.M., Carpenter, T. A., & Hall, L. D. (1997). Optimised diffusion-weighting for measurement of apparent diffusion coefficient (ADC) in human brain. *Magnetic Resonance Imaging, 15,* 771-784.

Xue, R., van Zijil, P. C. M., Vrain, B. J., Solaiyappan, M., & Mori, S. (1999). In vivo three-dimensional reconstruction of rat brain axonal projections by diffusion tensor imaging. *Magnetic Resonance in Medicine, 42,* 1123-1127.

Zhang, S., & Laidlaw, D. (2001). Elucidating neural structure in diffusion tensor MRI volumes using streamtubes and streamsurfaces. *Proceedings of International Society of Magnetic Resonance in Imaging,* (pp. 505), Glasgow, UK.

KEY TERMS

Brownian Motion: (named in honor of the botanist Robert Brown) is the random movement of particles suspended in a liquid or gas or the mathematical model used to describe such random movements, often called a particle theory.

Diffusion: The spontaneous movement of particles from an area of high concentration to an area of low concentration in a given volume of fluid. Diffusion MRI is a specific Magnetic Resonance Imaging (MRI) modality which produces in vivo images of biological tissues weighted by the local micro structural characteristics of water diffusion.

Diffusion Tensor Imaging: A magnetic resonance imaging (MRI) technique which enables the measurement of the restricted diffusion of water in tissue in order to produce neural tract images. Its common application is in the imaging of white matter where the location, orientation, and anisotropy of the tracts can be measured.

Echo Planar Imaging: A technique of planar imaging in which a complete planar image is obtained from one selective excitation pulse.

Fractional Anisotropy: One of the commonly used measures of deviation from isotropy and reflects the degree of alignment of cellular structures within fiber tracts, as well as their structural integrity.

Mean Diffusivity: A measure of the average molecular motion independent of any tissue directionality. It is affected by the cellular size and integrity.

Navigator Echoes: Additional spin or gradient echoes used to monitor changes in the position of the sample during the scan time.

Relative Anisotropy: The ratio of the anisotropic part of tensor D to its isotropic part.

Signal to Noise Ratio: Used to describe the relative contributions to a detected signal of the true signal and random superimposed signals (noise).

Volume Ratio: The ratio of the ellipsoid volume to the volume of a sphere.

Chapter XVI
Image Processing and Machine Learning Techniques for Facial Expression Recognition

Anastasios Koutlas
University of Ioannina, Greece

Dimitrios I. Fotiadis
University of Ioannina, Greece

ABSTRACT

The aim of this chapter is to analyze the recent advances in image processing and machine learning techniques with respect to facial expression recognition. A comprehensive review of recently proposed methods is provided along with an analysis of the advantages and the shortcomings of existing systems. Moreover, an example for the automatic identification of basic emotions is presented: Active Shape Models are used to identify prominent features of the face; Gabor filters are used to represent facial geometry at selected locations of fiducial points and Artificial Neural Networks are used for the classification into the basic emotions (anger, surprise, fear, happiness, sadness, disgust, neutral); and finally, the future trends towards automatic facial expression recognition are described.

INTRODUCTION

The face is the fundamental part of day to day interpersonal communication. Humans use the face along with facial expressions to denote consciously their emotional states (anger, surprise, stress, etc.) or subconsciously (yawn, lip biting), to accompany and enhance the meaning of their thoughts (wink) or exchange thoughts without talking (head nodes, look exchanges). Facial expressions are the result of the deformation in a human's face due to muscle movement. The importance of automating the task to analyse facial expressions using computing systems is apparent and can be beneficial to many different scientific subjects such as psychology, neurology, psychiatry, as well as, applications of everyday life such as driver monitoring systems, automated tutoring systems or smart environments and human-computer interaction. Although humans are able to identify changes in facial expressions easily and effortlessly even in complicated scenes, the same is not an easy task to be undertaken by a machine. Moreover, computing systems must share the same robustness and accuracy with a human so that these systems could be used in a real-world scenario and provide adequate aid.

Advances in topics such as face detection, face tracking and recognition, psychological studies as well as the processing power of modern computer systems make the automatic analysis of facial expressions possible for use with real world examples where responsiveness (i.e. real time processing) is required along with sensitivity (i.e. being able to detect various day to day emotional states and visual cues) and the ability to tolerate head movements or sudden changes.

For an effective automatic facial expression recognition (AFER) system there are several characteristics that must be present so that it can be efficient. These are outlined in the Figure 1.

Face detection and identification of prominent features is a crucial step for an AFER system. It is the first step for any system that carries the automatic tag and the performance of this step in terms of accuracy is crucial for the overall accuracy of the system. Various approaches are presented in the literature in terms of static or temporal identification of the face or identification of prominent features such as eyes in contrast to identifying the presence of a face in a scene.

When the face is located it must be modeled so that it can be represented in an appropriate manner. The facial representation could be based on the facial geometry that encompasses some unique features of homogeneity and diversion across humans. It could also be based in characteristics that appear after some transformation with mathematical expressions modeling texture, position and gray-level information. After that the feature vector is built by extracting features. It can be represented either holistically or locally. Holistic approach treats the face as a whole, i.e. the processing of the face and the mathematical information applies to the whole face without considering any special prominent features of it. On the other hand the local approach treats each prominent feature of the face in a different way and the feature extraction process is applied in selected locations in the image which are often called fiducial points. Lastly, there are systems which are related to the processing of image sequences or static images which combine the two approaches, treating the face in a hybrid manner. There is also a distinction in terms of the presence of temporal information or not.

Classification is the last step for an AFER system. The facial actions or the deformations

Figure 1. Structure of an automatic facial expression recognition system

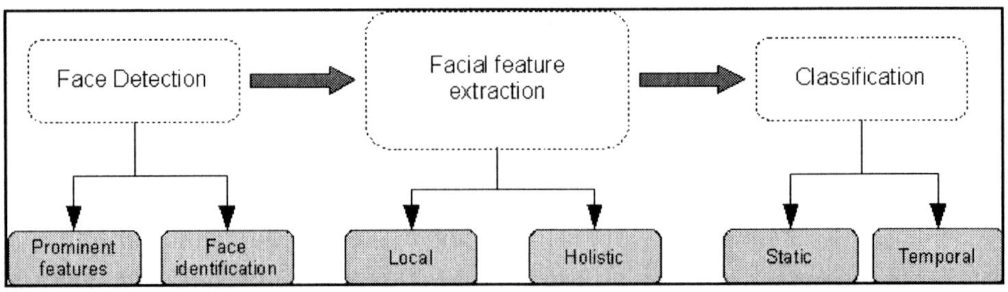

due to facial movement are categorized either as basic emotions or as Action Units (AUs). In what follows depending on the use of temporal characteristics or not the classification process is considered temporal or static for this chapter.

This chapter introduces recent advances in automatic facial expression recognition. The first part contains an introduction to the automatic facial expression recognition systems, including their structure, their objectives and their limitations. In the second part a review of recent work, is presented related to face identification, acquisition and recognition, facial feature transformation, feature vector extraction and classification. In part three a particular approach is described along with quantitative results.

BACKGROUND

Introduction

Most systems try to recognize a small set of prototypic emotions which share characteristics of universality and uniformity across people with different ethnic background or cultural heritage. The six basic emotions were proposed by Ekman and Friesen (1971) and are: disgust, fear, joy, surprise, sadness and anger. The neutral position inherits most of the characteristics that are shared across basic emotions and could be considered a seventh basic expression. Diversity of the neutral position arises mainly due to variations in pose and not muscle movement.

In every day life basic emotions occur rather infrequently. Emotions that are more frequent to occur in everyday life are due to subtle changes in certain specific areas such as the eyebrows or eyelids and so on. For example the tightening of the lips in case of anger or the lowering the lips in case of sadness. These changes in the appearance of facial expression are subtle and systems that recognize such changes are required to be more precise. The Facial Action Coding System (FACS) (Ekman & Friesen, 1978) provides the mechanisms to detect facial movement by human coders. When a coder is viewing a sequence of the facial behaviour of a human subject can decode Action Units (AU). Action Units are a set of actions that correspond either to muscle movement in facial expressions such as raising upper lip or blinking or some miscellaneous actions such as bite lip or blow. FACS consists of 44 action units. There is also a scale of intensity that can describe each action unit in a scale of 5.

Even though Ekman and Friesen proposed certain combinations of action units as descriptive of certain emotions, FACS itself does not contain any emotion-specific information. These are coded in separate systems such as the Emotional Specific FACS (EMFACS) (Friesen & Ekman, 1983). By converting action units from FACS to EMFACS or other emotion-specific systems, expressions can be coded, such as sadness or surprise.

It is reported in the literature that there is a distinction between facial expressions that are spontaneous and those that are initiated by request often referred to as posed (Ekman, 1991,2003). From a physiological point of view it is perfectly justified since spontaneous actions and posed actions originate from different parts of the brain; namely the subcortical areas of the brain and the cortical motor strip, respectively (Meihle, 1973). Major differences between spontaneous and posed facial expressions are the actual movement that is initiated from facial muscles and the dynamics of the expression (Ekman & Rosenberg, 2005). Subcorticaly initiated facial expressions (spontaneous) are characterized by synchronized, smooth, symmetrical, consistent and reflex-like facial muscle movement. On the other hand facial expressions that are cortically initiated (posed) tend to be less smooth, with more varying dynamics (Ekman & Rosenberg, 2005).

To develop and evaluate systems that are subject to the above conditions reliable annotated databases must be used. There are several attempts in the literature for the development of such databases but it is difficult to comprehend all different variability issues in a single database. An example is the Japanese Female Facial Expression Database (JAFFE) (Lyons et al. 1999). It features ten different Japanese women posing 3 or 4 examples for each basic emotion containing a total of 213 still images. The Cohn-Kanade database (Kanade et al. 2000) is another database but differs from JAFFE since it contains temporal information and is used widely for facial expression analysis (Tian et al. 2001). It contains image sequences of 100 subjects posing a set of 23 facial displays and contains FACS annotation in addition to basic emotion tags. Although it is used widely for the evaluation of AFER systems it has certain drawbacks. The image sequences in order to be complete and fully functional should contain 3 states for the dynamics of each expression; the onset which is the initialization of the expression, the apex which is the peak of the expression and the offset where the expression declines. Unfortunately, the Cohn-Kanade database contains information that excludes the offset of the expression. Another shortcoming of the Cohn-Kanade database is that the images contain a timestamp that is overlapping with the subject's expression certain times. The MMI database (Pantic et al., 2005) contains both posed and spontaneous facial actions. Furthermore, it contains over 4000 videos as well as 600 static images. The images are coded based on FACS, either single action units or combinations, and basic emotions. Furthermore apart from frontal views, profile views are included. Another recently developed database is the Yin Facial Expression Database (Yin et al. 2006) which contains 3D facial expression information. The expression data includes 3D models, texture information and raw model data. It also provides a landmark point set for evaluating facial features segmentation techniques. It also features 6 basic emotions plus the neutral position.

Most research groups that are working with AFER systems either use the available databases or collect their own signals to evaluate the methods. This slight fragmentation on the evaluation of such systems does not make possible the comperative evaluation of all methods proposed in the literature.

Face Detection

Face detection and identification of prominent features is a crucial step for an AFER system. This is the first step of any system that operates automatically and the overall performance of the system mainly depends on the correct identification of the face or certain facial features such as eyes, eyebrows, mouth and so on. The task of locating the face or the prominent features of a face in a scene should be independent of any occlusions in the scene, variations of lightening conditions and should tolerate changes in face pose. There are various approaches to detect faces or prominent characteristics of the face using appearance based methods and statistical techniques, or template based methods (Hjelmas & Low 2001; Yang et al. 2002; Li & Jain 2005).

The most commonly employed face detection algorithm in automatic facial expression recognition systems is the real-time face detector proposed by Viola and Jones (2001,2004). The face detector does not work directly with image intensities but there is a set of features extracted related to Haar basis functions. The Haar-like features can be computed at different scales and locations. For each set of features Adaboost is used to choose the most important features from the large set of potential features (Freund & Schapire, 1995). The classifiers are combined in a cascade, successive manner to speed up the detector's performance. The face detector is able to detect faces very rapidly. There are other works that have adapted the proposed methodology. Fasel et al. (2005) used Gentleboost (Friedman et al., 2000) instead of Adaboost. Gentleboost instead of using the binary output of each filter, uses the output in a continuous manner.

Statistical learning techniques combined with appearance features are usually used to detect faces in images. Rowley et al. (1998) used a neural network to detect face regions from non face regions using as a feature vector pixel intensities and spatial relationships between pixels. Sung and Poggio (1998) used a neural network also but as the feature vector they have used distance measures. A real-time method proposed by Petland et al. (1994) detects faces by using a view-based eigenspace method that incorporates prominent features of the face such as eyes and mouth. Apart from real-time processing the method can handle head positions which vary. Another method that can handle varying head motion was proposed by Schneiderman and Kanade (2000) which utilises a 3D object detection and appearance features such as object or non object features using a product of histograms which contains object statistics based on wavelets coefficients and their position on the object.

Template based methods are simple to implement but are usually prone to failure when large variations in pose or scale exist (Yang et al., 2002). In part the above problem can be tackled by deformable models. Kass et al. proposed the Active Contour Models or snakes (Kass et al., 1987). The snake is initialized at the proximity of the structure and is fitted onto nearby edges. The evolution of the snake relies in the minimization of an energy function. Cootes et al. has proposed Active Shape Models (ASM) (Cootes et al. 1995) and Active Appearance Models (AAM) (Cootes et al. 1998). Active Shape Models differ from snakes mainly due to global shape constrains that are enforced on the deformable model, ensuring this way that the model deforms according to the variations of the landmark points found in the training set. Moreover, a statistical gray-level model is built around landmark points which assume a Gaussian and unimodal distribution. Active Appearance Models extend the functionality of ASM capturing texturing information along with shape information. Recently variations of the ASM method have been introduced. Optimal Features ASM (OF-ASM) (Van Ginneken et al. 2002) allow for multimodal distribution of the intensities while high segmentation accuracy is reported but it is more computationally expensive. Sukno et al. (2007) extended OF-ASM to allow application in more complex geometries using Cartesian differential invariants.

Readers are referred to Hjelmas and Low (2001), Yang et al. (2002) and Li & Jain (2005) for a more thorough analysis concerning developments in detecting faces in images or image sequences.

Facial Features Extraction

The facial feature extraction step aims at modeling the face using some mathematical representation in such a way so that it could later form the feature vector and be fed into a classifier. There are two approaches to represent the face and subsequently facial geometry. Firstly, the face can be processed as a whole often referred to as holistic or analytic approach and secondly it can be represented at the location of specific regions or at the location of fiducial points often referred to as local approach.

Essa and Petland (1997) treated the face holistically using optical flow and measured deformations based on the face anatomy. Black and Yacoob (1998) also utilized an optical flow model of image motion for facial expression analysis. Their work explores the use of local parameterized optical flow models for the recognition of the six basic emotional expressions. Donato et al. (1999) has used several methods for facial expression recognition. They have used holistic Principal Component Analysis, EigenActions, where the principal components were obtained on the dataset by using difference images. A set of topographic local kernels were used for Local Feature Analysis that were matched to the second-order statistics of the input ensemple. They have used also Fisher linear discriminates (FLD) to project the images in a space that provided the maximal separability between classes and Independent Component Analysis (ICA) to preserve higher order information.

The other approach referred to as local approach, tries to symbolize the geometry of prominent features in a local manner. The local approach can be either based on the geometric properties of the features or some appearance based methods that transform the image with a mathematical representation. Pantic and Rothkrantz (2000) used geometric features to categorize in different action units as well as combinations of action units and basic emotions. Tian et al. (2001) detected and tracked changes in facial components. The models that they produced included a lip model with 3 states (open, close, tightly closed), an eye model with 2 states (open and closed), brow and cheek models and transient facial features model with 2 states (present or not present). Their categorization is based on action units.

Gabor based transformations are widely used to extract facial appearance changes. It has been shown that simple cells in the primary visual cortex can be modeled by Gabor functions (Daugman 1980, 1985). This solid physiological connection between Gabor functions and human vision has yielded several approaches to feature extraction (Ye et al. 2004) and facial expression recognition (Zhang et al. 1998; Lyons & Akamatsu 1998; Lyons et al. 1999; Gu et al. 2005; Guo & Dyer 2005; Liu & Wang 2006). Moreover, Gabor functions are optimal for measuring local spatial frequencies (Shen & Bai, 2006). Zhang et al. (1998) compared the Gabor function coefficients at the fiducial points location with the coordinates of the fiducial points and concluded that the first represent the face better than the latter. Donato et al. (1999) reported that Gabor functions performed better than any other method used in both analytic and holistic approaches.

Fiducial points are used around the prominent features of the face, the location of which are used to extract the feature vector. The number of fiducial points used varies and mainly depends on the desired representation, as it is reported that different positions hold different information regarding the expressions (Lyons et al. 1999). The way that these fiducial points are identified in an image can either be automatic (Gu et al. 2005) or manual (Zhang et al. 1998; Lyons et al. 1999; Guo & Dyer 2005).

For a more elaborate approach related to facial expression recognition the reader can refer to Pantic and Rothkrantz (2000) and Fasel and Luettin (2003).

Classification

The last step of an AFER system is the classification of the feature vectors into meaningful categories. The distinction between classification methods used in the literature depends on whether or not temporal information is used. Moreover, there is another distinction in terms of the categories that the classifiers classify into being basic emotions, single action units based on FACS or action units combinations that are used to form broader notions of emotions such as fear or stress and so on.

A Hidden Markov Model (HMM) describes the statistical behaviour of a process that generates time series data having certain statistical characteristics. Lien et al. (2000) used the temporal characteristics and HMM to classify into action units or combinations of action units. A comparative study of the performance of different classifiers is provided by Cohen et al. (2003). They have used both static and dynamic classifiers such as Naïve-Bayes based classifiers and Hidden Markov Models (HMM), respectively, to classify into basic emotions. The static classifiers used were, a modified Naïve-Bayes which assumed the distribution to be Cauchy not Gaussian and a Tree-Augmented Naïve Bayes classifier. They have also employed a multi-level HMM which allowed to segment long video sequences to different expression segments using temporal information.

Static classifiers do not use any temporal information that is available in image sequences. They use the information of a single image. Several methods can be found in the literature including neural networks, support vector machines (SVM), etc. Guo and Dyer (2005) provide a comparative study of different classifiers using the simplified Bayes, SVM and combinations of these classifiers using Adaboost. They also proposed a Linear Programming classifier. They categorized into basic emotions using the JAFFE database. Neural Networks have been deployed in various studies as well known classifiers for multi-class problems (Zhang et al. 1998).

Temporal classifiers are more suitable for person-depended tasks due to their higher degree of variability in expression in humans as well as the variation in the dynamics of each expression. They are considered more difficult to train since they need a larger training set and more parameters in order to train them adequately. Static classifiers can be problematic when they are used in sequences where each frame is categorized. When the expression is not at its peak it is likely that the static classifier can perform poorly. On the other hand static classifiers are easily using a smaller number of parameters

APPLICATION

On this section an approach for automatic facial expression recognition is presented. The proposed methodology includes four stages: (a) automatic discovery of prominent features of a face, such as the eyes, and subsequent discovery of fiducial points, (b) construction of the Gabor Filter Bank, (c) extraction of the Feature vector at the location of the fiducial points and (d) classification (Figure 2).

Active Shape Models

Active Shape Models (Cootes et al. 1995) utilize information from points around prominent features of the face which are called landmarks. A Point Distribution Model (PDM) and an image intensity profile are computed around the landmarks. For a total of S landmark points a single vector is represented as

$$\mathbf{x} = (x_1, \cdots, x_s, y_1, \ldots, y_s)^T. \quad (1)$$

The shapes collected from the training stage are aligned to the same coordinate frame. The dimensionality of the aligned data is reduced by applying Principal Component Analysis and the mean shape is computed, thus forming the PDM. Any shape of the training set can be approximated by the mean shape, $\bar{\mathbf{x}}$, the eigenvector matrix $\mathbf{P}$ and b_i, which defines the shape parameters for the ith shape,

$$\mathbf{x}_i = \bar{\mathbf{x}} + \mathbf{P}b_i, \quad b_i = \mathbf{P}^T(\mathbf{x}_i - \bar{\mathbf{x}}). \quad (2)$$

The dimensionality is reduced by selecting only the eigenvectors that correspond to the largest eigenvalues. Depending on the number of excluded eigenvectors there is an error introduced in Equation (2). Furthermore, the parameter b_i is constrained to deform in ways that are found in the training set:

$$|b_i| \leq \beta\sqrt{\lambda_i}, \quad 1 < i < M, \quad (3)$$

where β is a constant, usually, from 1-3, λ_i is the ith eigenvalue and M is the total number of the selected eigenvectors. This is done to ensure that only allowable shapes are represented by Equation (2).

At the training stage, for each point a profile that is perpendicular to the shape boundary is investigated to obtain information regarding the gray-level structure above and below each point. A vector is computed using the intensity derivatives along the profile. This is done to ensure some tolerance to global intensity changes. Each sample is then normalized using the statistical model gathered from all training images for that

Figure 2. Flow Chart of the proposed method

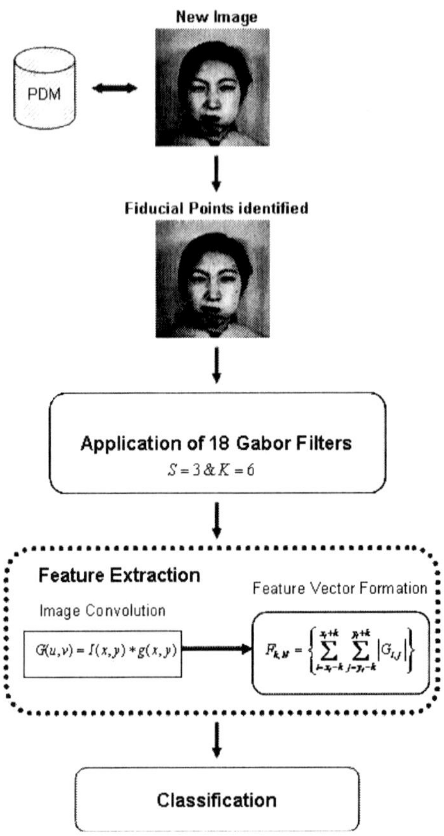

point. Under the assumption that the samples are part of a Gaussian distribution the mean and the covariance are calculated. The above procedure is repeated for all landmark points thus forming a statistical gray-level structure model. The correct deformation and convergence of a shape in a new image is done recursively. First, the mean shape is initialized. The goal is to deform each point of the shape so that its correct position is located. In order to identify the correct position for any given point a profile perpendicular to the shape model is investigated. This is the same procedure as in the training stage. The displacement for each landmark point is estimated by minimizing the Mahalanobis distance between the training model and the test model. The shape parameters are updated and the procedure is repeated until the point converges to a correct location. This procedure is repeated for all points until convergence to correct locations.

For each image a total number of 74 points are chosen to locate the landmark points. The number of fiducial points that are used in the feature extraction process is reduced to 20. The points that are chosen are near the places of interest in the face which contain information about the muscle movement. Figure 2 shows two examples of images that the prominent features were (a) correctly identified and (b) incorrectly identified and the set of the 20 fiducial points proposed for the feature vector extraction.

Gabor Function

A two dimensional Gabor function $g(x, y)$ is the product of a 2-D Gaussian-shaped function referred to as the envelop function and a complex exponential (sinusoidal) known as the carrier and can be written as (Dougman 1980,1985; Manjunathan & Ma 1996)

$$g(x,y) = \left(\frac{1}{2\pi\sigma_x\sigma_y}\right)\exp\left[-\frac{1}{2}\left(\frac{x^2}{\sigma_x^2}+\frac{y^2}{\sigma_y^2}\right)+2\pi jW\right], \tag{4}$$

where x, y are the image coordinates, σ_x, σ_y are the variances in the x, y coordinates respectively and W is the frequency of the sine wave. The above representation combines the even and odd Gabor functions which are defined in (Dougman, 1980).

Gabor Filter Bank

A Gabor filter bank can be defined as a series of Gabor filters at various scales and orientations. The application of each filter on an image produces a response for each pixel with different spatial-frequency properties.

Let $g(x, y)$ be the mother function, the Filter bank derives by scaling and rotating the mother function:

$$g'(x,y) = g(x',y'), \quad \begin{pmatrix} x' \\ y' \end{pmatrix} = \begin{pmatrix} \cos\theta & -\sin\theta \\ \sin\theta & \cos\theta \end{pmatrix}\begin{pmatrix} x \\ y \end{pmatrix}, \tag{6}$$

where $\theta = n\pi / K$, K is the total number of orientations and $n = 0, 1,..., K-1$.

Manjunathan and Ma showed that Gabor filters include redundant information in the images produced by the filter (Manjunath & Ma, 1996; Guo & Dyer, 2005). By selecting certain scaling parameters the constructed filters are not overlapping with each other thus avoiding redundant information. This leads to the following equations for the filter parameters a, σ_u and σ_v:

$$a = \left(\frac{U_h}{U_l}\right)^{\frac{1}{S-1}}, \quad W = a^m U_l, \tag{7}$$

$$\sigma_u = \frac{(a-1)W}{(a+1)\sqrt{2\ln 2}}, \tag{8}$$

$$\sigma_v = \tan\left(\pi/2K\right)\sqrt{\frac{W^2}{2\ln 2} - \sigma_u}, \tag{9}$$

where a is the scaling factor, S is the number of scales, $m = 0, 1,..., S-1$, U_h and U_l are the high and low frequency of interest. In this work $U_h = \sqrt{2}/4$, $U_l = \sqrt{2}/16$ are chosen with three scales and six orientations differing by $\pi/6$. A total of 18 different Gabor Filters are defined which are used to extract the feature vector.

Feature Extraction

The Gabor decomposition of any given image at any scale and orientation is produced by convolving the image with a particular filter. The magnitude of the resulting complex image is used to define the features that will form the feature vector. The feature vector is formed according to the following equation:

$$F_{k,l} = \left\{\sum_{i=x_l-k}^{x_l+k}\sum_{j=y_l-k}^{y_l+k}\left|G_{i,j}\right|\right\}, \quad l = 0,1,\ldots,N, \quad k = 0,1,\ldots,5, \tag{10}$$

where N is the number of the fiducial points used, and k is the number of neighboring pixels used to form the regions.

A total of 20 fiducial points are used to form the feature vector and regions of different size are employed to evaluate the methodology.

Artificial Neural Networks

A feed forward back propagation ANN is employed. The architecture of the ANNs is shown schematically in the Figure 3.

The first layer referred to as input layer consists of t inputs which is the dimension of the feature vector. The second layer referred to as hidden layer consists of $t + c/2$ neurons, where c is the number of classes used for classification. Finally, the output layer consists of the basic emotions and the neutral position. The sigmoid function is used as activation function for these hidden neurons. The third layer (output layer) consists of c neurons. The activation function of the output neurons is the linear function. In order to train the ANN the mean square error function is used and the number of epochs is 500.

Dataset

The JAFFE database (Lyons et al. 1999) is used for the evaluation of the proposed method. It features ten different Japanese women posing 3 or 4 examples for each basic emotion containing a total of 213 images. Neutral position inherits all characteristics of a basic emotion and it is included in the annotation of the database as a seventh basic emotion.

Results

Seven sets of experiments are conducted using automatic identification of fiducial points and are compared with seven sets of experiments conducted when 34 fiducial points are manually identified. Table 1 presents the accuracy of the methodology for both sets of points and all different regions which are used. In the tables presented below the abbreviations correspond to the 7 categories that are used for the classification (SU for surprise, DI for disgust, FE for fear, HA for happy, NE for neutral, SA for sadness and finally AN for anger). For the evaluation the ten fold stratified cross validation method is used. The gradual increase, points out that the when the region gets broader it utilizes more information that describe better facial geometry. It should be noted that the dimension of the feature vector when the 20 points are used is 360 whereas when 34 points are used the dimension is 612.

The best accuracy is reported when a region of 9x9 pixels is used for the 20 fiducial points set. In Table 2 below the confusion matrix of the best performing region is presented. Fear and sadness have the poorest performance amongst all emotions while neutral has the highest. There are a few misclassifications of sadness that are classified as fear. Zhang et al. (1998) have excluded fear from their experiments due to the difficulty of expressing the emotion from the subjects and some evidence that fear is processed differently by the human brain. Yin et al. (2006) reported

Figure 3. Artificial Neural Network Architecture

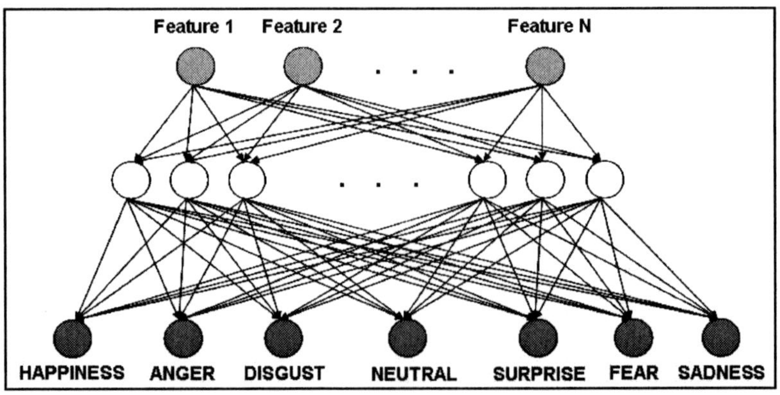

difficulties even among human experts to distinguish certain emotional states, namely sad with fear and disgust with anger.

Zhang et al. (1998) performed a set of experiments extracting the feature vector by single pixels at the location of 34 fiducial points manually identified and a modified ANN. When they used the full annotation of JAFFE they reported less than 90% accuracy. They repeated the experiments excluding fear and reported accuracy of 92.3%. Guo and Dryer (2005) compared the performance of different classifiers on the JAFFE database using 34 fiducial points manually identified. They extracted the feature vector using the magnitude of the pixel values of the 34 fiducial points proposed by Zhang et al. (1998) which were manually selected. Three classifiers were compared and the accuracy of each are presented. When the Simplified Bayes was used the reported accuracy was 63.3%, when the linear Support Vector Machines (SVM) was used the reported accuracy was 91.4% and when the non linear (Gaussian Radial Basis function kernel) SVM was used the reported accuracy was 92.3%. The methodologies presented above construct the feature vector utilizing information from a single pixel, the pixel that the fiducial point corresponds. This pixel-based approach can be modified to accommodate information from neighboring pixels at the location of each fiducial point forming a neighborhood, named region. The advantage of this modification is twofold: first artefacts that are introduced due to imprecise identification of prominent features of the face are avoided; an automatic methodology is more likely to vaguely identify the exact location of a fiducial point than a human expert. Second, a larger region is utilised which carries more information at certain areas of the face that contain important information on the facial muscle movement, allowing the reduction of the number of the fiducial points used to 20 (14 less that previous approaches). This is a 42% dimensionality reduction at the feature vector allowing for faster computation. The methodology has an accuracy of 90.2% and can be compared with methods that use single-pixel information and more fiducial points that are manually identified.

CONCLUSION

Automatic facial expressions recognition is a vital issue in human interpersonal communication. Systems that are able to perform well and analyse facial expressions in real world examples

Table 1. Accuracy obtained for different region sizes

Neighborhood size	Accuracy	
	Automatic 20 points	Manual 34 points
Single Pixel	67.6%	72.8%
3x3	77.0%	81.7%
5x5	84.0%	84.0%
7x7	83.1%	85.0%
9x9	90.2%	87.3%
11x11	89.7%	87.8%
13x13	87.3%	87.0%

Table 2. Confusion matrix of the best performing region (9x9) for the 20 points set.

	SU	DI	FE	HA	NE	SA	AN
SU	28	0	1	0	1	0	0
DI	0	26	2	0	0	1	0
FE	1	2	26	0	1	2	0
HA	0	0	1	29	1	0	0
NE	0	0	0	0	30	0	0
SA	0	1	4	1	0	25	0
AN	0	1	0	0	0	0	28

are advantageous for scientific applications as well as everyday real world applications.

In this chapter an approach to automatic facial expression recognition system is presented. The identification of the prominent features is done automatically and the feature vector is extracted using a specially constructed Gabor Filter bank that avoids redundant information. A region based methodology that ensures some flexibility on the identified points and avoids artefacts is employed. Moreover, a 20 fiducial point set is used that models facial geometry adequately for facial expression recognition. The methodology presented does not perform very well when trying to classify sadness or fear and reports the biggest losses between the two emotions but has been reported in the literature that these emotions often are troubling for human experts also and cannot be adequately distinguished (Zhang et al., 1998;Yin et al., 2006).

FUTURE TRENDS

Automatic facial expression systems will steadily move towards real world applications. In terms of research there are still fields that must be investigated in order to allow the transition of AFER systems to real world applications.

A very persistent requirement is often defined in terms of speed and accuracy of the system. The AFER systems should be developed to operate in real time and to be fully automated without manual intervention. Modern computer systems are close to allow this kind of processing overhead and there are system, usually embedded, that allow to operate in real time. More efficient methods for face identification, recognition and acquisition in terms of speed and accuracy would facilitate the application of AFER systems in real world examples.

An active research field concerning the AFER systems is the categorization of such systems not only in basic, global emotions that are limited in nature, but also in facial actions or deformations that would allow more diversity in terms of the categorized emotions. Basic emotions cover a small set of the emotions that are present in a human face in every day life. Scientific subjects that would benefit from an active fully working AFER system are very little concerned with basic emotions and study different states and emotions such as pain, stress, fatigue and so on. This will also be beneficial moving towards real-world applications since there is a distinction between posed expressions and spontaneous expressions. The databases that are currently in use in the scientific community do not include data for spontaneous expressions.

ACKNOWLEDGMENT

This work was partly funded by the General Secretariat for Research and Technology of the Hellenic Ministry of Development (PENED 2003 03OD139).

REFERENCES

Black, M. J., & Yacoob, Y. (1998). Recognising facial expressions in image sequences using local parameterised models. *Int'l J Computer Vision, 25*(1), 23-48.

Cohen, I., Sebe, N., Garg, A., Chen, L. S., & Huang, S. T. (2003). Facial expression recognition from video sequences: temporal and static modelling. *Computer Vision and Image Understanding, 91*, 160-187.

Cootes, T. F., Edwards, G., & Taylor, C. J. (1998). Active appearance models. *Proc. European Conf. Computer Vision, 2*, 484-498.

Cootes, T. F., Taylor, C. J., Cooper, D. H. & Graham, J. (1995). Active shape models – Their training and application. *Computer Vision and Image Understanding, 61*(1), 38-59.

Daugman, J. (1980). Two-dimensional spectral analysis of cortical receptive field profiles. *Vision Research, 20*, 846-856.

Daugman, J. (1985). Uncertainty relation for resolution in space, spatial frequency and orientation optimized by two-dimensional visual cortical fields. *J Optical Society of America A, 2*(7), 1160-1171.

Donato, G., Bartlett, M. S., Hager, J. C., Ekman, P., & Senjowski, T. J. (1999). Classifying facial actions. *IEEE Trans. Pattern Analysis and Machine Intelligence, 21*(10), 974-989.

Ekman, P. (1991). *Telling Lies: Clues to deceit in the Marketplace, Politics, and Marriage*. New York, USA: W. W. Norton.

Ekman, P., & Friesen, W. V. (1971). Constants across cultures in the face and emotion. *Journal of Personality and Social Psychology, 17*(2), 124-129.

Ekman, P., & Friesen, W. V. (1978). *The Facial Action Coding System: A technique for the measurement of facial movement.* San Francisco: Consulting Psychologist Press.

Ekman, P., & Rosenberg, E. L. (2005). *What the face reveals: Basic and applied studies of spontaneous expression using the FACS.* Oxford, UK: Oxford University Press.

Ekman, P. (2003). Darwin, deception and facial expression. *Annals New York Academy of sciences, 100*, 205-221.

Essa, I., & Petland, A. (1997). Coding, analysis, interpretation, recognition of facial expressions. *IEEE Trans. Pattern Analysis and Machine Intelligence, 19*(7), 757-763.

Fasel, B., & Luettin, J. (2003). Automatic facial expression analysis: a survey. *Pattern Recognition, 36*, 259-275.

Fasel, I. R., Fortenberry, B., & Movellan, J. R. (2005). A generative framework for real time object detection and classification. *Int'l J Computer Vision and Image Understanding, 98*(1), 181-210.

Freund, Y., & Schapire, R. E. (1995). A decision-theoretic generalization of on-line learning and an application to boosting. *Computational Learning Theory: Eurocolt, 95*, 23–37.

Friedman, J., Hastie, T., & Tibshirani, R. (2000). Additive logistic regression: a statistical view of boosting. *The Annals of Statistics, 28*(2), 337-374.

Friesen, W. V., & Ekman, P. (1983). *Emfacs-7: emotional facial action coding system.* Unpublished Manuscript, University of California at San Francisco

Gu, H., Zhang, Y., & Ji, Q. (2005). Task oriented facial behavior recognition with selective sensing. *Computer Vision and Image Understanding, 100*, 385-415.

Guo, G., & Dyer, C. R. (2005). Learning From Examples in the Small Sample Case: Face Expression Recognition. *IEEE Trans. Sys. Man and Cybernetics–PART B: Cybernetics, 35*(3), 477-488.

Hjelmas, E., & Low, B. K. (2001). Face detection: A survey. *Computer Vision and Image Understanding, 83*, 236-274.

Kanade, T., Cohn, J. F., & Tian, Y. (2000). Comprehensive database for facial expression analysis. *Proc. IEEE Int'l Conf. Face and Gesture Recognition,* (pp. 46-53).

Kass, M., Witkin, A., & Terzopoulos, D. (1987). Snakes: Active contours models. *Proc Int'l Conference Computer Vision*, (pp. 259-269).

Li, S. Z., & Jain, A. K. (2005). *Handbook of face recognition.* New York, USA: Springer.

Lien, J. J., Kanade, T., Cohn, J. F. & Li, C. C. (2000). Detection, tracking and classification of action units in facial expression. *Robotics and Autonomous Systems, 31*, 131-146.

Liu, W., & Wang, Z. (2006). Facial Expression Recognition Based on Fusion of Multiple Gabor Features. *Int'l Conf Pattern Recognition,* (pp. 536-539).

Lyons, M., & Akamatsu, (1998). Coding Facial Expressions with Gabor Wavelets. *Int'l Conf Automatic Face and Gesture Recognition,* (pp. 200-205).

Lyons, M. J., Budynek, J., & Akamatsu, S. (1999). Automatic classification of single facial images. *IEEE Trans. Pattern Analysis and Machine Intelligence, 21*(12), 1357-1352.

Manjunath, B. S., & Ma, W. Y. (1996). Texture features for browsing and retrieval of image data. *IEEE Trans. Pattern Analysis and Machine Intelligence, 18*(8), 837-842.

Meihle, A. (1973). *Surgery of the facial nerve.* Philadelphia, USA: Saunders.

Pantic, M., & Rothkrantz, L. (2000). Automatic analysis of facial expressions: The state of the art. *IEEE Trans. Pattern Analysis and Machine Intelligence, 22*(12), 1424-1445.

Pantic, M., & Rothkrantz, L. (2000). Expert system for automatic analysis of facial expressions. *Image and Vision Computing, 18*(11), 881-905.

Pantic, M., Valstar, M. F., Rademaker, R., & Maat, L. (2005). Web-based database for facial expression analysis. *Proc. IEEE Int'l Conf. Multimedia and Expo,* (pp. 317-321).

Petland, A., Moghaddam, B., & Starner, T. (1994). View-based and modular eigenspaces for face recognition. *Proc IEEE Conf. Computer Vision and Pattern Recognition,* (pp. 84-91).

Rowley, H., Baluja, S., & Kanade, T. (1998). Neural network-based face detection. *IEEE Trans. Pattern Analysis and Machine Intelligence, 20*(1), 23-38.

Schneiderman, H., & Kanade, T. (2000). A statistical model for 3d object detection applied to faces and cars. *Proc. IEEE Int'l Conf. Computer Vision and Pattern Recognition*, (pp. 746-751).

Shen, L., & Bai, L. (2006). A review on Gabor wavelets for face recognition. *Pattern Analsysis and Applications, 9*, 273-292.

Sung, K. K., & Pogio, T. (1998). Example-based learning for view-based human face detection. *IEEE Trans. Pattern Analysis and Machine Intelligence, 20*(1), 39-51.

Sunko, F. M., Ordaas, S., Butakoff, C., Cruz, S., & Frangi, A. F. (2007). Active shape models with invariant optima features: Application to facial analysis. *IEEE Trans. Pattern Analysis and Machine Intelligence, 29*(7), 1105-1117.

Tian, Y., Kanede, T., & Cohn J.F. (2001). Recognizing action units for facial expression analysis. *IEEE Trans. Pattern Analysis and Machine Intelligence, 23*(2), 97-115.

Tian, Y. L., Kanade, T., & Cohn, J. F. (2001). Recognizing action units for facial expression analysis. *IEEE Trans. Pattern Analysis and Machine Intelligence, 23*(2), 97-115.

Van Ginneken, B., Frangi, A. F., Staal, J. J., Ter Har Romeny, B. M., & Viergever, M. A. (2002). Active shape model segmentation with optimal features. *IEEE Trans. Medical Imaging, 21*(8), 924-933.

Viola, P., & Jones, M. (2001). Rosubt real-time object detection. *Int'l Workshop on Statistical and Computational theories of Vision - Modeling, Learning, Computing and Sampling.*

Viola, P., & Jones, M. (2004). Robust real-time face detection. *J. Computer Vision, 57*(2), 137-154.

Yang, M. H., Kriegman, D. J., & Ahuja, N. (2002). Detecting faces in images: a survey. *IEEE Trans. on Pattern Analysis and Machine Intelligence,* 24(1), 34-58.

Ye, Z., Zhan, Y., & Song, S. (2004). Facial expression features extraction based on Gabor wavelet transformation. *IEEE Int'l Conf Systems, Man and Cybernetics*, (pp. 2215-2219).

Yin, L., Wei, X., Sun, Y., Wang, J., & Rosato, M. (2006). A 3D facial expression database for facial behavior research. *Proc. IEEE Int'l Conf. Face and Gesture Recognition*, (pp. 211-216).

Zhang, Z., Lyons, M., Schuster, M., & Akamatsu, S. (1998). Comparison Between Geometry-Based and Gabor-Wavelet-Based Facial Expression Recognition Using Multi-Layer Perceptron. *Int'l Conf Automatic Face and Gesture Recognition*, (pp. 454-459).

KEY TERMS

Action Unit (AU): The key element of FACS, each action unit describes facial deformation due to each facial muscle movement. There are a total of 44 AUs where the majority involves contraction or relaxation of facial muscles and the rest involve miscellaneous actions such as "tongue show" or "bite lip".

Basic Emotions: They are a small set of prototypic emotions which share characteristics of universality and uniformity across people with different ethnic background or cultural heritage. The six basic emotions were proposed by Ekman and Friesen (1971) and are: disgust, fear, joy, surprise, sadness and anger.

Classification: The task that categorizes feature vectors into appropriate categories. Each category is called a class.

Facial Action Coding System (FACS): It is a system developed by Ekman and Friesen (1978) to categorize human expressions. Using FACS human coders can categorize all possible facial deformation into action units that describe facial muscle movement.

Feature Vector Extraction: The task of providing a feature vector that describes facial geometry and deformation. There are two ways to model facial geometry and deformation: first by using prominent features of the face and second by using a mathematical transformation so that changes in appearance are modeled.

Image Processing: The analysis of an image using techniques that can identify shades, colors and relationships which cannot be perceived by the human eye.

Machine Learning: The purpose of machine learning is to extract information from several types of data automatically, using computational and statistical methods. It is the use of computer algorithms which improve automatically using experience.

Point Distribution Model (PDM): It is a model that tries to form a distribution of sample points from the training set. When the PDM is constructed it can approximate the position of each model point in a new image without manual intervention.

Chapter XVII
Developments and Advances in Biomedical Functional Infrared Imaging

Arcangelo Merla
Institute of Advanced Biomedical Technologies (ITAB), Foundation G. d'Annunzio University, Chieti, Italy & G. d'Annunzio University, Chieti-Pescara, Italy

ABSTRACT

This chapter presents an overview on recent developments in the field of clinical applications of the functional infrared imaging. The functional infrared imaging is a relatively recent imaging methodology introduced for the study of the functional properties and alterations of the human thermoregulatory system for biomedical purposes. The methodology is based on the modeling of the bio-heat exchange processes and the recording of thermal infrared data by means of advanced technology. Some innovative applications of functional infrared imaging to diagnostics, psychometrics, stress measurements and psycho-neurophysiology will be presented, with special emphasis to the potentialities and the capabilities that such technique may bring to biomedical investigations.

INTRODUCTION

Objects are characterized by a variety of physical parameters such as shape, weight, and size. However, one of the most frequently measured physical properties is temperature. Temperatures may be measured with either a contact or non-contact device. The thermal infrared imaging systems create electronic picture of the scene. Such non-contact systems allow the representation of the surface thermal distribution of an object by detecting the thermal infrared emission spontaneously emitted by the object itself. Early use of thermal infrared imaging in medicine dates back to early '60s. Several studies have been performed so far to assess the contribution that such information may provide to the clinicians. The physiological basis for using thermal infrared imaging in medicine is the fact that the skin temperature distribution of the human body depends on the complex relationships defining the heat exchange processes between skin tissue, inner tissue, local vasculature, and metabolic activity. All of these processes are mediated and regulated by the sympathetic and parasympathetic activity to maintain the thermal homeostasis. The presence of a disease may affect both at a local or systemic level, the heat balance or exchange processes, resulting in an increase or a decrease of the skin temperature. Therefore, the detection of skin temperature abnormalities may provide diagnostic criteria for a variety of diseases interfering with the regular control of the skin temperature.

Unfortunately, such a simplistic approach, combined with early and not enough mature technology, did not provide adequate and effective results for supporting routinely use of thermal infrared imaging in diagnostics. Therefore, thermal infrared imaging has been substantially discarded as a diagnostic tool until the middle '90s.

At the beginning of '90s, the evolution of technological advances in infrared sensor technology, image processing, computer architecture, knowledge-based databases, and their overall system integration has resulted in new methods of research and use in medical infrared imaging. The development of infrared cameras with focal plane arrays added a new dimension to this imaging modality (Roganski, 2002). New detector materials with improved thermal sensitivity are now available and the production of high-density focal plane arrays (up to 640 x 480) has been achieved. Read-out circuitry using on-chip signal pre-processing is now in common use. These breakthroughs led to the availability of commercial and user-friendly camera systems with thermal sensitivity less than 30 mK (20 mK for nitrogen cooled cameras), as well as spatial resolution of 25-40 microns, given the appropriate optics. Furthermore, time resolution has been greatly improved, being now possible to acquire up to 100 full frame images per second (Bronzino, 2007).

The last-generation camera systems allow effective monitoring and studying the dynamics of the local control of the skin temperature and in which manner diseases or external stimuli may influence it (Diakides, 2002). This means that the characteristic parameters modeling the activity of the skin thermoregulatory system can be retrieved and used as quantitative and effective diagnostic parameters (Merla, 2002). Therefore, modeling the activity of the skin thermoregulatory system can provide specific parameters from which to infer diagnostic criteria (Merla, 2007).

As a consequence, there is an emerging interest in the development of smart image processing algorithms and bio-heat transfer models to enhance the interpretation of thermal signatures. In the clinical area, new researches are underway to achieve quantitative clinical data interpretation in standardized diagnostic procedures and protocols (Diakides, 2002).

In the past 10 years, significant progress has been made internationally by advancing a thrust for new initiatives worldwide for clinical quantification, international collaboration, and providing a forum for coordination, discussion, and publication. As a result of this process, three IEEE Engineering in Medicine and Biology Magazines, Special Issues dedicated to biomedical thermal imaging have been published (Diakides, 1998, 2000, 2002) in addition to a growing number of papers published on top international medical journals.

Developments of new quantitative approaches and methods in modern thermal infrared imaging have been proposed to re-visit classical applications of thermal imaging in medicine. The approaches so far proposed include among the others: quantitative active dynamic thermal-IR imaging (Novakowsky, 2007), dynamic thermal assessment (Anbar, 2007), advanced image processing (Wiecek, 2007). Even early detection of breast cancer by means of thermal imaging based on the new methodologies has been re-proposed (Keyserlingk, 2007, Qi, 2007).

A detailed review of such approaches and methodologies can be found in Bronzino (2006, 2007).

Among the other techniques, the functional infrared (fIR) imaging has been proposed (Merla, 2002). The functional Infrared Imaging is the study for diagnostic purposes of the local functional properties of the thermoregulatory system through extensive use of in vivo bio-heat transfer models (Merla, 2002, 2006). This approach is aimed at a quantitative assessment of functional properties of tissues, vascularisation and processes involved in the local control of the temperature. The use of bio-heat transfer models allows for obtaining functional information on bio-physics quantities involved in local thermoregulation (like tissue thermal capacity or heat exchange coefficients) from which to infer diagnostic parameters.

In this chapter we will focus on fIR imaging. Some of the most important recent clinical applications of the fIR imaging will be presented to highlight the typology of the approach. In addition, some innovative applications of thermal imaging to psychometrics, stress measurements and neuro-psycho-physiology will be presented with the general goal of showing future and interesting potentialities of the methodology.

UNDERSTANDING FUNCTIONAL INFRARED IMAGING THROUGH EXAMPLES OF BIOMEDICAL APPLICATIONS

For long time, medical infrared imaging (medical thermography) has been mostly associated with early detection of breast cancer. Thermal effects secondary to neoplastic-related angiogenesis have been used as a possible early detector of malignant lesions. The approach generally followed was based on the individuation of asymmetric thermal patterns or features, often subjectively interpreted (Keyserlingk, 2007). There is a general consensus that such an approach provides a screening tool, which may result, highly sensitive, but poorly specific. As the medical community moved toward other more anatomic screening techniques, like mammography, the general interest for medical thermal imaging soon decreased.

Thanks to the technological advancement and a better understanding of the physiology of the human thermal signal, thermal infrared imaging has been used in areas different from breast cancer detection. Such area cover diagnosis of a variety of diseases related to the following systems: micro/macro circulatory, peripheral nervous, autoimmune, muscle-skeletal, and cutaneous.

The capability of extracting quantitative parameters, in addition or conjunction to the temperature dynamics, from bio-heat models has open the medical thermal imaging to the use in several fields like immunology, dermatology, neurology, and many others. Such a functional approach has completely re-designed the use of thermal imaging in medicine. A complete ad exhaustive review of the applications of the functional approach to the medical infrared imaging cannot be allocated within this chapter. An exhaustive and detailed list of applications and references can be found in Bronzino (2007).

In order to show the approach proposed with functional infrared imaging, two examples of its application to diagnostic, respectively from immunology and urology, are presented.

Raynaud's Phenomenon and Scleroderma

Raynaud's phenomenon (RP) is defined as a painful vasoconstriction - that may follow cold or emotional stress - of small arteries and arterioles of extremities, like fingers and toes. RP can be primary (PRP) or secondary to scleroderma (SSc). Scleroderma is an auto-immunological disease affecting the connective tissue and determining structural and morphological changes in the microvascular tissue. The early evaluation of the vascular damage is crucial in order to distinguish between PRP and SSc. Merla et al. (2002) proposed to model the response of the fingertips to a cold stress to get an effective diagnostic parameter depicting the actual physiology of the finger, being the finger temperature determined by the net balance of the energy input/output. The more significant contributes come from the input power due to blood perfusion and the power lost to the environment (Figure 1).

The authors have demonstrated that, integrating the temperature curve T over time, it is possible to compute the amount of heat stored in the finger, namely Q. The latter quantity is intrinsically related to the finger thermal capacity. The Q parameter has been used to discriminate and classify PRP, SSc and healthy subjects (Merla et al., 2002). The grand average Q values for PRP, SSc and healthy subjects groups are in shown in Figure 1, lower panel. The sensitivity of the method in order to distinguish patients from

Figure 1. (a) Experimental re-warming curves after cold stress in normal subjects. The continuous curve represents the recorded temperature finger. The outlined curve represents the exponential temperature pattern exhibited by the finger in absence of thermoregulatory control. In this case, the only heat source for the finger is the environment. (b) One- way ANOVA test applied to the Q parameter calculated for each group (PRP, SSc, and healthy). The Q parameter clearly discriminates among the three groups (from Merla et al., 2002).

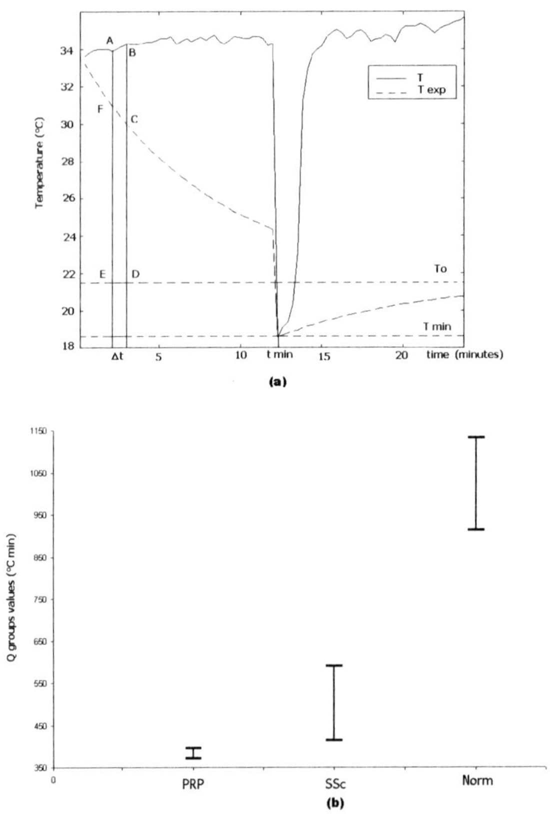

normal is 100%. The specificity in distinguishing SSc from PRP is 95%. Q clearly highlights the difference between PRP, SSc, and normal subjects. The method is actually used to monitor the clinical evolution of the disease and to follow-up the pharmacological treatment.

Varicocele, Scrotal Hyperthermia, and Infertility

Varicocele is a widely spread male disease consisting into a dilatation of the pampiniform venous plexus and of the internal spermatic vein. Consequences of such a dilatation are an increase of the scrotal temperature and a possible impairment of the potential fertility (Miusset, 1991; Merla, 2002).

The study of the scrotal thermoregulatory processes, together with scrotal thermal imaging data, allows for revealing secondary-to-varicocele abnormal thermoregulation after an induced cold stress (Figure 2). Affected testicles return to pre-stress equilibrium temperatures faster than do normal testicles (Merla, 2002). A series of studies conducted by the authors has shown that functional infrared imaging allows the accurate detection of asymptomatic varicocele and that the semen properties (especially spermatozoa motility) are related to the scrotal thermoregulatory dynamics as measured by the time constant of the thermal recovery after a controlled cold stress (Merla, 2002, 2006). The sensitivity and specificity of fIR imaging for detecting asymptomatic varicocele are actually 100% and around 95%, respectively.

The control of the scrotum temperature should improve after varicocelectomy as a complementary effect of the reduction of the blood reflux.

Figure 2. (a) Second grade right varicocele. The temperature distribution all over the scrotum clearly highlights significant differences between affected and unaffected testicles. (b) The same scrotum after varicocelectomy. The surgical treatment reduced the increased temperature on the affected hemiscrotum and restored the symmetry in the scrotal temperature distribution. (c) Third grade left varicocele. (d) The same scrotum after varicocelectomy. The treatment was unsuccessful into repairing the venous reflux, as documented by the persisting asymmetric scrotal distribution. (From Merla et. al, 2004).

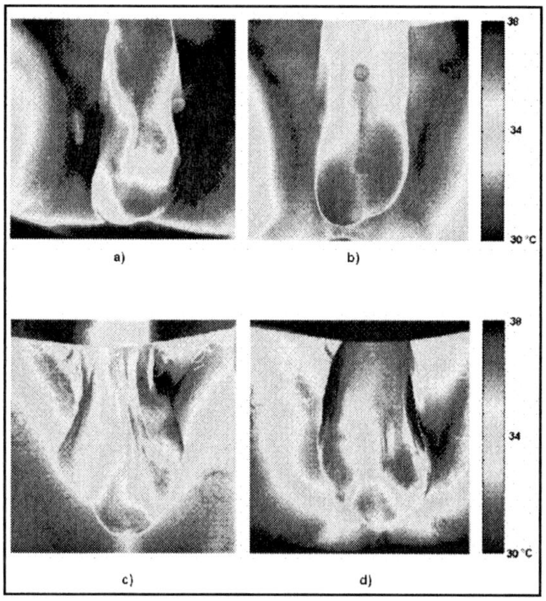

Moreover, follow-up of the changes in scrotum thermoregulation after varicocelectomy (Figure 2) may provide early warning on the presence of relapsing or persistence of the disease after incomplete or improper treatment and it may be used as a suitable complementary follow up tool (Merla, 2004).

COMPUTATIONAL NEURO-PSYCHO-PHYSIOLOGY BASED ON FIR IMAGING

One of the most important and innovative potentiality that fIR imaging may offer is the capability of providing data of neuro-psycho-physiology relevance in unobtrusive and non invasive way. Studying emotional reactions using thermal infrared imaging and fIR imaging is becoming a reality and several applications have been developed so far in very diversified fields, like psychometrics, human-computer interfaces, continuous healthy monitoring, and even security, with the last generation of deception detection systems based on thermal imaging (Pavlidis, 2002).

Emotional reactions constitute the response to a wide variety of external stimuli, like alarms, psychological pressure, as also pleasant situations, etc. Codification of other individual's emotional status and responses plays a fundamental role for the strategies of the inter-individual interactions. It is extremely interesting and challenging to transfer to an artificial intelligence system the interpretation of emotional states and responses. In fact, an automatic computerized system, which would be able "to read" the emotions, could be applied in many and diversified basic and applied research fields, up to revolutionizing several aspects of daily life. Preliminary efforts for developing automated monitoring system for emotion recognition have regarded mainly virtual reality, human-computer interaction, and, with the intensification of the war on terror after September 11th, deception detection. Conventional approaches for emotion recognition are based on the measurements of several physiological parameters expressing autonomic sympathetic nervous system (ANS) activity, like skin sympathetic response (SSR), hand palm temperature, heart beat and/or breath rate modulations, peripheral vascular tone (i.e., blood perfusion), facial expression and electromyography activity. Monitoring these parameters is, in a certain sense, invasive because it requires contact between the subject and the sensors. It requires the voluntary and cooperative participation of the subjects. Finally, the time required for placing sensors, performing measurements and analyzing data is not negligible. Therefore, traditional channels for monitoring ANS activity do not allow non-invasive, non-contact and quick measurement of emotional responses or physiological vital signs. On the contrary, neuropsychology, security surveillance systems based on psychophysiological response of suspects, and sustained health care monitoring during daily life activity requires the "true" spontaneous emotional response recorded in a contact-less fashion. Since ANS activity regulates cutaneous blood perfusion, local tissue metabolism, and sudomotor response, sympathetic cutaneous thermal effects are expected as side results of emotional responses or arousal. Therefore, sympathetic thermal effects of emotional responses can be recorded non-invasively and at distance by means of infrared thermal (IR) imaging (Merla, 2004, 2007). Adequate bio-heat modeling of IR data could then allow for the characterization of each specific ANS physiological signals, as already demonstrated for some of them, at a preliminary level – (Garbey, 2007; Pavlidis, 2007). The researches in the above-mentioned fields unlock the more general possibility of monitoring human physiological vital signs at a distance and in a non-invasive fashion throughout the integrated use of advanced thermal imaging, bioheat transfer modeling and computational physiology. Thermal data for bioheat-based computations and monitoring of vital signs are usually performed on the subject's face. The face is usually exposed and – given the proper optics -within the field of view of the thermal camera. Many physiological variables, such as superficial blood flow and cardiac pulse, are related in some way to the heat transfer mechanism of the human body. Due to this interrelationship, it is possible to compute such physiological variables from the raw thermal imagery. Relatively little work exists in the literature towards this direction. The models are based on partial differential equations (PDE). The time evolution of 2D blood flow, cardiac pulse, and breath rate can reveal important clues about many health problems. The screening allowed is automated, continuous, and it permits a rigorous mathematical modeling (Pavlidis, 2003). Following, the state of the art in the field of infrared imaging-based computational physiology is reviewed and described.

Blood Flow Computation

Superficial blood flow on the face can be computed by using a pair of bioheat models. One model computes blood perfusion in homogeneous tissue regions that are void of large superficial vessels (perfusion model) (Figure 3).

The other model computes directional blood flow in a major superficial vessel, like the external carotid (directional model). The perfusion model has been reported in a number of papers (Pavlidis et al., 2001, 2002, 2003) and tested extensively in human experiments with excellent results. The directional model has been briefly reported in the 2004 CVPR Proceedings (Garbey, 2003). Since the model measures directional blood flow in a major vessel, it is related to the heart output and can yield the cardiac pulse waveform. In general, bioheat modelling on the surface of the body starts with the construction of the energy balance equation on a control volume that extends several millimetres in depth.

The dynamic form of this equation is a PDE with boundary conditions that are determined by environmental and other factors, including the sensor output (skin temperature). A major term in the energy balance equation is convective heat produced by blood flow. The solution of the PDE form of the equation yields the evolution of the blood flow variable. Specifically, the directional blood flow model assumes that the vessel acts as a heat source for the surrounding four-layer control volume tissue. These layers are successively, in positive z direction, the skin, the fat, the muscle, and the core (see Figure 4(a)).

It is assumed that each layer is isotropic with respect to thermal conductivity K(z), metabolic heat rate $q_M(z)$, density ρ, and specific heat c of the tissue. The heat effect of the vessel on the skin temperature depends on the vessel's depth and shape as well as the blood temperature and flow rate. Let consider a single large vessel running along a direction x parallel to the skin layer (see Figure 4(a)). The heat conduction in the tissue surrounding the vessel is dominant in directions parallel (x) and perpendicular (z) to the skin. In the remaining y direction we can neglect heat transfer because of the presence of other vessels, which are assumed being quasi-periodically arranged and similar to that considered. Therefore, the following 2D PDE model has been introduced:

$$\rho c \frac{\partial \Theta}{\partial t} - \frac{\partial}{\partial x}\left(K(z)\frac{\partial \Theta}{\partial x}\right) - \frac{\partial}{\partial z}\left(K(z)\frac{\partial \Theta}{\partial z}\right)$$

$$= q_{BL}(x,t) + q_M(x,z), (x,z) \in (0,L) \div (0,D)$$

where q_M is the volumetric metabolic heat while q_{BL} is the heat due to blood flow speed u_{BL} in a vessel assimilated to a line source z = S(x). Θ(x,z,t) is the temperature distribution function in the control volume tissue over time, K(z) is the thermal conductivity of a particular layer within the volume, while ρ and c are the tissue density and specific heat, respectively. Given the proper boundary conditions, the mathematical problem is to retrieve the blood flow speed $u_{BL}(t)$ from the

Figure 3. Cutaneous blood perfusion rate visualization while watching neutral-content (left) and erotic-content (right) movies. Specific cutaneous distributions appear to be evoked by emotional stimuli. (From Merla, 2007).

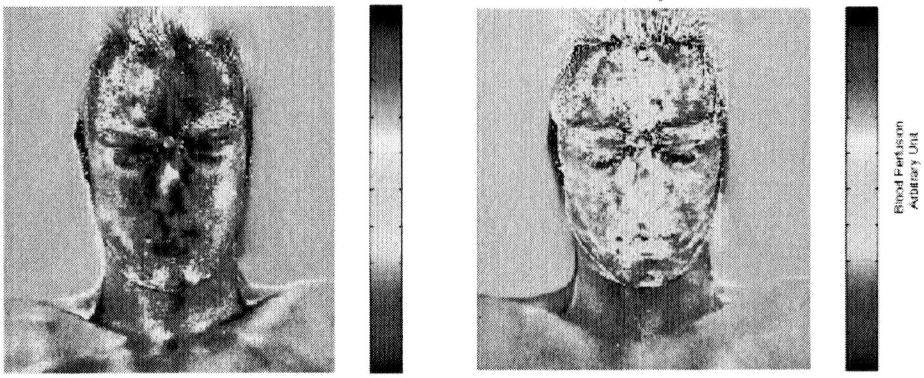

Figure 4. (a) Four-layer tissue structure hypothesized by our model along with the coordinate system convention. The red curve represents the assumed position and shape of the vessel. (b) The graph at the top shows the time variation of the blood flow speed in a major superficial vessel, as the PDE model computes it. The graph at the bottom shows the corresponding input to the model, that is, the time variation of the skin temperature (from Pavlidis, 2007).

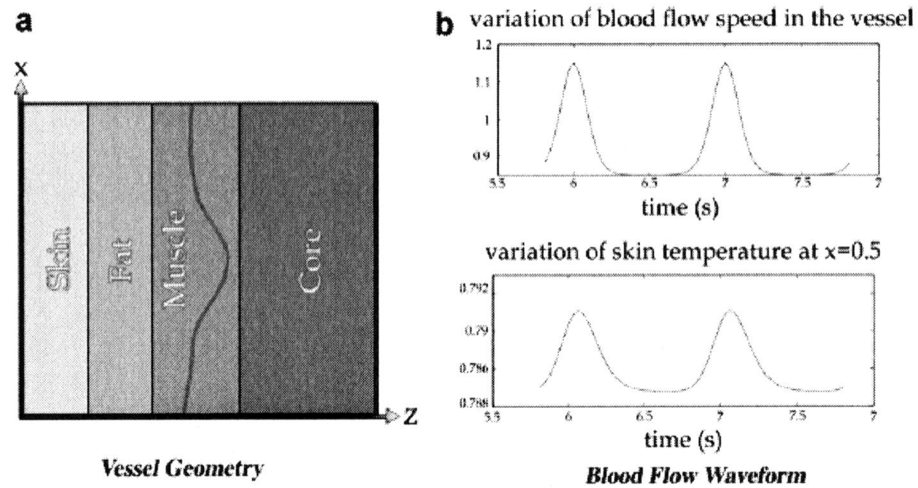

skin temperature obtained with a thermal infrared camera. In extensive direct simulation and limited application of the inverse solution on real data the model behaved excellently (Pavlidis, 2007) (see Figure 4(b)). The inverse solution correlated very well with ground-truth data collected through a standard contact blood flow meter (Pavlidis, 2007).

Cardiac Pulse Computation

In addition to the amplitude of the blood flow-waveform as computed above, it is possible to compute the frequency of the blood flow pulsation (cardiac pulse). Both amplitude and frequency are important in potential applications of this technology. The method is based on the assumption that temperature modulation due to pulsating blood flow produces the strongest thermal signal on a superficial vessel. This signal is affected by physiological and environmental thermal phenomena. Therefore, the resulting thermal signal that is being sensed by the infrared camera is a composite signal, with the pulse being one of its components. Research efforts are directed into recovering the frequency of the component signal with the highest energy content. A contact-free pulse measurement methodology has been proposed by Sun et. al. (2005). Based on the outcome of Fourier analysis, an estimation function computes the cardiac pulse. Figure 5 illustrates the general steps of the proposed methodology. Considering that the blood vessel is a long, narrow structure, the pulse propagation phenomenon causes slight phase shift on the temperature profiles along the blood vessel. This may weaken the signal if conventional signal recovery methods in the time domain are used. Each pixel along the blood vessel has a unique periodical temperature profile, which is shifted with respect to the others. Averaging these temperature profiles may weaken the signal. Although, the temperature profiles of the pixels along the blood vessel are shifted in the time domain, their frequency should remain the same (un-shifted). Therefore, by operating on the frequency domain and combining appropriately the power spectra of these temperature profiles it is possible to reinforce the signal instead of weakening it.

Breath Rate Computation

Human breathing consists of expiration and inspiration phases. In expiration, air that was heated through its contact with the lungs flows via the nostrils to the environment. Conversely, in inspiration environmental air flows via the nostrils to the lungs. This creates a periodic thermal signal in the vicinity of the nostrils that oscillates between high (expiration) and low (inspiration) values. In traditional pulmonary studies, a thermistor is attached near the nostrils to capture this phenomenon and produce a representative breath signal. The thermal imager can be viewed as a virtual thermistor, since it captures the same phenomenon, but at a distance (Pavlidis, 2007). Figure 6 shows a thermal snapshot of a subject during the expiration phase. One can observe the contrast between the hot expired air, next to the nasal area and the lower intensity surrounding background. During the inspiration phase, the hot expired air is absent. As a periodic signal, the breath signal can be analyzed through Fourier transformation on sliding segments (windows) of the normalized breath thermal signal.

Sudomotor Response and Galvanic Skin Response

The Autonomic Nervous System (ANS) and particularly its sympathetic division has been the object of intense study in neurophysiology and psychophysiology. The sympathetic division readies the body for a crisis that may require sudden, intense physical activity. It is a primal survival mechanism. Therefore, interest on methodologies that scrutinize sympathetic responses is well founded and has many applications. When sympathetic activation occurs, an individual experiences increased activity in the cardiovascular and respiratory centres of the pons and medulla oblongata, leading to elevations in blood pressure, heart rate, breathing rate, and depth of respiration. These vital sign changes are mediated through adrenergic postganglionic fibres. Determination of sympathetic activation through vital sign monitoring is not always straightforward. As an alternative, researchers focused their efforts on sympathetic manifestations effected through cholinergic postganglionic fibres. These fibres innervate sweat glands of the skin and the blood vessels to skeletal muscles and the brain. They provide a pathway to stimulating sweat gland secretion and selectively enhancing blood flow to muscles. In this context, Electro-Dermal Activity (EDA) has been the gold standard for peripheral monitoring of sympathetic responses. EDA is measured through the Galvanic Skin Response (GSR), which is a simple and reproducible method for quantifying sweat gland activation in the palm.

Alternatively, EDA can be captured through a palm thermistor, which registers the full thermo-regulatory phenomenon including changes both in blood flow and sweat gland activation. Indeed, in recent years, it has been demonstrated that during arousal additional physiological signs materialize on the face. Specifically, it has been shown that sudomotor responses associated to EDA can be appreciated, recorded and quantified by means of thermal camera (Merla et al., 2004, Pavlidis, 2007) (see Figure 7). Concomitantly to the palm area, strong sweat gland activation is manifested in the maxillary area. This is one more sympathetic

Figure 5. Pulse measurement methodology (from Garbey, 2007).

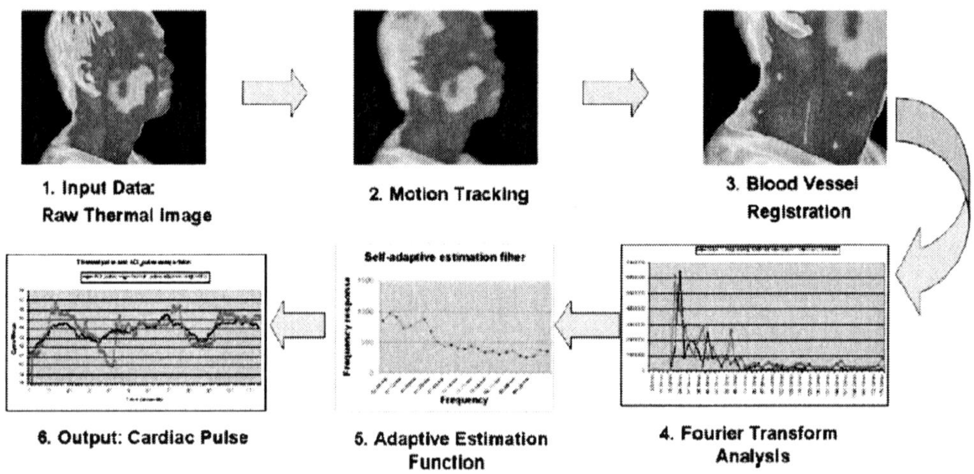

Figure 6. Breathing rate measurement methodology. The thermal signal (upper panel) is delayed with respect to the signal obtained through standard belt respiratory device

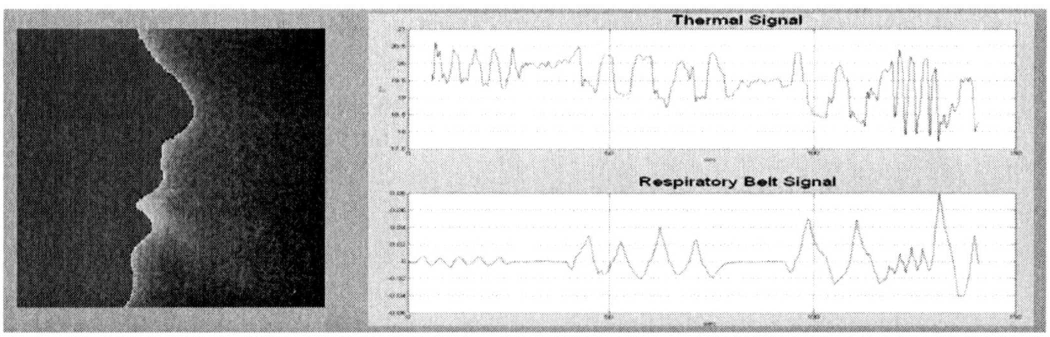

Figure 7. Sudomotor response activated by a startle stimulus. Discontinuous thermal pattern around the mouth highlights the arousal activation of the sweat glands

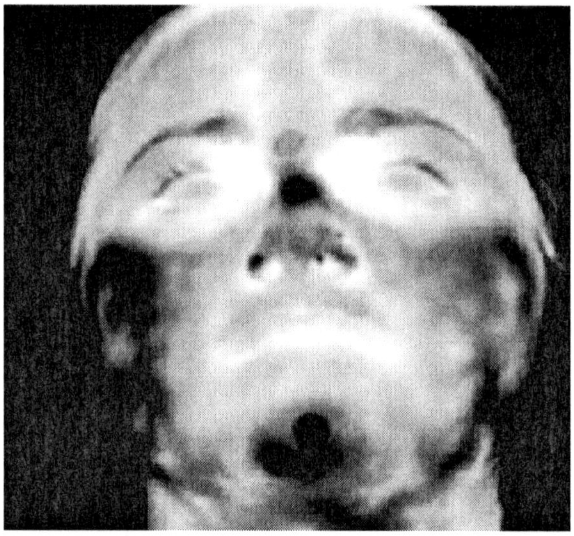

Figure 8. Coronary bypass. Thermal imaging documents blood re-perfusion after de-clamping of the anastomosis. (a) closed clamp; (b) just after de-clamping; (c) at regime. The temperature increase along the artery is used to compute arterial blood flow and myocardial tissue perfusion.

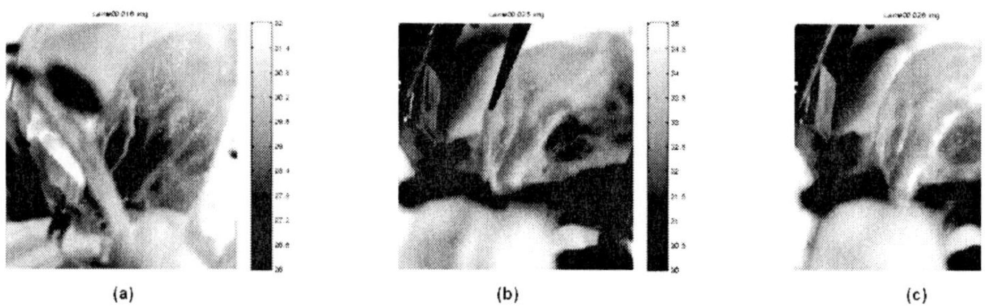

thermoregulatory phenomenon manifested on the face. Therefore, it can be sensed and computed through thermal imaging and multi-resolution analysis (Coli, 2007). The results reveal tonic (baseline) and phasic (event related) component of the GSR and of the associated sympathetic thermal response.

FUTURE TRENDS

The functional infrared imaging has great potentialities for establishing itself as a useful functional and parametric imaging modality in the next future. The ongoing research is mainly devoted for developing new algorithms for sustained and unobtrusive monitoring of individuals, both in terms of health monitoring and neuro-psychological investigation. Improved bio-heat transfer models and solving algorithms are also needed for faster and more effective computation of functional parameters of interest for diagnosis and monitoring.

Diseases manifesting themselves through impairment of the skin thermoregulation are the best candidates to be studied through the proposed approach.

Moreover, the functional infrared imaging has been proposed as an adjunctive tool for imaging-based assistance to microsurgery (Campbell, 2006) and cardiac surgery aimed at assessing correct arterial blood re-perfusion after anastomosis de-clamping (Figure 8) (Merla, 2001). Arm re-implantation, local sympathectomy and coronary bypass surgeries were considered. In addition, the technique has been used to follow up the restoration of the neurovascular functions through the evaluation thermoregulatory processes related to the treated region. The preliminary results from the conducted studies have proved that the functional infrared imaging can be advantageously used in imaging-assisted surgery thanks to its non-invasiveness and its high informative content on re-vascularization and re-perfusion processes.

CONCLUSION

Functional infrared imaging is a biomedical imaging technique that relies on high-resolution infrared imaging and on the modeling of heat exchange processes. Functional infrared imaging is aimed at providing quantitative diagnostic parameters through the functional investigation of the local thermoregulatory processes. The potential biomedical applications of functional infrared imaging are numerous, ranging from those described here, to psychometrics, cutaneous blood flow modeling, activity of the peripheral nervous system, and angiopathies. For the studies reported here, the technique is sensitive as the corresponding gold standard techniques. In some cases, it represents a useful follow-up tool (like in varicocelectomy, to promptly assess possible relapses) or even an elective diagnostic tool, as in the scleroderma and Raynaud's phenomenon. In neuro-psycho-physiology, it offers the capability of monitoring individuals without requiring their cooperation and without limiting their spontaneous activity. A strong and continuous research is going on to reinforce and spread out these innovative biomedical imaging techniques.

REFERENCES

Anbar, M. (2007). Dynamic thermal assessment. In J. D. Bronzino & N. A. Diakides (Ed.), *Medical Infrared Imaging* (pp. 8.1 – 8.23).Boca Raton, FL: CRC Press.

Bronzino, J. D. (2006). *The Biomedical Engineering Handbook*. CRC Press, 3rd ed. Boca Raton, FL: CRC Press.

Bronzino, J. D., & Diakides, N. A. (2007). *Medical Infrared Imaging*. Boca Raton, FL: CRC Press.

Campbell, P., & Roderick, T. (2006). Thermal imaging in surgery. In J. D. Bronzino & N. A. Diakides (Ed.), *Medical Imaging Devices and Systems, The Biomedical Engineering Handbook* (pp. 19.1 – 19.18).Boca Raton, FL: CRC Press.

Coli, M., Fontanella, L., Ippoliti, L., & Merla. A. (2007). Multiresolution KLE of psycho-physiological signals. In *Proceedings of S.Co.2007, Fifth Conference on Complex Models and Computational Intensive Methods for Estimation and Prediction, Book of Short Papers,* ISBN 978-88-6129-114-0, (pp. 116-121).

Diakides, N. A. (Guest Editor). (1998). Special Issue on Medical Infrared Imaging. *IEEE Engineering in Medicine and Biology*, 17, July/August.

Diakides, N. A. (Guest Editor). (2000). Special Issue on Medical Infrared Imaging. *IEEE Engineer-*

ing in Medicine and Biology, 19, May/June.

Diakides, N. A. (Guest Editor). (2002). Special Issue on Medical Infrared Imaging. *IEEE Engineering in Medicine and Biology, 21*, November/December.

Di Romualdo, S., Merla, A., & Romani, G. L. (2007). Superimposition of thermal imaging to visual imaging using homography. In *Proceedings of the 2007 IEEE Engineering Medicine Biology Society,* (pp. 3365-8).

Garbey, M., Merla, A., & Pavlidis I. (2004). Estimation of blood flow speed and vessel location from thermal video. In *Proceedings of the IEEE Computer Society Conference on Computer Vision and Pattern Recognition, 1*, 356–363.

Garbey, M., Sun, N., Merla, A., & Pavlidis, I. (2007). Contact-free measurement of cardiac pulse based on the analysis of thermal imagery. *IEEE Transactions Biomedical Engineering, 54*(8), 1418-26.

Keyserlingk, J. R., Ahlgren, P. D., Yu, E., Belliveau, N., & Yassa, M. (2007). Functional infrared imaging of the breast: Historical perspectives, current applications, and future considerations. In J. D. Bronzino & N. A. Diakides (Ed.), *Medical Infrared Imaging* (pp. 10.1 – 10.30).Boca Raton, FL: CRC Press.

Merla, A., Di Donato, L., & Romani, G. L. (2001). Assistance to surgery by means of infrared functional imaging: preliminary results. In *Proceedings of the 2001 IEEE Engineering Medicine Biology Society*, Proceedings CD track 1264.

Merla, A., Di Donato, L., Di Luzio, S., & Romani, G. L. (2002). Quantifying the Relevance and Stage of Disease with the Tau image Technique. *IEEE Engineering in Medicine and Biology Magazine, 21*(6), 86 – 91.

Merla, A., Di Donato, L., Salsano, F., & Romani, G. L. (2002). Raynaud's Phenomenon: infrared functional imaging applied to diagnosis and drugs effects. *International Journal of Immunopathology and Pharmacology, 15*(1), 41-52.

Merla, A., Ledda, A., Di Donato, L., & Romani, G. L. (2002). Use of infrared functional imaging to detect impaired thermoregulatory control in men with asymptomatic varicocele. *Fertility and Sterility, 78*(1), 199-200.

Merla, A., Di Donato, L., Rossini, P. M., & Romani, G. L. (2004). Emotion detection through Functional Infrared Imaging: preliminary results. *Biomedizinische Technick, 48*(2), 284-286.

Merla, A., Ledda, A., Di Donato, L., & Romani, G. L. (2004). Assessment of the effects of the varicocelectomy on the thermoregulatory control of the scrotum. *Fertility and Sterility, 81*(2), 471-2.

Merla, A., & Romani, G. L. (2006). Functional Infrared Imaging in Clinical Applications. In J. D. Bronzino & N. A. Diakides, (Ed.), *Medical Imaging Devices and Systems, The Biomedical Engineering Handbook* (pp. 32.1 – 32.13).Boca Raton, FL: CRC Press.

Merla, A., & Romani, G. L. (2006). Functional infrared imaging in medicine: a quantitative diagnostic approach. In *Proceedings of the 2006 IEEE Engineering Medicine Biology Society, 1*, 224-7.

Merla, A. (2007). Computational physiology in a thermal image setting. In: *Proceedings of S.Co.2007, Fifth Conference on Complex Models and Computational Intensive Methods for Estimation and Prediction*, Book of Short Papers, ISBN 978-88-6129-114-0, (pp. 338-343).

Merla, A., Di Romualdo, S., Di Donato, L., Proietti, M., Salsano, F., & Romani, G. L. (2007). Combined thermal and laser Doppler imaging in the assessment of cutaneous tissue perfusion. In: *Proceedings of the 2007 IEEE Engineering Medicine Biology Society,* (pp. 2630-3).

Merla, A., & Romani, G. L. (2007). Thermal signatures of emotional arousal: a functional infrared imaging study. In *Proceedings of the 2007 IEEE Engineering Medicine Biology Society,* (pp. 247-9).

Merla, A., & Romani, G. L. (2007). Biomedical applications of functional infrared imaging. In J. D. Bronzino & N. A. Diakides (Ed.), *Medical Infrared Imaging* (pp. 15.1 – 15.20). Boca Raton, FL: CRC Press.

Mieusset, R., Bujan, L., Plantavid, M., Mansat, A., Grandjean, H., & Pontonnier, F. (1991) Scrotal hyperthermia: frequency in an infertile population and associated alterations in testicular function. *Advanced Experimental Medicine and Biology, 286*, 203-9.

Nowakowski, A. (2007). Quantitative active dynamic thermal IR-imaging and thermal topography in medical diagnostics. In J. D. Bronzino, & N. A. Diakides (Ed.), *Medical Infrared Imaging* (pp. 7.1 – 7.29).Boca Raton, FL: CRC Press.

Pavlidis, I., & Cooper, M. (2001). The face of fear. *The Lancet, 357,* 1757.

Pavlidis, I., Levine, J., & Baukol, P. (2001). Thermal image analysis for anxiety detection. In: *Proceedings of the 2001 IEEE International Conference on Image Processing, 2*, 315–318.

Pavlidis, I., Eberhardt, N. L., & Levine, J. A. (2002). Human behaviour: Seeing through the face of deception. *Nature, 415,* 35.

Pavlidis, I. (2003). Continuous physiological monitoring. In: *Proceedings of the 25th Annual International Conference of the IEEE Engineering in Medicine and Biology Society, 2,* 1084–1087.

Pavlidis, I., Dowdall, J., Sun, N., Puri, C., Fei, J., & Garbey, M. (2007): Interacting with human physiology. *Computer Vision Image Understanding,* doi:10.1016/j.cviu.2006.11.018

Qi, H., Kuruganti, P. T., & Snyder, W. E. (2007). Detecting beast cancer from thermal infrared images by asymmetry analysis. In J. D.Bronzino & N. A. Diakides (Ed.), *Medical Infrared Imaging* (pp. 11.1 – 11.14).Boca Raton, FL: CRC Press.

Roganski, A. (2002). Infrared Detectors: an overview. *Infrared Physics and Technology, 43*(5), 187- 210.

Shastri, D., Merla, A., Tsiamyrtzis, P., & Pavlidis, I. (2007). Imaging facial signs of neuro-physiological responses. In *Proceedings of the 10th International Conference on Medical Image Computing and Computer-Assisted Intervention-MICCAI,* Brisbane, Australia, October 29 – November 2.

Sun, N., Garbey, M., Merla, A., & Pavlidis, I. (2005). Imaging the cardiovascular pulse. In: *Proceedings of the IEEE Computer Society Conference on Computer Vision and Pattern Recognition, 1,* 416-421.

Wiecek, B., Strzelecki, M., Jakubowska, T., & Wysocki, M. (2007). Advanced thermal image processing. In J. D. Bronzino, & N. A. Diakides, (Ed.), *Medical Infrared Imaging* (pp. 12.1 – 12.13). Boca Raton, FL: CRC Press.

KEY TERMS

Autonomic Nervous System: The autonomic nervous system (ANS) (or visceral nervous system) is the part of the peripheral nervous system that acts as a control system, maintaining homeostasis in the body. These maintenance activities are primarily performed without conscious control or sensation. The ANS has far reaching effects, including: heart rate, digestion, respiration rate, salivation, perspiration, diameter of the pupils, micturition (the discharge of urine), and sexual arousal.

Bioheat: Heat amounts generated within *in vivo* tissues and vasculature.

Infrared Imaging: Graphical representation of the superficial temperature distribution of bodies obtained through its thermal emission.

Perfusion: Amount of blood for volume unity of tissue.

Sympathetic Activity: The activity of nervous system that takes over where an immediate and effective response is required. The sympathetic nervous system works alongside the parasympathetic nervous system and is known as the involuntary system because the actions caused by it are not consciously executed.

Thermal Emission: Photonic emission of energy by bodies due to their temperature. The thermal emission is described by Stefan-Boltzmann, Planck and Wien laws.

Thermoregulation: The complex of the processes involved into maintaining the human body temperature at stationary ranges.

Chapter XVIII
DNA Microarrays:
Analysis and Interpretation

Aristotelis Chatziioannou
National Hellenic Research Foundation, Greece

Panagiotis Moulos
National Hellenic Research Foundation, Greece

ABSTRACT

The completion of the Human Genome Project and the emergence of high-throughput technologies at the dawn of the new millennium, are rapidly changing the way we approach biological problems. DNA microarrays represent a promising new technological development, widely used for the investigation and identification of genes associated with important biological processes. The chapter is divided in two parts: the first discusses current methods for the acquisition and quantitation of the microarray image while the second focuses in the analysis and interpretation of the microarray signals (standardization, normalization, statistical analysis etc.)

INTRODUCTION

DNA molecules encode the total information regarding cellular proteinosynthesis. Understanding cellular processes and the association between cells of dissimilar functionality, is essential for biological sciences. The ever increasing number of available fully or partially sequenced species across the evolutionary scale, fruit of the latest technological and computing advancements (shotgun sequencing, explosion of computational and storing capacity) have reshaped modern biological research, shifting it towards a systems approach rather than focusing in individual genes (Ideker, Galitski, & Hood, 2001).

DNA microarrays constitute part of these new biotechnological developments which allow the simultaneous monitoring of the expression of whole genomes. Since its introduction, there has been a deluge of papers presenting experimental outcomes from a broad range of biological and clinical domains including: i) identification and categorization of diagnostic or prognostic biomarkers, ii) classification of diseases, e.g. tumours with different prognosis microscopically indistinguishable, iii) monitoring the response to different treatments or therapies, iv) understanding of the mechanisms involved in disease genesis (Tarca, Romero, & Draghici, 2006), v) discovery of key nodes-promising drug targets- in biological pathways at several pathological states (Maynard et al., 2003) and vi) better understanding of several biological functions among different organisms.

BACKGROUND

A DNA microarray is normally a slide made of silica or synthetic materials where on top an ordered array of oligonucleotide clones is imprinted, corresponding to regions of all discovered or putative genes of an organism's genome, at sufficient quantities to ensure evasion of saturation effects, which allows the specific binding of genes or gene products (Schena, 2003). DNA microarrays are composed of thousands of DNA sequences (probes), each representing a gene. The DNA sequences can be long (500-2500bp) cDNA sequences or shorter (25-70bp) oligonucleotide sequences. Oligonucleotide sequences can be pre-synthesized and deposited with a pin or piezoelectric spray, synthesized in situ by photolithographic (Affymetrix) or inkjet (Agilent) technologies, or be attached to microscopic beads (Illumina) which are then randomly dispersed over the wells of the microarray slide.

Relative quantitative detection of gene expression can be carried out between two samples on a single array or by single samples using multiple arrays. The first approach entails (at least) two sample sources which are labelled with different fluorescent molecules, usually Cy3 (green fluorescence) and Cy5 (red fluorescence) Conventionally Cy3 represents the 'control' state whereas Cy5 represents the state under examination. These samples are hybridized together on the same array, a scanner laser-excites the dyes and an image is produced for each dye. The relative intensities of each channel represent the relative abundance of the RNA or DNA product in each sample. In the second approach, each sample is labelled with the same dye and hybridized onto separate arrays (Bajcsy, Liu, & Band, 2007). The absolute fluorescent values of each spot may then be scaled and compared to detect possible alterations in gene expression.

The resulting images are used to generate a dataset where pre-processing is performed prior to the analysis and interpretation of the results, in order to ensure the same level of comparison within and across slides, as well as to mitigate the role of noise. The pre-processing step entails useful transformations and assessment of the signal quality of the gene probes, in order to extract or enhance reliable signal characteristics which render the dataset amenable to the application of various data analysis methods.

The quantification of gene expression implies that the amount of fluorescence measured at each sequence specific location is proportional to the amount of mRNA hybridized onto the gene probes on the array. Processing of the images maps the arrayed gene spots and quantifies their expression, to the relative fluorescence intensities, measured for each spot. Microarray experiments do not directly provide insight on the absolute level of expression of a particular gene; nevertheless, they are useful to compare the expression level among conditions and genes (e.g. health vs. disease, treated vs. untreated) (Quackenbush, 2002; Tarca et al. 2006).

After pre-processing, normalization is applied to compensate for systematic differences among genes or arrays. Among others, it addresses issues such as unequal quantities of RNA, differences in labelling dyes, systematic bias of the measured expressions stemming either from the image acquisition part with different PMT or laser gains or from flaws in the washing/dilution procedure. It can be performed either on a per chip basis or/and across chips.

Another hindering factor is the absence of expression values usually for hundreds of probes within a microarray, due to several unpredictable factors (e.g. array scratches, scanner improper configuration, spot light saturation etc.). Reliable missing value imputation has therefore significant implications regarding the successful conduct of a microarray experiment and requires special consideration.

The statistical selection stage provides significantly differentially expressed gene lists but this represents nothing but a first step. Transforming information into knowledge and gaining insight over specific biological questions are daedalean tasks. Available biological databases, can contribute in revealing biological pathways or more generally processes underlying the biological mechanism investigated. The use of sophisticated statistical learning and data mining techniques for the identification of important genes, as classifiers among different experimental conditions (e.g. healthy tissue from cancer tissue or two different tumour types) and the derivation of disease specific molecular genetic signatures (biomarkers) can pave the way for rational drug design. This exhaustive course is termed as 'meta-analysis' and includes pathway analysis to uncover genes with a certain expression profile, potentially regulated by common transcription factors, exploration for common regulatory elements among groups of genes and functional analysis based on biological ontologies.

The rest of the chapter is organized as follows: firstly, information regarding the image related methodologies of microarrays is given as it constitutes an important aspect with a large impact on subsequent analysis steps (Yang, Buckley, & Speed, 2001). Then a brief overview of the various steps of microarray data analysis and interpretation is provided.

MICROARRAY IMAGE ANALYSIS

Three major tasks that have to be carried out for the transition of scanner acquired raw images to quantitative arithmetic data used for further experimental assessment (Yang et al., 2001): i) *addressing* or *gridding*, which is the process of assigning coordinates to each of the spots for a spotted or bead array or the alignment of a rectangular lattice for the mapping of pixels to specific probes in Affymetrix arrays, ii) *segmentation*, which allows the classification of pixels either as foreground, or background and iii) *information exctraction* which involves calculating foreground and background intensities.

Gridding

Grid alignment arranges a set of unevenly spaced, parallel and perpendicular lines (a template) to the image representing a 2D array of spots. The objective is to find all template descriptors (e.g. line coordinates and their orientations), so that pairs of intersecting perpendicular lines define the signal area of 2D array spots in a microarray scan (Bajcsy et al., 2007). Although the basic structure of arrays is usually known and can be provided as feedback to the gridding algorithm, there is a number of parameters that have to be properly estimated: such as the dimensions of grid rows and columns, the slight variation on print positions, the area enclosed between rows and columns within each grid and overall position of the array in the image (e.g. array rotation) (Yang et al., 2001). Generally, the gridding procedures can be distinguished in three main categories (Bajcsy et al., 2007): i) manual gridding, where the user specifies dimensions and spot radius to form a template and the rest of the alignment is performed manually, ii) semi-automated gridding, where the user provides basic data (e.g. corner spots and grid dimensions) and the algorithm performs the rest using image correlation techniques and iii) fully-automated gridding, where the user provides any prior knowledge regarding microarray layout and the algorithm uses data driven methods to optimize internal parameters for the optimal grid layout. Most microarray image analysis packages (GenePix, Spot, ScanArray) support several gridding algorithms with varying results. Other automated algorithms perform optimal alignment by multiple template matching and finalization criteria based on pixel locations and distances among them (Galinsky, 2003), using Markov random fields (Brandle, Bischof, & Lapp, 2003), or local minimization of each row, and column pixel intensity sums, using sliding windows with size approximating a typical spot size. Bajcsy et al., 2007 provides an extensive description of gridding methods for cDNA microarrays. Concerning gridding on Affymetrix arrays, it is performed through bi-linear interpolation between the 4 corners of the array, identified by checkerboard-like sequences manufactured for this purpose (Arteaga-Salas, Zuzan, Langdon, Upton, & Harrison, 2008).

Segmentation

Image segmentation can be generally defined as partitioning the image to several different regions of certain properties (Soille, 1999). There exist several segmentation algorithms. The most widely used in spotted microarrays are the *fixed circle*, *adaptive circle*, *seeded region growing* and *histogram* segmentations. The fixed circle algorithm simply fits a constant radius circle to each spot on the array. The background can be estimated by extending the radius of the circles and averaging the intensity of the pixels lying between the outer part of the inner circle and the inner part of the outer circle. Although simple in its implementation, it works nicely when all spots are circular and around the same size but proves unsatisfactory for spots of various diameters. Adaptive circle algorithm partially tackles this as the diameter of each circle is tuned for each spot separately. An arising problem is the automaticdetection of spot edges, as manual diameter adjustment can be extremely time-consuming (each array contains several thousands of spots). Dapple software (Buhler, Ideker, & Haynor, 2000) addresses this by calculating the Laplacian of the image and locating pixels with high values in the transformed image. These should correspond to spot edges. Even though adaptive circle is more sophisticated, it is still not suitable for irregularly shaped spots (e.g. doughnut shaped or scratched), as it may not detect accurately their precise shape (Figure 1). Seeded region growing (Adams & Bischof, 1994) use specified starting points as spot centers and proper thresholds to create an adapted polygon that encloses as much of the spot's shape as possible. A different approach is implemented in the histogram segmentation, where a mask larger than any spot on the array is applied to each spot. Then, a histogram of pixel intensities within each mask is constructed and predefined percentile thresholds determine the foreground and background areas (Yang et al., 2001). Variations of this method include statistical testing (Chen et al., 2002) or k-means clustering (Bajcsy et al., 2007; Li, Fraley, Bumgarner, Yeung, & Raftery, 2005) to classify pixel intensities as foreground or background. Other approaches for image segmentation utilize the theory of *mathematical morphology* (Angulo & Serra, 2003; Soille, 1999) and introduce image filters such as the *morphological opening* and *closing* and morphological operators such as *erosion* and *dilation*.

Segmentation in Affymetrix microarrays is easier in many ways than spotted arrays, as the gene probes are synthesized in strictly predefined coordinates. Taking into account possible misalignment during the gridding procedure which affects mostly the pixels around the perimeter of a probe cell and that the signal of a probe cell tends to be weakest around its edges, the 5×5 array of pixels attributed to a probe cell is reduced to a 3×3 array of central pixels (Arteaga-Salas et al., 2008). Segmentaton in Illumina microarrays is performed using incomplete Voronoi diagrams (Galinsky, 2003). Image segmentation algorithms and software packages that support them are summarized in Table 1.

Information Extraction

This step in microarray image analysis transforms the preceding procedures into useful arithmetic values to be used in subsequent analysis steps. Two main values have to be estimated for each spot: the foreground intensity so as to have a measure of mRNA hybridization for each gene and the background intensity which reflects several non-specific hybridizations, owed to numerous biochemical (non-specific binding, cross hybridization, washing protocol) or technical (presence of dust, scratches or other artefacts on the glass, scanner miscalibration) reasons. Background estimation enables background correction for the derivation of more robust gene expression estimates.

Figure 1. A small portion of a scanned spotted microarray image displaying nine spots on gray-scale where the dark and bright pixels represent low and high pixel values respectively. The variability in spot sizes and shapes can be easily noticed (image adapted from (Yang et al., 2001)).

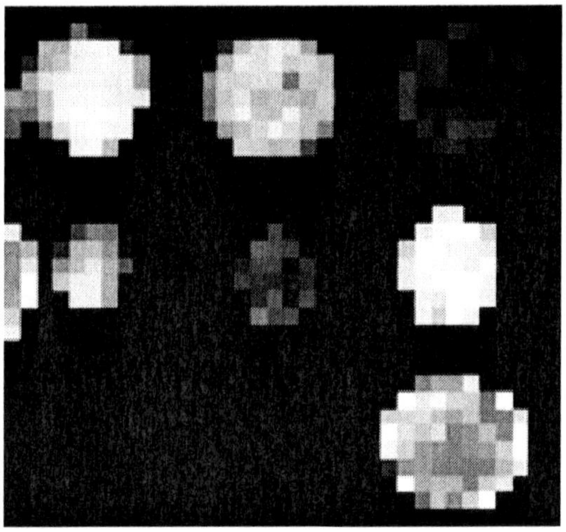

Table 1. Segmentation algorithms and indicative software packages, where the respective methods are implemented.

Segmentation algorithm	Software packages
Fixed circle	ScanAlyze, GenePix, QuantArray, ScanArray
Adaptive circle	GenePix, Dapple
Adaptive shape	Spot, GenePix
Histogram method	QuantArray, ScanArray, DeArray, ImaGene
Affymetrix segmentation	GCOS
Illumina segmentation	BeadStudio, R Bioconductor package: beadarray (Dunning, Smith, Ritchie, & Tavare, 2007)

Foreground Intensity

As each pixel value in a scanned image represents the hybridization level for a particular cDNA sequence (Yang et al., 2001), a natural measure of expression is the mean intensity over all pixels that define a spot in spotted arrays. An alternative estimate is the median of spot pixels which is more robust to outliers than the mean. In Affymetrix arrays, the 75th percentile of the reduced pixel set is reported as the estimate of the probe cell intensity, along with the standard deviation (Arteaga-Salas et al., 2008). Concerning Illumina bead arrays, intensities are extracted followin the algorithm of (Galinsky, 2003) where bead centers are supplied as virtual pixel centers. Individual bead signals are computed based on a 3x3 pixel area around each of four real pixels covering the virtual one (Kuhn et al., 2004).

Background Intensity

Background estimation algorithms for spotted microarrays can be classified in three main categories (Yang et al., 2001): (1) local background, where background intensities are estimated using several regions surrounding the spot (Figure 2). (2) constant background, where background is estimated based in a set of negative controls (plant genes that should not hybridize with human mRNA samples) and (3) no background estimation at all, as the proper background correction method for spotted microarrays remains a debatable issue (Scharpf, Iacobuzio-Donahue, Sneddon, & Parmigiani, 2007). Background correction in Affymetrix microarrays is based both in pixels surrounding the reduced pixel set, as well as on the mismatch probe pairs which reflect effects such as non-specific or cross hybridization. Concerning Illumina bead arrays, background correction is based both in local background estimated by the area defined by the surrounding spot pixels as well as negative controls (Kuhn et al., 2004).

MICROARRAY DATA PROCESSING AND INTERPRETATION

Having derived the raw expression signal for each gene probe from the microarray images, the need for further processing arises in order to render these indexes of gene expression comparable as much within the same slide as across different slides. The tens of thousands of probes existing in every microarray slide, as well as the pronounced noise impact render imperative the use of systematic methodologies for the mathematically reliable and computationally effective processing of tens or hundreds of thousands of values.

Pre-Processing

The initial step in this direction is the pre-processing which comprises the following actions:

- Signal background correction
- Logarithmic transformation of the signal channel values and calculation of their ratio in the case of two channel experiments
- Filtering procedures to eliminate non-informative genes

Regarding background correction, the intention is to adjust for hybridization of sample transcripts whose sequences do not perfectly match those of the probes on the array, and for other systematic or haphazard sources of error (scanner artefacts, technical setbacks, washing issues or quantum fluctuations) (Speed, 2003). Depending on the type of microarray technology adopted, each slide contains specific spots for estimation of the background (empty spots, exogenous negative control spots, spiked-in genes)) which permit the application of various methods for the background estimation. Concerning Affymetrix arrays, background can be estimated through the 'mismatch probes' which cover all slide surface. Spot background correction, when applied, can be effected either by subtracting the background

Figure 2. This image depicts several local background estimation methods. The region inside the dashed circle corresponds to the spot mask from which the foreground intensity is estimated. The solid circles represent pixel regions that are used by QuantArray for background intensity estimation while the dotted square is used on ScanAlyze. The dashed diamond shapes depict regions which are used for background estimation by Spot (image adapted from (Yang et al., 2001)).

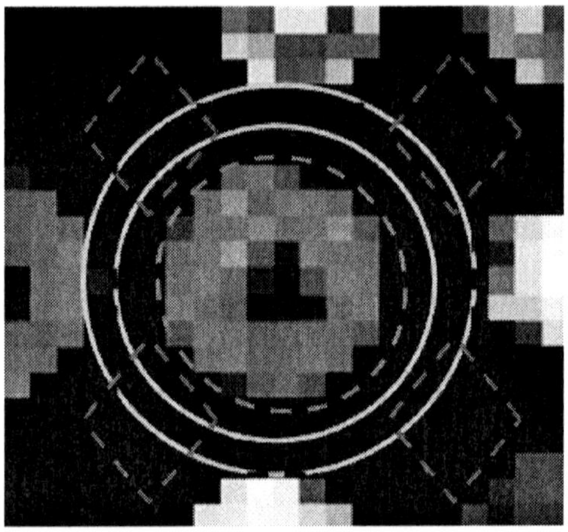

value from the signal value for each probe, or by dividing the background value from the signal value for each probe that is, subtraction of the log transformed values of the background from the signal respectively or by providing model based corrected signal estimations. For the estimation of the signal and the background, the mean or the median of the spot signal and background can be utilized. Regarding weak signal datasets(a majority of spot signals is close or below background levels), dividing rather than subtracting the signal by the background, (signal-to-noise ratio), an established notion in systems theory, is tacitly adopting the perception of the experimentalist about the quality of a signal. Signal quality is considered good when its strength is some orders of magnitude greater than that of the background, namely its ratio compared to noise, is big enough, according to criteria set by the expert or inferred statistically (Chatziioannou & Moulos, 2007b).

Logarithmic transformations transform the data population in order, torender it compliant with the normality assumptionand amenable to the utilization of parametric statistics. In the case of ratio values, the logarithm base 2 transformation of the expression ratio (i.e. Cy5/Cy3 in cDNA microarray experiments or Signal_condition(x)/ Signal_control(x)) is advocated. This has the major advantage that it treats differential up-regulation and down-regulation equally (Quackenbush, 2002) while at the same time projects data on a continuous mapping space. For example, if the expression ratio is 1, then $\log_2(1)$ equals 0 and represents no change in expression. If the expression ratio is 4, then $\log_2(4)$ equals +2 and for expression ratio of $\log_2(1/4)$ equals -2. Besides the advantages of using expression ratios here, the pitfalls of working with ratios should also be stressed. For example, genes with the same R/G ratios of 400/100 and 4/1 but whose values lie at a completely different range with different error thresholds for the respective regions will end up having the same expression ratio of 4, a fact that raises significant concerns, regarding the validity of the results.

Finally, the filtering procedures aim at excluding problematic or unreliable, array spots. They are usually based in processes which utilize either the estimation of the probe's background or the detection of possible outlier values, to locate candidate genes to be removed from further analysis. In this way, both the computational efficiency of the processing of the whole dataset is increasing by limiting useless calculations, and the impact of noise is decreasing, as erroneous values are excluded from the derivation of the normalized values. Some gene filtering methods are cited here (Chatziioannou & Moulos, 2007b):

- A signal-to-noise threshold filter: Signal(x)/Background(x) < T, where T represents a threshold below which noisy spots are filtered out.
- A distance based filter between the signal and background distributions. A spot is robust if their signal and background means diverge from each other a fixed distance determined by the respective standard deviations. Spots with signal features smaller than this distance are filtered out.
- A filter test for the reproducibility of measurements where parametric or non-parametric statistical tests are used to examine for each spot, if the derived values of all replicates within a condition follow a normal (or more generally a continuous symmetrical) distribution with mean (median) equal to the respective one derived by the respective replicates, thus excluding outliers among the replicate signal values of a specific condition.

Data Normalization

Typical normalization methods are global mean or median normalization (Bilban, et al., 2002), rank invariant normalization (Tseng et al., 2002) and LOWESS/LOESS methods (Cleveland, Grosse, & Shyu, 1992). Normalization methods tacitly assume that the total level of RNA expression in a microarray slide through varying conditions is roughly constant. Actually housekeeping gene expression (around 10% of the total gene population and responsible for the greatest - around 90% - of the total RNA expression) does not exhibit significant variation among conditions, an assumption though that might be proven refutable for certain housekeeping genes. Rank invariant normalization methods are based exclusively on signal intensities and they do not use all genes during the normalization procedure. Instead, a statistical algorithm determines a subset of genes which are found to be non-differentially expressed across different slides (Tseng et al., 2002; Hoffmann, Seidl, & Dugas, 2002). However, they do not account for systematic dependencies of the log ratio statistics to signal intensity (Quackenbush, 2002). The need for normalization and its impact on the dataset values is depicted in Figure 3.

There exist several methods for normalizing cDNA (Hedge et al., 2000; Finkelstein et al., 2002; Yang, Dudoit et al., 2002) as well as oligonucleotide (i.e. Affymetrix, Illumina, Nimblegen) microarray data (Irizarry et al., 2003; Wu et al., 2004; Lin et al., 2008). There has been a seminal effort, to propose a framework for the comparison of normalization algorithms scoping to provide a checklist to the researcher on which algorithm to pick for his dataset. In brief, the algorithm that is associated with the less over-normalization potential (smaller reduction of the total signal entropy), smaller bias (greater accuracy) and variance (greater precision) is the optimal one for the dataset at hand (Argyropoulos et al., 2006).

Imputation of Missing Values

During a microarray experiment, expression measurements may become unavailable for several probes due to several reasons, a phenomenon which might affect a significant part of the total probe values population. This problem further hinders the application of automated procedures since it affects different genes in each microarray image. Therefore the issue of missing value imputation, based on certain statistical or geometrical criteria is imperative. A naïve solution is to estimate missing data for a probe by the mean expression of the remaining probes over the rest of the slides. However, this strategy demonstrates poor performance (Troyanskaya et al. 2001) and does not account for the correlation among genes. More sophisticated methods have been proposed using matrix Singular Value Decomposition and k-Nearest Neighbors (Troyanskaya et al. 2001; Nguyen, Wang & Carrol, 2004).

Statistical Selection

Target of a microarray experiment is the identifcation of differentially expressed genes between two or more states (time points, phenotypic categories, biological specimen from different tissues, species etc.) Thus, for each gene on the array, the "null" hypothesis is that this gene is not differentially expressed among different states and the "alternative" is that there is indeed difference in the gene's expression among the different states. Several types of statistical tests are used, parametric (t-test, ANOVA) (Kerr, Martin, & Churchill, 2000; Ideker et al., 2000; Dudoit et al., 2002) or non-parametric (Wilcoxon sign-rank, Kruskal-Wallis) (Conover, 1980) which can be applied to cDNA

*Figure 3. (a) An MA plot for a cDNA microarray slide. It displays the log2(R/G) for each element of the array as a function of the ½*log2(R*G) product intensities and can reveal systematic intensity dependent effects on the log2 ratio values. R and G correspond to corrected Cy5 and Cy3 signal intensities respectively. The upper panel of (a) depicts the MA plot before normalization while the bottom panel, after LOESS normalization. The bright line on the upper panel draws the normalization curve. After normalization, the cloud is centered around zero (b) A boxplot for 19 cDNA arrays. The upper panel of (b) presents the systematic trends in microarray slides briefly mentioned in sections 2.1-2.4. Direct comparisons in ratios cannot be made since data are not centered around a common reference value. Bias is removed after normalization, as depicted in the bottom panel of (b) (borrowed from the normalization analysis of the dataset of Tzouvelekis et al., 2007).*

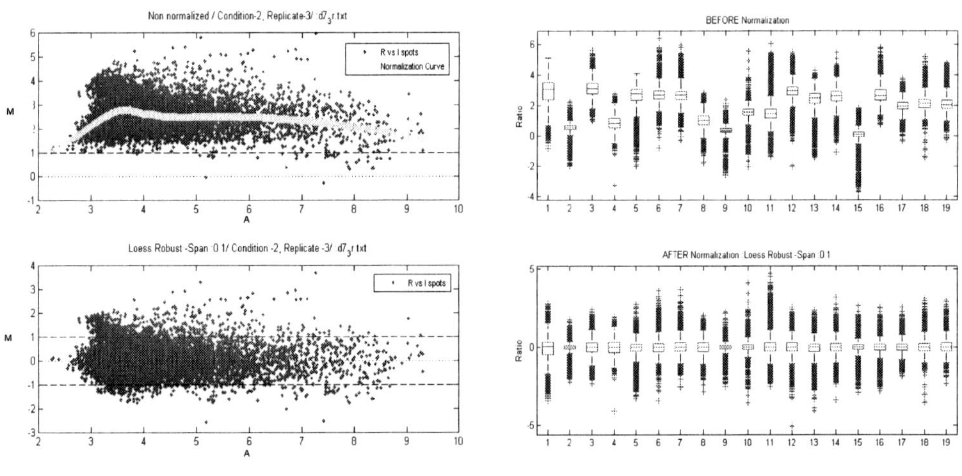

(a) (b)

or oligonucleotide arrays (Tusher, Tibshirani, & Chum 2001). A comparison of several statistical selection methods can be found in (Pan, 2002). However, strong statistical significance does not necessarily mean biological significance as it is not coupled with the notion of a strong fold change or absolute intensity. On the other hand, many genes might not reach the threshold simply because of the small number of replicates used to define each state.

As in general there is no golden standard method for microarray data statistical analysis whereas the results of several methods might present limited overlap (Kim et al., Lee, & Sohn, 2006), a fact which does not appear to depend on different microarray platform technologies (; Canales et al., 2006), a recent study (Guo et al., 2006) suggests that the overlap among results, is increasing, when a less stringent statistical threshold together with a reasonable fold-change cut-off is adopted.

In microarray experiments, even for a strict statistical threshold like 0.01, a large number of false positives (100 in 10000 genes) can be observed. Instead of using FWER methods, which adjust p-values by dividing them with the number of hypotheses tested (Dudoit et al., 2003), FDR methods seek to minimize the proportion of errors committed by falsely rejecting null hypotheses (Benjamini, & Hochberg, 1995; Storey, & Tibshirani, 2003). As they are less stringent than they are considered more suitable for microarray data (Tarca et al., 2006; Allison, Cui, Page, & Sabripour, 2006).

Meta-Analysis

In microarray experiments, researchers usually find themselves bewildered by a myriad of findings (Allison et al., 2006), with no evident pattern of correlation among them. Transforming information into knowledge about specific biological functions is by all means a self-evident task. The use of sophisticated statistical learning and data mining techniques can highlight important groups of genes, which are able to act as disease-specific molecular genetic signatures, or belong to the same pathways or more generally biological processes. This exhaustive search process can be termed as 'meta-analysis'.

Classification

One of the targets of meta-analysis is to assign genes or biological samples to classes on the basis of their expression measurements (Speed, 2003). Such problems are mainly classified into two categories: unsupervised and supervised learning. In unsupervised learning, the algorithm attributes objects into classes without any prior knowledge of these classes (Newton, 2002). This task is accomplished through proper metrics, which estimate the relative distance between objects and linkage algorithms that perform the clustering of the closest objects (Kaufman & Rousseeuw, 1990). Examples of unsupervised learning techniques are k-means clustering, hierarchical clustering (Speed, 2003), gene-shaving (Hastie et al., 2002), self-organizing maps (Torkkola et al.,2001) and FLAME (Fu, & Medico, 2007).

Principal Component Analysis

Principal Component Analysis (PCA) can identify a core set of genes, out of the thousands, able to distinguish the dataset among different experimental conditions and thus simplify the analysis and visualization of multidimensional data sets (Raychaudhuri, Stuart, & Altman, 2000; Jolliffe, 2002).

Given m observations on n variables on an m by n data matrix, PCA reduces the dimensionality of the data matrix by finding r new variables, termed Principal Components, ($r \leq n$) accounting for a fixed significant percentage of the total original variance, while remaining mutually uncorrelated and orthogonal. In microarray data analysis, the genes can be considered as variables and the conditions as observations, the opposite or even both (Parmigiani et al., 2003). PCA has been used for outlier genes (Hilsenbeck, et al., 1999), in the optimization of clustering (Yeung, & Ruzzo, 2001) and generally classification techniques (Liu et al., 2002).

Gene Shaving

Gene shaving (Hastie et al., 2002) identifies subsets of genes with coherent expression patterns and large variation across conditions. It differs from hierarchical clustering and other analysis methods in that genes may belong to more than one cluster and the clustering may be supervised by an outcome measure. It performs an iterative PCA process on genes (rows) to obtain nested gene clusters and then uses a statistic to determine the optimum cluster size.

k-Nearest Neighbours (k-NN) Classification

The k-NN classification is a very simple, yet powerful classification method. The key idea behind k-NN is that similar observations belong to similar classes. The weighting scheme of the class numbers is often a majority rule, but other schemes are conceivable. The class assessment is usually performed according to the distance of the new instant from the majority of the instances that belong to different classes. One major drawback of k-NN classifiers is the requirement of all available data, something incurring significant overhead, for a large training dataset. The k-NN algorithm can be naturally expanded to treat multiclass problems since the only difference is that there are more than two data clouds in the data space.

RankGO

RankGO (Chatziioannou & Moulos, 2007a) is an application for the derivation of groups of genes related to Gene Ontology (GO) Terms, which do not only have a high statistical score (high gene enrichment, namely a high proportion of genes annotated to a specific GO term from the significant gene list, to the total number of genes assigned to this GO term within the total genes of the whole microarray) but at the same time comprise a biologically significant number of genes as this significance is derived from the mapping of genes to specific GO terms. In brief, RankGO assigns each GO term a statistical score, through a proper statistical test (hypergeometric, Fisher exact test), groups together GO terms with the same score, sorts the distribution of GO term scores according to their frequency, and finally GO terms corresponding to scores above the cutoff threshold after bootstrapping, represent both statistically and biologically significant pathways.

GOALIE

GOALIE (Ramakrishnan, et al., 2005) is an application that uses clustered numerical microarray gene expression measurements to reconstruct the cluster analysis based on time windows, proper statistical measures and temporal logic methods. It results in a temporal logic model connecting gene with their GO terms across different time points.

Gene Set Enrichment Analysis (GSEA)

GSEA (Subramanian et al., 2005) uses a ranked gene list, depicting the whole array for all samples (phenotypic classes) instead of the top scoring portion of it, together with gene sets (derived from prior biological knowledge, GO etc.). The goal of the algorithm behind GSEA is to determine whether a gene set is enriched with members of the gene list primarily found at the top or bottom for the various classes.

Bayesian Analysis for Time Series Microarray Experiments (BATS)

BATS (Angelini et al., 2007) is a new software equipped with a friendly GUI for Bayesian Analysis of Time Series microarray experiments. It implements a fully functional Bayesian software which permits the user to automatically identify and estimate differentially expressed genes, in time course microarray experiments. BATS can carry out both simulations and analysis on real data experiments from different platforms.

FUTURE TRENDS

Certain recent studies (Allison et al., 2006; Draghici, Khatri, Eklund, & Szallasi, 2006; Dupuy & Simon, 2007) raise some skepticism regarding certain aspects of microarray analysis methodologies performance, with the scope to highlight any problematic approaches used so far or to consider properly inconsistencies among results derived from different microarray platforms. A comparative study published in 2004 using microarrays for cancer studies (Dupuy & Simon, 2007) focuses on 3 basic analysis misconceptions: (1) in outcome-related gene findings where there is no clear or inadequate control for multiple statistical testing, (2) when clustering gene expression values, it is considered that clusters are meaningful for distinguishing outcomes whereas the clustering procedure itself is based on genes selected for their correlation with outcome, and (3) in studies using supervised learning methods for prediction, there is bias in the estimation of prediction accuracy through an inaccurate cross-validation procedure (e.g. not proper setup of a training and test dataset). Some more general considerations are proposed in (Allison et al., 2006). Thus, apart from the fact that more accurate methods for microarray quality-control assessment need to be developed together with approaches for their validation, more attention should be drawn to the scrutiny of sets of analysis outcomes and their correlation to well known functionalities in order to evaluate complex multi-component biological hypotheses. Additionally, as the assumption of statistical independence regarding the expression among genes is generally not valid, this imposes caution to the statistical procedures that should be applied and how, together with an extended attention in the evaluation of current techniques for normalization, statistical selection procedures and clustering methodologies, rather than to the development of novel ones. Finally, the existence of certain limitations in current microarray platforms should be recognized, resulting to the inability of detecting expression changes of specific genes. Problems of such nature should be resolved in the future by research in the areas of nucleic acid hybridization, and technological advances in detection methods and hybridization conditions (Draghici et al., 2006) moving microarrays towards becoming an accurate diagnostic tool rather than a high-throughput tool used in biological research.

CONCLUSION

It is now widely accepted that DNA microarrays have become an invaluable tool to modern biological research. Their usefulness can be easily verified by the deluge of papers published during the last years, either exploring several biological systems in a more systematic way using microarrays, or introducing novel tools and statistical algorithms for the extraction or grouping of valuable information. Although their use might raise certain problems of systematic nature, if such issues as those described in section 5 will be taken into account during the analysis procedure, microarrays can provide useful results in various aspects of biological research.

REFERENCES

Adams, R., & Bischof, L. (1994). Seeded region growing. *IEEE Trans. Pattern Anal. Machine Intell., 16*, 641-647.

Allison, D. B., Cui, X., Page, G. P. (2006). Sabripour, M., Microarray Data Analysis: from Disarray to Consolidation and Consensus, *Nat. Rev. Genet. 7*, 55-65.

Angelini, C., De Canditiis, D., Mutarelli, M., Pensky M, (2007). A Bayesian Approach to Estimation and Testing in Time-course Microarray Experiments, *Statistical Applications in Genetics and Molecular Biology*: *6*(1), 24.

Angulo, J., & Serra, J. (2003). Automatic analysis of DNA microarray images using mathematical morphology. *Bioinformatics, 19*(5), 553-562.

Argyropoulos, C., Chatziioannou, A. A., Nikiforidis, G., Moustakas, A., Kollias, G., & Aidinis, V. (2006). Operational criteria for selecting a cDNA microarray data normalization algorithm. *Oncology reports,15*(4), 983-996.

Arteaga-Salas, J. M., Zuzan, H., Langdon, W. B., Upton, G. J., & Harrison, A. P. (2008). An overview of image-processing methods for Affymetrix GeneChips. *Brief Bioinform, 9*(1), 25-33.

Bajcsy, P., Liu, L., & Band, M. (2007). DNA microarray image processing. In G. Kamberova (Ed.), *DNA array image analysis*: Nuts & Bolts.

Benjamini, Y., & Hochberg, Y. (1995). Controlling the False Discovery Rate: a Practical and Powerful Approach to Multiple Testing. *J. R. Statist. Soc., 57*, 289-300.

Bilban, M., Buehler, L. K., Head, S., Desoye, G., & Quaranta, V. (2002). Normalizing DNA Microarray Data. *Curr. Issues Mol. Biol. 4*, 57-64.

Brandle, N., Bischof, L., & Lapp, H. (2003). Robust DNA microarray image analysis. *Machine Vision and Applications, 15*, 11-28.

Buhler, J., Ideker, T., & Haynor, D. (2000). *Improved techniques for finding spots on cDNA microarrays*: University of Washington.

Canales, R. D., Luo, Y., Willey, J. C., Austermiller, B., Barbacioru, C. C., Boysen, C., Hunkapiller, K., Jensen, R. D., Knight, C. R., Lee, K. Y., Ma, Y., Maqsodi, B., Papallo, A., Peters, E. H., Poulter, K., Ruppel, P. L., Samaha, R. R., Shi, L., Yang, W., Zhang, L., & Goodsaid, F. M. (2006). Evaluation of cDNA Microarray Results with Quantitative Gene Expression Platforms. *Nat. Biotech., 24*, 1115-1122.

Chatziioannou, A., & Moulos, P. (2007a). Extending the Interpretation of Gene Profiling Microarray Experiments to Pathway Analysis Through the Use of Gene Ontology Terms. *ICCS 2007 Proceedings (22-27 July, Sheffield), QA-Gen Workshop.*

Chatziioannou, A., & Moulos, P. (2007b). ANDROMEDA: A MATLAB automated cDNA microarray data analysis platform. *IFIP International Federation for Information Processing, 247*, (pp. 127-136).

Chen, Y., Kamat, V., Dougherty, E. R., Bittner, M. L., Meltzer, P. S., & Trent, J. M. (2002). Ratio statistics of gene expression levels and applications to microarray data analysis. *Bioinformatics, 18*(9), 1207-1215.

Cleveland, W. S., Grosse, E., & Shyu, W. M. (1992). *Local Regression Models, Statistical Models in S*. In J. M. Chambers & T. J. Hastie (Eds.), *Practical Nonparametric Statistics* Wadsworth & Brooks/Cole Dormand, J.R. Conover, W.J., (1980)., Wiley.

Draghici, S., Khatri, P., Eklund, A. C., & Szallasi, Z. (2006). Reliability and reproducibility issues in DNA microarray measurements. *Trends Genet, 22*(2), 101-109.

Dudoit, S., Yang, Y. H., Speed, T., & Callow, M. J. (2002). Statistical Methods for Identifying

Differentially Expressed Genes in Replicated cDNA Microarray Experiments. *Statistica Sinica 12*, 111-139.

Dudoit, S., Shaffer, J. P., & Boldrick, J. C. (2003). Multiple Hypothesis Testing in Microarray Experiments. *Statistical Science, 18*, 71-103.

Dunning, M. J., Smith, M. L., Ritchie, M. E., & Tavare, S. (2007). beadarray: R classes and methods for Illumina bead-based data. *Bioinformatics, 23*(16), 2183-2184.

Dupuy, A., & Simon, R. M. (2007). Critical review of published microarray studies for cancer outcome and guidelines on statistical analysis and reporting. *J Natl Cancer Inst, 99*(2), 147-157.

Finkelstein, D. B., Ewing, R., Gollub, J., Sterky, F., Somerville, S., & Cherry, J. M. (2002). *Iterative Linear Regression by Sector, Methods of Microarray Data Analysis,* S. M. Lin & K. F. Johnson (Eds.). Cambridge, MA: Kluwer Academic (pp. 57-68).

Fu, L., & Medico, E. (2007). FLAME, a Novel Fuzzy Clustering Method for the Analysis of DNA Microarray Data. *BMC Bioinformatics, 8*(3).

Galinsky, V. L. (2003). Automatic registration of microarray images. I. Rectangular grid. *Bioinformatics, 19*(14), 1824-1831.

Guo, L., Lobenhofer, E. K., Wang, C., Shippy, R., Harris, S. C., Zhang, L., Mei, N.,Chen, T., Herman, D., Goodsaid, F. M., Hurban, P., Phillips, K. L., Xu, J., Deng, X., Sun, Y. A., Tong, W., Dragan, Y. P., & Shi, L. (2006). Rat Toxigonecomic Study Reveals Analytical Consistency Across Microarray Platforms. *Nat. Biotech., 24*, 1162-1169.

Hastie, T., Tibshirani, R., Eisen, M. B., Alizadeh, A., Levy, R., Staudt, L., Chan, W. C., Botstein, D., & Brown, P. (2002). 'Gene Shaving' as a Method for Identifying Distinct Sets of Genes with Similar Expression Patterns. *Genome Biology, 1,* research0003.1-0003.21.

Hilsenbeck, S. G., Friedrichs, W. E., Schiff, R., O'Connell, P., Hansen, R. K., Osborne, C. K., & Fuqua, S. A. W. (1999). Statistical Analysis of Array Expression Data as Applied to the Problem of Tamoxifen Resistance. *J. Natl. Cancer Institute, 91*, 453-459.

Hoffmann, R., Seidl, T., & Dugas, M. (2002). Profound effect of normalization on detection of differentially expressed genes in oligonucleotide microarray data analysis. *Genome Biology, 3*(7). research 0033.1-0033.11.

Ideker, T., Thorsson, V., Siehel, A. F., & Hood, L. E. (2000). Testing for Differentially Expressed Genes by Maximum Likelihood Analysis of Microarray Data. *J. Comput. Biol., 7*, 805-817.

Ideker, T., Galitski, T., & Hood, L. (2001). A new approach to decoding life: systems biology. *Annu Rev Genomics Hum Genet, 2*, 343-372.

Irizarry, R. A., Hobbs, B., Collin, F., Beazer-Barclay, Y. D., Antonellis, K. J., Scherf, U., & Speed, T. P. (2003). Exploration, Normalization, and Summaries of High Density Oligonucleotide Array Probe Level Data. *Biostatistics, 4*, 249-264.

Jolliffe, I. T. (2002). *Principal Component Analysis*. Springer.

Kaufman, L., & Rousseeuw, P. J. (1990). *Finding Groups in Data: An Introduction to Cluster Analysis*. New York: Wiley.

Kerr, M. K., Martin, M., & Churchill, G. A. (2000). Analysis of Variance for Gene Expression Microarray Data. *J. Computational Biol. 7*, 819-837.

Kim, S. Y., Lee, J. W., Sohn, I. S. (2006). Comparison of Various Statistical Methods for Identifying Differential Gene Expression in Replicated Microarray Data. *Statistical Methods in Medical Research, 15*, 3-20.

Kuhn, K., Baker, S. C., Chudin, E., Lieu, M. H., Oeser, S., Bennett, H., et al. (2004). A novel, high-performance random array platform for quantitative gene expression profiling. *Genome Res, 14*(11), 2347-2356.

Li, Q., Fraley, C., Bumgarner, R. E., Yeung, K. Y., & Raftery, A. E. (2005). Donuts, scratches and blanks: robust model-based segmentation of microarray images. *Bioinformatics, 21*(12), 2875-2882.

Lin, S. M., Du, P., Huber, W., & Kibbe, W.A. (2008). Model-based variance-stabilizing transformation for Illumina microarray data. *Nucleic Acids Res., 36*(2), e11. Epub 2008.

Liu, A., Zhang, Y., Gehan, E., & Clarke, R. (2002). Block Principal Component Analysis with Application to Gene Microarray Data Classification. *Stat. Med. 21*, 3465-3474.

Maynard, S. E., Min, J. Y., Merchan, J., Lim, K. H., Li, J., Mondal, S., et al.(2003). Excess placental soluble fms-like tyrosine kinase 1 (sFlt1) may contribute to endothelial dysfunction, hypertension, and proteinuria in preeclampsia. *J Clin Invest, 111*, 649-58.

Newton, J. (2002). *Analysis of Microarray Gene Expression Data Using Machine Learning Techniques*. Technical Report, University of Alberta, Canada.

Nguyen, D. V., Wang, N., & Carrol, R. J. (2004). Evaluation of Missing Value Estimation for Microarray Data. *Journal of Data Science, 2*, 347-370.

Pan, W. (2002). A Comparative Review of Statistical Methods for Discovering Differentially Expressed Genes in Replicated Microarray Experiments. *Bioinformatics, 18*, 546-554.

Parmigiani, G., Garett, E. S., Irizarry, R. A., & Zeger, S. L. (2003). *The Analysis of Gene Expression Data: Methods and Software*. Springer.

Quackenbush, J. (2002). Microarray Data Normalization and Transformation. *Nat. Genetics, 32*, 496-501.

Ramakrishnan, N., Antoniotti, M., & Mishra, B. (2005). Reconstructing Formal Temporal Models of Cellular Events using the GO Process Ontology. *Bio-Ontologies SIG Meeting, ISMB 2005*, Detroit, U.S.A..

Raychaudhuri, S., Stuart, J. M., & Altman, R. B. (2000). Principal Component Analysis to Summarize Microarray Experiments: *Application to Sporulation Time Series, Pac. Symp. Biocomput., 5*, 452-463.

Scharpf, R. B., Iacobuzio-Donahue, C. A., Sneddon, J. B., & Parmigiani, G. (2007). When should one subtract background fluorescence in 2-color microarrays? *Biostatistics, 8*(4), 695-707.

Schena, M. (2003). *Microarray analysis*. New Jersey: John Wiley & Sons.

Soille, P. (1999). *Morphological image analysis: principles and applications*. Berlin, Heidelberg: Springer Verlag.

Speed, T. (2003). *Statistical Analysis of Gene Expression Microarray Data*. Chapman & Hall/CRC.

Storey, J. D., & Tibshirani, R. (2003). Statistical significance for genomewide studies. *Proc. Nat. Acad. Sci., 100*, 9440-9445.

Subramanian, A., Tamayo, P., Mootha, V. K., Mukherjee, S., Ebert, B. L., Gillette, M. A., Paulovich, A., Pomeroy, S. L., Golub, T. R., Lander, E. S., & Mesirov, J. P. (2005). Gene Set Enrichment Analysis: A Knowledge-Based Approach for Interpreting Genome-Wide Expression Profiles. *Proc. Nat. Acad. Sci. 102*, 15545-15550.

Tarca, A. L., Romero, R., & Draghici, S. (2006). Analysis of microarray experiments of gene expression profiling. *Am J Obstet Gynecol, 195*(2), 373-388.

Torkkola, K., Gardner, R. M., Kaysser-Kranich, T., & Ma, C. (2001). Self-Organizing Maps in Mining Gene Expression Data. *Information Sciences, 139*, 79-96.

Tseng, G. C., Oh, M. K., Rohlin, L., Liao, J. C., & Wong, W. H. (2001). Issues in cDNA Microarray Analysis: Quality Filtering, Channel Normalization, Models of Variations and Assessment of Gene Effects. *Nucleic Acids Research, 29,* 2549-2557.

Troyanskaya, O., Cantor, M., Sherlock, G., Brown, P., Hastie, T., Tibshirani, R., Botstein, D., & Altman, R. B., (2001). Missing Value Estimation Methods for DNA Microarrays. *Bioinformatics 17,* 520-525.

Tusher, V. G., Tibshirani, R., & Chum, G. (2001). Significance Analysis of Microarrays Applied to the Ionizing Radiation Response. *Proc. Nat. Acad. Sci., 98,* 5116-5121.

Tzouvelekis, A., Harokopos, V., Paparountas, T., Oikonomou, N., Chatziioannou, A., Vilaras, G., Tsiambas, E., Karameris, A., Bouros, D., & Aidinis, V. (2007). Comparative expression lprofiling in pulmonary fibrosis suggests a role of hypoxia-inducible factor-1α in disease pathogenesis. *American Journal of Respiratory and Critical Care Medicine, 176*(11), 1108-1119.

Wu, Z., Irizarry, R., Gentleman, R. C., Murillo, F. M., & Spencer, F. (2004). A Model Based Background Adjustment for Oligonucleotide Expression Arrays. *Collection of Biostatistics Research Archive, 1.*

Yang, Y. H., Buckley, M. J., & Speed, T. P. (2001). Analysis of cDNA microarray images. *Brief Bioinform, 2*(4), 341-349.

Yang, Y. H., Dudoit, S., Luu, P., Lin, D. M., Peng, V., Ngai, J., & Speed, T. P. (2002). Normalization for cDNA Microarray Data: A Robust Composite Method Addressing Single and Multiple Slide Systematic Variation. *Nucleic Acids Research, 30*(15).

Yeung, K. W., & Ruzzo, W. L. (2001). Principal Component Analysis for Clustering Gene Expression Data. *Bioinformatics, 9,* 763-774.

KEY TERMS

Addressing or Gridding: The process of assigning coordinates to each of the spots for a spotted or bead array or the alignment of a rectangular lattice in order to map pixel elements to specific probes in Affymetrix arrays.

DNA Microarray: Normally a slide made of silica or synthetic materials where on top an ordered array of oligonucleotide clones is imprinted, corresponding to regions of all discovered or putative genes of an organism's genome, which allows the specific binding of genes or gene products.

Meta-Analysis: The exhaustive search process which comprises numerous and versatile algorithmic procedures to exploit the gene expression results by combining or further processing them with sophisticated statistical learning and data mining techniques coupled with annotated information concerning functional properties of these genes residing in large databases.

Missing Value Imputation: The estimation of missing probe values for a gene by the expression of other probes over the rest of the slides, based on certain statistical or geometrical criteria.

Normalization: The set of processes applied to compensate for systematic errors among genes or arrays in order to derive meaningful biological comparisons.

Segmentation: The process of classification of the area regarding a specific spot on the array to permit the distinction of the spot pixels either as foreground, or background.

Signal Information Exctraction: The process of calculating foreground and background intensities, based on the respective pixel distributions derived from the segmentation step.

Chapter XIX
Image Processing and Machine Learning Techniques for the Segmentation of cDNA Microarray Images

Nikolaos Giannakeas
University of Ioannina, Greece

Dimitrios I. Fotiadis
University of Ioannina, Greece

ABSTRACT

Microarray technology allows the comprehensive measurement of the expression level of many genes simultaneously on a common substrate. Typical applications of microarrays include the quantification of expression profiles of a system under different experimental conditions, or expression profile comparisons of two systems for one or more conditions. Microarray image analysis is a crucial step in the analysis of microarray data. In this chapter an extensive overview of the segmentation of the microarray image is presented. Methods already presented in the literature are classified into two main categories: methods which are based on image processing techniques and those which are based on Machine learning techniques. A novel classification-based application for the segmentation is also presented to demonstrate efficiency.

INTRODUCTION

Several types of microarrays have been developed to address different biological processes: (i) cDNA microarrays (Eisen, 1999) are used for the monitoring of the gene expression levels to study the effects of certain treatments, diseases, and developmental stages on gene expression. As a result, microarray gene expression profiling can be used to identify disease genes by comparing gene expression in diseased and normal cells. (ii) Comparative genomic hybridization application assesses genome content in different cells or closely related organisms (Pollack et al., 1999). (iii) SNP detection arrays identify single nucleotide polymorphism among alleles within or between populations (Moran & Whitney, 2004). (iv) Finally, Chromatin immunoprecipitation (chIP) technologies determine protein binding site occupancy throughout the genome, employing ChIP-on-chip technology (Buck & Lieb, 2004).

The experiment of cDNA microarrays typically starts by taking two biological tissues and extracting their mRNA. The mRNA samples are reverse transcribed into complementary DNA (cDNA) and labelled with fluorescent dyes resulting in a fluorescence-tagged cDNA. The most common dyes for tagging cDNA are the red fluorescent dye Cy5 (emission from 630-660 nm) and the green-fluorescent dye Cy3 (emission from 510-550 nm). Next, the tagged cDNA copy, called the sample probe, is hybridized on a slide containing a grid or array of single-stranded cDNAs called probes. Probes are usually known genes of interest which were printed on a glass microscope slide by a robotic arrayer. According to the hybridization principles, a sample probe will only hybridize with its complementary probe. The probe-sample hybridization process on a microarray typically occurs after several hours. All unhybridized sample probes are then washed off and the microarray is scanned twice, at different wavelengths corresponding to the different dyes used in the assay. The digital image scanner records the intensity level at each grid location producing two greyscale images. The intensity level is correlated with the absolute amount of RNA in the original sample, and thus, the expression level of the gene associated with this RNA.

Automated quantification of gene expression levels is realized analyzing the microarray images. Microarray images contain several blocks (or subgrids) which consist of a number of spots, placed in rows and columns (Fig. 1). The level of intensity of each spot represents the amount of sample which is hybridized with the corresponding gene. The processing of microarray images (Schena et al., 1995) includes three stages: initially, spots and blocks are preliminarily located from the images (gridding). Second, using the available gridding information, each microarray spot is individually segmented into foreground and background. Finally, intensity extraction,

Figure 1. A Block of a Typical Microarray Image

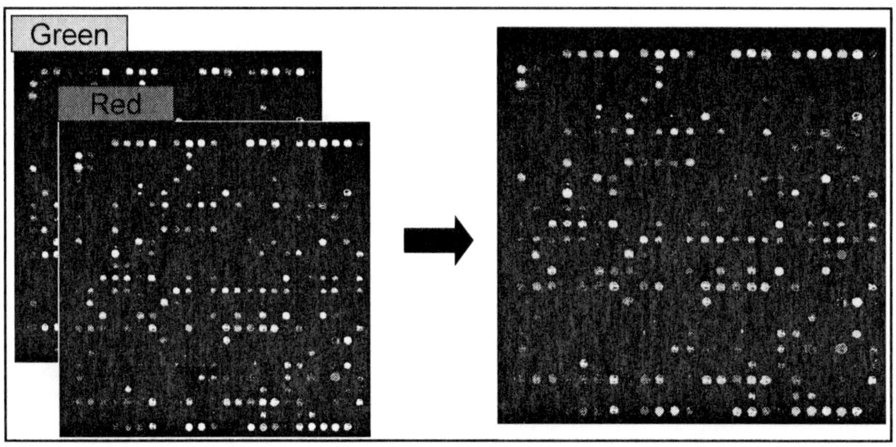

calculates the foreground fluorescence intensity, which represents each gene expression level, and the background intensities. Ideally, the image analysis would be a rather trivial process, if all the spots had circular shape, similar size, and the background was noise and artefact free. However, a scanned microarray image has none of the above characteristics, thus microarray image analysis becomes a difficult task. In this chapter, we describe several microarray segmentation algorithms based on image processing and machine learning techniques.

BACKGROUND

Resent studies in microarrays have been shown that segmentation methods can significantly influence microarray data precision (Ahmed et al., 2004). Several methods have been proposed for the segmentation of microarray images. These methods can be classified into four categories: (i) Fixed and adaptive circle, (ii) histogram-based, (iii) adaptive shape, (iv) clustering. The first three categories are based on image processing techniques, while the fourth is based on machine learning. Fig. 2 shows an overview of the already developed methods for microarray image segmentation. Earliest approaches fit a circle (with fixed or adaptive size) around each spot, characterizing the pixels in the circle as signal pixels and the pixels out of the circle as background pixels. Such an approach is used by Scanalyse (Eisen, 1999) and Dapple (Buhler et al., 2000). Histogram-based techniques estimate a threshold (GSI Lumonics, 1999; Chen et al., 1997), such that pixels with intensity lower than the calculated threshold are characterized as background pixels, whereas pixels with higher intensity as signal pixels. The adaptive shape segmentation methods are usually based on the Watershed Transform (Siddiqui et al., 2002) and the Seed Region Growing algorithm (Buckley, 2000; Wang et al., 2001). The most recent techniques employ clustering algorithms such as K-means (Bozinov & Rahnenführer, 2002; Ergüt et al., 2003; Wu & Yan, 2004), Fuzzy C-Means (FCM) (Ergüt et al., 2003), Expectation-Maximization (EM) (Blekas et al., 2005) and Partitioning Around Medoid (PAM) (Nagarajan, 2003). A hybrid method (Rahnenführer & Bozinov, 2004) which engages Image Processing and Machine learning techniques has been proposed. In this chapter we address a pixel by pixel classification approach for the segmentation of microarray images. The current application, which is presented in section 4, classifies the pixels of the image into two categories (foreground and background) using the Bayes classifier. Already developed clustering techniques generate groups of pixels, characterizing these pixels as signal or background using a set of rules, i.e. the group with the maximum mean intensity value is characterized as signal. Instead of this, the current approach directly classifies each pixel to the designated category.

MICROARRAY SEGMENTATION METHODS

Image Processing Techniques

Fixed or Adaptive Circle Segmentation

Fixed circle segmentation is the earliest method developed for microarray image analysis. This algorithm is implemented by Eisen et al, (Eisen, 1999) and it is included in the ScanAnalyze software tool. The method assumes that all the spots are circular with a constant radius. A circular mask of a fixed radius, called target mask, is placed on each spot location, considering all the pixels inside the mask as foreground pixels. On the other hand, background contains any external pixel which is close to the corresponding spot. Fig. 3 shows the way that masks are placed on each spot using the ScanAlyze software.

The elimination of the constant radius assumption was the next step in microarray image analysis studies, generating the adaptive circle algorithm. Assuming that the shape of all spots is circular, the radius for each spot is automatically estimated or manually adjusted by the user, for each spot. For instance, Dapple (Buhler et al., 2000) estimates the radius of the spot using the Laplacian-based edge detection. The manual approaches are extremely difficult and time consuming due to the large amount of microarray spots contained in a single image.

Histogram-Based Segmentation

The methods inn this category are based on the histogram of the image. Histogram-based approaches fix a circular mask on each spot, which is larger than the spot size, and then a threshold value of the pixel intensity is computed to seperate the foreground and background pixels within the mask. QuantArray software (GSI Lumonics, 1999) calculates the threshold globally from the

Figure 2. Current status of microarray image segmentation methods.

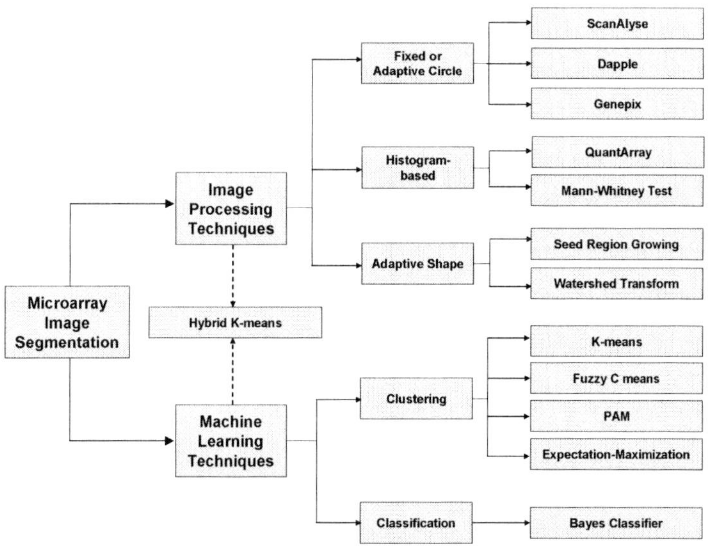

Figure 3. ScanAlyze image segmentation

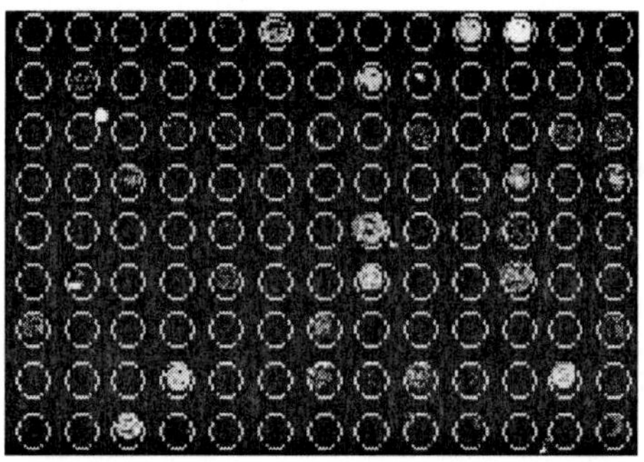

histogram for all pixels within the masked area, while UCSF Spot software (Jain et al., 2002) estimates locally the threshold using the percentile cut-off. These methods can be unstable since the circular mask could be too large and it can cover neighbouring spots. In addition, adaptive thresholding segmentation methods do not provide the expected results when the signal is weak because there is no marked transition between foreground and background.

To overcome these difficulties, Chen et al. proposed a pixel selection method based on the Mann-Whitney test (Mann & Whitney, 1947). The Mann-Whitney test is a non-parametric statistical test for assessing the statistical significance of the difference between two distributions. The method associates a confidence level with every intensity measurement based on the significance level of the test. Each iteration of the algorithm calculates the threshold value between foreground and background pixels. At the first step, a circular target mask is placed in order to enclose all possible foreground pixels separating them from the background. A set of pixels from the background is randomly selected and compared against the pixels with the lowest intensity within the target mask. If the difference between the two sets is not significant, the algorithm discards some predetermined number of pixels from the target area and selects new pixels for investigation. Each iteration ends when the two sets significantly differ from each other, and the signal pixels are considered as the pixels remaining inside the target mask.

Adaptive Shape Segmentation

More sophisticated image processing techniques comprise the adaptive shape segmentation. These methods include no assumption on the size and the shape of the spot. The Seed Region Growing (SRG) algorithm (Adams & Bischof, 1994) selects randomly a small set of pixels, called seeds, as the initial points of a region in the area of each spot. At each iteration, the algorithm considers simultaneously the neighbouring pixels of every region grown from a seed. The neighbouring pixels are ordered under several criteria. The most common criterion uses only the intensity of the neighbouring pixels and the mean intensity of the growing region. This criterion C is defined as:

$$C(i) = \left| I(i) - \overline{I_s} \right|, \qquad (1)$$

where S refers to the growing region, $I(i)$ is the intensity of the pixel i which is neighbour to the region S, and $\overline{I_s}$ is the mean intensity of the growing region S at the current iteration.

Next, the algorithm finds the region's neighbouring pixel m which corresponds to the minimum criterion C and labels it as a region pixel or as a boundary pixel between two regions. If all the neighbours of m belong to a single region, m is also labelled to the region. Therefore if m has only one neighbour that belongs to another region, m is marked as boundary pixel. The algorithm iterates until all pixels have been assigned to a region or labelled as boundary pixels.

Another adaptive shape segmentation method is based on the Watershed Transform (WT) (Roerdink & Meijster, 2000). WT is a popular segmentation method which originates from mathematical morphology. The image is considered as a topographical relief, where the height of each point is related to its grey level, resulting to a topological relief with many wells in the position where spots are located, as it is shown in Fig. 4.

Imaginary rain falls on the terrain. The watersheds are the lines separating the catchment basins. The output of the watershed algorithm is a tessellation of the input image into its different catchment basins, each one characterized by a unique label. The pixels that belong to the watershed lines are assigned a special label. Siddiqui et al. (Siddiqui et al., 2002) had implemented a segmentation method where the watershed transform is applied to the gradient of the image (Serra, 1982) and not to the original one. The gradient operator is very sensitive to grayscale variation

Figure 4. A microarray image represented as a topographical relief

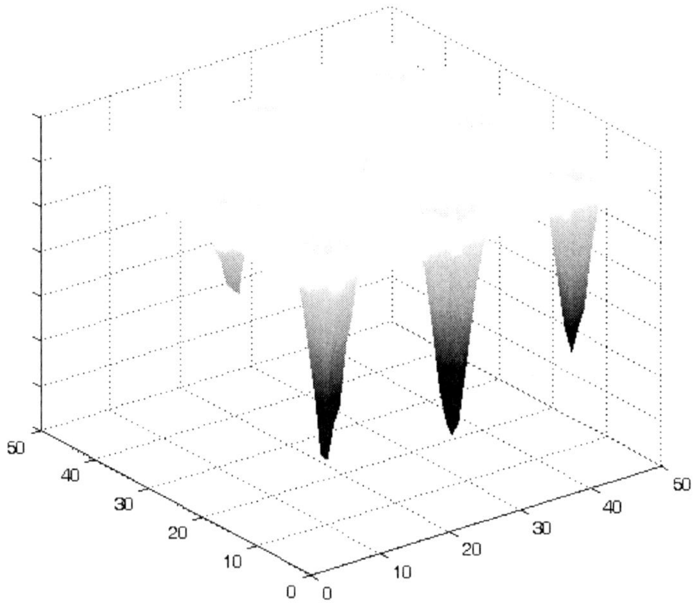

and noise and it can cause development of a large number of irrelevant catchment basins. However, these oversegmentation problems can be overcome using watershed transform techniques without any additional computational effort.

Machine Learning Based Segmentation

Nowadays, traditional image processing techniques have to cope with more complex problems in the fields of medical informatics and bioinformatics. The integration of machine learning in image processing is very likely to have a great benefit to the field, which will contribute to a better analysis of medical and biological data. Microarray image analysis methods have already employed several machine learning techniques in order to segment the image. Clustering is the most common technique that is used for the segmentation of the microarray images. The idea of the clustering application is to divide the pixels of the image into several clusters (usually two clusters) and then to characterize these clusters as signal or background. Clustering algorithms, such as K-means, Fuzzy C-Means, Expectation-Maximization etc. have been employed in several microarray imaging segmentation studies.

The K-means segmentation algorithm is based on the traditional K-means clustering (MacQueen, 1967). It employs a square-error criterion, which is calculated for each of the two clusters. The square error criterion for the two clusters is given as:

$$E^2 = \sum_{k=1}^{2} e_k^2, \qquad (2)$$

where

$$e_k^2 = \sum_{i=1}^{n_k} \left(x_{ik} - M_k\right)^2, \qquad k = 1,2 \qquad (3)$$

and x_{ik} is the feature vector of the ith pixel , n_k is the number of pixels which belong to the kth cluster and M_k are the centroids of the kth cluster, respectively:

$$M_k = \left(\frac{1}{n_k}\right)\sum_{i=1}^{n_k} x_{ik}. \quad (4)$$

K-means is commonly fed with the intensity of each pixel in the microarray image as features. However, there is already developed segmentation methods based on the K-means algorithm, which use more intensity features of each pixel (such as mean intensity of the neighbourhood of the pixel, or spatial features). For instance, Ergüt et al. (Ergüt et al., 2003) employed the K-means algorithm using only the intensity of the pixel as a feature, while Wu et al. (Wu & Yan, 2004) used three intensity-based features as well as the Euclidean distance between the pixel and the center of the spot, as the fourth feature. Both the channels of the microarray image are segmented simultaneously. Thus, for each pixel the intensities from both channels are combined to one feature vector. The number of cluster centres K is set usually to two, due to the fact that the segmentation is used for characterizing the pixels of the image as foreground or background pixels.

A number of studies employ the Fuzzy C-Means (FCM) (Bezdek, 1981), instead of the crisp K-means algorithm. FCM is a data clustering technique in which a dataset is grouped into K clusters with each data point in the dataset belonging to a cluster to a certain degree. For example, a certain pixel that lies close to the centroid of a signal cluster will have a high degree of belonging or membership to that cluster and another pixel that lies far away from the centroid of a cluster will have a low degree of membership to that cluster.

The FCM algorithm is based on the minimization of the following objective function:

$$J_m = \sum_{i}^{n_k}\sum_{k=1}^{3}(u_{ik})^{\gamma}\left\|x_{ik} - M_k\right\|^2, \quad (5)$$

where, x_{ik} is the feature vector of the ith pixel, M_k is the centroid of each cluster, u_{ik} is the degree of membership of x_{ik} in each cluster, $\left\|x_{ik} - M_k\right\|^2$ is the Euclidean distance between x_{ik} and M_k, n_k is the number of the pixels that belong to the kth cluster. The parameter γ is the weighting exponent for u_{ik} which controls the fuzziness of the resulting clusters. Each pixel is classified in the cluster with the maximum calculated membership function.

A more robust than K-means and FCM clustering technique is the Partition Around Medoids (PAM) (Kaufman & Rousseeuw, 1989) clustering. PAM minimizes a sum of dissimilarities instead of a sum of squared Euclidean distances. The algorithm first computes a number of representative objects, called medoids. A medoid can be defined as that object of a cluster, whose average dissimilarity to all the objects in the cluster is minimal. In the classification literature, such representative objects are called centrotypes. After finding the set of medoids, each object of the dataset is assigned to the nearest medoid. Nagarajan et al. (Nagarajan, 2003) developed a segmentation method based on the PAM to extract the target intensity of the spots. The distribution of the pixel intensity in a grid containing a spot is assumed to be the superposition of the foreground and the local background. The partitioning around medoids is used to generate a binary partition of the pixel intensity distribution. The medoid (PAM) of the cluster members are chosen as the cluster representatives.

According to the assumption that the pixels of the image could be grouped in several clusters in order to extract the signal and background of a microarray image, more sophisticated methods had been proposed in the literature. Blekas et al. (Blekas et al., 2005) proposed a Gaussian Mixture Model (GMM) approach for the analysis of the microarray images using the Expectation-Maximization (EM) (Dempster et al., 1977) algorithm. EM is an ideal candidate for solving parameter estimation problems for the GMM or other neural networks. This methodology provides modelling, flexibility and adaptability to the data, which are well-known strengths of GMM. The maximum likelihood and maximum a posteriori approaches are used to estimate the GMM parameters via the expectation-maximization algorithm. The approach has the ability to detect and compensate for artefacts that might occur in microarray images. This is accomplished by a model-based criterion that selects the number of the mixture components.

Hybrid K-Means Segmentation

Finally, it is meaningful to refer a work presented by Rahnenführer et al. (Rahnenführer & Bozinov, 2004) who tried to engage both the image processing and the machine learning techniques. The hybrid K-means algorithm is an extended version of the K-means segmentation approach (Bozinov & Rahnenführer, 2002). The machine learning contribution includes repeated clustering in order to increase the number of foreground pixels. As long as the minimum amount of foreground pixels is not reached, the remaining background pixels are clustered into two groups and the group with pixels of higher intensity is assigned as foreground. After the clustering, the number of outlier pixels in the segmentation result is reduced with mask matching.

CLASSIFICATION-BASED APPLICATION

Segmentation Using the Bayes Classifier

In this section a novel segmentation method that classifies the pixels of the image into two categories (foreground and background) using classification techniques is presented. This classification-based approach directly classifies each pixel to the designated category. More specifically, the Bayes classifier (Gonzalez et al., 2004) is employed to classify the pixels of the image into different classes. The Bayes Classifier is fed with an informative set of 11 features (Table 1) (Giannakeas & Fotiadis, 2007) to deal with the artefacts of the image. Thus, the method can classify the pixels of the image into signal, background and artefacts.

Table 1. Features for the classification segmentation

FEATURE TYPE	CHANNEL		DESCRIPTION
Intensity features	GREEN	1	Intensity of the pixel
		2	Mean intensity value of the 3x3 neighbourhood of the pixel
		3	Intensity standard deviation of the 3x3 neighbourhood of the pixel
	RED	4	Intensity of the pixel
		5	Mean intensity value of the 3x3 neighbourhood of the pixel
		6	Intensity standard deviation of the 3x3 neighbourhood of the pixel
Spatial Features		7	x-coordinate of the pixel in the image
		8	y-coordinate of the pixel in the image
		9	Euclidean distance between the pixel and the centre of the spot
Shape features	GREEN	10	Correlation of the neighbourhood of the pixel and the Gaussian template
	RED	11	Correlation of the neighbourhood of the pixel and the Gaussian template

The concept of the Bayes classifier is to estimate the a posteriori probability of a sample (pixel) to belong in a class. The a posteriori probability is given by the Bayes theorem:

$$P(w_i \mid x) = \frac{p(x \mid w_i)P(w_i)}{\sum_{i=1}^{2} p(x \mid w_i)P(w_i)} = \frac{p(x \mid w_i)P(w_i)}{p(x)}, \quad (6)$$

where, $x \in R^{11}$ is the feature vector, w_i: $i = 1,2$ are the two classes, $P(w_i)$ is the a priori probability that an arbitrary sample belongs to class w_i, $P(w_i \mid x)$ is the a posteriori conditional probability that a specific sample belongs to a class, $p(x)$ is the density distribution of all samples, and $p(x|w_i)$ is the conditional density distribution of all samples belonging to w_i.

The Gaussian density function is often used to model the distribution of feature values of a particular class. The general multivariate Gaussian density function is given as:

$$p(x) = \frac{1}{(2\pi)^{D/2}\left|\Sigma_i\right|^{1/2}} e^{-\frac{1}{2}(x-\mu_i)^T \Sigma_i^{-1}(x-\mu_i)}, \quad (7)$$

where D is the dimension of the feature vector (D=11 in our case). μ_i and Σ_i are the mean vector and the covariance matrix of the features of the corresponding class respectively:

$$\mu_i = \frac{1}{N_i}\sum_{x \in w_i} x, \qquad \mu_i \in R^{11}, \quad (8)$$

$$\Sigma_i = \frac{1}{N_i}\sum_{x \in w_i} xx^T - \mu_i\mu_i^T, \qquad \Sigma_i \in R^{11\times 11}, \quad (9)$$

where N_i is the number of pixels belonging to class w_i.

In the training stage, the proposed approach estimates the mean vector and the covariance matrix for each class. Given the mean vector, the covariance matrix and the gaussian density distribution, the a posteriori probability is estimated for each sample and each class in the testing stage. The pixel is classified to the class with the maximum a posteriori probability.

Results

To quantify the effectiveness of the classification-based approach an image from the Stanford Microarray Database (SMD) (Gollub et al., 2003) is used. This image includes 16 blocks and each block consists of 576 spots, forming 24x24 rows and columns. Two of the blocks are used for the training (1152 spots and ~350000 pixels) and 14 blocks for the testing (5184 spots and ~3500000 pixels). In order to extract pixel by pixel information from the annotation, we simulate the fixed circle segmentation that is used by Scanalyse. For this task, the known radius of the fixed circle and the coordinates of the centres of each spot are used. Thus, a binary map is generated for the whole block, characterizing the pixels inside the circle as signal pixels and the pixel outside of the circle as background.

Table 2 presents the overall accuracy, specificity and selectivity of classification based methodology while the Table 3 shows the results of the Bayes classification in each individual spot. The accuracy, the specificity and the sensitivity of the proposed method is defined as:

Table 2. Accuracy results for the classification-based segmentation

Images	Training	Training	Acc %	Sp %	Se %
Experiment lc4b007rex2	2 Blocks (1152 spots)	14 Blocks (8050 spots)	86.28	90.21	82.21

Table 3. Results of the classification-based segmentation in individual spots

Description	Red	Green	Annotation	Result
Expressed spot	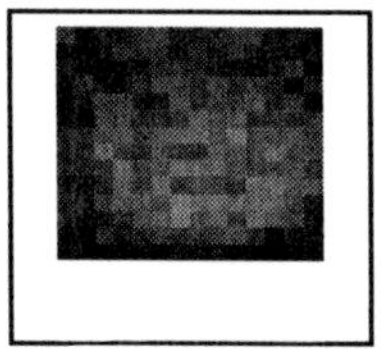	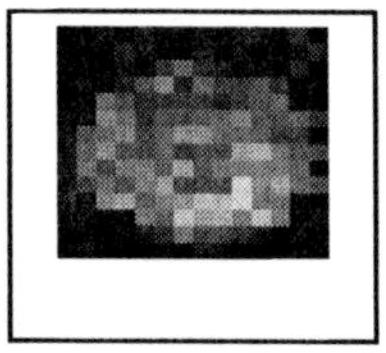	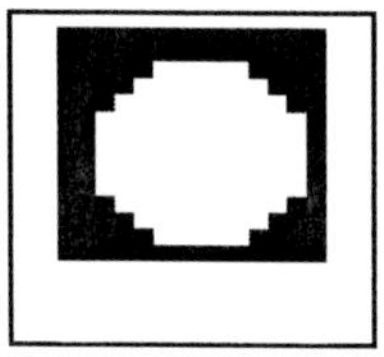	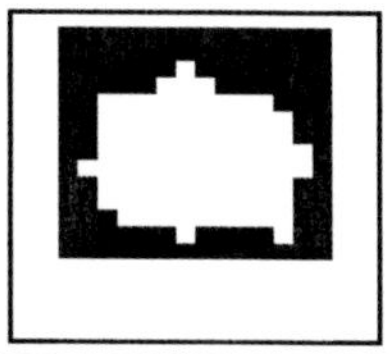
Low expressed spot	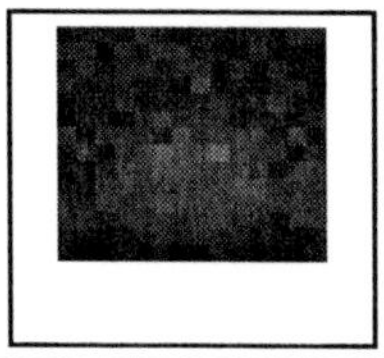	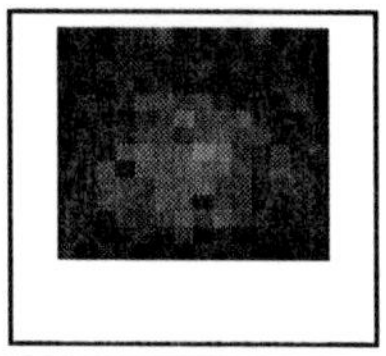	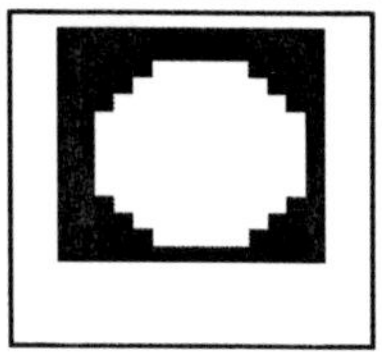	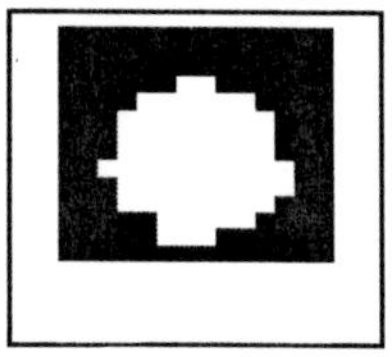
High expressed spot	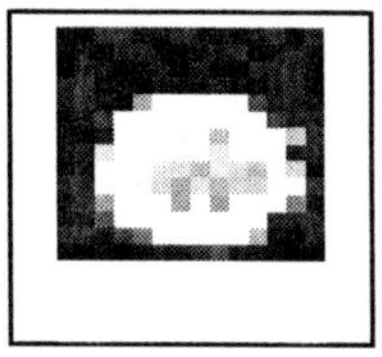	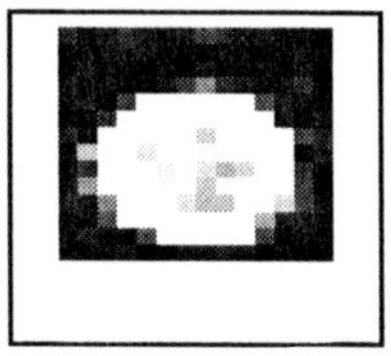	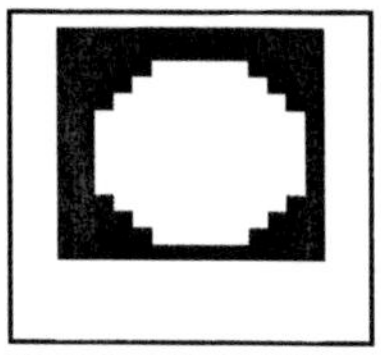	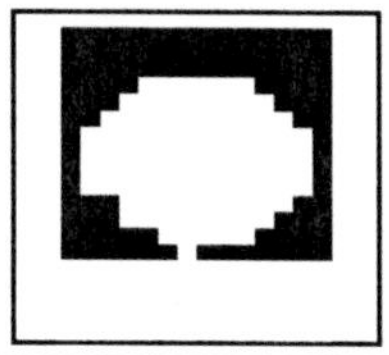

$$Acc = \frac{\#\ of\ correctly\ detected\ pixels}{total\ \#\ of\ pixels\ in\ the\ image}, \quad (10)$$

$$Sp = \frac{\#of\ correctly\ identified\ signal\ pixels}{total\ \#\ of\ signal\ pixels}, \quad (11)$$

$$Se = \frac{\#of\ correctly\ identified\ background\ pixels}{total\ \#\ of\ background\ pixels}. \quad (12)$$

In Table 3, three different types of spot are selected for illustration, expressed, low expressed and high expressed spot.

The current classification-based method detects efficiently the signal and the background pixels as it is shown in Table 2. We also have to stress that better results are reported for specificity as it is shown in Table 3. The main reason for this is the imbalanced dataset, i.e. it contains a large number of background pixels compared to the signal ones.

To compare the clustering-based techniques versus the classification based one four clustering approaches based on the K-means and the FCM algorithms are employed. Initially, both of these algorithms are fed with only the intensity of the two channels of the image. Then all the features of Table 1 are used. The accuracy results are shown in Table IV. As it is shown in this Table, the reported accuracy of the Bayes classifier is quite better than the other four approaches. In addition, the specificity (Sp) of the background class is extremely increased using the supervised classification-based segmentation.

FUTURE TRENDS

Future trends in the field of microarray technology could include: (1) The manufacturing and use of simpler arrays for quick and more-accurate-clinical diagnoses. (2) The acceptance of national (if not international) standards for array manufacturing, scanning, and analysis, and (3) The emergence and increasing use of smaller nano-arrays.

Accordingly, investigation and future challenges are generated for the computer-based

Table 4. Comparison of clustering and classification-based methods

Method	Acc %	Signal Sp %	Background Sp %
K-means (2 features)	65.49	88.14	41.95
K-means (11 features)	73.85	91.36	55.66
FCM (2 features)	65.88	87.21	43.71
FCM (11 features)	74.20	**90.94**	56.79
Bayes (11 features)	**86.28**	90.21	**82.21**

analysis of the microarrays. The development of new intelligent image processing techniques to eliminate the noise sources inherent in the DNA microarray process becomes more challenging. Additionally, the development of advanced image processing methodologies is significant to speed up the real-time diagnosis and implementation procedures of the next generation of system-on-a-chip devices. The extension of the machine leaning applications in the field of microarray image processing could provide more robust and effective tools for these purposes. Those methods can ultimately provide a new generation of diagnostic systems that can help to unlock the unknown patterns of complex diseases and their molecular phenotypes and allow rapid and responsive treatment mechanisms for these diseases.

CONCLUSION

An overview of the already developed methods for microarray is presented in this chapter. We categorized all the methods into two main categories, earlier approaches which use image processing techniques and approaches which use Machine learning techniques such as clustering. Image processing is an important stage in the circle of life of a microarray experiment. Reliability of this stage strongly influences the results of data analysis performed on extracted gene expressions. Several methods related to image processing or Machine learning techniques have been developed in this area. In this chapter we emphasized to the significance of the classification-based techniques for the segmentation of microarray image analysis. A Bayes classifier is presented to demonstrate the effectiveness of the classification techniques. According to the promising accuracy results, the precision of the microarray data during the next steps of the experiment might be significantly influenced.

REFERENCES

Adams, R., & Bischof, L. (1994). Seeded region growing. *IEEE Trans. on Pat. Anal. and Mach. Intell., 16*, 641–647.

Ahmed, A. A., Vias, M., Iyer, N. G., Caldas, C., & Brenton J. D. (2004). Microarray segmentation methods signifficantly influence data precision. *Nucleic Acids Research, 32*, e50.

Bezdek, J. C. (1981). Pattern Recognition with Fuzzy Objective Function Algorithms. *Plenum Press.* New York.

Blekas, K., Galatsanos, N., Likas, A., & Lagaris, I. E. (2005). Mixture Model Analysis of DNA

Microarray Images. *IEEE Transactions on Medical Imaging, 24*(7), 901-909.

Bozinov, D., & Rahnenführer, J. (2002). Unsupervised Technique for Robust Target Separation and Analysis of DNA Microarray Spots Through Adaptive Pixel Clustering. *Bioinformatics, 18*(5), 747-756.

Buck, M. J., & Lieb, J. D. (2004). ChIP-chip: considerations for the design, analysis, and application of genome-wide chromatin immunoprecipitation experiments. *Genomics, 83*, 349-360.

Buckley, M. J. (2000). Spot User's Guide. *CSIRO Mathematical and Information Sciences,* Australia,. from http://www.cmis.csiro.au/iap/Spot/spotmanual.htm

Buhler, J., Ideker, T., & Haynor D. (2000). Dapple: improved techniques for finding spots on DNA microarrays. (UWCSE Tech Rep). Washington: *UWTR Dept. of Computer Science and Eng.,* University of Washington.

Chen, Y., Dougherty, E. R., & Bittner, M. L. (1997). Ratio-Based Decisions and the Quantitative Analysis of cDNA Microarray Images. *Journal Of Biomedical Optics*, *2*(4), 364–374.

Dempster, A., Laird, N., & Rubin, D. (1977). Maximum likelihood from incomplete data via the EM algorithm. *Journal of the Royal Statistical Society, 39*(1), 1-38.

Eisen, M. B. (1999). *ScanAlyse.* form http://rana.Stanford.EDU/software/

Eisen, M. B., & Brown, P. O. (1999). DNA Arrays for Analysis of Gene Expression. *Methods Enzymol, 303*, 179-205.

Ergüt, E., Yardimci, Y., Mumcuoglu, E., & Konu, O. (2003). Analysis of microarray images using FCM and K-means clustering algorithm. *In IJCI 2003*, (pp. 116-121).

Giannakeas, N., & Fotiadis, D. I. (2007). Multichannel Segmentation of cDNA Microarray Images using the Bayes Classifier. *In 29th Annual International Conference of the IEEE Engineering in Medicine and Biology Society.* Lyon, France.

Gollub, J., Ball, C. A., Binkley, G., Demeter, K., Finkelstein, D. B., Hebert, J. M., Hernandez-Boussard, T., Jin, H., Kaplper, M., Matese, J. C., Schroeder, M., Brown, P. O., Botstein, D., & Sherlock, G. (2003). The Stanford Microarray Database: data access and quality assessment tools. *Nucleic Acids Res., 31*, 94-96.

Gonzalez, R. C., Woods, R. E., & Eddins, S. L. (2004). Digital image processing using MATLAB. *Prentice Hall, Upper Saddle River,* NJ.

GSI Lumonics (1999). *QuantArray Analysis Software*. Operator's Manual.

Jain, A. N., Tokuyasu, T. A., Snijders, A. M., Segraves, R., Albertson, D. G., & Pinkel, D. (2002). Fully automatic quantification of microarray image data. *Genome Research, 12*, 325–332.

Kaufman, L., & Rousseeuw, P. J. (1989). Finding Groups in Data - An Introduction to Cluster Analysis. *Wiley,* NY.

MacQueen, J. B. (1967). Some Methods for classification and Analysis of Multivariate Observations. *In 5-th Berkeley Symposium on Mathematical Statistics and Probability, 1,* 281-297. Berkeley: University of California Press.

Mann, H. B., & Whitney, D. R. (1947). On a test of whether one of two random variables is stochastically larger than the other. *Annals of Mathematical Statistics, 18*, 50-60.

Moran, G., Stokes, C., Thewes, S., Hube, B., Coleman, D. C., & Sullivan, D. (2004). Comparative genomics using Candida albicans DNA microarrays reveals absence and divergence of virulence-associated genes in Candida dubliniensis. *Microbiology, 150*, 3363-3382.

Nagarajan, R. (2003). Intensity-Based Segmentation of Microarray Images. *IEEE Trans. On Medical Imaging, 22*(7), 882–889.

Pollack, J. R., Perou, C. M., Alizadeh, A. A., Eisen, M. B., Pergamenschikov, A., Williams, C. F., Jeffrey, S. S., Botstein, D., & Brown, P. O. (1999). Genome-wide analysis of DNA copy-number changes using cDNA microarrays. *Nat Genet, 23*, 41-46.

Rahnenführer, J., & Bozinov, V. (2004). Hybrid clustering for microarray image analysis combining intensity and shape features. *BMC Bioinformatics, 5*, 47.

Roerdink, J. B. T. M., & Meijster, A. (2000). The watershed transform: definitions, algorithms and parallelization strategies. *Fundamenta Informaticae, 41*(1-2), 187-228.

Schena, M., Shalon, D., Davis, R. W., & Brown, P. O. (1995). Quantitative motoring of gene expression patterns with a complementary DNA Microarray. *Science, 270*, 467-470.

Serra, J. (1982). *Image Analysis and Mathematical Morphology*. London, England: Academic Press.

Siddiqui, K. I., Hero, A., & Siddiqui, M. (2002). Mathematical Morphology applied to Spot Segmentation and Quantification of Gene Microarray Images. *In. Asilomar Conference on Signals and Systems.*

Wang, X., Ghosh, S., & Guo, S. W. (2001). Quantitative quality control in microarray image processing and data acquisition. *Nucleic Acids Research, 29*(15), e75.

Wu, H., & Yan, H. (2003). Microarray Image Processing Based on Clustering and Morphological Analysis. *In First Asia Pacific Bioinformatics Conference*, (pp. 111-118).

KEY TERMS

Block: Blocks are also known as grids or subgrids. These are areas of the microarray slide (and relatively of the microarray image) in which a number of spots are located.

Classification: It is a procedure in which individual items are placed into groups based on quantitative information on one or more characteristics inherent in the items and based on a training set of previously labelled items.

Clustering: It is the task of decomposing or partitioning a dataset into groups so that the points in one group are similar to each other and are as different as possible from the points in the other groups.

Image Processing: The analysis of an image using techniques that can identify shades, colours and relationships that cannot be perceived by the human eye. In the biomedical field, image processing is used to produce medical diagnosis or to extract data for further analysis.

Machine Learning: It refers to the design and development of algorithms and techniques that allow computers to "learn". The purpose of machine learning is to extract information from several types of data automatically, using computational and statistical methods.

Microarray: Sets of miniaturized chemical reaction areas that may also be used to test DNA fragments, antibodies, or proteins, by using a chip having immobilised target and hybridising them with a probed sample.

Spot: It is a small and almost circular area in the microarray image whose mean intensity represents the expression level of the corresponding gene.

Chapter XX
Recent Advances in Automated Chromosome Image Analysis

Petros S. Karvelis
University of Ioannina, Greece

Dimitrios I. Fotiadis
University of Ioannina, Greece

ABSTRACT

Automated chromosome analysis is now becoming routine in most human cytogenetics laboratories. It involves both processing and analysis of digital images and has been developed because of the demand by cytogeneticists. Over the years, many techniques have been introduced for the automatic segmentation and classification of chromosome images, of which only a few are included in the available commercial systems. Today, advances in chromosome imaging techniques, especially in multispectral imaging, lead the way for the development of new and improved methods for the location, segmentation and classification of chromosome images by exploiting the color information. In this chapter the authors describe methods which have been already developed for automated chromosome analysis.

INTRODUCTION

Chromosomes

Chromosomes are structures that contain genes, which store in strings of DNA all the data necessary for an organism's development and maintenance. They contain vast amounts of information; in fact each cell in a normal human being contains 46 chromosomes which have 6×10^9 bits of information (Thompson, 1992). Chromosomes can only be examined visually during cell division (mitosis). They are extremely long and thin which make them essentially invisible. However, during the metaphase stage of mitosis, they contract and become much shorter (around 2–10μm) and wider (around 1–2 μm diameter), (Fig. 1(a)). At this stage, they can be stained to become visible and can be imaged by a microscope.

Chromosome analysis is the procedure from which chromosomes are photographed during cell division and then are assigned to each class. This procedure is called karyotyping, where chromosomes are aligned in pairs in a tabular array as it is shown in Fig. 1(b). Karyotyping is a useful tool to detect deviations from normal cell structure. Examples include peripheral blood, bone marrow, amniotic fluid, and products of conception. Normal human somatic cells have 46 chromosomes: 22 pairs of autosomes (chromosomes 1-22) and two sex chromosomes. Females carry two X chromosomes (46, XX), while males have a X and a Y (46, XY). Germ cells (egg and sperm) have 23 chromosomes: one copy of each autosome plus a single sex chromosome. This is referred to as the haploid number. One chromosome from each autosomal pair plus one sex chromosome is inherited from each parent. Mothers can contribute only an X chromosome to their children, while fathers can contribute either an X or a Y. Abnormal cells may have an excess or a deficit of chromosomes and/or structural defects which depict an exchange of genetic material.

Chromosome Abnormalities

Chromosome abnormalities can be very complex. There are two basic types of abnormalities: numerical and structural and both types can occur simultaneously. The most obvious abnormality is an unusual number of chromosomes. Having only one type of chromosome is a monosomy, such as Turner's syndrome, in which there is only one X chromosome and no Y. Having three chromosomes is a trisomy, such as Down's syndrome, in which there are three Type-21 chromosomes.

There can also be duplications of genetic material within a chromosome and translocations where two chromosomes exchange genetic information. The Philadelphia chromosome results from a translocation in the 9th and 22nd chromosomes. This is often associated with chronic myelogenous leukemia (Nowell, 1960). Detecting these abnormalities is vital because they are reliable indicators of genetic disease and damage. Chromosome abnormalities are particularly useful in cancer diagnosis and the related research (Gray, 1992).

Digital imaging has contributed to cytogenetics instrumentation reducing the workload in clinical labs and producing quantitative data for both research and diagnosis. The last few

Figure 1. (a) A slide of grayscale banded chromosomes and (b) their karyotype.

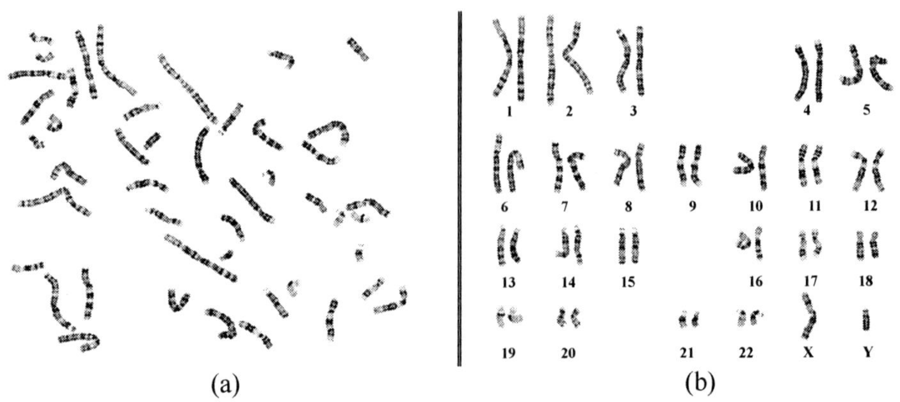

decades we have seen continuous endeavors in (a) the development of innovative image acquisition and enhancement methods on technologies that exploit our knowledge of the molecular basis of cancer or other diseases, and (b) the integration of these emerging genomic technologies with traditional imaging methods for more effective solutions for health care delivery. In this chapter we introduce the reader to the state of the art for automated methods in chromosome analysis.

BACKGROUND

The methods presented below are divided into two main categories based on the type of the image which is used.

Methods Based on Grayscale Chromosome Images

Grayscale chromosome imaging techniques developed in early 60s (Human Ch., 1960) and they were able to distinguish seven groups of chromosomes. This type of classification was known as Denver classification. On 1971, Giemsa staining technique was proposed and finally a unique banding pattern appeared on each chromosome type so that all 22 pairs of chromosomes and the X and Y chromosomes could be uniquely identified (Summer, 1971).

Segmentation

By the term segmentation we mean the segmentation of the image into background and objects of interest (which are the chromosomes). Although image segmentation could be automatic: the segmentation of touching and overlapping clusters of chromosomes (Ji, 1989) prevent this. These often consist of two or more chromosomes, either touching or overlapping with each other. Therefore, these objects must be further divided into the consisting chromosomes.

The methods developed for automated segmentation can be classified into three categories:

- **Thresholding methods** (Lundsteen, 1987; Piper, 1989): These methods choose automatically a threshold *T*. Pixels with intensity above or equal of *T* are considered as chromosome pixels and pixels with intensity lower of *T* are considered as background pixels. These methods cannot handle touching or overlapping chromosomes.
- **Valley or Pale path searching methods** (Ji, 1989; Vossepoel, 1987; Ji, 1994; Popescu, 1999): Valley searching methods try to find "valleys" of gray values called pale paths that represent separations of chromosomes. They are complex methods which depend on several parameters. Ji (Ji, 1989) was the first who introduced pale paths. The chromosome image is searched for clusters of chromosomes and then the pale path usually starts from a point of high curvature – cut point. When the pale path reaches the opposite side of the boundary of the cluster the procedure is terminated and the cluster is cut using the pale path. An example of a pale path is shown in Fig. 2. Later, Ji (Ji, 1994) used the concepts of skeletons and convex hulls to decompose overlaps. Vossepoel (Vossepoel, 1987) defined a set of rules to find candidate cut points and then to link points with a minimum-cost algorithm. This method often works well at finding accurate boundaries, but does not handle overlaps.
- **Model based methods** (Agam, 1997; Lerner, 1998; Carters, 1999; Carters, 2002): These methods first find all the touching chromosomes and then determine all lines starting from points of high curvature. These lines are used to cut the touching chromosomes and the objects derived are compared to prototypes. Agam et al. (Agam, 1997) used minsets to decompose touching and overlapping grayscale chromosomes. In

their work, they determined minsets using (rectangular) shape-based hypothesis testing to choose cut points for dividing clusters of chromosomes. Their method was successful in many cases but its application is limited to grayscale chromosome images.

- **Watershed based methods** (Graham, 1989; Karvelis 2005): Watershed based methods use the watershed algorithm (Vincent 1991) to decompose touching chromosomes. Graham et. al. (Graham 1989) proposed a split-and-merge technique to oversegment the image and combine segments only if they satisfy certain criteria, such as convexity. These methods are useful for decomposing touching chromosomes but they cannot handle overlaps.

Classification

Once the chromosome image is segmented, classification of the segmented regions follows. The goal of this step is to arrange the chromosomes into a karyotype such the one shown in Fig. 1(b) to be examined by the cytogeneticists. Features of the segmented regions are used to classify each region to a chromosome class. These features usually include: chromosome length, centromere index, and banding pattern.

Figure 2. Pale path separating two chromosomes

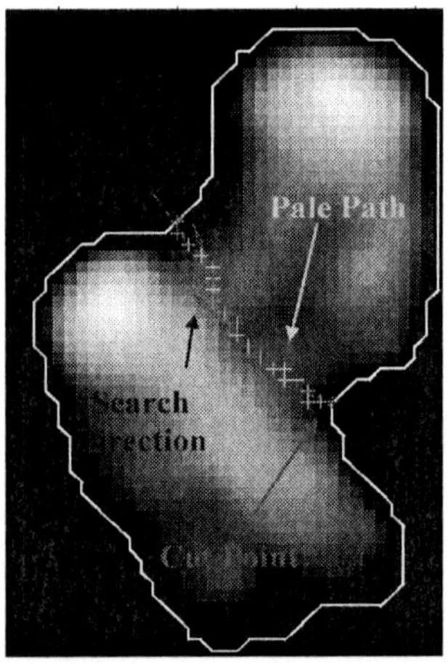

Chromosome length is simple to measure for properly segmented chromosomes. The centromere is the region in the middle of the chromosome involved in cell division and the control of gene expression (Moradi, 2003). The centromere divides the chromosome into two arms the *p-arm* and the *q*-arm. The centromere index is defined as the ratio of the length of the p-arm divided by the length of the q-arm.

$$Centromere\_Index = CI = \frac{length of\ p - arm}{length of\ q - arm}. \tag{1}$$

This ratio divides the 24 chromosome classes into three groups: (a) Submetacentric ($CI < 1$), (b) Acrocentric ($CI \cong 0$) and (c) Metacentric ($CI \cong 1$), (Fig. 3). However, centromeres are subtle and sometimes difficult to locate. The length and the centromere index by themselves cannot be used to classify chromosomes reliably into their 24 classes.

A very powerful and popular feature for manual and automated chromosome classification is the banding pattern of each chromosome class. However, banding patterns are often difficult to extract automatically. Often a medial axis transform (Lerner, 1995) is performed to measure a density profile by integrating the intensities along sections perpendicular to the medial axis.

Several transforms have been proposed for representing chromosome banding patterns. Fourier descriptors have been used as global descriptors of the chromosome's density profile, and the first eight components of the Fourier transform were found to be the most useful for discrimination (Moller, 1970). Another transform proposed in (Granum, 1981) describes a set of weighted density distribution functions which serve as a set of basis functions. Each chromosome's density profile was correlated with these functions, and the correlations served as a representation of that chromosome, rather than the profile itself.

Several classifiers have been used as well. These include neural networks (Sweeney, 1994; Errington, 1993; Lerner, 1998)and support vector machines, achieving high classification rates (Kou, 2002). Another popular approach is homologue matching (Zimmerman, 1986; Stanley 1998). This technique classifies chromosomes based on the assumption, that every chromosome class is represented by two identical chromosomes. This technique is useful for detecting chromosome abnormalities.

Fuzzy classifiers (Vanderheyydt, 1980) have also been employed. The output of these classifiers is a numerical measure of similarity to a chromosome class. While notable success has been achieved with these methods, they all suffer from the same drawback. They rely on features, such as centromere position and banding pattern, which is difficult to measure and depend on the segmentation.

Combined Segmentation and Classification Methods

Although traditional image analysis methods have considered segmentation and classification as separate processes they can be combined. The result of this combination is that often information of classification could be passed to segmentation and vice versa. Indeed in the case of chromosome segmentation, this has been realized and suggested by Ji (Ji, 1994). Agam et. al. (Agam, 1997) also combined the two stages.

Methods Based on Multichannel Chromosome Images

New imaging techniques started to appear in mid 90s with the most promising technique the Multiplex Fluorescent In Situ Hybridization (M-FISH, Speicher, 1996). Using M-FISH, it is possible to create a combination of fluorophores, where each class of chromosomes absorbs a different combination of these fluorophores. Since each fluorophore has a different emission spectrum, each chromosome class appears as a different color visually distinguishable from all other classes without the aid of banding patterns. An image of each fluorophore can be obtained using appropriate optical filters. An example of an M-FISH image is shown in Fig. 4.

This new imaging technique introduces several advantages:

1. The chromosome classification is simplified (Speicher, 1996). Only the spectral information from the multispectral image

Figure 3. The three categories of chromosomes according to the centromeric index

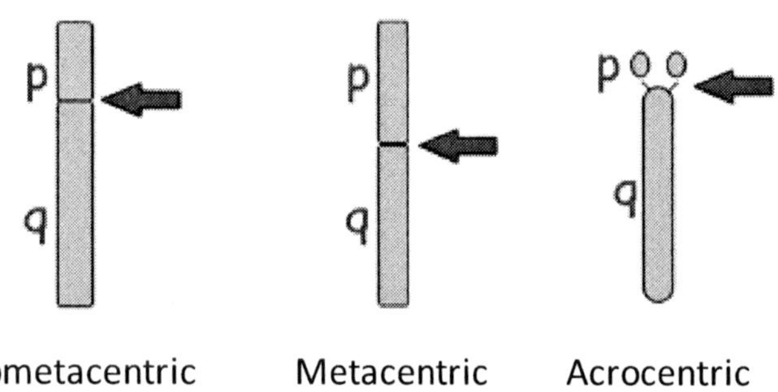

is estimated and no features such as length, centromere position and band pattern are used.

2. Subtle chromosomal aberrations are detected (Veldman, 1997). Traditional monochrome imaging techniques failed to detect rearrangements of genetic material such as the translocation of telemetric chromatin, because it is difficult to detect them with banding alone. M-FISH (color karyotyping) is able to sufficiently depict these anomalies.
3. It can be used for the identification of small genetic markers which remain elusive after banding (Ried, 1997).

To date there is little work on image analysis of M-FISH chromosomes images. Methods developed for the classification of human chromosomes are mainly based on pixel-by-pixel classification algorithms (Sampat, 2002; Choi, 2004; Wang, 2005; Schwartzkopf 2005). A typical M-FISH set consists of 6 images. Hence each pixel can be viewed as a 6 feature vector in a 6 dimensional space where each element represents the response of the dye. The classification procedure is modeled as a 6 feature 24 class pattern recognition problem. Each of the 24 chromosomes classes is modeled by a Gaussian density probability. The parameters (mean vectors and covariance matrixes) of the densities are learned through a training set using standard Maximum Likelihood Estimation.

Then for any given pixel, described by the feature vector $x \in \Re^6$, can be classified by using the Bayes Decision Rule, which is:

$$Decide\, c_i \text{ if } P(c_i \mid x) > P(c_j \mid x), \forall i \neq j, \quad (2)$$

where c_i is the ith chromosome class and $P(c_i|x)$ is the a posteriori probability of the class c_i.

Region based classification approaches have also been proposed (Eils, 1998; Saracoglu, 2001). The method of Eils et al. consisted of two stages: (i) spectral calibration and (ii) adaptive region classification. During the calibration stage a five-dimensional optimal vector called adaptive feature vector, representing each class, was found by minimizing an energy term. The region classification stage was based on a Voronoi image tessellation algorithm. Then the closest adaptive feature was computed determining the class for each region. Neighboring regions were merged if they belong to the same class or alternatively, when their color distance was below a preset threshold.

ADVANCES IN AUTOMATED CHROMOSOME ANALYSIS USING MULTICHANNEL CHROMOSOME IMAGING (M-FISH)

Most of the methods for automated chromosome classification problem are based on pixel-by-pixel classification techniques; without taking into account neighborhood information. Therefore, segmentation information provided by a multichannel segmentation method followed by a region-based classification could be employed in order to more accurately segment M-FISH images and thus improve the classification accuracy.

Segmentation

In order to segment the M-FISH image into regions the Watershed Transform (Vincent, 1991) is employed. However in order to compute the watershed transform first the gradient magnitude of the multispectral image (Drewniok, 1994) is computed combining the contrast information from the different spectral channels.

Instead of separately computing the scalar gradient for each channel, DiZenzo (DiZenzo, 1986) introduced a tensor gradient while Drewniok extended this work to multispectral images. Suppose, an M-FISH $I(x, y): \Re^2 \rightarrow \Re^5$ since the M-FISH image consists of 5 image channels.

Figure 4. Five channel M-FISH image data: (a) Aqua fluor, (b) Far red fluor, (c) Green fluor, (d) Red fluor, (e) Gold fluor and (f) Color M-FISH image.

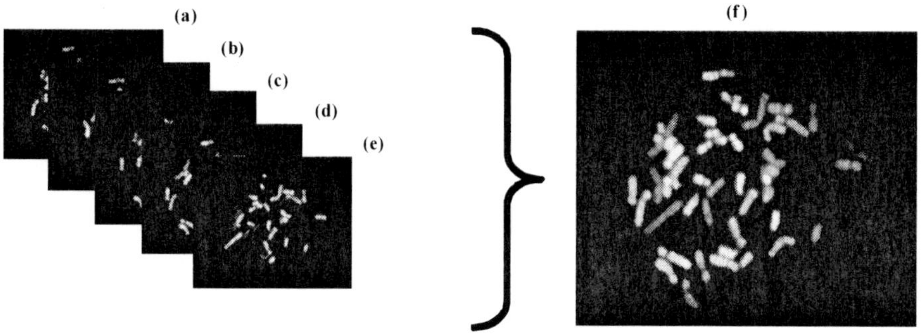

Each pixel of the image is represented by a 5-dimension vector:

$$I(x,y)=\left[I_1(x,y)\quad I_2(x,y)\quad \dots \quad I_5(x,y)\right]^T \tag{3}$$

where $I_i(x,y)$, $1 \le i \le 5$ are the components (channels) of the M-FISH image.

Let also the direction v defined by the angle ω:

$$v = [\cos\omega \quad \sin\omega]^T, \tag{4}$$

thus the directional derivative of the function $I(x, y)$ is:

$$\frac{\partial I}{\partial v}=\left[\frac{\partial I_1}{\partial v},\frac{\partial I_2}{\partial v},\dots,\frac{\partial I_m}{\partial v}\right]^T=\begin{bmatrix}\nabla I_1\cdot v\\ \nabla I_2\cdot v\\ \vdots\\ \nabla I_m\cdot v\end{bmatrix}=\begin{bmatrix}I_1^x & I_1^y\\ I_2^x & I_2^y\\ \vdots & \vdots\\ I_m^x & I_m^y\end{bmatrix}\cdot v=J\cdot v \tag{5}$$

where $\nabla I_i=\left[I_i^x \quad I_i^y\right]: 1 \le i \le 5$, J is the Jacobian matrix and I_i^x and I_i^y are the derivatives of the ith component in the x and y direction, respectively.

The direction v which corresponds to the maximum of the directional derivative $I(x, y)$ is found, by maximizing the Euclidean norm:

$$\|J\cdot v\|^2=(J\cdot v)^T(J\cdot v)=v^T(J^TJ)v \tag{6}$$

The extrema of the quantity $v^T(J^TJ)v$, are given by the eigenvalues of the matrix J^TJ (Drewniok, 1994).

A common problem of the direct application of the watershed transform on the gradient image is over-segmentation. To overcome this problem (Bieniecki, 2004) the grayscale reconstruction (Vincent, 1993) of the multichannel gradient magnitude was computed. Grayscale reconstruction reduces the number of unwanted minima, as it provides an intuitive selection scheme controlled by a single parameter.

The next step of the method is the computation of the watershed transform. The watershed transform is a powerful segmentation method which presents several advantages over other developed segmentation methods:

1. The watershed lines form closed and connected regions, where edge based techniques usually define disconnected boundaries that need post-processing to produce closed regions.
2. The watershed lines always correspond to obvious contours of objects which appear in the image.

The output of the WT is a tessellation T_n of the image into its different catchment basins, each one characterized by a unique label:

$$T_n = \{T_1, T_2, \ldots, T_n\}, \qquad (7)$$

where n is the number of the regions.

Only the pixels belonging to the watershed lines are assigned a special label to distinguish them from the catchment basins. The application of the WT to the grayscale reconstructed multi-channel gradient magnitude image is illustrated in Fig. 5.

Classification

Let ω_i, $i = 1,\ldots,24$ denote the 24 classes and $z \in \Re^5$ is a 5-dimensional random variable. The a priori probability that a feature z belongs to a class ω_i is $P(\omega_i)$. $p(z \mid \omega_i)$ is the class conditional probability distribution function, which represents the probability distribution function, for a feature vector z given that z belongs to class ω_i. $P(\omega_i \mid z)$ is the a posteriori probability, which represents the probability that the feature vector z belongs to class ω_i given the feature vector z. The above quantities are related through the Bayes theorem:

$$P(\omega_i \mid z) = \frac{p(z \mid \omega_i)P(\omega_i)}{\sum_{k=1}^{24} p(z \mid \omega_k)P(\omega_k)} \qquad (8)$$

Suppose that a segmented region R_i, $1 \le i \le Q$, where Q is the number of regions in the image, produced by the multispectral watershed segmentation, consists of ℓ pixels. Z is the set of (ℓ) vector values of each region in the image $Z = \{z_1, z_2, \ldots, z_\ell\}$. It can be observed that two pixels in spatial proximity to one another are unconditionally correlated with the degree of correlation decreasing as the distance between them increases. Assuming that the watershed transform segments the image into homogenous regions the likelihood $p(z \mid \omega_i)$ is computed as,

$$p(Z \mid \omega_i) = p(z_1, z_2, \ldots, z_\ell \mid \omega_i) = \prod_{k=1}^{\ell} p(z_k \mid \omega_i)$$
$$= \left(\frac{1}{(2\pi)^{d/2}\left|\Sigma_i\right|^{1/2}}\right)^{\ell} \exp\left(-\frac{1}{2}\sum_{k=1}^{\ell}(z_k - \mu_i)'\Sigma_i^{-1}(z_k - \mu_i)\right) \qquad (9)$$

where $\mu_i, \Sigma_i : 1 \le i \le 24$ is the mean vector and covariance matrix of the ith probability density function.

Working with the natural logarithm and dropping all terms that are the same for all classes, the Bayes decision rule assigns a region Z to class ω_i if:

$$\forall i \ne j,\ DS_i(Z) > DS_j(Z),$$
$$DS_i(Z) = -\frac{\ell}{2}\ln\left|\Sigma_i\right| - \frac{1}{2}\sum_{k=1}^{\ell}(z_k - \boldsymbol{\mu}_i)'\Sigma_i^{-1}(z_k - \boldsymbol{\mu}_i) + \ln P(\omega_i) \qquad (10)$$

The a priori class probabilities for each class $P(\omega_i)$, are computed using a training set. Then $P(\omega_i)$ is calculated as the percentage of all chromosome pixels in the training data that belong to the class ω_i:

$$P(\omega_i) = \frac{(\#\,pixels\,belong\,to\,class\,\omega_i)}{\sum_{k=1}^{24}(\#\,pixels\,belong\,to\,class\,\omega_k)} \qquad (11)$$

It is well known that the chromosome class reflects the size of each chromosome in descending order (i.e. chromosome 1 is the largest and chromosome 22 is the smallest). The application of the method in an M-FISH image is shown in Fig. 6. Initially the image is segmented using the multichannel watershed segmentation (Fig. 6(b)) and then the segmented regions are classified based on the region Bayes classification method (Fig. 6(c)). The final classification map after the region merging step is shown in Fig. 6(d). A separate colour was used to represent each chromosome class in the image.

Figure 5. M-FISH watershed segmentation. (a) Initial M-FISH image, and (b) watershed regions of the M-FISH image.

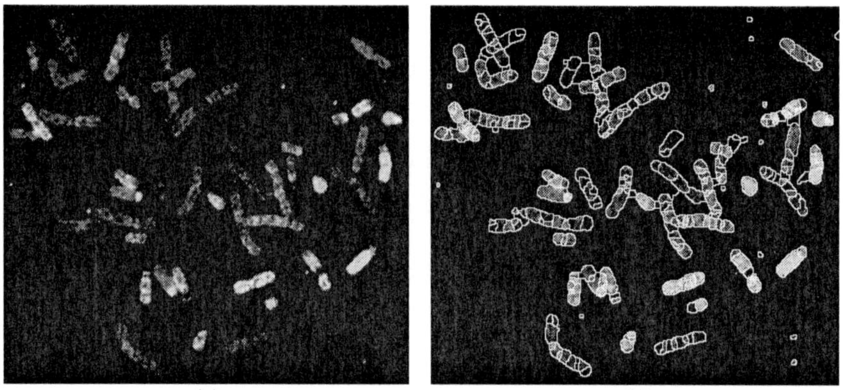

(a) (b)

Image Dataset

A public available database ADIR MFISH chromosome image database (ADIR, M-FISH) can be used to measure the classification accuracy. The database consists of 200 multispectral images having dimension 517x645 pixels. The database contains five-channel image sets recorded at different wavelengths. In addition, a DAPI image file is included for each M-FISH image. The specimens were prepared with probe sets from four different laboratories: Applied Spectral Imaging (Migdal HaEmek, Israel), Advanced Digital Imaging Research (ADIR; League City, Texas, USA), Cytocell Technologies (Cambridge, UK), and Vysis (Downers Grove, IL, USA).

Results

Four images were chosen randomly three times from the dataset and the test was performed with the remaining images. Thus, three different training subsets (Sub A, Sub B, Sub C) were created. The training dataset consists of all chromosome classes and no overlap between the training and testing data exists. Also pixels belonging to two or more chromosomes (chromosome overlaps) were not included for training and testing.

The proposed method was compared with a Bayes pixel-by-pixel classification technique (Sampat, 2002), which is the main classification scheme for several related works in the literature (Sampat, 2002; Choi, 2004; Sampat, 2005; Wang, 2005; Schwartzkopf, 2005). Pixel-by-pixel classification is performed for the pixels in the segmented regions of chromosomes. The training and evaluation of both methods was made using the same training and testing set. The average chromosome classification accuracy obtained for each M-FISH training subset: Sub A, Sub B, and Sub C is shown in Table 1.

FUTURE TRENDS

Automated chromosome analysis and recognition of microscopic images is undergoing active development. Methods based on high-resolution digitized imagery appear currently to be the only approach with the required discriminatory power. The field of microscopic chromosome image analysis demands competence in a wide range

Figure 6. Example of an M-FISH image segmentation and classification: (a) Original M-FISH mage, (b) the segmented image using the multichannel watershed segmentation, (c)the image after region classification, and (d) the final classification map using region merging.

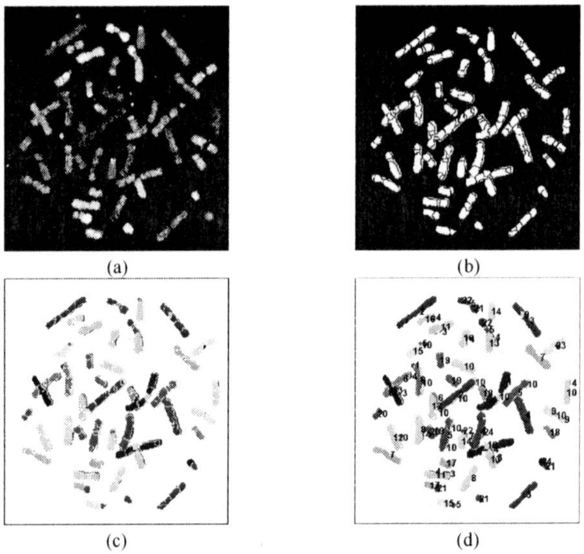

Table 1. Chromosome classification accuracy using the described method and a pixel-by-pixel classification method.

	Classification accuracy	
Subsets	**Region based**	**Pixel-by-pixel [35]**
Sub A	82.2%(± 14.9%)	70.8%(± 16.2%)
Sub B	82.4%(± 14.8%)	70.6%(± 16.8%)
Sub C	82.6%(± 14.4%)	70.4%(± 16.5%)
Overall	**82.4%**	**70.6%**

of disciplines, from the practical clinical situation to optics, electrooptical devices, computer architecture, software engineering, multivariate statistics, and decision theory.

CONCLUSION

Chromosome image analysis is an essential tool for detecting chromosome abnormalities, which can be indicators of radiation damage, cancer, and a wide variety of inherited diseases. Grayscale chromosome imaging techniques have been the golden standard for many years and a wide variety of automated classifications methods exist already in the literature. Although new imaging techniques developed to aid the cytoneticists in detecting those abnormalities, such as M-FISH, only few automated classification methods exploit these types of images.

If classification is performed on a pixel-by-pixel basis, the classification will be dominated by noisy painting inhomogeneities. This is obvious by the misclassification errors produced by the pixel-by-pixel algorithm. In contrary region-based classification avoids these types of errors, since pixels with similar spectral information contribute in the classification.

REFERENCES

ADIR M-FISH Image Database. Available at: http://www.adires.com/05/Project/MFISH_DB/MFISH_DB.shtml

Agam G., & Dinstein I., (1997). Geometric separation of partially overlapping nonrigid objects applied to automatic chromosome classification. *IEEE Transactions on Pattern Analysis and Machine Intelligence*, *19*, 1212-1222.

Bieniecki, W. (2004). Oversegmentation avoidance in watershed-based algorithms for color images. *In Proc. Of Modern Problems of Radio Engineering, Telecommunications and Computer Science*.

Carters, G., & Graham, J. (2002). Disentangling chromosome overlaps by combining trainable shape models with classification evidence. *IEEE Transactions on Signal Processing*, *50*, 2080-2085.

Carters G., & Graham J. (1999). Trainable grey-level models for disentangling overlapping chromosomes. *Pattern Recognition*, *32*, 1335-1349.

Choi, H., Castleman, K., & Bovik, A. (2004). Joint Segmentation and Classification of M-FISH Chromosome Images. In *Proc. 26th IEEE Ann. Intern. Conf (EMBS)*, San Francisco, (pp. 1636-1639).

DiZenzo, S. (1986). A note on the gradient of a multi-image. *Comput. Vis. Graph. Image Process*, *33*, 116-125.

Drewniok, C. (1994). Multi-spectral edge detection - Some experiments on data from Landsat-TM, *Intern. J. Remote. Sens.*, *15*, 3743-3765.

Eils, R., Uhrig, S., Saracoglu, K., Satzler, K., Bolzer, A., Petersen, I., Chassery, J., Ganser, M., & Speicher, M. (1998). An optimized fully automated system for fast and accurate identification of chromosomal rearrangements by multiplex-FISH (M-FISH), *Cytogenet. Cell Genet.*, *82*, 160-171.

Errington P., & Graham J. (1993). Application of artificial neural networks to chromosome classification. *Cytometry*, *14*, 627–639.

Graham, J. (1989). Resolution of composites in interactive karyotyping. In *Automation of Cytogenetics*, Berlin, Germany: Springer-Verlag, (pp. 191–203).

Granum, E., Gerdes, T., & Lundsteen, C. (1981). Simple weighted density distributions, WDD's for discrimination between G-banded chromosomes. *In Proc. Eur. Chrom. Anal. Workshop*, Edinburgh, U.K.

Gray, J., & Pinkel, D. (1992). Molecular cytogenetics in human cancer diagnosis. *Cancer*, *69*, 1536–1542.

Human Chromosome Study Group (1960). A proposed standard of nomenclature of human mitotic chromosomes. *Cereb. Palsy Bull.*

Ji, L. (1989). Intelligent Splitting in the chromosome domain. *Pattern Recognition*, *22*, 519-532.

Ji, L. (1994). Fully automatic chromosome segmentation. *Cytometry*, *17*, 196-208.

Karvelis, P., Fotiadis, D., Syrrou, M., & Georgiou, I., (2005). Segmentation of chromosomes images based on a recursive watershed transform. *3rd European Medical & Biological Engineering Conference*, (EMBEC 2005), (pp. 497-502, 20-25).

Karvelis, P., Tzallas, A., Fotiadis, D., & Georgiou, I. (2007). A Multichannel Watershed-Based Segmentation Method for Multispectral Chromosome Classification. *IEEE Trans. Med. Imaging.*

Kou, Z., Ji, L., & Zhang, X. (2002). Karyotyping of Comparative Genomic Hybridization Human Metaphases by Using Support Vector Machines. *Cytometry, 47*, 17-23.

Lerner, B. (1998). Toward a completely automatic neural-network-based human chromosome analysis. *IEEE Trans. Trans. Syst., Man, Cybern.*, pt. B, Cybern., *28*, 544–552.

Lerner, B., Guterman, H., & Dinstein, I. (1998). A Classification-driven Partially Occluded Object Segmentation (CPOOS) method with application to chromosome analysis. *IEEE Transactions on Signal Processing, 46*, 2841-2847.

Lerner, B., Guterman, H., Dinstein, I., & Romem, Y. (1995). Medial axis transform-based features and a neural network for human chromosome classification. *Pattern Recognition, 28*, 1673-1683.

Lundsteen, C., Gerdes, T., Maahr, J., & Philip, J., (1987) Clinical performance of a system for semiautomated chromosome analysis. *American Journal of Human Genetics, 41*, 493-502.

Moller, M., Nilsson, H., Caspersson, T., & Lomakka, G. (1970). Identification of human chromosome regions by aid of computerized pattern analysis. *Exp. Cell. Res., 70*, 475–478.

Moradi, M., Setarehdan, S., & Ghaffari, S. (2003). Automatic Locating the Centromere on Human Chromosome Pictures. *16th IEEE Symposium on Computer-Based Medical Systems (CBMS'03)*, (pp. 56-61).

Nowell, P., & Hungerford, D. (1960). A minute chromosome in human chronic granulocytic leukemia. *Science, 132*, 1197–1200.

Piper, J., & Granum, E. (1989). On fully automatic feature measurement for banded chromosome classification. *Cytometry, 10*, 242-255.

Popescu, M., Gader, P., Keller, J., Klein, C., Stanley, J., & Caldwell, C. (1999). Automatic karyotyping of metaphase cells with overlapping chromosomes. *Computers in Biology and Medicine, 29*, 61-82.

Ried, T., Liyanage, M., Manoir, S., Heselmeyer, K., Auer, G., Macville, M., & Schröck, E., (1997). Tumor cytogenetics revisited: comparative genomic hybridization and spectral karyotyping. *J. Mol. Med., 75*, 801-814.

Sampat, M., Bovik, A., Aggarwal, J., & Castleman, K. (2002). Pixel-by-Pixel classification of MFISH images. In *Proc. of the 24th IEEE EMBS Ann. Intern. Conf.*, (pp. 999-1000).

Sampat, M., Bovik, A., Aggarwal, J., & Castleman, K. (2005). Supervised parametric and nonparametric classification of chromosome images. *Pattern Recognit., 38*, 1209-1223.

Saracoglu, K., Brown, J., Kearney, L., Uhrig, S., Azofeifa, J., Fauth, C., Speicher, M., & Eils, R. (2001). New concepts to improve resolution and sensitivity of molecular cytogenetic diagnostics by multicolor fluorescence in situ hybridization. *Cytometry, 44*, 7-15.

Schwartzkopf, W., Bovik, A., & Evans, B. (2005). Maximum-likelihood techniques for joint segmentation-classification of multispectral chromosome images. *IEEE Trans. Med. Imag., 24*, 1593-1610.

Speicher, M., Ballard, S., & Ward, D. (1996). Karyotyping human chromosomes by combinatorial Multi-Fluor FISH. *Nat. Gen., 12*, 341-344.

Stanley, R., Keller, J., Gader, P., & Caldwell, C. (1998). Data-driven homologue matching for chromosome identification. *IEEE Trans. Med. Imag., 17*, 451–462.

Sumner, T., Evans, J., & Buckland, A. (1971). A new technique for distinguishing between human chromosomes. *Nature New Biol., 232*, 31-32.

Sweeney, W., Musavi, M., & Guigi, J. (1994). Classification of chromosomes using a probabilistic neural network. *Cytometry, 16*, 17–24.

Thompson, M., McInnes, R. & Willard, H. (1992). *Genetics in Medicine* 5th Edition, WB Saunders Company, Philadelphia.

Vanderheydt, L., Oosterlinck, A., Daele, J., & Berghe, H., (1980). Design of graph-representation and a fuzzy-classifier for human chromosomes. *Pattern Recognit., 12*, 201–210.

Veldman, T., Vignon, C., Schröck, E., Rowley, J., & Ried, T. (1997). Hidden chromosome abnormalities in haematological malignancies detected by multicolor spectral karyotyping. *Nat. Genet., 15*, 406-410.

Vincent, L., & Soille, P. (1991). Watershed in Digital Spaces: An Efficient Algorithm Based on Immersion Simulations. *IEEE Transactions on Pattern Analysis and Machine Intelligence, 13*, 583-598.

Vincent, L. (1993). Morphological grayscale reconstruction in image analysis: Applications and efficient algorithms. *IEEE Trans. Image Processing, 2*, 176-201.

Vossepoel, A. (1987). *Analysis of Image Segmentation for Automated Chromosome Identification*, Ph.D. dissertation, Univ. Leiden, Leiden, The Netherlands.

Wang, Y., & Castleman, K. (2005). Normalization of multicolor fluorescence in situ hybridization (M-FISH) images for improving color karyotyping. *Cytometry, 64*, 101-109.

Zimmerman, S., Johnston, D., Arrighi, F., & Rupp, M. E. (1986). Automated homologue matching of human G-banded chromosomes. *Comput. Biol. Med., 16*, 223–233.

KEY TERMS

Centromere: The centromere is a region, found in the middle of the chromosome, involved in cell division and the control of gene expression.

Centromere Index: The centromere index is defined as the ratio of the length of the short arm of the chromosome divided by the length of the other arm.

Chromosome: A chromosome is a continuous piece of DNA, which contains many genes, regulatory elements and other nucleotide sequences.

Classification: The process of deriving a mathematical function that can predict the membership of a class based on input data.

Machine Learning: As a broad subfield of artificial intelligence, machine learning is concerned with the design and development of algorithms and techniques that allow computers to "learn".

Watershed: The segmentation based on watershed designs is a family of segmentation methods that consider an image as a topographic relief the flooding of which is simulated.

Chapter XXI
Machine Learning in Morphological Segmentation

O. Lezoray
Université de Caen Basse-Normandie, France

A. Elmotataz
Université de Caen Basse-Normandie, France

G. Lebrun
Université de Caen Basse-Normandie, France

M. Lecluse
Centre Hospitalier Public du Cotentin, France

C. Meurie
INRETS-LEOST, France

H. Elie
Centre Hospitalier Public du Cotentin, France

C. Charrier
Université de Caen Basse-Normandie, France

ABSTRACT

The segmentation of microscopic images is a challenging application that can have numerous applications ranging from prognosis to diagnosis. Mathematical morphology is a very well established theory to process images. Segmentation by morphological means is based on watershed that considers an image as a topographic surface. Watershed requires input and marker image. The user can provide the latter but far more relevant results can be obtained for watershed segmentation if marker extraction relies on prior knowledge. Parameters governing marker extraction varying from image to image, machine learning approaches are of interest for robust extraction of markers. We review different strategies for extracting markers by machine learning: single classifier, multiple classifier, single classifier optimized by model selection.

INTRODUCTION

The visual evaluation of microscopic slides is a tedious task, which requires hard concentration of the pathologist screening the specimen under study. With the advent of image processing as an efficient way to extract objects of interest in images, the automatic analysis of images acquired from light microscopes has become an emerging and challenging image analysis application.

Microscopic image analysis schemes are usually threefold: image segmentation, objects features computation, objects classification. We propose to focus on the first part of this scheme for the segmentation of microscopic images of bronchial cytology stained by the international coloration standard of Papanicolaou and acquired in light microscopy. The aim of the segmentation is to extract cells in images; cells being composed of a nucleus and a cytoplasm. Segmentation being in general a difficult task, machine learning has emerged as a key component of intelligent computer vision programs when adaptation is needed (Arif, 2007). In this Chapter, we consider the segmentation of microscopic images by morphological methods and show how to integrate machine learning into a morphological segmentation scheme.

BACKGROUND

Mathematical Morphology is a very well established theory to process images (Serra, 1988). The watershed is the basic tool of Mathematical Morphology for segmentation. It has proved to be a powerful tool and it is used in a large number of applications, such as, medicine, remote sensing, robotics, and multimedia (Meyer, 2001). The parameters for a watershed are marker and input images (Soille, 2004). The watershed grows the markers based on a flooding simulation process by considering the input image as a topographic surface. The problem is to produce the divide-line image on this surface (Roerdink, 2000). Each marker is associated to a color. The topography is flooded from below by letting colored water rise from the holes with its associated color, at an uniform rate across the entire image. When the rising water of distinct colors would merge, a dam is built to prevent the merging. Figure 1 illustrates such a process on a color hematology image with two different sets of markers (provided by the user or by a machine learning algorithm). The most difficult problem when using watershed is of course the definition of appropriate markers with minimal efforts (Rivest, 1992; Meyer, 2001). User provided markers can be attractive for interactive segmentation but for automatic segmentation other techniques have to be considered. An accurate extraction of reliable markers requires prior knowledge on the latter (color, texture, shape, etc.). To incorporate such prior knowledge for the automatic extraction of markers, machine-learning techniques (Derivaux, 2007; Lezoray, 2002; Levner 2007) are the most natural candidates. Figure 2 provides a schematic view of all components involved in the design of a morphological segmentation scheme relying on machine learning algorithms for marker extraction. To perform morphological color image segmentation, a machine learning based classification of pixel feature vectors is done. The result is labeled in connected components and refined by a color watershed. To infer a proper machine learning based pixel classifier, an image database with an associated ground truth is constructed and pixel feature vectors are shared among classes as a basis for supervised learning. In the following Sections, conceiving of each one of these components is described.

MACHINE LEARNING IN MORPHOLOGICAL SEGMENTATION OF MICROSCOPIC IMAGES

Machine Learning

Far more relevant results can be obtained for watershed segmentation if marker extraction relies on prior knowledge. Parameters governing marker extraction varying from image to image, machine learning approaches are of interest for robust extraction of markers. However, with the use of machine learning algorithms for the extraction of seeds, one can consider either unsupervised or supervised learning approaches. Unsupervised approaches do not make use of any learning step

Figure 1. Segmentation by watershed: a) original hematology image, b) 3D view of the image as a topographic surface c) user-defined inner and outer marker after connected components labeling, d) user-defined markers superimposed, e) superimposed regions of color watershed with c) as markers, f) Machine Learning based marker extraction after connected components labeling, g) Machine Learning based markers superimposed, h) superimposed regions of color watershed with f) as markers. Regions colored in black in marker images ((c) and (f)) correspond to unlabeled pixels, other pixels correspond to region seeds.

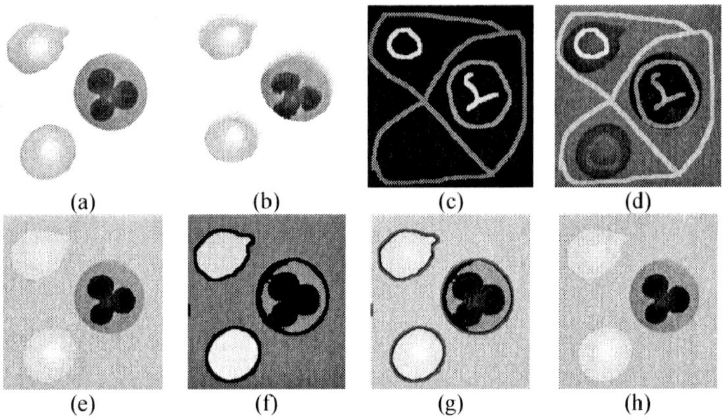

Figure 2. Schematic view of components involved in the design of a morphological segmentation scheme relying on machine learning algorithm for marker extraction.

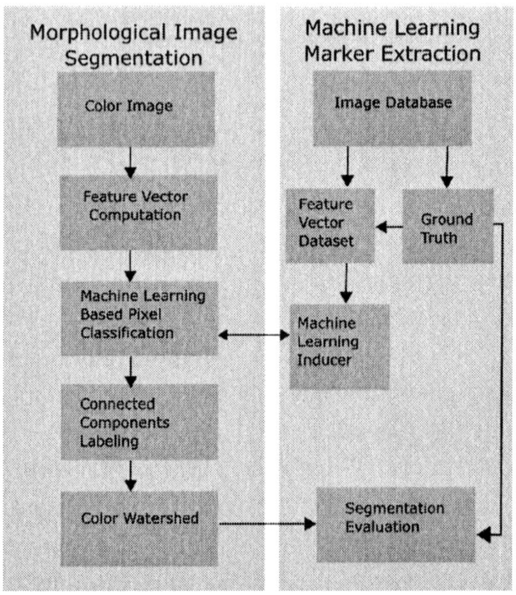

and supervised methods do need a learning step to infer an appropriate model of the data. The two approaches (unsupervised or supervised learning) have benefits and defects, and it is often difficult to make a choice between both. A machine learning algorithm is a recognition tool called a classifier that provides class memberships information for a vector received in input. Therefore, a classifier aims at building a function F that maps the input feature space to an output space. Each example (x, y) consists of an instance $x \in X \subset \mathbb{R}^p$ and a label $y \in Y = \{\omega_1,...,\omega_K\}$ where X is the feature vector input space and K the number of classes to be discriminated. A classifier can be considered as a mapping F from instances to labels $F: X \rightarrow Y$. Usually, classifiers provide class membership estimates $f(x, \omega_i)$ and the classification of an input feature vector x is performed by:

$$F(x) = \arg\min_{\omega_i} f\left(x, \omega_i\right)$$

We assume that a dataset D of n examples in a real-dimensional space $\mathbb{R}^p$ is provided. In the sequel, we review some classical unsupervised and supervised classifiers (Duda, 2000).

k-Means

Among unsupervised clustering formulations that are based on minimizing a formal objective function, the most widely used is probably k-means clustering (Linde, 1980). It consists in finding a set of k examples of $\mathbb{R}^p$ called centers, so as to minimize the mean squared distance from each data example to its nearest neighbor. To classify an input feature vector x, the class memberships are estimated in terms of Euclidean distance:

$$f\left(x, \omega_i\right) = \left\| x - c_{\omega_i} \right\|$$

where c_{ω_i} denotes the center of class ω_i and $\|.\|$ is the Euclidean distance.

Fisher Linear Discriminant Analysis (FLDA)

Fisher's linear discriminant is an unsupervised classification method that projects high-dimensional data onto a line (denoted by w) and performs classification in this one-dimensional space (Fisher, 1936). To find this projection, one maximizes the following objective:

$$J(w) = \frac{w^T S_B w}{w^T S_W w}$$

where S_B is the between classes scatter matrix and S_W the within classes scatter matrix. To classify an input feature vector x, the class memberships are estimated by:

$$f\left(x, \omega_i\right) = w^T x + b_i$$

where b_i is a threshold deduced from prior probabilities.

Bayesian Classifier

This classifier is based on the Bayesian decision theory (Duda, 2000). It is a supervised statistical approach to pattern classification that assumes that the decision problem is expressed in probabilistic terms. For multivariate distributions, mixtures of Gaussian distribution models are used. To classify an input feature vector x, the class memberships are estimated for each class by the equation in ,

$$f\left(x, \omega_i\right) = -\frac{1}{2}\left(x - \mu_{\omega_i}\right)^T \Sigma_{\omega_i}^{-1}\left(x - \mu_{\omega_i}\right) - \frac{1}{2}\log\left(\left|\Sigma_{\omega_i}\right|\right) - \log\left(p_{\omega_i}\right) + \frac{K}{2}\log(2\pi)$$

where μ_{ω_i} denotes mean attribute vector, Σ_{ω_i} is conditional covariance matrix of class ω_i (normally distributed) and p_{ω_i} prior probability of class ω_i.

k-NN

The k Nearest Neighbors method is a well known supervised algorithm in the field of machine learning (Michie, 1994). Given a training set and a distance defined in the feature space, the basic k-NN rule consists in searching for the k nearest neighbors of an input feature vector. The estimated class probabilities are proportional to the number of classes among the k nearest neighbors:

$$f(x,\omega_i) = \frac{|S(x,\omega_i,k)|}{k}$$

where $S(x, \omega_i, k)$ denotes the set of patterns among the k nearest neighbors to point x that belong to class ω_i and $|.|$ denotes the cardinal of a set.

Support Vector Machines (SVM)

SVM are supervised classifiers based on the structural risk minimization principle from statistical learning theory (Cristianini, 2000; Vapnik, 1998). SVM express predictions in terms of a linear combination of kernel functions on a subset of the training data, known as support vectors. SVM map an input vector x into a high-dimensional feature space H through some nonlinear mapping function $\phi(.)$ and builds an optimal separating hyper-plane in that space. The mapping is performed by a kernel function $k(.,.)$ that defines an inner product in H. A typical kernel is Gaussian kernel:

$$k(x_1,x_2) = \exp\left(-\frac{\|x_1 - x_2\|^2}{2\sigma^2}\right)$$

This reduces the training of a SVM to maximizing a convex quadratic form subject to linear constraints. The maximum margin separating hyper-plane can be represented as a linear combination of training points called support vectors (SV):

$$w = \sum_{i=1}^{n} \alpha_i^* y_i \phi(x_i)$$

An example of the training set is a support vector if $\alpha_i^* \geq 0$. Many specific algorithms can solve the convex quadratic problem of SVM, the most competitive being Sequential Minimal Optimization (Platt, 1998). The training algorithm produces a decision function where each support vector has a α_i value characterizing his weight on the hyper plane position. The output of a SVM for a given input feature vector x is:

$$f(x) = \sum_{i \in SV}^{n} \alpha_i^* y_i k(x_i, x)$$

The output of a SVM is not a probabilistic value, but non-calibrated distance measurement of an example to the separating hyper-plane. Platt proposed a method to map SVM outputs into positive class posterior probabilities by applying a sigmoid function to the SVM output (Platt, 1999):

$$f(x,\omega_i) = \frac{1}{1+\exp(Af(x)+B)}$$

where A and B are obtained by minimizing the negative log like hood under a test set. Finally, SVM are binary classifiers and multi-class decision functions are usually designed by combining several two-class SVM decision functions (Hsu, 2002).

Multi Layer Perceptrons (MLP)

A MLP is a supervised classifier expressed by a network of simple neurons called perceptrons. The perceptron computes a single output from multiple real-valued inputs by forming a linear combination according to its input weights and then possibly putting the output through some nonlinear activation function (Rosenblatt, 1958). A single perceptron is not very useful because of its limited mapping ability. The perceptrons can, however, be used as building blocks of a larger, much more practical structure. A typical multilayer perceptron (MLP) network consists of a set of source nodes forming the input layer, one or more hidden layers of computation nodes, and an output layer of nodes. The input signal propagates through the network layer-by-layer (Dreyfus, 2005). The computations performed by such a feed forward network with a single hidden layer are:

$$f(x,\omega_i) = g\left(\sum_{j=0}^{n_h} w_{ij} g\left(\sum_{k=0}^{n_d} w_{jk} x_k\right)\right)$$

Where w_{ij} denotes the weight between neurons i and j, n_h the number of hidden units, n_d the number of input units and g is a nonlinear activation function (e.g. a sigmoid). The supervised learning problem of the MLP can be solved with the back-propagation algorithm.

Image Database

When one wants to conceive a segmentation method for a given type of microscopic color images, it is essential to utilize a data set of representative images. This shows several key benefits for the conception and the evaluation of a complete segmentation scheme. For the considered class of microscopic images, a microscopy expert has to choose judicious images that well describe the whole segmentation problem: all the objects to be extracted (and further segmented) are present on at least one image. Once the representative images are determined, they are manually segmented in several classes and objects of interest are extracted. This enables the constitution of a database of segmented images (a ground truth). This ground truth is associated to a set of pixel feature vectors shared in several classes that a machine-learning algorithm has to learn to categorize. Therefore, a ground truth database can be used for the learning step of supervised machine-learning algorithms (Bayes, k-NN, SVM, MLP) and also as a reference segmentation to evaluate the relevance of an automatic segmentation. In the sequel, we will consider a publicly available database of 8 images from bronchial cytology that have been manually segmented (Meurie, 2005).

The use of machine-learning algorithms to extract seed from images comes to perform pixel feature vector classification. Each pixel of the ground truth is associated to a feature vector x and a class y. All the couples (x,y) associated to ground truth pixels define a dataset of examples and a machine learning algorithm has to infer a mapping function F as close as possible to ground truth. A machine-learning algorithm used to categorize pixels in images produces image classification and not image segmentation. In an image classification, classes are assigned to pixels that are not necessarily spatially connected. To obtain segmentation from an image classification result, one has therefore to perform a labeling of connected components. Figure 3 (a)-(b) show a microscopic color image from bronchial cytology and its ground truth where pixels have been classified into three classes (background, cytoplasm, nuclei). One the opposite, Figure 3 (c)-(d) show typical image segmentations where connected components have distinct labels.

Moreover, since color is the main information used to classify pixels, different feature vectors can be considered by using different color representations in different colors spaces (Lukac, 2006). This change of color representation can have high influence on final results. Figure 3(c)-(d) show two different segmentation results where the feature vector associated to pixels is either a vector in YCh_1Ch_2 color space (Figure 3(c)) or a vector in *RGB* color space (Figure 3(d)).

Classification and Segmentation Evaluation

An important issue when designing a segmentation method is the evaluation of results. Having

Figure 3. Morphological segmentation of a microscopic color image (a) with a Bayesian classifier for extracting seeds: in YCh_1Ch_2 (c) and RGB (d) color spaces. Figure 3(b) presents the ground truth of Figure 3(a) where three classes of pixels are shown (black for background, blue for cytoplasm, and green for nuclei). F-measures for the nuclei and cytoplasm classes are provided. Figure 3(e) and (f) respectively present results of a pixel classification by SVM and further refined by a watershed. q_{shape} and q_{seg} measures are provided to globally quantify the segmentation quality.

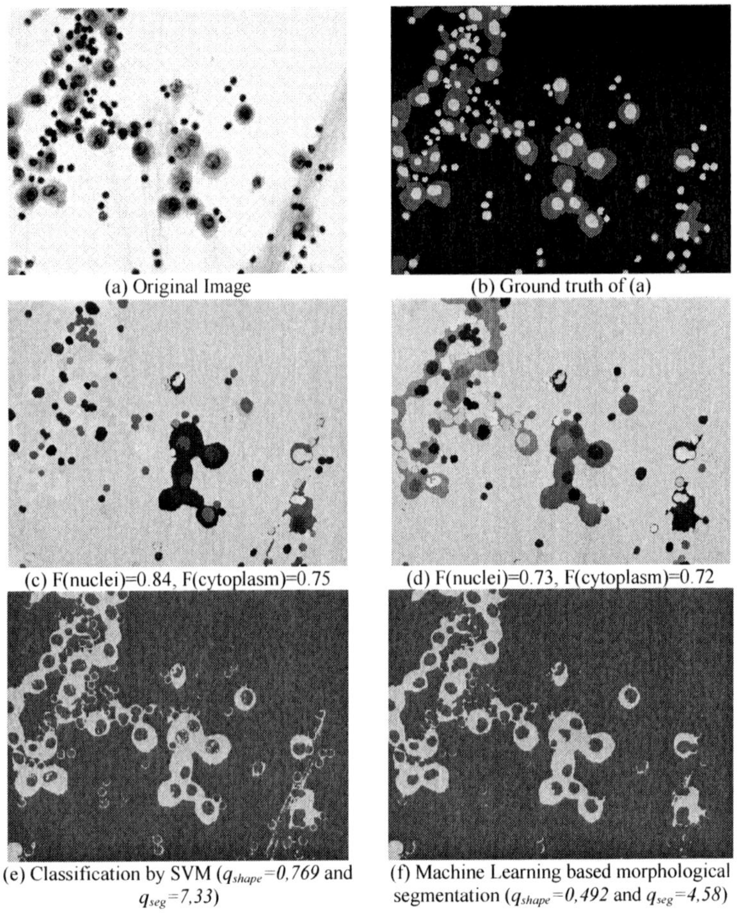

(a) Original Image

(b) Ground truth of (a)

(c) F(nuclei)=0.84, F(cytoplasm)=0.75

(d) F(nuclei)=0.73, F(cytoplasm)=0.72

(e) Classification by SVM (q_{shape}=0,769 and q_{seg}=7,33)

(f) Machine Learning based morphological segmentation (q_{shape}=0,492 and q_{seg}=4,58)

a ground truth obviously facilitates evaluation but several precautions have to be undertaken. A classical way to assess the performance of a classifier that produces a classification on image pixels is to compute a classification rate for each class.

Let F be a machine learning algorithm given feature vector inputs X and class outputs Y. To quantify the error rate of a machine-learning algorithm, a loss function is defined to assess if the prediction realized is close to the ground truth. The error rate (*ER*) is defined by (Duda, 2000):

$$ER(X,Y,F)=\frac{1}{n}\sum_{n} l\left(F(x_i),y_i\right)$$

and the loss function is usually defined by

$$l(x,y)=\begin{cases}0 & \text{if } x=y\\ 1 & \text{if } x\neq y\end{cases}$$

This involves counting the misclassification error if input feature vector x is wrongly classified. The classification (success) rate is then defined as $1\text{-}ER(X,Y,Z)$.

However, if the proportion of elements among classes is not well balanced, the classification rate is no more confident. This is generally the case for feature data sets coming from microscopic ground truth images where most of pixels belong to background in a very high proportion (higher than 80%). A classifier that classifies all pixels as background will have a classification rate close to 80% although it performs very badly. To correct this, it is recommended to use a Balanced Error Rate (BER) that computes the average of the error rates on each class. BER is defined by:

$$BER(X,Y,Z)=\frac{1}{|Y|}\sum_{\omega_i\in Y}\left(\frac{1}{|\omega_i|}\sum_{(x_j,y_j),y_j=\omega_i} l\left(F\left(x_j\right),y_j\right)\right)$$

Other measures to evaluate classification results exist. The most used are based on Precision and Recall measures. They are obtained from an analysis of the classification confusion matrix. Let TP denote *True Positives*, FP *False Positives*, and FN *False Negatives* that are defined for each class by:

$$TP(\omega_i)=\left|\{(x_i,y_i),y_i=\omega_i \text{ and } F(x_i)=\omega_i\}\right|$$

$$FN(\omega_i)=\left|\{(x_i,y_i),y_i=\omega_i \text{ and } F(x_i)\neq\omega_i\}\right|$$

$$FP(\omega_i)=\left|\{(x_i,y_i),y_i\neq\omega_i \text{ and } F(x_i)=\omega_i\}\right|$$

From the latter, Precision, Recall and F-measure, can be defined by:

$$\text{Precision}(\omega_i)=\frac{TP(\omega_i)}{TP(\omega_i)+FP(\omega_i)}$$

$$\text{Recall}(\omega_i)=\frac{TP(\omega_i)}{TP(\omega_i)+FN(\omega_i)}$$

$$\text{F-measure}(\omega_i)=\frac{2\text{Precision}(\omega_i)\text{Recall}(\omega_i)}{\text{Precision}(\omega_i)+\text{Recall}(\omega_i)}$$

For instance, a specific F-measure for the evaluation of microscopic image classification has been proposed in (Meurie, 2003). Figure 3(c)-(d) provides such a F-measure for nuclei and cytoplasm classes. One can see that this measure well reflects how good the classification is with respect to ground truth (the higher the F-measure, the better).

All previous methods are dedicated to pixel classification results evaluation: they do not take into account the spatial information in images. Therefore, for the case of segmentation evaluation, other specific measures have to be taken into account. An excellent review of segmentation evaluation methods can be found in (Chabrier, 2006). However, all these methods are not always suited for evaluating microscopic image segmentation results. A more specific method has been proposed in (Lebrun, 2007) to evaluate in a single measure the segmentation of cells in microscopic images. This cell segmentation quality criterion q_{seg} takes into account the adequacy q_{shape} between the shape of the objects produced by an automatic segmentation I_a and an expert segmentation I_e. That criterion also takes into account the number of missing objects $n_{missing}$ and the number of artifact objects $n_{artifact}$. Definition of that criterion is, with $\lambda \in [0,1]$:

$$q_{seg}=q_{shape}+\lambda n_{\text{missing}}+(1-\lambda)n_{\text{artifact}}$$

Constant λ makes it possible to favor a segmentation that limits the number of missing objects as compared to the number of artifact objects. In the case of cell segmentation, it is essential that no cell is lost, even if that forces to keep some artifacts, so a typical value is $\lambda = 0{,}9$. The shape adequacy q_{shape} is defined as following:

$$q_{shape}=\frac{1}{|I_a|}\sum_{I_a(p)\neq I_e(p)}\min\left(d_e\left(p,I_e\right),d_{\max}\right)^2$$

In the latter, $d_e(p,I_e)$ corresponds to the distance between the pixel p and its nearest pixel belonging to the shape edges in expert segmentation I_e. d_{max}

value aims at restricting the effect of weighting decrease when pixels are close to expert segmentation boundaries. In Figure 3, values of q_{seg} and q_{shape} are provided for two images obtained from image classification by SVM, and further refined by a watershed. Obtained values efficiently quantify segmentation results (the lower q_{seg} value, the better) as confirmed by visual analysis.

Multiple Classifier Fusion

In this Section, a complete morphological segmentation scheme based on machine learning techniques for marker extraction is designed for the automatic segmentation of bronchial color microscopic images. First, the abilities of different machine learning algorithms are studied for sole pixel classification. Given an image as input, each classifier processes an image by assigning a label to each pixel. Unsupervised classification directly treats each image without exploiting any model inferred from an image database whereas this is the case for supervised classification. Whatever the classifier, its hyper-parameters and feature vector used to represent a color pixel have serious influence on final results. It is therefore essential to choose the best representation and parameters. This is performed in cascade: first, each classifier has its parameters optimized, and second the best pixel color features are determined, both steps with respect to F-measure. Once this is done, a set of different classifiers is obtained, operating on different pixel representations and having different abilities to extract seeds. Table 1 presents, for each of the abovementioned classifiers, the retained color feature vector used to represent pixels so as to obtain the best results in terms of F-measure for the extraction of cytoplasm and nuclei. This F-measure is measured and averaged over all the comparisons with ground truth images. As shown in Table 1, the color representation has high influence on results and classifiers do not respond in the same way to similar feature vectors. Moreover, supervised classifiers (SVM, Bayes, MLP and kNN) tend to provide better pixel classification results in terms of F-measure. Figure 4 presents classification results for a color microscopic image with classifiers of Table 1.

Previous results have shown that pixel classification is a good candidate for marker extraction. However, it remains difficult to choose only one single classifier for extracting markers since results obtained by some of them are very close. Despite this, SVM, Bayes, kNN and k-means can be retained as the most reliable classifiers. Therefore, this first step of classifier evaluation was essential to retain the best machine-learning candidates for marker extraction regarding the problem under consideration.

Since it is difficult to choose a single classifier to perform a marker extraction task, an alternative lies in combining outputs of several classifiers. Figure 4(h) shows an intersection map of several pixel classifications obtained from different classifiers. In this image, pixels colored in yellow present cases where at least one classifier predicted a different class from the other classifiers. To alleviate these incoherencies, a classical way is to fuse the outputs of several classifiers to take a final decision. This comes to do multiple classifier fusion. Given a set of m classifiers, a combination rule g can be used to fuse results. This combination rule is used to estimate class membership estimates by (Kuncheva, 2004):

$$p(\omega = \omega_i \mid x) = g\left(\left\{\phi_j(\omega_i) f_j(x, \omega_i), \forall j \in [1, m[\right\}\right)$$

where $f_j(x,\omega_i)$ and $\phi_j(\omega_i)$ respectively denote class membership estimates by classifier j for class ω_i, and the confidence in the classification performed by classifier j for class ω_i. The confidence is a value assessing the reliability of a classifier in its recognition of a given class. Typical values for confidence are provided by evaluation measures. Table 2 presents results that show the interest in multiple classifier fusion with respect to using single classifiers. The confidence of each classifier is evaluated with F-measures and only three clas-

Table 1. Pixel classification results with different machine learning algorithms and feature vectors. The first four rows concern unsupervised classifiers and the last four rows supervised classifiers. Best F-measures are bold faced.

Classifier	Color feature vector	100*F(cytoplasm)	100*F(nuclei)
k-means	YCh_1Ch_2	69,5	74,4
FLDA	RGB	50,8	72,4
FLDA	$I_1I_2I_3$	57,3	71,9
FLDA	HSL	59,9	69,8
SVM	YCh_1Ch_2	77,4	74,2
Bayes	YCh_1Ch_2	72,2	**74,6**
MLP	YC_bC_r	56,9	73
kNN	HSL	**79,9**	70

Figure 4. Several pixel classifications ((c) to (g)) of an original image (a) and the intersection map of all these classifications (h) illustrating the way they agree altogether.

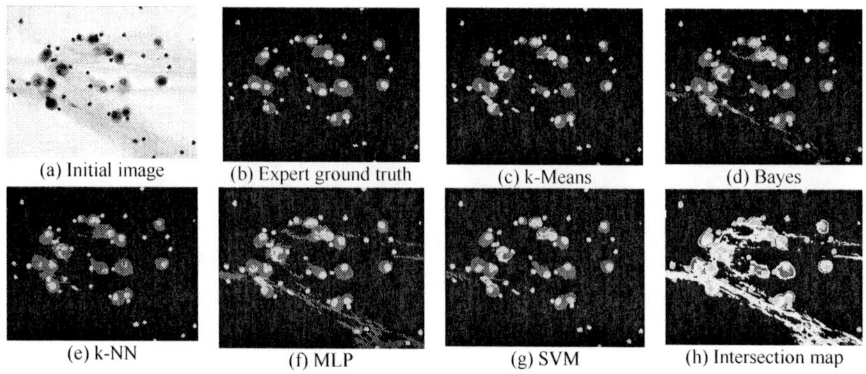

sifiers are combined (SVM, Bayes and k-means). Two combination rules *g* are considered (sum and majority vote). First, multiple classifier combination enables to obtain better final classification whatever the combination rule, sum combination rule outperforming majority vote. Therefore, multiple classifier combination is a simple and efficient method to merge the outputs of several classifiers with close accuracies.

As mentioned earlier, pixel classification is only one step in a machine-learning based morphological segmentation scheme. To assess the quality of marker extraction by machine-learning means, one needs evaluation of the whole segmentation scheme (classification followed by watershed) and not only of the sole pixel classification. These results are presented in Table 2. In this case, one evaluates the final segmentation obtained through the whole scheme of Figure 2. First, whatever the classifier, multiple classifier combination for marker extraction of a watershed performs always better than single classifier marker extraction. Second, spatial refinement by watershed enables increasing of the nuclei detection rate.

Finally, there are few differences between the obtained results. Even if one classifier performs slightly better than another one, this is not of high

Table 2. F-measures for cytoplasm and nuclei extraction by different combination rules of pixel classifications (k-means, Bayes, SVM) and by classification refined by watershed (i.e. a complete morphological segmentation making use of machine-learning algorithms for extracting markers).

Classification scheme	100*F(cytoplasm)	100*F(nuclei)
Classification by sum rule combination	78,3	74,9
Classification by majority vote rule combination	78,1	74,8
Classification refined by Watershed	**100*F(cytoplasm)**	**100*F(nuclei)**
k-means + Watershed	72,8	76,2
SVM + Watershed	73,2	75,8
Bayes + Watershed	71,1	76,3
Sum rule combination + Watershed	76,5	76,4

importance for the next morphological segmentation step, watershed. However, the previous scheme has pointed out which classifier performs the best in average: Support Vector Machines. In next Section, we show one can globally optimize such a single supervised classifier.

Single Classifier Optimization

Working with machine learning algorithms for pixel classification involves taking into account not only the recognition rate of the base inducer but also the processing time needed to perform a single pixel classification (Lebrun, 2008). SVM are powerful classifiers having high generalization abilities, but the decision function build by SVM has a complexity that increases with training set size (Steinwart, 2004). As a consequence, using SVM directly on a huge pixel dataset is not directly tractable to produce fast and efficient pixel classifier (Lebrun, 2008). Therefore, it is essential to perform an efficient model selection of SVM that achieves a trade-off between recognition rate and low complexity of the inducer (the decision function). Such a trade-off can be expressed via a criterion to optimize (Lebrun, 2007) that will be called Decision Function Quality (DFQ) in the sequel. A natural way to reduce the complexity of decision functions produced by SVM is to control the number of support vectors. Since the latter is related to training set size, one can control complexity by modifying training set size through Vector Quantization (Gersho, 1991). As opposed to the approach described in previous Section that operates in cascade, it is more natural to choose for a SVM, in a single optimization process, the values of the SVM hyper-parameters, and the simplification level of the training set, in order to optimize the proposed DFQ criterion. Such an optimization process is usually named model selection. Exhaustive search for model selection being not tractable, meta-heuristic have to be used, e.g. taboo search (Glover, 1999). Such a model selection for pixel classification has been proposed in (Lebrun, 2007) to design SVM decision function of high recognition rates while being parsimonious. To perform pixel classification, three different binary decision functions are induced, each one discriminating one class of pixel against the others. This is called a one-against-all decomposition.

Results obtained with this methodology are shown in Table 3. Recognition rate is determined using a balanced error rate. Results show that training time stays tractable in all cases. Mean classification time per image is also tractable (only few seconds) as compared with no dataset quantization (classification time higher than 1 hour). If we compare this to results presented in previous Section, SVM was probably the best pixel classifier

*Table 3. Recognition rate (**1-BER**), total number of support vectors |SV|, training time and mean classification time (in seconds) per image are given for multi-class decision functions produced with nine different color spaces.*

Color space	1-BER	|SV|	Training time	Mean classification time
RGB	86.55%	479	2639	10.32
XY_lZ	86.80%	1364	12017	29.22
L*a*b*	86.74%	745	3856	16.80
L*u*v*	86.35%	2680	5761	61.98
LCH_l	85.97%	1239	6785	27.40
YCh_1Ch_2	**87.09%**	**303**	**6404**	**6.58**
$I_1I_2I_3$	86.85%	2589	4760	54.11
HSL	86.02%	2520	2899	55.52
YC_bC_r	86.67%	519	2668	11.08
Average	86.56%	1382	5310	30.34

Table 4. Cell segmentation quality (q_{seg}), shape quality (q_{shape}) and missed artifact trade-off quality ($q' = q_{seg} - q_{shape}$) with 8 microscopic images for pixel classification and pixel classification refined by watershed.

	Pixel classification			Pixel Classification refined by watershed		
Image	q_{seg}	q_{shape}	q'	q_{seg}	q_{shape}	q'
0	17.24	1.04	16.20	**4.60**	**0.80**	**3.80**
1	6.11	1.01	5.10	**4.36**	**0.96**	**3.40**
2	11.00	0.90	10.10	**6.26**	**0.66**	**5.60**
3	24.59	2.19	22.40	**4.89**	**1.49**	**3.40**
4	6.34	0.24	6.10	**2.30**	**0.20**	**2.10**
5	6.42	0.52	5.90	**2.45**	**0.45**	**2.00**
6	7.33	0.73	6.60	**4.58**	**0.68**	**3.90**
7	13.99	0.79	13.20	**3.17**	**0.57**	**2.60**
average	11.63	0.93	10.70	**4.08**	**0.73**	**3.35**

but also the slowest. A careful model selection is therefore essential. As attended, color space has also an impact on recognition rate.

Moreover, one can see that high confidence in class memberships is obtained. Classification result is close to ground truth but with processing times largely lower than for classifiers described in previous Section. Finally, to obtain image segmentation from image classification, a watershed is performed with as markers the classification result of a SVM-based pixel classification after model selection. Table 4 shows benefits of refining image segmentation obtained by pixel classification: better results are always obtained regarding sole pixel classification. Figure 5 shows segmentation results with this segmentation scheme in comparison with expert segmentation. Globally, automatic segmentations have good matchings with expert segmentations.

Figure 5. Cell microscopic images (first row), segmentations produced by SVM after model selection refined by watershed (middle row) and expert segmentation (last row).

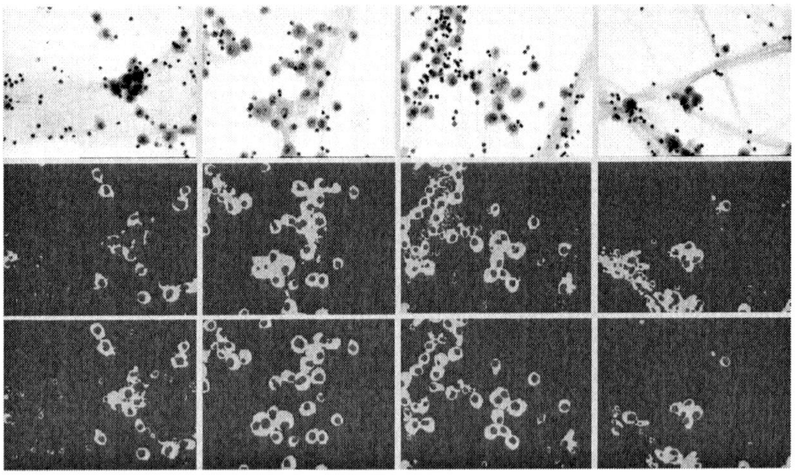

FUTURE TRENDS

Future works will concern the adaptation of machine-learning based algorithms to the classification of regions. It is much more natural, and presumably more efficient, to work with perceptually meaningful entities obtained from low-level grouping process. This will transform the problem of pixel classification into a problem of region classification. However, even if this can be attractive in terms of complexity reduction, this introduces other problems in terms of region description that have to be studied in depth.

CONCLUSION

Machine Learning algorithms have emerged as powerful techniques to introduce adaptation into the conception of image processing algorithms. For the special case of Mathematical Morphology making use of watershed from markers, far more relevant results can be obtained with markers extracted by pixel classification by machine learning algorithms. In this chapter, we described how to exploit machine learning for morphological segmentation.

ACKNOWLEDGMENT

This work was partially supported under a research grants of the ANR Foundation (ANR-06-MDCA-008-01/FOGRIMMI), FEDER and FNADT funds, and doctoral grants of the Conseil Régional de Basse-Normandie and of the Cœur et Cancer association.

REFERENCES

Arif, M., & Rajpoot, N. M. (2007). Detection of nuclei by unsupervised manifold learning. *Proceedings of Medical Image Understanding and analysis.*

Chabrier, S., Emile, B., Rosenberger, C., & Laurent, H. (2006). Unsupervised performance evaluation of image segmentation. *EURASIP Journal on Applied Signal Processing*, (pp. 1-12).

Cristianini, N., & Shawe-Taylor, J. (2000). *Introduction to Support Vector Machines and other kernel-based learning methods*. Cambridge University Press.

Derivaux, S., Lefèvre, S., Wemmert, C., & Korczak, J. J. (2007). On machine learning in watershed segmentation. *IEEE International Workshop on Machine Learning in Signal Processing* (pp. 187-192).

Dreyfus, G. (2005). *Neural Networks, Methodology and Applications*. Springer.

Duda, R., Hart, P., & Stork, D. (2000). *Pattern Classification*, Second Edition.

Fisher, R. A. (1936). The Use of Multiple Measurements in Taxonomic Problems. *Annals of Eugenics*, *7*, 179-188.

Gersho, A., & Gray, R. M. (1991). *Vector Quantization and Signal Compression*. Kluwer Academic edition.

Glover, F., & Lagun, M. (1999). *Tabu search*. Boston, MA: Kluwer Academic Publishers.

Hsu, C.-W., & Lin, C.-J. (2002). A comparison of methods for multiclass support vector machines. *IEEE Transactions on Neural Networks*, *13*, 415-425.

Kuncheva, L. (2004). *Combining Pattern Classifiers - Methods and Algorithms*. Wiley.

Lebrun, G., Charrier, C., Lezoray, O., & Cardot H. (2007). A fast and efficient segmentation scheme for cell microscopic image. *Cellular and Molecular Biology, Biomedical Signal and Image Processing*, *53*(2), 51-61.

Lebrun, G., Charrier, C., Lezoray, O., & Cardot, H. (2008) Tabu search model selection for SVM. *International Journal of Neural Systems*, *18*(1), 19-31.

Levner, I., & Zhang, H. (2007). Classification-Driven Watershed Segmentation. *IEEE Transactions on Image Processing*, *16*(5), 1437-1445.

Lezoray, O., & Cardot, H. (2002). Cooperation of color pixel classification schemes and color watershed : a study for microscopical images. *IEEE transactions on Image Processing*, *11*(7), 783-789.

Linde, Y., Buzo, A., & Gray, R. M. (1980). An Algorithm for Vector Quantizer Design. *IEEE Transactions on Communications*, (pp. 702-710).

Lukac, R., & Plataniotis, K. (2006). *Color Image Processing: Methods and Applications*. Boca Raton, FL: CRC Press / Taylor & Francis.

Meurie, C., Lebrun, G., Lezoray, O., & Elmoataz, A. (2003). A supervised segmentation scheme for cancerology color images. *IEEE ISSPIT* (pp. 664-667).

Meurie, C., Lezoray, O., Charrier, C., & Elmoataz, A. (2005). Combination of multiple pixel classifiers for microscopic image segmentation. *International Journal of Robotics and Automation*, *20*(2), 63-69.

Meyer, F. (2001). An Overview of Morphological Segmentation. *IJPRAI*, *15*(7), 1089-1118.

Michie, D., Spiegelhalter, D., & Taylor, C. (1994). *Machine learning, neural and statistical classification*.

Platt, J. (1998). Sequential minimal optimization: A fast algorithm for training support vector machines. In *Advances in Kernel Methods - Support Vector Learning*, (pp. 185-208).

Platt, J. (1999). Probabilistic outputs for support vector machines and comparisons to regularized likelihood methods. In *Advances in Large Margin Classifiers*, (pp. 61-74).

Rivest, J.-F., Beucher, S., & Delhomme, J. P. (1992). Marker-controlled segmentation: an application to electrical borehole imaging. *Journal of Electronic Imaging*, *1*(2), 136-142.

Roerdink, J. B. T. M., & Meijster, A. (2000). The watershed transform: definitions, algorithms, and parallellization strategies. *Fundamenta Informaticae, 41*, 187-228.

Rosenblatt, F. (1958). The Perceptron: A Probabilistic Model for Information Storage and Organization in the Brain. *Psychological Review, 65*(6), 386-408.

Serra, J. (1988). *Image Analysis and Mathematical Morphology: Theoretical Advances.* London: Academic Press.

Soille, P. (2004). *Morphological Image Analysis: Principles and Applications*, Springer-Verlag, Berlin and New York, corrected 2nd printing of the 2nd edition.

Steinwart, I. (2004). Sparseness of support vector machines -some asymptotically sharp bounds. *Proceedings of NIPS* (pp. 169-184).

Vapnik, V.N. (1998). *Statistical Learning Theory.* Wiley.

KEY TERMS

Classification: The process of deriving a mathematical function that can predict the membership of a class based on input data.

Classifier Combination: Classifier combination consists in combining results obtained from a set of classifiers to achieve higher performance than each single classifier.

Ground Truth: A ground-truth database is a database that provides a list of the objects in each image.

Machine Learning: As a broad subfield of artificial intelligence, machine learning is concerned with the design and development of algorithms and techniques that allow computers to "learn".

Mathematical Morphology: Mathematical morphology (MM) is a theoretical model for digital images built upon lattice theory and topology. It is the foundation of morphological image processing, which is based on shift-invariant (translation invariant) operators based principally on Minkowski addition.

Model Selection: Selection of an optimal model to predict outputs from inputs by fitting adjustable parameters.

Support Vector Machines: SVM map input vector to a higher dimensional space where a maximal hyperplane is constructed.

Watershed: Segmentation by watershed designs a family of segmentation methods that consider an image as a topographic relief the flooding of which is simulated.

Chapter XXII
Pit Pattern Classification Using Multichannel Features and Multiclassification

Michael Häfner
Medical University of Vienna, Austria

Alfred Gangl
Medical University of Vienna, Austria

Michael Liedlgruber
Salzburg University, Austria

A. Uhl
Salzburg University, Austria

Andreas Vécsei
St. Anna Children's Hospital, Austria

Friedrich Wrba
Medical University of Vienna, Austria

ABSTRACT

Wavelet-, Fourier-, and spatial domain-based texture classification methods have been used successfully for classifying zoom-endoscopic colon images according to the pit pattern classification scheme. Regarding the wavelet-based methods, statistical features based on the wavelet coefficients as well as structural features based on the wavelet packet decomposition structures of the images have been used. In the case of the Fourier-based method, statistical features based on the Fourier-coefficients in ring filter domains are computed. In the spatial domain, histogram-based techniques are used. After reviewing the various methods employed we start by extracting the feature vectors for the methods from one color channel only. To enhance the classification results the methods are then extended to utilize multichannel features obtained from all three color channels of the respective color model used. Finally, these methods are combined into one multiclassifier to stabilize classification results across the image classes.

INTRODUCTION

Today, the third most common malignant disease in western countries is colon cancer.. For that reason a regular examination of the colon is recommended, especially for people at an age of 50 years and older. *Colonoscopy* is currently the best test available to identify colon cancer.

Colonoscopy is a medical procedure which allows a physician to investigate the inside of the colon. This is done by using a colonoscope, a flexible instrument equipped with a CCD chip for visualisation of the organ and controlled by the physician. In case a lesion is detected, tissue samples can be taken and relevant lesions can be removed, avoiding thus surgery.

Modern colonoscopies allow the acquisition of digital images and video sequences from inside the colon during the colonoscopy. This makes it easier for the physician to review the results from a colonoscopy and to document the growth and spreading of an eventually tumorous lesion. To obtain images which are as detailed as possible a magnifying colonoscope is used. This type of colonoscope provides images which are up to 150-fold magnified and thus are very detailed as they uncover the fine surface structure of the mucosa as well as small lesions.

A common procedure to visually enhance the structure of the mucosa is to spray indigo carmine or methylen blue onto the mucosa. While dyeing with indigo carmine causes a plastic appearance of the mucosa, dyeing with methylen blue helps to highlight the boundary of a lesion. Cresyl violet is often used to actually stain the margins of the pit structures, which is also referred to as staining.

In this work we document the good performance of several texture classification techniques to perform an automated classification of pit pattern images acquired by a magnifying colonoscope. Based on these methods, we show the benefit of using features based on three color channels. Finally, we present one possible way to combine several methods and classifiers to build a multiclassifier.

Note that the developed techniques are not meant to replace the physicians' diagnosis but are designed to act as a decision support system for the human operator during colonoscopy – here a reliable and immediate diagnosis is a significant advantage since a second colonoscopy required in many cases can be avoided as there is no need to wait for the histological classification of eventually extracted biopsies.

PIT PATTERN CLASSIFICATION

Polyps of the colon are a frequent finding and are usually divided into metaplastic, adenomatous, and malignant. As resection of all polyps is time-consuming, it is imperative that those polyps which warrant endoscopic resection can be distinguished: polypectomy of metaplastic lesions is unnecessary and removal of invasive cancer may be hazardous. For these reasons, assessing the malignant potential of lesions at the time of colonoscopy is important.

To be able to differentiate between the different types of lesions a classification method is needed.

The most commonly used classification system for distinguishing between non-neoplastic and neoplastic lesions in the colon is the pit pattern classification originally reported by Kudo, Hirota et al. (1994) and Kudo, Tamura et al. (1996).

This system allows a differentiation between normal mucosa, hyperplastic lesions (non-neoplastic), adenomas (a pre-malignant condition), and malignant cancer based on the visual pattern of the mucosal surface. Hence, this classification scheme is a convenient tool to decide which lesions need not, which should, and which most likely can't be removed endoscopically. The mucosal pattern as seen after dye staining and by using magnification endoscopy shows a high agreement with the histopathologic diagnosis. Furthermore, due to the fact that this method is based on the histopathologic (and therefore visual) structure of the mucosa, it is a convenient choice for a classification using image processing methods.

As illustrated in Figure 1, this classification method differentiates between the five main types I to V according to the mucosal surface of the colon. Type III is divided into two sub-types, III-S and III-L, designating the size of the pit structure. The higher the number of the pit type is, the higher is the risk that the lesion under investigation is malignant.

It has been suggested that pattern of type I and II are characteristic of non-neoplastic lesions, type III and IV are found on adenomatous polyps, and type V are strongly suggestive of invasive carcinoma.

Lesions of type I and II are benign, representing the normal mucosa or hyperplastic tissue, and in fact are non-tumorous. Lesions of type III and IV in contrast represent lesions which are neoplastic. Type V lesions usually are highly indicative for cancer. Thus a coarser grouping of lesions into two instead of six classes is also possible.

Using a magnifying colonoscope together with indigo carmine dye spraying, the mucosal crypt pattern on the surface of colonic lesions can be observed (Kudo et al., 1996). Several studies found a good correlation between the mucosal pit pattern and the histological findings, where especially techniques using magnifying colonoscopes led to excellent results (Hurlstone et al., 2004).

As depicted in Figure 1 pit pattern types I to IV can be characterized fairly well, while type V is a composition of unstructured pits. Table 1 contains a short overview of the main characteristics of the different pit pattern types.

Although at a first glance this classification scheme seems to be straightforward and easy to be applied, it needs some experience and exercising to achieve fairly good results (Hurlstone, 2002; Tung, Wu, & Su, 2001) – here, an automated decision support system for the physician conducting the colonoscopy would improve the situation. To illustrate this, Figure 2 contains images out of the training set used throughout this work.

FEATURE EXTRACTION AND CLASSIFICATION

The task of automated image classification consists of two major parts: the extraction of relevant features from images and the classification based on these features. These parts are outlined in the following section.

Wavelet-Based Methods

Previous work has already shown that wavelet-based methods can be used successfully for the classification of colon cancer. In (Karkanis et al., 2001) frames of an endoscopic video are transformed to the wavelet domain using the discrete pyramidal *wavelet transform*. Based on the resulting wavelet coefficients, second order statistics are computed from co-occurrence matrices for the wavelet subbands. These statistical values are used as input for an artificial neural network. An implementation along with results is documented in (Maroulis et al., 2003).

The approaches described in (Karkanis et al., 1999; Karkanis et al., 2000) are very similar, but instead of using all subbands, only the subband with the highest variance in the coefficient histogram is used to obtain features.

In (Häfner et al., 2006a; Liedlgruber & Uhl, 2007) different wavelet-based methods in conjunction with different classifiers have been used successfully for *pit pattern classification*. Six distinct methods have been investigated to obtain features based on the wavelet transform. The types of features include statistical features as well as structural features.

Statistical Features

In previous work (Häfner et al., 2006a) we have already presented results using two classical feature sets generated from the discrete wavelet packets transform (DWP). The DWP transform domain contains the pyramidal wavelet transform

Figure 1. Pit pattern classification according to Kudo et al.

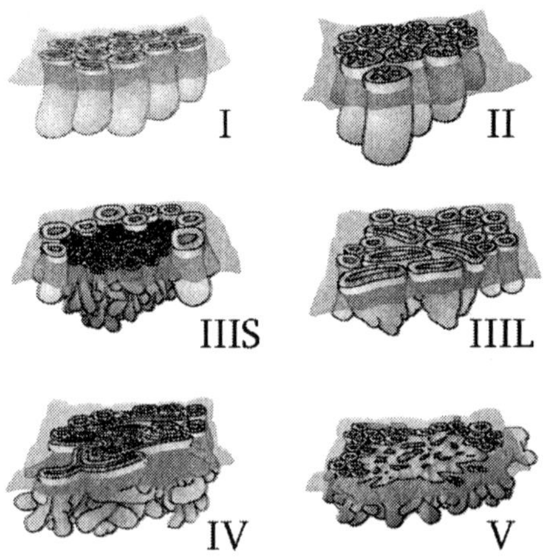

Table 1. The characteristics of the different pit pattern types.

Pit type	Characteristics
I	roundish pits, which designate a normal mucosa
II	stellar or papillary pits
III-S	small roundish or tubular pits which are smaller than the pits of type I
III-L	roundish or tubular pits which are larger than the pits of type I
IV	branch-like or gyrus-like pits
V	non-structured pits

Figure 2. Images taken with a colonoscope showing the different types of pit pattern.

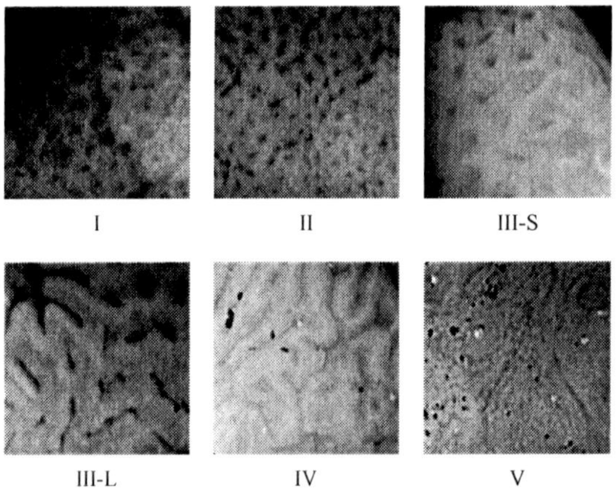

(WPC) as a subset of the subbands which are used to extract the corresponding first type of feature vector. Possible features computed are based on the coefficients in the subbands (e.g. the Energy, Logarithm of energy, Variance, Entropy, or the l-Norm).

The Local discriminant bases algorithm (LDB) (Saito & Coifman, 1995; Saito, 1997; Rajpoot, 2003) is used to generate the second type of feature vectors considered in previous work. Contrasting to the previous technique this method is already highly focused on discrimination between different classes. Here, a wavelet packet basis optimal for discrimination between images of different classes is constructed. Once this basis has been identified all training images are decomposed into this basis. The resulting subbands are then used in the subsequent feature extraction step.

Wavelet packets can be used in two additional ways to extract statistical features from the DWP domain (Liedlgruber & Uhl, 2007). Both rely on the best-basis algorithm (Coifman & Wickerhauser, 1992) which decomposes a given image into an optimal wavelet packet basis according to a specified cost function (e.g. like Logarithm of energy, Entropy, L_p-Norm and the Threshold cost function). The resulting subband structure usually concentrates the energy of the image in an optimal way.

The Best-basis method (BB) decomposes each training image into an optimal wavelet packet basis with respect to the chosen wavelet family. The resulting subbands are used to extract features from. Since however the resulting decomposition structures are different among the images, we employ a voting procedure, which assures, that the feature vectors for the different images are based on the same subbands and that the subband ordering within the feature vectors is the same. After all training images are decomposed into their respective best basis subband structures, we count the occurrence of each subband of a fully decomposed DWP decomposition quadtree in the set of all training images' best basis subband structures. The subbands used to extract features from (also for the images to be subsequently classified) are those with the highest occurrence count.

The Best-basis centroid (BBCB) method also decomposes each training image into an optimal wavelet packet basis according to the best-basis algorithm. Subsequently, a common decomposition structure – a so-called centroid – is determined, into which all images are being subsequently decomposed and which is used to extract features from. This centroid is obtained by determining the subband structure which has the smallest average distance to all best-basis decomposition trees of the training images according to some quadtree distance metric.

Structural Features

In contrast to the feature extraction methods presented in the previous section, the methods presented in this section rely on the best-basis subband structures.

In the best-basis structural method (BBS) we use two different ways to create a feature vector (Liedlgruber & Uhl, 2007). The first method creates a feature vector for a given image, which contains the so-called unique node values of the respective decomposition quadtree. These unique node values uniquely identify each possible node in a quadtree. To ensure, that the feature vectors among all images contain the same node positions, for each node present in a tree a zero is inserted into the feature vectors for those images, which do not contain the according node in their decomposition structures. Having obtained these feature vectors, the euclidean distance is used to calculate the similarity between two images.

The second feature extraction method uses the decomposition trees directly as features. Using a quadtree distance metric the distance between two images can then be calculated. These distances are subsequently used to classify an unknown image using the k-NN classifier (see below).

Fourier-Based Approach

Contrasting to the feature extraction methods presented above, also the discrete Fourier transform (DFT) can be used for feature extraction resulting in excellent classification results (Häfner et al., 2007). This approach is based on the *Fast Fourier Transform* (FFT), which is an efficient algorithm to compute the DFT. Using the 2D-FFT, all training images are transformed to the Fourier domain. Based on the resulting Fourier coefficients, the power spectrum is computed for each image. Several non-overlapping rings of different starting offsets and widths are chosen from the power spectrum (ring filters, band-pass filters). These rings are then used to extract features such as the mean and the standard deviation of the coefficients' magnitudes contained in each of the rings. This yields a feature vector consisting of n entries for n distinct rings in the filter. Figure 3 shows two examples of ring filters.

In (Häfner et al., 2007) the entire information contained in the RGB color model has been chosen to create feature vectors from. Therefore a single feature vector is created from each of the three color channels (R, G and B). These feature vectors are then concatenated to form one large feature vector. Then the Bayes classifier (see below) is used for classification.

One major problem is the huge number of possible ring configurations to choose from. As a consequence, in (Häfner et al., 2007) a genetic algorithm is proposed to perform a search for optimal ring configurations. We follow this strategy but use all types of classifiers considered in this work (see below).

Spatial Domain Approach

Pit pattern classification can also be performed in the spatial domain using a selection of different *histograms* (Häfner et al., 2006b).

The experiments in (Häfner et al., 2006b) have been conducted using 1D, 2D and 3D histograms. The classical intensity 1D histograms are created for all channels of the RGB color model. The 2D histograms (co-occurrence histograms) are created for the luminance channel of the YUV color model. The 3D histograms are created for all channels of the RGB color model concurrently per definition.

For the classification process the k-NN classifier (see next section) is used. The distance measure used to compute the distance between two normalized histograms H_a and H_b for images I_a and I_b, respectively, is based on the so-called histogram intersection. For 1D histograms the distance is defined as

$$d(H_a, H_b) = 1 - \sum_{i=1}^{n} \min(H_a[i], H_b[i]) \quad (1)$$

where n is the number of bins in each histogram. The equivalents for the 2D and 3D case are

$$d(H_a, H_b) = 1 - \sum_{i=1}^{n}\sum_{j=1}^{n} \min(H_a[i,j], H_b[i,j]) \quad (2)$$

and

$$d(H_a, H_b) = 1 - \sum_{i=1}^{n}\sum_{j=1}^{n}\sum_{k=1}^{n} \min(H_a[i,j,k], H_b[i,j,k]) \quad (3)$$

The experiments in (Häfner et al., 2006b) consider the RGB color model and the luminance channel of the YUV color model only. In this work we examine the information of all color channels of the YUV and HSV color model too.

Classification

In (Häfner et al., 2006a) we employed two distinct classifiers, namely the *k-Nearest Neighbors classifier* (k-NN) and *Support Vector Machines* (SVM). Using the k-NN classifier classification is done by finding the k closest neighbors of an input feature vector $\mathbf{x}$ in the feature space according to some distance metric (e.g. euclidean). The unknown sample $\mathbf{x}$ is then assigned

Figure 3. Two examples of possible ring configurations

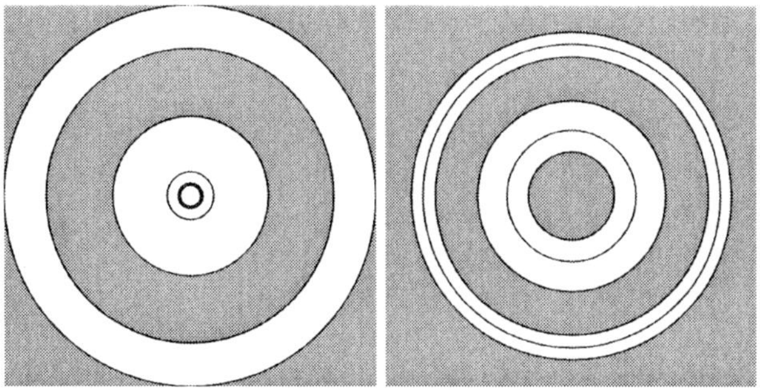

to the dominating class among the k nearest neighbors.

The SVM classifier, presented in more detail in (Chang & Lin, 2001; Hsu, Chang, & Lin; Burges, 1998), is another, recently developed classifier, which has already been successfully used to classify texture using wavelet features (Rajpoot & Rajpoot, 2004). The basic idea behind SVM is to construct classifying hyperplanes, which are optimal for separation of given data. These hyperplanes divide the feature space into two distinct classes. For the 6-classes case a voting procedure, combining the two classes classification steps, is employed.

In addition to these two classifiers, we also use the *Bayes classifier*, which is explained in more detail in (Fukunaga, 1990). This is a probabilistic classifier based on the Bayes theorem. During classification each unknown image is a assigned to that class, to which the image belongs to most probably or which causes minimal costs with respect to some cost function.

MULTICHANNEL FEATURES AND THE MULTICLASSIFIER

As already mentioned above, the experiments presented in (Häfner et al., 2007) have been carried out by using all color channels for feature extraction. Since this improved the results, hope is raised that this will also apply to the wavelet-based methods. Therefore we extended the wavelet-based methods using non-structural features to use all color channels.

Multiclassifier for Two Classes

Although the methods presented above deliver a very promising classification accuracy already, we now describe how these methods have been combined in the 2-classes case to improve the accuracy.

The *multiclassifier* mainly relies on two pieces of information: method ranking and method reliability. The ranking expresses how accurately a method classifies images mostly misclassified. Based on a list containing the x most misclassified images for class c the rank for each method is updated for all x images. The rank for the most accurate method for the given image is incremented by N, which denotes the total number of methods combined. The rank for the second-best method is incremented by $N-1$, and so on. Finally, the ranking $R_{m,c}$ for each method m and class c is normalized and transformed to lie between -1 and 1. This computation is repeated for each image class c to get the ranking information for all classes.

The method reliability is telling us how much we can rely on the classification result of a specific method. The computation of the reliability A_m for a method m is based on the Bayesian a posteriori probability:

$$A_m = \left(\sum_{i=1}^{C} N_i \frac{b_i r_i}{(1-b_i)(1-r_i)+b_i r_i} \right) / \frac{N}{2} - 1 \qquad (4)$$

where C is the number of classes used, N_i is the number of images in class i, N is the total number of images, b_i is the a priori probability for class i and r_i is the classification rate for class i. Multiplying the inner part of the sum by N_i produces a weighted measure, which accounts for the unbalanced training set. Finally, the value is normalized and transformed to lie between *-1* and *1*.

Two allow controlling the strength of influence the ranking and the reliability have on the result of the multiclassifier, these values are remapped by

$$V_f(x) = \operatorname{sign}(x)|x|^{\ln(f)/\ln(0.5)} \qquad (5)$$

where f is the parameter controlling the shape of the remapping function. The effect of choosing different values for f is depicted in Figure 4. Obviously $f=0.5$ corresponds to a linear mapping. The resulting image class c_i for an image i is calculated by

$$c_i = \sum_{j=1}^{M} D_{i,j} V_f(A_j) V_f(R_{j,p}) \qquad (6)$$

where M is the number of methods combined, $D_{i,j}$ is the remapped value of the previously assigned class p for image i by method j (*-1* for class *1* and *1* for class *2*), A_j is the reliability of method j and $R_{j,p}$ is the ranking for method j and class p. The resulting class is then

$$resultclass = \begin{cases} 1, & \text{if } c_i < 0 \\ 2, & \text{else} \end{cases} \qquad (7)$$

Multiclassifier for Six Classes

Due to the binary nature of the *multiclassifier* introduced by Equation (6), the 6-classes case needs to be handled slightly different. The computation of the ranking and the reliability remain almost the same, just the transformation to the range between -1 and 1 has been omitted. Additionally the reliability is computed for each class which reflects the reliability of a method for a specific class.

The final classification result is obtained by a weighted majority voting, based on value x_c which is calculated for each image i and class c as follows:

$$x_c = \sum_{j=1}^{M} \alpha_{i,j} V_f(A_{j,c}) V_f(R_{j,c}) \qquad (8)$$

where $A_{j,c}$ is the reliability of method j for class c, $R_{j,c}$ is the ranking for method j and $\alpha_{i,j}$ is

$$\alpha_{i,j} = \begin{cases} 1, & \text{if } D_{i,j} = c \\ 0, & \text{else} \end{cases} \qquad (9)$$

The final class C for the unknown image is obtained by

$$C = \arg\max_c x_c \qquad (10)$$

Methods which perform poor for a class c, are filtered out on a per-class basis. Thus only the X_c most reliable methods are considered for class c. Furthermore, to reduce the worsening effect of unreliable methods, we apply a threshold function to the reliability of a class c. The result is a modified version of Equation (8):

$$x_c = \sum_{j=1}^{M} \alpha_{i,j} \beta_{j,c,k} B_t(A_{j,c}) V_f(R_{j,c}) \qquad (11)$$

where $\beta_{j,c,k}$ is set to *1* if method j is among the k most reliable methods for class c. Otherwise $\beta_{i,j,k}$ is set to *0* and therefore method j is ignored. B_t is the threshold function using threshold t.

To consider the low sample count for class III-S, different threshold values are used for this class and all other classes (empirical values 0.1 and 0.4, respectively). This is necessary since the reliability is based on a priori knowledge, which leads to very low reliabilities for class III-S - even if a method performs equally well or better than for another class.

EXPERIMENTS AND RESULTS

Settings

In our experiments we use 484 images acquired in 2005 and 2006 at the Department of Gastroenterology and Hepatology (Medical University of Vienna) using a zoomcolonoscope (Olympus Evis Exera CF-Q160ZI/L) with a magnification factor set to 150. Lesions found during colonoscopy have been examined after application of dye-spraying with indigo carmine as routinely performed in colonoscopy. Biopsies or mucosal resection have been performed in order to get a histopathological diagnosis. Biopsies have been taken from type I, II, and type V lesions, as those lesions need not to be removed or cannot be removed endoscopically. Type III and IV lesions have been removed endoscopically. Out of all acquired images, histopathological classification resulted in 198 non-neoplastic and 286 neoplastic cases. The detailed classification results, which are used as ground truth for our experiments, are shown in Table 2.

Due to the rather limited set of images available for our experiments, we use leave-one-out cross-validation. Thus, 483 out of 484 images are used as training set. The remaining image is then classified. This process is repeated for each image.

Results

Multichannel Features

Figure 5 shows the differences between the overall classification results (percentage of correctly classified images) we obtain using features from single color channels and multichannel features in the 2-classes case using the RGB color model. Figure 6 depicts the same comparison, but for the 6-classes case. In Tables 5 and 6 the respective results are presented in a more detailed fashion (especially with respect to results for each single class).

As we can see from Figure 5, regarding the 2-classes case, using multichannel features im-

Figure 4. The effect of different choices for f in the value remapping function

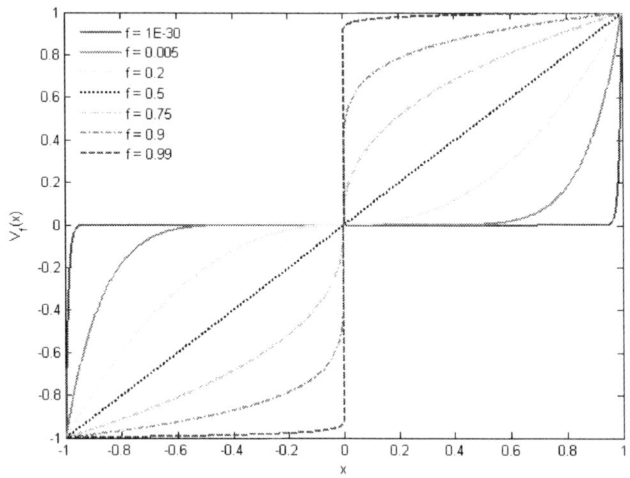

Table 2. Number of images per class used in our experiments

Pit Pattern	I	II	III-S	III-L	IV	V
# of Images	126	72	18	62	146	60

Figure 5. Comparison of the different methods using single channel (SC) and multichannel (MC) features in the 2-classes case

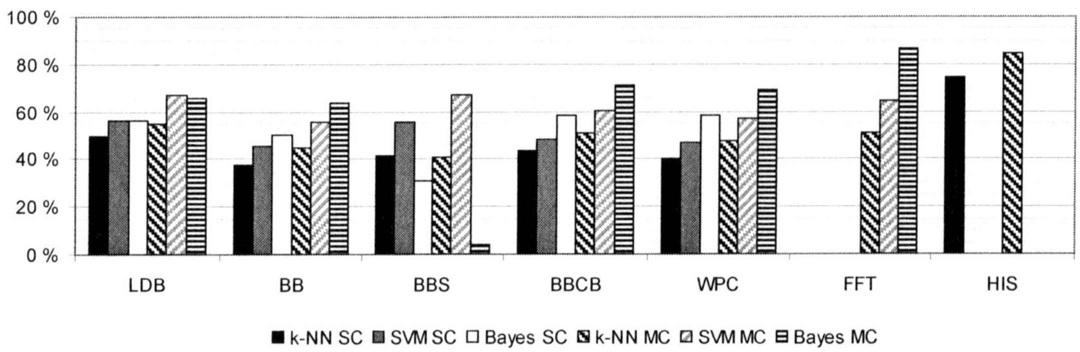

proves the results for nearly all methods. The result improvements lie between 5 % and 17 % for the BB method with the k-NN classifier and BBCB with the Bayes classifier, respectively. Only the result for the BBS method used with the Bayes classifier drops by 4 %. Concerning classifiers, the Bayes classifier gives the best results, followed by SVM and k-NN (except for the BBS method which performs best using SVM).

Regarding the 6-classes case, the improvements are very similar, as shown in Figure 6. Using multichannel features the results are improved by values between 5 % and 13 % for the LDB method with the k-NN classifier and the BB and BBCB methods using the Bayes classifier, respectively. Again the results drop considerably using the BBS method.

While the result drops by 1 % only when using BBS in conjunction with the k-NN classifier, the result decreases by 27 % for the combination of BBS and the Bayes classifier. Again, the Bayes classifier provides the best overall results but again BBS behaves significantly different compared to the rest of the feature extraction methods.

The best classification results given in Tables 3 to 6 have been found by large scale experimentation testing a significant amount of different parameter settings for each technique considered (e.g. by using different feature vector lengths, different color channels or k-values when using the k-NN classifier).

During our experiments it turned out that regarding the single channel tests most of the best results have been achieved using the red channel of the RGB color model. The other color channel often yielding good results is the luminance channel of the YUV color model. Regarding the multichannel tests the best results have always been achieved using the RGB color model.

Apart from that, it has been observed that some of the feature vector lengths in the multichannel case are considerably higher compared to their single channel counterparts. In the 2-classes case the feature vector lengths vary between 3 and 100, and 3 and 261, in the single channel and

Figure 6. Comparison of the different methods using single channel (SC) and multichannel (MC) features in the 6-classes case

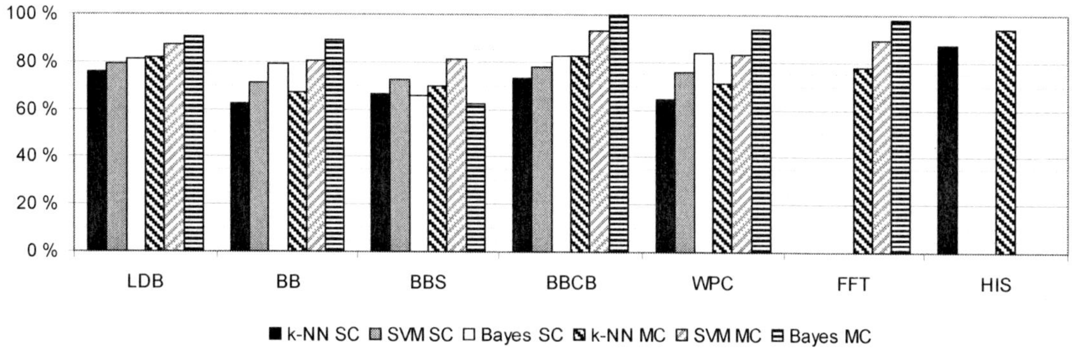

Table 3. Percentage of correctly classified pit pattern images using single channel features in the 2-classes case

	I - II	III-S - V	Total
LOCAL DISCRIMINANT BASES			
k-NN	66	83	**76**
SVM	65	89	**79**
Bayes	73	86	**81**
BEST BASIS METHOD			
k-NN	42	76	**62**
SVM	56	81	**71**
Bayes	71	84	**79**
STRUCTURAL BEST BASIS METHOD			
k-NN	47	79	**66**
SVM	73	73	**73**
Bayes	53	75	**66**
BEST BASIS CENTROID METHOD			
k-NN	70	76	**73**
SVM	60	90	**78**
Bayes	77	87	**83**
PYRAMIDAL WAVELET TRANSFORM			
k-NN	56	71	**65**
SVM	63	85	**76**
Bayes	77	88	**84**
HISTOGRAM METHOD			
k-NN	83	90	**87**

Table 4. Percentage of correctly classified pit pattern images using multichannel features in the 2-classes case

	I - II	III-S - V	Total
LOCAL DISCRIMINANT BASES			
k-NN	73	88	**82**
SVM	78	93	**87**
Bayes	89	92	**91**
BEST BASIS METHOD			
k-NN	37	88	**67**
SVM	67	90	**81**
Bayes	84	92	**89**
STRUCTURAL BEST BASIS METHOD			
k-NN	62	75	**70**
SVM	54	100	**81**
Bayes	44	74	**62**
BEST BASIS CENTROID METHOD			
k-NN	82	84	**83**
SVM	92	95	**94**
Bayes	100	100	**100**
PYRAMIDAL WAVELET TRANSFORM			
k-NN	56	81	**71**
SVM	77	87	**83**
Bayes	91	95	**94**
HISTOGRAM METHOD			
k-NN	94	93	**94**
FOURIER METHOD			
k-NN	74	81	**78**
SVM	85	92	**89**
Bayes	97	98	**98**

multichannel case, respectively. In the 6-classes case we observe lengths between 7 and 91, and 3 and 150, when using single channel features and multichannel features, respectively. This resulted in notedly higher computational demand.

The k-values for the k-NN classifier used to get the best results in the 2-classes case are rather low compared to the number of samples in each class (between 1 and 11, and 1 and 29, in the single channel and multichannel case,

Table 5. Percentage of correctly classified pit pattern images using single channel features in the 6-classes case

	I	II	III-S	III-L	IV	V	Total
LOCAL DISCRIMINANT BASES							
k-NN	69	42	28	45	57	10	**49**
SVM	65	51	0	50	64	48	**56**
Bayes	67	49	0	65	55	55	**56**
BEST BASIS METHOD							
k-NN	52	18	0	42	53	0	**38**
SVM	59	43	0	47	53	17	**46**
Bayes	63	29	39	65	43	57	**50**
STRUCTURAL BEST BASIS METHOD							
k-NN	53	31	0	44	52	15	**42**
SVM	100	0	0	3	98	0	**56**
Bayes	94	0	0	3	10	22	**31**
BEST BASIS CENTROID METHOD							
k-NN	54	35	11	45	42	43	**43**
SVM	61	47	11	39	51	38	**49**
Bayes	68	54	6	68	53	62	**58**
PYRAMIDAL WAVELET TRANSFORM							
k-NN	59	32	0	27	47	22	**40**
SVM	63	26	0	8	73	30	**47**
Bayes	68	60	6	71	48	65	**58**
HISTOGRAM METHOD							
k-NN	71	61	67	81	84	67	**74**

Table 6. Percentage of correctly classified pit pattern images using multichannel features in the 6-classes case

	I	II	III-S	III-L	IV	V	Total
LOCAL DISCRIMINANT BASES							
k-NN	61	38	6	58	73	33	**55**
SVM	71	51	11	76	76	63	**67**
Bayes	75	60	6	52	77	60	**66**
BEST BASIS METHOD							
k-NN	55	26	0	45	67	8	**45**
SVM	94	6	6	2	100	0	**56**
Bayes	68	51	0	65	71	68	**63**
STRUCTURAL BEST BASIS METHOD							
k-NN	54	4	0	6	67	42	**41**
SVM	92	92	0	8	95	0	**67**
Bayes	0	0	100	0	0	0	**4**
BEST BASIS CENTROID METHOD							
k-NN	56	43	17	56	53	53	**51**
SVM	60	51	0	53	76	60	**61**
Bayes	75	51	0	65	79	95	**71**
PYRAMIDAL WAVELET TRANSFORM							
k-NN	64	44	6	48	53	17	**48**
SVM	53	51	6	61	69	52	**57**
Bayes	84	56	0	47	90	47	**69**
HISTOGRAM METHOD							
k-NN	81	82	83	87	89	80	**84**
FOURIER METHOD							
k-NN	53	47	11	52	59	43	**51**
SVM	70	53	0	61	77	60	**64**
Bayes	87	81	28	89	94	88	**86**

respectively). Regarding the 6-classes case, the values are rather high compared to the number of samples of class III-S (between 1 and 10, and 1 and 22, in the single channel and multichannel case, respectively).

In the case of the wavelet-based tests we tried different statistical features of which no dominating one has been observed. For structural features, in most cases using the unique node IDs delivers the best results. This is due to the fact that the underlying implementation is not able to use quadtrees as features for the SVM and Bayes classifier.

Figures 7 and 8 show the ring configurations used for the Fourier method in the 2-classes and 6-classes case, respectively. From these figures it seems that mostly low frequency components contain important coefficients for the classification regarding the 2-classes case as well as the 6-classes case.

Multiclassifier

Since the multichannel features outperformed the single channel features as pointed out above, the multiclassifier has been tested using the multichannel feature based methods only.

From Table 7 we see that in the 2-classes case the multiclassifier outperforms all methods except the Fourier method and the BBCB method. Both superior methods are using the Bayes classifier in this case and reach 98 % and 100 %, respectively, compared to 98 % overall classification accuracy reached by the multiclassifier.

Regarding the 6-classes case, the multiclassifier delivers a considerably better overall classification result of 94 % compared to the single

Figure 7. The Fourier filters in the 2-classes case for the R, G and B channel (from left to right)

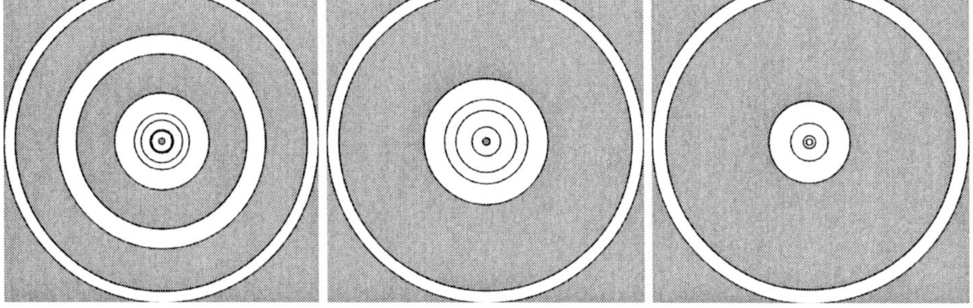

Figure 8. The Fourier filters used in the 6-classes case for the R, G and B channel (from left to right)

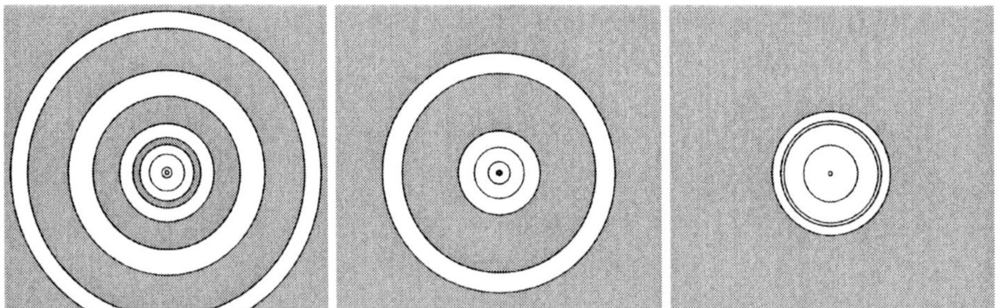

methods, which reach an overall classification result between 4 % and 86 % for the BBS method and the Fourier method, respectively, both using the Bayes classifier.

DISCUSSION AND FUTURE TRENDS

To highlight the clinical relevance of the results obtained throughout this work, a comparative meta-study of Kato, Fu et al. (2006) should be mentioned. This study showed, that regarding the 2-classes case, the overall (human) classification accuracy of magnifying colonoscopy based on the pit pattern scheme varies between approximately 80 % and 99 %. The multiclassifier presented in this work delivers a classification accuracy of 98 % in the 2-classes case which ranges among the top-values achieved by physicians documented in this study. The Fourier method in the multichannel case is able to deliver almost the same accuracy as well. This clearly shows that the discussed approach can be a valuable decision support technique in clinical usage.

One possible way to further improve the classification results would be to map features into another, better suitable feature space using Linear discriminant analysis or Principal component analysis. Apart from that, additional preprocessing to the images may be applied. Up to now no particular preprocessing has been performed except for the histogram method, where a Gaussian blur has been used. Although this has been tried with the rest of the methods too, there was no significant gain in classification performance.

Table 7. Overall classification results in percent using the multiclassifier based on methods using multichannel features

Pit Type	I	II	III-S	III-L	IV	V	Total
2 classes	94		100				**98**
6 classes	100	94	83	81	97	92	**94**

CONCLUSION

In this work we show that automated pit pattern classification is feasible using general purpose texture classification techniques. However, optimal results are achieved after careful selection and optimization of classification parameters only, except for the histogram-based techniques which deliver satisfying results in an almost ad-hoc manner. It has turned out that classification results can be enhanced when considering all the color information stored in an image.

Apart from that we showed one possible way to combine different methods into one multiclassifier. The proposed multiclassifier is able to yield significantly better results in the 6-classes case as compared to the single classification techniques (while in the 2-classes case a slight degradation of the best results is found). The classification accuracy observed for the best standalone multichannel techniques and the multiclassifier already qualify the approach as an interesting choice for a decision support system for clinical usage.

ACKNOWLEDGMENT

This work is partially funded by the Austrian Science Fund (FWF) under Project No. L366-N15 and by the Austrian National Bank "Jubiläumsfonds" Project No. 12514.

REFERENCES

Burges, C. J. C. (1998). A Tutorial on Support Vector Machines for Pattern Recognition. *Data Mining and Knowledge Discovery, 2*(2), 121-167.

Chang, C., & Lin, C. (2001). LIBSVM: A Library for Support Vector Machines. Retrieved April 1, 2005, from http://www.csie.ntu.edu.tw/~cjlin/

Coifman, R. R., & Wickerhauser, M. V. (1992). Entropy-based algorithms for best basis selection. *IEEE Transactions on Information Theory, 38*(2), 713-719.

Fukunaga, K. (1990). *Statistical Pattern Recognition*. Morgan Kaufmann.

Hsu, C., Chang, C., & Lin, C. A Practical Guide to Support Vector Classification.

Häfner, M., Liedlgruber, M., Wrba, F., Gangl, A., Vécsei, A., & Uhl, A. (2006a). Pit pattern classification of zoom-endoscopic colon images using wavelet texture features. *Proceedings of the International Conference on Advances in Medical Signal and Image Processing (MEDSIP 2006).*

Häfner, M., Kendlbacher, C., Mann, W., Taferl, W., Wrba, F., Gangl, A., Vécsei, A., & Uhl, A. (2006b). Pit pattern classification of zoom-endoscopic colon images using histogram techniques. *Proceedings of the 7th Nordic Signal Processing Symposium (NORSIG 2006)*, 58-61.

Häfner, M., Brunauer, L., Payer, H., Resch, R., Wrba, F., Gangl, A., et al. (2007). Pit pattern classification of zoom-endoscopical colon images using evolved Fourier feature vectors *Proceedings of the 2007 IEEE Machine Learning for Signal Processing Workshop (MLSP'07)*, 99 - 104.

Hsu, C., & Lin, C. (2002). A Comparison of Methods for Multi-Class Support Vector Machines. *IEEE Transactions on Neural Networks*, *13*(2), 415-425.

Hurlstone, D. P. (2002). High-Resolution Magnification Chromoendoscopy: Common Problems Encountered in "Pit Pattern" Interpretation and Correct Classification of Flat Colorectal Lesions. *American Journal of Gastroenterology*, *97*, 1069-1070.

Hurlstone, D. P., Cross, S. S., Adam, I., Shorthouse, A. J., Brown, S., Sanders, D. S., & Lobo, A. J. (2004). Efficacy of High Magnification Chromoscopic Colonoscopy for the Diagnosis of Neoplasia in Flat and Depressed Lesions of the Colorectum: a Prospective Analysis. *Gut*, *53*, 284-290.

Karkanis, S., Iakovidis, D., Maroulis, D., Theofanous, N., & Magoulas, G. (2000). Tumor Recognition in Endoscopic Video Images using Artificial Neural Network Architectures. *Proceedings of the 26th EUROMICRO Conference (EUROMICRO'00)*, 423-429.

Karkanis, S., Iakovidis, D., Karras, D., & Maroulis, D. (2001). Detection of Lesions in Endoscopic Video using Textural Descriptors on Wavelet Domain supported by Artificial Neural Network Architectures. *Proceedings of the. International Conference on Image Processing (ICIP'01)*, 833-836.

Karkanis, S., Magoulas, G., Grigoriadou, M., & Schurr, M. (1999). Detecting Abnormalities in Colonoscopic Images by Textural Description and Neural Networks. *Proceedings of the Workshop on Machine Learning in Medical Applications, Advance Course in Artificial Intelligence (ACAI'99)*, 59-62.

Kato, S., Fu, K., Sano, Y., Fujii, T., Saito, Y., Matsuda, T., et al. (2006). Magnifying colonoscopy as a non-biopsy technique for differential diagnosis of non-neoplastic and neoplastic lesions. *World journal of gastroenterology : WJG*, 12(9), 1416-20.

Kudo, S., Hirota, S., Nakajima, T., Hosobe, S., Kusaka, & H., Kobayashi, T. (1994). Colorectal tumours and pit pattern. *Journal of Clinical Pathology*, *47*(10), 880-885.

Kudo, S., Tamura, S., Nakajima, T., Yamano, H., Kusaka, H., & Watanabe, H. (1996). Diagnosis of colorectal tumorous lesions by magnifying endoscopy. *Gastrointestinal endoscopy*, *44*(1), 8-14.

Liedlgruber, M., & Uhl, A. (2007). Statistical and structural wavelet packet features for Pit pattern classification in zoom-endoscopic colon images (P. Dondon, V. Mladenov, S. Impedovo, & S. Cepisca, Hrsg.). *Proceedings of the 7th WSEAS International Conference on Wavelet Analysis & Multirate Systems (WAMUS'07)*, 147-152.

Maroulis, D., Iakovidis, D., Karkanis, S., & Karras, D. (2003). CoLD: a versatile detection system for colorectal lesions in endoscopy video-frames. *Computer methods and programs in biomedicine*, 70(2), 151-66.

Rajpoot, N. (2003). Local Discriminant Wavelet Packet Basis for Texture Classification. *Proceedings of the International Society for Optical Engineering SPIE Wavelets: Applications in Signal and Image Processing X*, 774-783.

Rajpoot, K., & Rajpoot, N. (2004). Wavelets and support vector machines for texture classification. *Multitopic Conference, 2004. Proceedings of INMIC 2004. 8th International*, 328-333.

Saito, N. (1997). Classification of Geophysical Acoustic Waveforms and Extraction of Geological Information Using Time-Frequency Atoms. *1996 Proceedings of the Computing Section of the American Statistical Association*, 322-327.

Saito, N., & Coifman, R. R. (1995). Local Discriminant Bases and their Applications. *J. Mathematical Imaging and Vision*, *5*(4), 337-358.

Tung, S., Wu C-S, & Su, M. (2001). Magnifying Colonoscopy in Differentiating Neoplastic From Nonneoplastic Colorectal Lesions. *American Journal of Gastroenterology*, *96*, 2628-2632.

KEY TERMS

Classification Feature: A numerical or syntactical value used to describe an observed property of an object (e.g., size, color, shape, …).

Classification Feature Vector: A collection of classification features describing the properties of an object.

Classifier: An algorithm to assign unknown object samples to their respective classes. The decision is made according to the classification feature vectors describing the object in question.

Colonoscope: A flexible, lighted instrument used to examine the inside of the colon.

Colonoscopy: A medical procedure during which a physician is examining the colon for polyps using a colonoscope.

Color Histogram: A graphical representation of a distribution of colors within an image. The data contained in a histogram is obtained by counting the occurrence of each possible color of the respective color model within the image.

Fourier Transform: An algorithm used to decompose a signal (e.g., an image) into its frequency components and to compute the frequency spectrum for a given signal.

Wavelet Transform: A transform used to decompose a signal into its frequency components, similar to the Fourier transform. But the time-frequency resolution of the wavelet transform can be adjusted since basis functions with compact support are used, in contrast to the Fourier transform, where sine and cosines are used as basis functions.

Chapter XXIII
Automatic Identification and Elastic Properties of Deformed Objects Using their Microscopic Images

C. Papaodysseus
National Technical University of Athens, Greece

M. Panagopoulos
National Technical University of Athens, Greece

P. Rousopoulos
National Technical University of Athens, Greece

P. Loumou
National Technical University of Athens, Greece

D. Arabadjis
National Technical University of Athens, Greece

G. Theodoropoulos
Agricultural University of Athens, Greece

ABSTRACT

In this chapter the state of the art is presented in the domain of automatic identification and classification of bodies on the basis of their deformed images obtained via microscope. The approach is illustrated by means of the case of automatic recognition of third-stage larvae from microscopic images of them in high deformation instances. The introduced methodology incorporates elements of elasticity theory, image processing, curve fitting and clustering methods; a concise presentation of the state of the art in these fields is given. Combining proper elements of these disciplines, we first evaluate the undeformed shape of a parasite given a digital image of a random parasite deformation instance. It is demonstrated that different orientations and deformations of the same parasite give rise to practically the same undeformed shape when the methodology is applied to the corresponding images, thus confirming the consistency of the approach. Next, a pattern recognition method is introduced to classify the unwrapped parasites into four families, with a high success rate. In addition, the methodology presented here is a powerful tool for the exact evaluation of the mechano-elastic properties of bodies from images of their deformation instances.

INTRODUCTION

There are numerous applications, where bodies suffer deformation due to elastic forces (stresses). In these cases, one frequently encounters two important problems: (a) to make a consistent and reliable estimation of the deformed body's mechano-elastic properties from images of random instances of body deformation and (b) to identify the deformed body automatically from these very images. We would like to emphasize that, as a rule, automatic classification of bodies on the basis of images of their deformation, is practically prohibited by the randomness of the deformation. One encounters such problems in various disciplines applications, such as automatic identification of highly deformed parasites, cells or large molecules from their images obtained via microscope, in strength of materials, elastography (Manduca et al. 1998, Washington and Miga, 2004) in civil engineering in general, etc.

In the present chapter, we present the following new approach to tackle the aforementioned problems: We estimate the mechano-elastic properties of a body suffering an equivalent to 2D deformation from an image of it at an arbitrary deformation instance. Knowledge of these mechano-elastic properties allows unwrapping/straightening the deformed body image, a fact that in turn permits the application of pattern recognition techniques for the body automatic classification/identification. We have applied the introduced approach to an important and some times crucial veterinary problem, namely the automatic identification of domestic animal parasites, from their images obtained via microscope.

BACKGROUND

Some Necessary Notions and Relations from Elasticity Theory

We now proceed to state some notions that are commonly used in most approaches of Elasticity theory (Chandrasekharaiah and Debnath, 1994). These will later be used in the analysis on which the unwrapping of the parasite is based.

Definition of the Stress and the Strain Tensor

Consider a one-to-one correspondence between all points of the deformed and the undeformed parasite states. Thus, let us consider two arbitrary points, say $A(x,y)$ and $B(x+dx,y+dy)$ of an undeformed parasite element and let A' and B' be their unique images in the deformed parasite body. In other words, due to the deformation, point A moves to $A'(x+u_x, y+u_y)$ and point B to $B'(x+dx+u_x+du_x, y+dy+u_y+du_y)$. We consider the lengths of $\overline{AB}$ and $\overline{A'B'}$:

$$ds = \left|\overrightarrow{AB}\right| = \sqrt{dx^2+dy^2} \quad \text{and}$$

$$ds' = \left|\overrightarrow{A'B'}\right| = \sqrt{(du_x+dx)^2+(du_y+dy)^2}$$

$$= \sqrt{\left(\frac{\vartheta u_x}{\vartheta x}dx + \frac{\vartheta u_x}{\vartheta y}dy + dx\right)^2 + \left(\frac{\vartheta u_y}{\vartheta x}dx + \frac{\vartheta u_y}{\vartheta y}dy + dy\right)^2}$$

Now one defines the relative elongations along the x- and y-axes:

Along the x-axis, we set $dy = 0$, in which case, ds and ds' above become ds_x and ds_x', respectively. Thus, the relative elongation is defined to be

$$\varepsilon_{xx} = \frac{ds_x' - ds_x}{ds_x}$$

$$= \sqrt{\left(\frac{\vartheta u_x}{\vartheta x}\right)^2 + 2\frac{\vartheta u_x}{\vartheta x} + 1 + \left(\frac{\vartheta u_y}{\vartheta x}\right)^2} - 1 \qquad (1)$$

Similarly, along the y-axis we set $dx = 0$ and thus the relative elongation ε_{yy} is defined to be:

$$\varepsilon_{yy} = \frac{ds_y' - ds_y}{ds_y}$$

$$= \sqrt{\left(\frac{\vartheta u_y}{\vartheta y}\right)^2 + 2\frac{\vartheta u_y}{\vartheta y} + 1 + \left(\frac{\vartheta u_x}{\vartheta y}\right)^2} - 1 \qquad (2)$$

If the relative elongations are small, after expanding the square roots of (1) and (2) in Taylor series, we obtain

$$\varepsilon_{xx} = \frac{\partial u_x}{\partial x}, \quad \varepsilon_{yy} = \frac{\partial u_y}{\partial y} \qquad (3)$$

Moreover, using the same assumption, the tangent of the angle of deformation of the *x*-axis, $\tan\phi_1$, and the y-axis, $\tan\phi_2$, become $\frac{\vartheta u_y}{\vartheta x}$ and $\frac{\vartheta u_x}{\vartheta y}$ respectively (Figure 1). Also, the hypothesis of small relative elongations results that $\tan\varphi_1 \cong \varphi_1$, $\tan\varphi_2 \cong \varphi_2$ implying that the initially right angle is deformed by

$$\delta\varphi = \varphi_1 + \varphi_2 = \frac{\partial u_y}{\partial x} + \frac{\partial u_x}{\partial y} \qquad (4)$$

Therefore, after using the shear stress definition $t_{xy} = t_{yx} = \frac{1}{2}\delta\varphi = \frac{1}{2}\left(\frac{\vartheta u_y}{\vartheta x} + \frac{\vartheta u_x}{\vartheta y}\right)$, we adopt thestandard strain tensor definition: $\hat{\varepsilon} = \begin{bmatrix} \varepsilon_{xx} & \tau_{xy} \\ \tau_{yx} & \varepsilon_{yy} \end{bmatrix}$.

Next, in order to study the elastic forces' distribution throughout the parasite body, we proceed by considering an arbitrary differential element in the parasite body, starting at point (*x*, *y*) with vertices *A*(*x*,*y*), $B(x+dx, y)$, $C(x+dx, y+dy)$, $D(x, y+dy)$ (Figure 2). Let the force per unit area/length acting on the side *AD* be $\vec{\sigma}_x = \sigma_{xx}\vec{i} + \sigma_{xy}\vec{j}$, where the first subscript denotes the axis to which the side is vertical, while the second subscript denotes the vector component axis. Similarly, $\vec{\sigma}_y = \sigma_{yx}\vec{i} + \sigma_{yy}\vec{j}$. It is evident that the four functions $\sigma_{xx}, \sigma_{xy}, \sigma_{yx}, \sigma_{yy}$, suffice to determine the stress condition of the considered differential element. Hence, we define the standard stress tensor

$$\hat{\sigma} = \begin{bmatrix} \sigma_{xx} & \sigma_{xy} \\ \sigma_{yx} & \sigma_{yy} \end{bmatrix}$$

Hypothesis on the Parasite Constitutive Equation

The parasite constitutive equation relates the stress tensor $\hat{\sigma}$ with the strain tensor $\hat{\varepsilon}$. These two tensors can be related through any functional form, i.e. $\hat{\sigma} = f(\hat{\varepsilon})$. However, in many practical circumstances, this functional form can be considered to be linear, namely $\hat{\sigma} = \hat{A} \cdot \hat{\varepsilon}$, where $\hat{A}$ is a constant matrix (generalized Hooke 's law).

Presentation of Vector Quantization and Clustering Methods and Algorithms

In many practical applications, one encounters the problem of classifying kindred objects into different groups, according to a set of criteria. Usually, these criteria are quantitatively expressed by means of characteristics; the ensemble of the values of these characteristics form vectors. Thus, the classification problem transforms into collecting similar vectors in separate clusters. For this reason this problem is often called "vector quantization" or "clustering". Many different clustering methods have been developed so far, which are distinguished to the hierarchical methods and the partitional ones.

Partitional Algorithms

Suppose we have N-distinct groups and that the mean value (the centroid) of the members of each group is C_i, $i = 1...N$. Then each new member is classified to the group from the centroid, C_o, of which it has the minimum distance. Partitional algorithms based on this approach are called centroid-based. One of the first centroid-based algorithms is the K-Means (Jain and

Figure 1. Element differential deformation

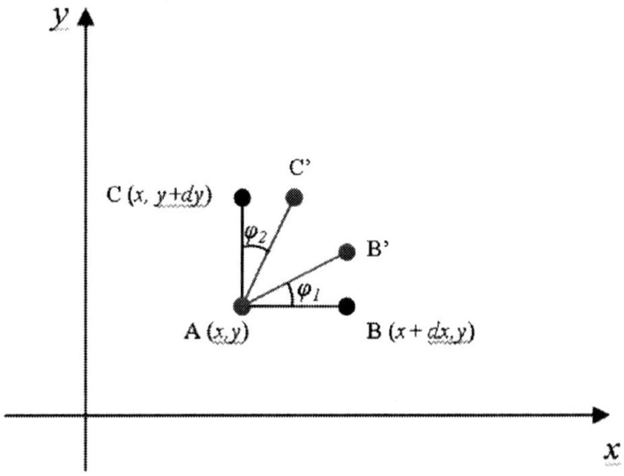

Figure 2. Differential element strain forces

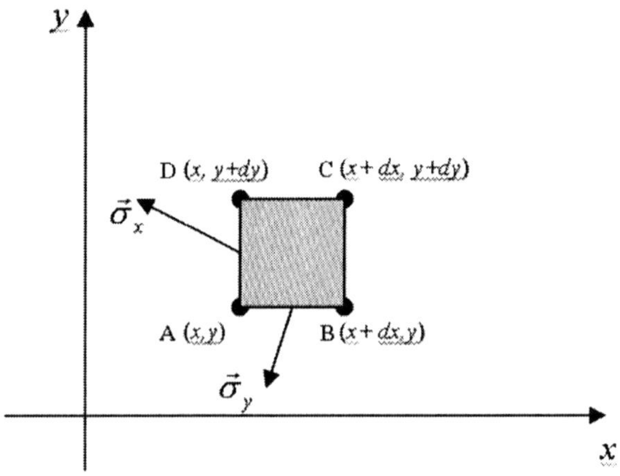

Dubes, 1988) where the data are classified into K clusters according to the Euclidean distance of each member from the centroid vector of each cluster. The member is attributed to the cluster of minimum distance, while the centroid vector is dynamically computed. Another well-known centroid-based algorithm, called ISODATA, employs the same approach reformulating the choice of distance function between the members and the centroids.

Other algorithms (PAM Kaufman and Rousseeuw 1990, CLARANS Ng and Han 1994), called medoid-based, replace groups' mean values with other reference points inside the groups (medoids). The medoid of a group is calculated so as its mean distance from the group members is minimal. Although these algorithms perform a more reliable classification than centroid-based ones, they fail to deal with clusters significantly different in size, or with clusters with convex borders. Specifically, medoid-based algorithms are less noise-sensitive than the centroid-based ones but they can reliably classify only data sets with groups of round borders and similar sizes.

Hierarchical Algorithms

This class of algorithms is conceptually different to the partitional ones. Initially, they attribute a different group to each member of the data set. They proceed by merging the pairs of groups of minimum distance. This merging process is repeated until a desired number of groups or a threshold distance between them is achieved. In general, hierarchical algorithms comprise the following steps:

- A proper distance function (Euclidean, Minkowski, Manhattan) is chosen to evaluate the similarity between two groups.
- Based on this distance, the algorithm creates a similarity matrix, **S**, containing the relative distances between all pairs of groups.
- When two groups manifest strong dissimilarity, then the corresponding entry in matrix **S** is close to zero, thus creating a sparse matrix **S'**.
- Next, this sparse matrix is represented by a graph, where the graph nodes are data groups and the graph weighted vertices are the similarity values between data groups.

This approach has been realized by means of various algorithms, where each algorithm employs a different distance and/or a different merging process. Thus we have the following variations of hierarchical algorithms.

- In the first class of algorithms (Jain and Dubes, 1988), a representative of each group is defined, e.g. its centroid. Subsequently, proper thresholds are defined both for the computation of the sparse matrix and the merging of similar data groups.
- *Single link method*: The distance of all elements of a group A from all elements of a group B is computed and the minimum of these distances, d_m, is spotted. Then, similarity between A and B is expressed via d_m; clearly the smaller d_m the grater the similarity between A and B.
- *The CURE method* (Guha et al., 1998): This is a combination of the previous two methods, in the sense that a class of representatives for each group is separately defined and the distance of the representatives of group A from the representatives of group B is calculated. These distances express the similarity of A and B and determine if groups A and B must be merged. When two groups get merged a new class of representatives of the resulting group is dynamically computed. These algorithms satisfactory deal with the classification of noisy groups of irregular size and shape.
- *group-average method*: This algorithm differs from the *single link* method in the sense that it normalizes distances between group elements of A and B with the sizes of the groups, to cope with substantial group size variability.
- *ROCK* (Guha et al., 1998): This algorithm is actually the *group-average* method, where the user interactively performs normalization.
- *The class of CHAMELEON algorithms*: The basic idea behind these algorithms is that the similarity between two groups A and B is based not only on the distance between their elements, but also on the internal similarity of the elements of each group. Thus, the notion of closeness of each group A is introduced, that measures a kind of average distance between the elements of A. It also introduces the concept of interconnectivity to be a kind of average distance between two clusters or sub-clusters. The similarity between A and B is expressed via the product of interconnectivity and closeness.

Finally a clustering algorithm that performs best for the problem in hand is more analytically presented in the Section entitled "The employed method of automatic identification of parasites".

DETERMINATION OF MECHANO-ELASTIC PROPERTIES AND AUTOMATIC CLASSIFICATION OF OBJECTS USING IMAGES OF THEM IN HIGH DEFORMATION

One of the main ailments of the livestock industry is related to the threat of strongyles, which are common endoparasitic nematodes of domestic animals. The correct identification of the parasite population that has infected a particular organism would allow for quick and efficient treatment of the disease, thus minimizing economic losses.

Usually, to diagnose the presence of such a parasitic infection, a coprological examination is required, where eggs produced by the strongyles are identified. Most of the commonly encountered parasitic strongyles, such as *Haemonchus* and *Osteragia* spp., produce similarly sized and shaped eggs that are hard to identify. However, the third-stage larvae, obtained after coproculture of the corresponding eggs, are sufficiently different (McMurtry et al., 2000, Theodoropoulos et al., 2000). To the best of our knowledge, automated identification of third stage larvae from their digital images has not been previously achieved.

One major difficulty in the automatic parasite identification, is that many quantitative features explicitly depend on the shape of the deformed parasite. The identification process can be greatly improved if the images of the larvae were straightened digitally, so that all quantitative features could be used irrespectively of larva deformation.

In this section, we formulate an integrated solution to the problem of the automatic identification of parasites from their microscopic images representing the parasite at a highly deformed stage. The presented methodology can be extended so as to tackle the general problem of automatic identification of objects suffering an equivalent to 2D elastic deformation. To achieve this, we first use digitised parasite images, in which the motile parasite is oriented in a random fashion and may have assumed any shape. Proper image segmentation algorithms are employed and a suitable edge detection algorithm is used to extract the parasite contour line. For the unwrapping, or straightening, of the contour line, concepts of curve fitting and elasticity theory are used. Once the parasites are straightened, we automatically classify them by means of a novel algorithm, which employs a set of quantitative features such as parasite perimeter, area etc.

Determination of the Body Mechano-Elastic Properties

Assumptions for the mechano-elastic properties of the parasite

We will now state some hypotheses concerning general elastic properties of the parasite, whose validity will be confirmed by the subsequent analysis and the performed experiments.

- All parasite parts are isotropic, homogeneous and continuous.
- The static equation of balance holds for the deformed element too (1st order Theory)
- The longitudinal axis of the undeformed parasite is a straight line and an axis of symmetry.
- The plane parasite surfaces, the cross sections, which are initially perpendicular to its symmetry axis, remain plain and perpendicular to a proper corresponding line after the deformation.
- The cross dimensions are small compared to the parasite length.
- The stress plane is either vertical to or includes the symmetry axis.
- The generated stresses and displacements along the parasite body are linearly related. More specifically, Hooke's law is valid,

namely the displacement tensor is linearly associated with the stress tensor.

The adopted symmetry assumptions allow us to study the elastic behavior of the parasite in two dimensions. As a result, the information extracted from the parasite images may be sufficient for this study, as well as for unwrapping the parasite.

Properties of the Parasite Elastic Deformation

In the following, we will compute the strains the deformed parasite suffers at an arbitrary instance. All these strains on the deformed plain section, initially perpendicular to the symmetry axis, are expressed by means of the strains that the center of the section suffers. Using these results, we will, for the first time, prove an important property of the tangents along parasite contour.

The Parasite Element Deformation. The Strains on the Undeformed Cross Sections

Without any loss of generality, we assume that the undeformed parasite is placed so as to have its symmetry axis parallel to the x-axis. Consider a differential element $AB\Gamma\Delta$ on the undeformed parasite, with $A\Delta$ and $B\Gamma$ normal to the axis of symmetry, which, after the completion of the parasite deformation, is transformed to $A'B'\Gamma'\Delta'$. Let point M, the middle of section $A\Delta$, have coordinates $(x,0)$. Consequently, point N, the middle of section $B\Gamma$, has coordinates $(x+dx,0)$, while an arbitrary point P at section $A\Delta$ is at (x,y). Moreover, we let (u,w) be the displacement of M, meaning that point M' of the deformed element has coordinates $(x+u,w)$.

Now, we want to find the displacement of P, namely $\overrightarrow{PP'}$ under the aforementioned deformation; we emphasize that according to our hypothesis cross section $A\Delta$ remains plain and undeformed in all parasite wrapping instances (Figure 3).

Let ε'_1 be a straight line parallel to the x-axis passing through P'. $\overrightarrow{\Lambda'M'}$ defines a straight line ε'_2 parallel to the y-axis and $\overrightarrow{K'N'}$ is vertical to it. In addition, we consider $\overrightarrow{N'M'}$ to be vertical to the line segment $A'\Delta'$. Thus, the coordinates of K' are $(x+u, w+dw)$ and $\tan\phi = \frac{K'M'}{K'N'} = \frac{dw}{du+dx}$.

Since u is only x-dependent, it holds that $\frac{du}{dx} = \frac{\vartheta u}{\vartheta x}$.

Consequently,

$$\tan\phi = \frac{dw}{dx}\frac{1}{1+\frac{du}{dx}} \tag{5}$$

The coordinates of P' are $(x + u - y\sin(\phi), w + y\cos(\phi))$. So, the coordinates of $\overrightarrow{PP'}$ become

$$\overrightarrow{PP'} = \left(u - y\sin(\phi), w + y\left(\cos(\phi)-1\right)\right)$$

Since u and w are only x-dependent quantities, strains ε_{xx}, ε_{yy}, ε_{xy} and ε_{yx} are given by the following expressions:

$$\varepsilon_{xx} = \frac{du}{dx} - y\cos(\phi)\frac{d\phi}{dx} = \frac{du}{dx} - \frac{y\cos^3(\phi)}{1+\frac{du}{dx}}\left[\frac{d^2w}{dx^2} - \tan(\phi)\frac{d^2u}{dx^2}\right],$$

$$\varepsilon_{yy} = \cos(\phi) - 1,$$

$$\varepsilon_{xy} = \varepsilon_{yx} = \frac{1}{2}\left(\frac{dw}{dx} - y\sin(\phi)\frac{d\phi}{dx}\right) = \frac{1}{2}\frac{dw}{dx}\left(1 - y\cos^3(\phi)\left[\frac{d^2w}{dx^2} - \tan(\phi)\frac{d^2u}{dx^2}\right]\right) \tag{6}$$

According to the adopted assumptions, the expression connecting stresses and strains is

$$\hat{\sigma} = E\,\hat{\varepsilon} \tag{7}$$

Figure 3. Completed differential element deformation

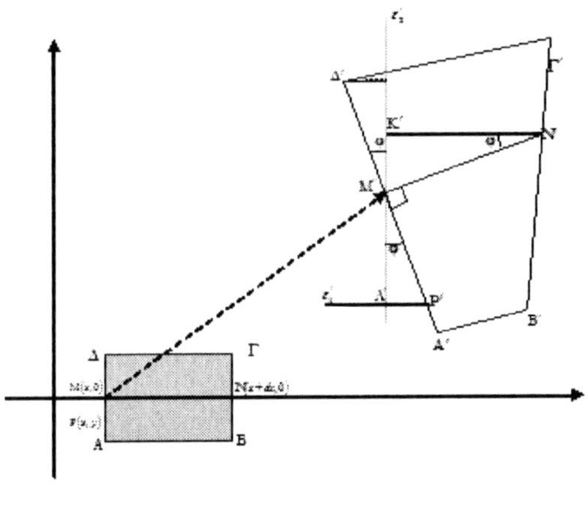

Equation (11).

$$N = E_{11}\frac{du}{dx}A + \frac{E_{12}}{2}\frac{dw}{dx}A - \left[\frac{E_{11}}{1+\frac{du}{dx}} + \frac{E_{12}}{2}\frac{dw}{dx}\right]\cos^3(\phi)\left[\frac{d^2w}{dx^2} - \tan(\phi)\frac{d^2u}{dx^2}\right]\int_A y\,dA$$

$$N = E_{11}\frac{du}{dx}A + \frac{E_{12}}{2}\frac{dw}{dx}A$$

where $\hat{\varepsilon}$ is the strain tensor formed by the relations (6), $E = \begin{bmatrix} E_{11} & E_{12} \\ E_{21} & E_{22} \end{bmatrix}$ a constant matrix, $\hat{\sigma}$ the corresponding stress tensor.

Parasite Equilibrium Equations

Consider a section A normal to the x-axis in the undeformed parasite's state. Then, the bending moment M about the y-axis and the vertical shear force V are given by the following expressions:

$$M = \int_A y\sigma_{xx}dA \tag{8}$$

and

$$V = \int_A \sigma_{xy}dA \tag{9}$$

In addition, the stress component σ_{xx} also results in a force N normal to A and in the x-direction given by

$$N = \int_A \sigma_{xx}dA \tag{10}$$

We assume that the parasite is in an equilibrium position each time a photograph is taken. Then, equilibrium along the x-axis implies that $N = 0$, $V = 0$. Since we have considered the x-axis to be the symmetry axis of the parasite and since we have adopted the assumption that the generalized Hooke's law holds, Equation (11) follows.

Combining (11) and N = 0, we deduce that

$$E_{11}\frac{du}{dx} + \frac{E_{12}}{2}\frac{dw}{dx} = 0 \tag{12}$$

and Equation (13).

Equation (13).

$$V = E_{12}\left(1-\cos(\phi)\right)A + \frac{E_{11}}{2}\frac{dw}{dx}A - \left[\frac{E_{11}}{2}\frac{dw}{dx}\right]\cos^3(\phi)\left[\frac{d^2w}{dx^2} - \tan(\phi)\frac{d^2u}{dx^2}\right]\int_A ydA$$

$$V = E_{12}\left(1-\cos(\phi)\right)A + \frac{E_{11}}{2}\frac{dw}{dx}A$$

Box 1.

$$\vec{r}'_{\Lambda'} - \frac{d}{dx}\overrightarrow{OM}' = \left(\frac{d\ell(x)}{dx}\sin(\phi) + \ell(x)\cos^3(\phi)\frac{d^2w}{dx^2}\right)\vec{i} + \left(-\frac{d\ell(x)}{dx}\cos(\phi) + \ell(x)\sin(\phi)\cos^2(\phi)\frac{d^2w}{dx^2}\right)\vec{j}$$

$$\vec{r}'_{U'} - \frac{d}{dx}\overrightarrow{OM}' = \left(-\frac{d\ell(x)}{dx}\sin(\phi) - \ell(x)\cos^3(\phi)\frac{d^2w}{dx^2}\right)\vec{i} + \left(\frac{d\ell(x)}{dx}\cos(\phi) - \ell(x)\sin(\phi)\cos^2(\phi)\frac{d^2w}{dx^2}\right)\vec{j}$$

Combining (13) and $V = 0$, we deduce that

$$E_{12}\left(1-\cos(\phi)\right) + \frac{E_{11}}{2}\frac{dw}{dx} = 0 \qquad (14)$$

(12) and (14), imply that

$$\sigma_{xx} = -y\cos^3(\phi)\left[\frac{E_{11}}{1+\frac{du}{dx}} + \frac{E_{12}}{2}\frac{dw}{dx}\right]\left[\frac{d^2w}{dx^2} - \tan(\phi)\frac{d^2u}{dx^2}\right]$$

$$\sigma_{xy} = -y\cos^3(\phi)\left[\frac{E_{11}}{2}\frac{dw}{dx}\right]\left[\frac{d^2w}{dx^2} - \tan(\phi)\frac{d^2u}{dx^2}\right]$$

i.e. linear expressions of y. Therefore, the middle of the deformed cross section suffers no stress; the curve formed by all these unstressed middle points, usually called the neutral line, has the following properties:

- It is the curve to which the symmetry axis is transformed due to the elastic deformation process.
- No stress is exerted along it.
- As a consequence, the neutral line and the parasite symmetry axis are of the same length.
- The undeformed cross sections initially perpendicular to the symmetry axis, remain perpendicular to the neutral line even after the parasite deformation.

An Important Property of the Deformed Parasite Contour Tangents

Let $\ell(x)$ be the upper boundary of the parasite in its two-dimensional image; hence $-\ell(x)$ is the lower contour bound. Let AD be an arbitrary parasite cross section, intersecting the x-axis at the point $M(x,0)$. Then this cross section, moves to a section $A'D'$, perpendicular to neutral line, where A' is $(x+u+\ell(x)\sin(\phi), w-\ell(x)\cos(\phi))$ and D' is $(x+u-\ell(x)\sin(\phi), w+\ell(x)\cos(\phi))$. The upper and lower parasite boundaries now correspond to two curves, say U' and L' respectively. The vector x-parametric equation of U' in the 2D image parasite representation is,

$$\vec{r}_{U'} = \left(x+u-\ell(x)\sin(\phi)\right)\vec{i} + \left(w+\ell(x)\cos(\phi)\right)\vec{j} \qquad (15)$$

while the corresponding one for the deformed lower boundary is

$$\vec{r}_{\Lambda'} = \left(x + u + \ell(x)\sin(\phi)\right)\vec{i} + \left(w - \ell(x)\cos(\phi)\right)\vec{j} \tag{16}$$

Next we compute the inner products of tangent vector $\vec{r}'_{U'}$ and cross section $\overrightarrow{D'A'}$ and $\vec{r}'_{\Lambda'}$ and $\overrightarrow{D'A'}$. Thus (see Box 1).

Since, we have assumed that neutral line tangent is perpendicular to the rotated and translated cross section

$$\frac{d}{dx}\left(\vec{r}_{U'} - \overrightarrow{OM'}\right)\cdot\overrightarrow{D'A'} = \vec{r}\,'_{U'}\cdot\overrightarrow{D'A'} = -2\ell(x)\frac{d\ell(x)}{dx} \tag{17}$$

$$\frac{d}{dx}\left(\vec{r}_{\Lambda'} - \overrightarrow{OM'}\right)\cdot\overrightarrow{D'A'} = \vec{r}\,'_{\Lambda'}\cdot\overrightarrow{D'A'} = 2\ell(x)\frac{d\ell(x)}{dx} \tag{18}$$

It also holds that

$$\left|\vec{r}\,'_{U'} - \frac{d}{dx}\overrightarrow{OM'}\right| = \left|\vec{r}\,'_{\Lambda'} - \frac{d}{dx}\overrightarrow{OM'}\right| \tag{19}$$

Now, if we let γ be the angle between $\vec{r}\,'_{U'}$ and $\overrightarrow{D'A'}$ and θ the one between $\vec{r}\,'_{\Lambda'}$ and $\overrightarrow{D'A'}$, then, combining (17), (18) and (19) we obtain

$$\frac{\left(\vec{r}\,'_{U'} - \frac{d}{dx}\overrightarrow{OM'}\right)\cdot\overrightarrow{D'A'}}{\left(\vec{r}\,'_{\Lambda'} - \frac{d}{dx}\overrightarrow{OM'}\right)\cdot\overrightarrow{D'A'}} = \frac{\cos\gamma}{\cos\theta} = -1 \tag{20}$$

and, as a consequence, $\cos\gamma = -\cos\theta$, which gives us

$$\gamma + \theta = \pi \tag{21}$$

This last relation proves to be fundamental in defining and obtaining the cross section's coordinates, as well as those of the neutral line. Knowledge of the coordinates of the neutral line allows us to "unwrap", or straighten, the outline of the parasite, as is shown in the following Section.

Unwrapping the Parasite: Evaluation of the Method

Polynomial Approximation of the Deformed Parasite Contour: State of the Art

The next step is to determine if there are specific mathematical curves that optimally fit the parasite contour in the obtained images. First, parasite contour has to be extracted. To achieve this, initially we have performed segmentation of the image of the deformed parasite by the method introduced in Papaodysseus et al., 2004. Next, the contour of the parasite has been determined via dedicated software.

In order to determine polynomial curves that best fit the contour, we have tentatively applied techniques introduced in Craig, 1999, Papaodysseus et al., 2005, Papaodysseus et al., 2008. For the present application the following method proved quiet satisfactory:

The curve parameter is chosen to be the contour length s, calculated via the distance of the successive pixels that form it. Subsequently, we approximate the variables x and y of the parasite by polynomials up to 21 degree:

$$x(s) = a_n s^n + a_{n-1}s^{n-1} + a_{n-2}s^{n-2} + \ldots + a_1 s^1 + a_0$$
$$y(s) = b_n s^n + b_{n-1}s^{n-1} + b_{n-2}s^{n-2} + \ldots + b_1 s^1 + b_0 \tag{22}$$

Suppose now, that one wants to test if the upper parasite contour corresponds to the aforementioned curve and at the same time to compute the parameters of this optimal curve: Let $\overrightarrow{r_i^P}, i = 1,2,\ldots,N^P$ be the centers of the pixels forming the upper contour and let $\Pi = \{a_n, a_{n-1}, \ldots, a_1, a_0, b_n, b_{n-1}, \ldots, b_1, b_0\}$. Hence the parametric vector equation of the prototype curve is $\overrightarrow{r^M}(s \mid \Pi) = x(s)\vec{i} + y(s)\vec{j}$.

Next, we compute the optimal set of parameters Π^O and the corresponding sequence of values of the independent variable s_i, $i = 1, 2, ..., N^P$, so that $\overrightarrow{r^M}(s_i \mid \Pi^O)$ best fits $\overrightarrow{r_i^P}$ according to the chosen quadratic norm $E_2 = \sum_{i=1}^{N^P} \left(\overrightarrow{r_i^P} - \overrightarrow{r_i^M}\right)^2$.

Algorithms that can minimize E_2 are the conjugate gradient and/or the Nelder – Mead method (Nelder and Mead, 1965). Both these algorithms start from a tentative initial position Π^1 and each time generate a new set of parameter values Π^2, Π^3, etc, so that E_2 eventually converges to its minimum value, in which case the optimal set of parameters Π^0 is obtained.

In order that this approximation is good enough, the minimum value of E_2, say $E_{2(\min)}$, that corresponds to the theoretical curve generated by Π^0, must be smaller than a small threshold common for all parasites (Figures 4a and 4b).

Figure 4a. Outer and inner polynomial curves that best fit this parasite's contour

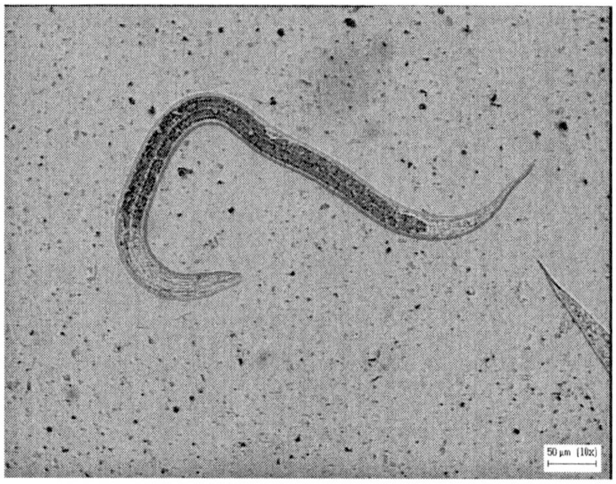

Figure 4b. Polynomial curves that best fit another parasite's contour

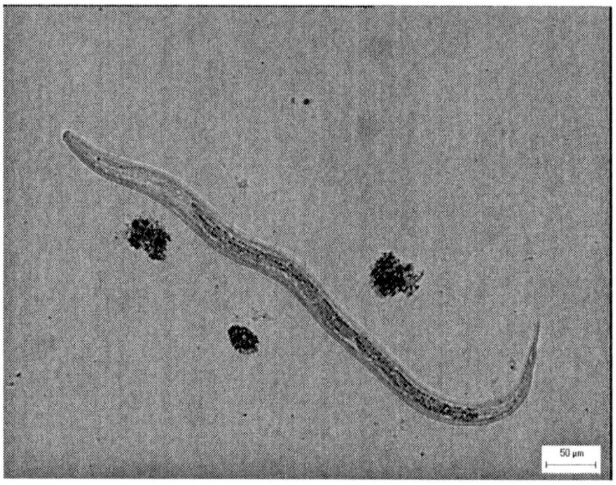

Determining the Deformed Body's Neutral Line

In this section, we will analytically describe the methodology we have introduced and applied for determining the exact position of the neutral line in the deformed parasite, as well as the positions of the cross sections that, by hypothesis, always remain undeformed and normal to the neutral line. This methodology comprises the following steps:

Step 1: We, first, extract the parasite contour. Next, we spot the head and the tail of the parasite as follows: First, to spot the tail, for each contour pixel p we consider the sets of pixels P_L that lie on its left and P_R that lie on its right and we approximate both P_L and P_R with line segments in the Least Squares sense. We let the tail T be the pixel where these two line segments form the most acute angle.

Second, we spot the parasite "head" H: We move away from the tail and we locally approximate the contour by polynomials of fifth degree, of which we compute the curvature. We let the "head" be the point of maximum curvature which also lies between 0.4 and 0.6 of the whole contour length.

Step 2: We divide the whole contour into two parts I and II (arbitrarily upper and lower), that both end at the parasite "head" and "tail". Then we approximate both parts with polynomials of type (22). All performed experiments indicate that this approximation is excellent. We form a dense sequence M_j^{II} , $j = 1...N^{II}$ of points belonging to the polynomial curve best fitting part II and a less dense sequence M_i^{I} , $i = 1...N^{I}$ on curve fitting part I; let $\vec{\tau}_i^{\,I}$ and $\vec{\tau}_j^{\,II}$ be the unit tangent vector to these model curves at each M_i^I and M_j^{II} respectively.

Step 3: Subsequently we spot parasite's neutral line as follows.

We move away from tail T along part I and we connect M_1^I with each point of set M_j^{II} , $j = 1...K$, where K is a predefined number of pixels, say 5% of the whole contour length. We form vectors $\vec{r}_{1,j} = \overline{M_j^{II} M_1^{I}}, j = 1,...,K$. We keep only those vectors $\vec{r}_{1,j}$ that lie entirely within the parasite body and for these we compute the angles $\varphi_{1,j}^{I}$ and $\varphi_{1,j}^{II}$ formed by each vector $\vec{r}_{1,j}$ and the tangent vectors $\vec{\tau}_1^{\,I}$ and $\vec{\tau}_{1,j}^{\,II}$ respectively. Then, we define the sequence $\Delta\varphi_{1,j} = \left|\varphi_{1,j}^{I} + \varphi_{1,j}^{II} - \pi\right|$ and we let N_1^{II} be that point where the minimum value of the sequence $\Delta\varphi_{1,j}$ occurs, say the d_1-th of sequence M_j^{II}; we consequently define $\overline{M_1^I N_1^{II}}$ to be a cross section of the parasite that remains undeformed and normal to the neutral line.

Next we compute the second cross section as follows: We move away from the tail vertex T and M_1^I at M_2^I and once more, we define the set of points $M_{d_1+j}^{II}$, $j = 1,...,K$. Proceeding as before we define the vectors, $\vec{r}_{2,j} = \overline{M_{d_1+j}^{II} M_2^{I}}, j = 1,...,K$. We compute the corresponding angles $\varphi_{2,j}^{I}$ between $\vec{r}_{2,j}$ and $\vec{\tau}_2^{\,I}$, as well as $\varphi_{2,j}^{II}$ between $\vec{r}_{2,j}$ and $\vec{\tau}_{d_1+j}^{\,II}$. We spot the minimum of the sequence $\Delta\varphi_{2,j} = \left|\varphi_{2,j}^{I} + \varphi_{2,j}^{II} - \pi\right|$ which occurs at point N_2^{II}, say the d_2-th point of sequence M_j^{II}. We let $\overline{M_2^I N_2^{II}}$ be the second cross section that remains undeformed and normal to the neutral line.

Finally we proceed in obtaining all cross sections $\overline{M_i^I N_i^{II}}$ passing from M_i^I , $i = 1...N^I$ by the same method (Figures 5a,b). The middle points of these cross sections belong to the neutral line and the unit vector normal to these sections is tangent to the neutral line.

Description of the Unwrapping Process

We have shown in the Section entitled "Properties of the parasite elastic deformation" that under the adopted assumptions the neutral line undertakes no stress and it is found in the middle of the corresponding cross section. Consequently, we define the neutral line of the deformed parasite to be the locus of the middle points K_v of the cross sections $M_v^I N_v^{II}$ as they are determined

Figure 5a. Determination of the cross sections of the parasite in Figure 4a

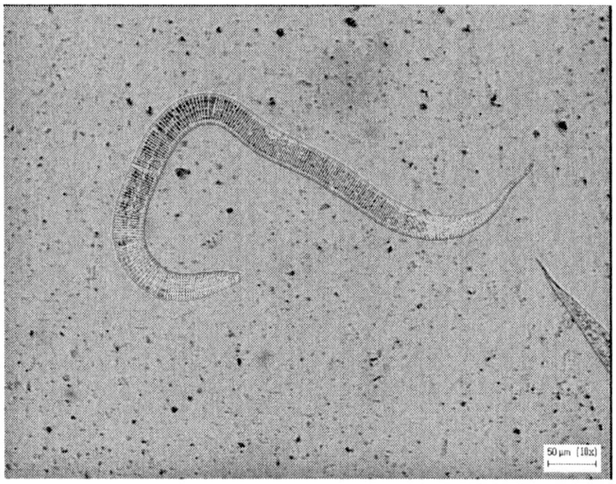

Figure 5b. Determination of the cross sections of the parasite in Figure 4b

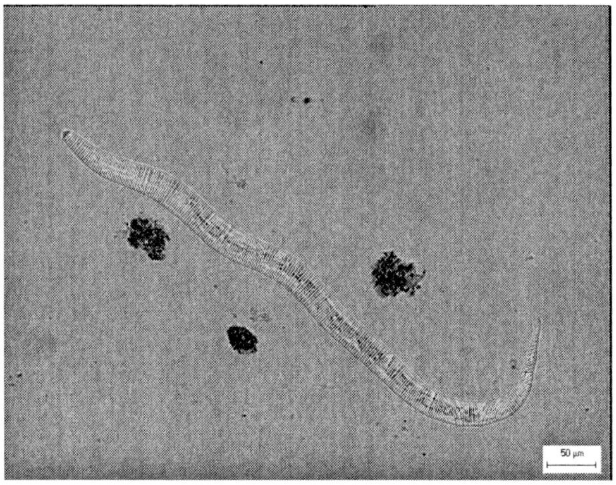

in the previous section. Clearly, the length of the neutral line remains unchanged during the various phases of the parasite deformation and it coincides with the length of the undeformed parasite's symmetry axis.

Therefore, in order to unwrap the parasite and find its undeformed shape, we proceed as follows:

- We compute the distance of all successive middle points K_i and K_{i+1}, say δ_i.
- Along the x-axis we form a sequence of points Λ_i of equal number with K_i, as follows: Λ_1 is placed at the axis origin; Λ_2 in the positive x-axis, so that the distance between points Λ_1 and Λ_2 is equal to the distance between middle points K_1 and K_2. We continue this process so that Λ_i and Λ_{i+1} are equidistant

Figure 6. The unwrapped contour versions for 6 parasites of the same gender with the one in Figure 4a

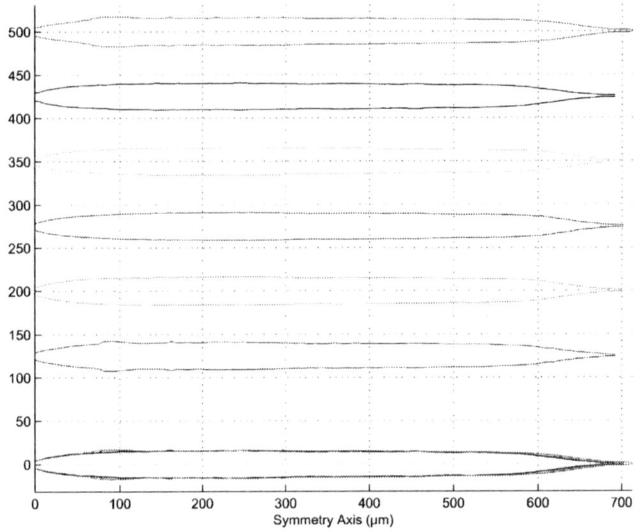

Figure 7. The unwrapped contour versions for 6 parasites of the same gender with the one in Figure 4b

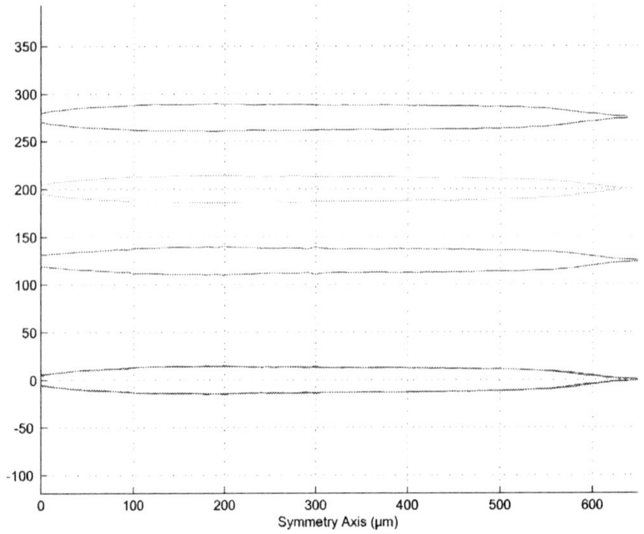

with $K_i K_{i+1}$, until all middle points are exhausted.

- Moving in a direction perpendicular to the x-axis at each point Λ_i we choose two points: A_i with y-coordinate equal to $\lambda_i / 2$, namely half the length of the cross section $M_i^I N_i^{II}$ and point B_i with y-coordinate $-\lambda_i / 2$. We set points A_i to form the one part of the parasite, while points B_i form the other parasite part (Figures 6, 7).

Evaluation of the Parasite Unwrapping Results

If the assumptions made and the introduced methodology are correct, one expects that different phases of the parasite deformation will generate the same undeformed parasite version, at least with an acceptable approximation. Figures 6, 7 demonstrate that this is indeed the case. In fact, the undeformed parasite borders have a difference that might be considered negligible in respect to the parasite dimensions. We have employed five different measures to describe the differences between the shapes of the unwrapped parasite that resulted from different phases. These measures are:

I. $a_{1,i} = \frac{\left(\ell_i^P - \bar{\ell}^P\right)}{\bar{\ell}^P} \cdot 100\%$, where ℓ_i^P is the length of the unwrapped parasite obtained from the ith wrapped larva phase and $\bar{\ell}^P$ its mean value.

II. $a_{2,i} = \frac{\left(E_i^P - \bar{E}^P\right)}{\bar{E}^P} \cdot 100\%$, where E_i^P is the area of the unwrapped parasite obtained from the ith wrapped larva phase and $\bar{E}^P$ its mean value.

III. $a_{3,i} = \frac{\underset{j}{mean}\left(y_{i,j} - \bar{y}_j\right)}{\underset{j}{mean}\left(\bar{y}_j\right)} \cdot 100\%$, where $y_{i,j}$ is the width of the unwrapped parasite that corresponds to the ith phase at point x_j; hence, we define $\bar{y}_j = \underset{i}{mean}\left(y_{i,j}\right)$.

IV. $a_{4,i} = \frac{\left(\Pi_i^P - \bar{\Pi}^P\right)}{\bar{\Pi}^P} \cdot 100\%$, where Π_i^P is $\bar{\Pi}^P$ the perimeter of the unwrapped parasite obtained from the ith wrapped larva phase and $\bar{\Pi}^P$ its mean value.

V. $a_{5,i} = \frac{\left(C_i^P - \bar{C}^P\right)}{\bar{C}^P} \cdot 100\%$, where C_i^P is the maximum cross section diameter of the unwrapped parasite obtained from the ith wrapped larva phase and $\bar{C}^P$ its mean value.

The mean value and standard deviation of quantities $a_{1,i}$, $a_{2,i}$, $a_{3,i}$, $a_{4,i}$, $a_{5,i}$ are shown in Table 1.

The Employed Method of Automatic Identification of Parasites

Description of the Introduced Classification Algorithm

In the previous sections, we have deduced a number of reasonable and justifiable mechano-elastic properties of the considered parasites and we have exploited them in order to virtually unwrap the parasites from the corresponding initial wrapped instances.

In order to classify the unwrapped parasite curves to the proper family, we have employed an original identification algorithm presented in this Section. This algorithmic scheme is in a sense a more complicated version of the k-means algorithm, however, at the same time differs from the other partitional algorithms, e.g. Lee et al. 1997, Jain and Dubes, 1988, Ng and Han 1994, since it does not require a predefined number of clusters, while it also dynamically estimates the cluster centers by exploitation of the entire data set and not only of the group. This method comprises the following steps:

- **Step 1:** We divide the available set of unwrapped parasite curves into a Training and a Test Set, by means of a random number generator. We also enumerate the individuals of the Training Set, randomly. Finally we define a set of characteristics upon which automatic identification will be based.
- **Step 2:** We determine a set of useful quantities that will be employed throughout the automatic identification process.

Table 1. Negligible dissimilarities between unwrapped versions of the same parasite are computed from images of radically different deformation stages of the same individual.

	Evaluation the discrepancy between the unwrapped versions of Figure 6.		Evaluation the discrepancy between the unwrapped versions of Figure 7.		Average discrepancy of all experimental results	
	Mean value	**Standard Deviation**	**Mean value**	**Standard Deviation**	**Mean value**	**Standard Deviation**
a_1 (Length):	0.82	0.29	1.04	0.73	0.91	0.56
a_2 (Area):	2.30	1.18	1.41	0.62	1.73	1.01
a_3 (Width):	1.87	1.06	1.32	0.60	1.68	0.94
a_4 (Perimeter):	0.84	0.34	1.07	0.74	0.95	0.59
a_5 (Max cross section diameter):	2.63	1.68	2.62	1.63	2.71	1.72

- **Step 3:** We perform an initial classification of the Training Set samples to groups where we stress that the parasite family may incorporate various different groups. We also compute the center of each such group.
- **Step 4:** We correct the clustering performed in Step3, as well as the groups' centers estimation, for the Training Set in hand.
- **Step 5:** We attribute the parasites of the Test Set in corresponding groups and hence families.

A detailed presentation of the aforementioned steps follows.

Step 1: First, the available set of unwrapped parasite curves is randomly divided in two subsets, a Training Set and a Test Set. The elements of the Training Set are also randomly enumerated.

Subsequently we define a number of characteristics upon which we will base the automatic parasite classification. Specifically:

CH1. The length of the axis of symmetry of the unwrapped parasite.
CH2. The maximum length of the sections normal to the parasite's neutral line.
CH3. The average parasite width.
CH4. The standard deviation of the parasite widths
CH5. The area defined by the upper and lower contour of the unwrapped parasite.
CH6. The perimeter of the unwrapped parasite.
CH7. The ratio of perimeter/area.
CH8. The average curvature of the contour of the parasite, computed directly by means of the explicit form of the contour polynomial approximation of the wrapped parasite in its initial image.
CH9. The standard deviation of the curvature computed above.
CH10. The average curvature of the contour of parasite, computed numerically on its unwrapped version.
CH11. The standard deviation of the curvature computed above.

Next, we define the a vector $\vec{x}$ in R^{11} such that its first component x^1 is the value of CH1 characteristic for a single individual, its second component is the value of CH2 for the same parasite instance, etc. To avoid unbalanced distances between different components of two parasites characteristics' vectors, we normalize $\vec{x}$ as follows: For each one of the aforementioned characteristics, say the j-th, we compute its average value for all parasites of the Training Set. If this mean value is $\bar{x}^j$, we substitute the j-th component of $\vec{x}$ with $\frac{x^j - \bar{x}^j}{\bar{x}^j}$ for all individuals in both Training and Test Set.

Step 2: Now, we will estimate the values of a number of parameters that will be proved useful in the automatic classification of parasites in the proper group. First, we compute the value of a parameter $D\max$, so as to ensure an as great as possible separability between the groups' centers. Therefore, for each family of individuals of the Training Set, say the j-th, we compute the mean value $\vec{\mu}(j)$ of its characteristic vectors; moreover let $I(j)$ be the set of individuals of the j-th family and $I^C(j)$ the set of samples belonging in other families. Next, we estimate $D\max$ via maximization of quantity shown in Box 2.

Second, we define a weight function of each characteristic vector on the basis of the distance of $\vec{x}$ from the center of each group. In fact, if $\vec{c}$ is the center of an arbitrary group, then this weight function is given by the formula $\beta(\vec{x},\vec{c}) = \exp\left(-A\|\vec{x}-\vec{c}\|^2\right)$. The constant A appearing in this formula is estimated using $D\max$ and the assumption that values of each characteristic inside the same group follows a normal distribution. We note that application of both Kolmogorov and Chi2 Tests does not contradict this hypothesis ($a = 0.0001$). Thus, the goal of achieving separation between groups at a confidence level 99.9% leads to the value of A:

$$A = \frac{3}{D\max\sqrt{2}}$$

Step 3: In order to achieve a first automatic classification of the Training Set parasites, we consider the first sample of this set $\vec{x}(1)$ and we let it be an initial estimation of the center of the first group $\vec{c}_1(1) = \vec{x}(1)$. Next, we consider the second sample of the Training ensemble with characteristic vector $\vec{x}(2)$ and we compute its Euclidean distance from $\vec{c}_1(1)$, say:

$$d(\vec{c}_1(1),\vec{x}(2)) = \sum_{i=1}^{11}\left(c_1^i(1) - x^i(2)\right)^2$$

If $d(\vec{c}_1(1),\vec{x}(2)) \geq D\max$, then $\vec{x}(2)$ becomes the center of a new group letting $\vec{c}_2(1) = \vec{x}(2)$. Simultaneously the value of center $\vec{c}_1(1)$ is updated via formula $\vec{c}_1(2) = \frac{\vec{c}_1(1)+\beta_1(2)\vec{x}(2)}{1+\beta_1(2)}$, $\beta_1(2) = \exp(-A\cdot d(\vec{c}_1(1),\vec{x}(2))^2)$; we also define quantity $S_1(1) = 1$ and we update $S_1(2) = 1 + \beta_1(2)$. Simultaneously, to avoid dependence of the groups' centers value on the order of choice of samples, we update the value of $\vec{c}_2$, employing $\vec{x}(1)$, by means of the formula $\vec{c}_2(2) = \frac{\vec{c}_2(1)+\beta_2(1)\vec{x}(1)}{1+\beta_2(1)}$ similarly defining $S_1(1) = 1$ and updating $S_1(2) = 1 + \beta_1(2)$; in the notation $\vec{c}_2(2)$ the subscript indicates the cardinal number of the group while the argument is used to indicate the number of the iteration.

Box 2.

$$S = \sum_{j=1}^{4}\left[\frac{1}{N_{I^C}(j)}\sum_{\nu\in I^C(j)}\left(\|\vec{x}(\nu)-\vec{\mu}(j)\| - D\max\right)^2 - \frac{1}{N_I(j)}\sum_{i\in I(j)}\left(\|\vec{x}(i)-\vec{\mu}(j)\| + D\max\right)^2\right]$$

We continue this recursive process and suppose that at the (j-1)-th step, k centers have been generated $\vec{c}_1(j-1),\ldots,\vec{c}_k(j-1)$. Let $\vec{x}(j)$ be the characteristic vector of the new incoming sample of the Training Set; then we compute distances

$$d(\vec{c}_i(j-1),\vec{x}(j)) = \sum_{l=1}^{11}\left(c_i^l(j-1)-x^l(j)\right)^2$$

If the maximum of these distances is greater than Dmax, we generate a new group center, $\vec{c}_{k+1}(1)=\vec{x}(j)$. In addition we update the value of previously estimated centers via formulas

$$\vec{c}_m(j)=\frac{S_m(j-1)\vec{c}_m(j-1)+\beta_m(j)\vec{x}(j)}{S_m(j)},$$

$S_m(j)=S_m(j-1)+\beta_m(j)$ where

$$\beta_m(j)=\exp(-A\cdot d(\vec{c}_m(j-1),\vec{x}(j))^2)$$

for $m = 1...k$.

Again, to minimize dependence on the order of choice of the characteristics vectors, we compute the whole sequence $\vec{c}_{k+1}(2),\ldots,\vec{c}_{k+1}(j)$ of updates of center $\vec{c}_{k+1}(1)$ via the following process: we consider that for the updating of $\vec{c}_{k+1}(1)$ only, the characteristics vector $\vec{x}(1)$ is a newcomer, in which case $\vec{c}_{k+1}(2)$ is computed via $\vec{c}_{k+1}(2)=\dfrac{\vec{c}_{k+1}(1)+\beta_{k+1}(1)\vec{x}(1)}{1+\beta_{k+1}(1)}$. Next we consider that $\vec{x}(2)$ comes and consequently the centre of the k+1 group is updated as before, etc. until $\vec{c}_{k+1}(j)$ is evaluated.

At the end of Step3, a number of distinct centers $\vec{c}_k\ k=1\ldots M$, is generated. To correspond these centers to parasite families, we compute the distances of each $\vec{c}_k$ from all characteristics vectors $\vec{x}(j)$; let $\vec{x}(j_k)$ be the vector of minimum distance from $\vec{c}_k$. Then $\vec{c}_k$ is attributed to the family from which $\vec{x}(j_k)$ is generated. We emphasize that this computation of the centers is not irrevocable and it must be readjusted using the entire information the Training Set offers. This will be realized in the next step.

Step 4: We attribute each individual of the Training Set with characteristic vector $\vec{x}$ to the group with center $\vec{c}_k$ from which $\vec{x}$ has the minimum distance. After having classified all samples of the Training Set to a family by means of this method, we compare this classification with the actual one, the expert has made. In practice, the procedure described in Step 3 offers an initial classification of the Training Set samples, which has a success rate of at least 75%. Let W_1 be the subset of individuals of the Training Set that have been erroneously classified so far; we will employ the samples of W_1 to readjust the proper parasite groups' centers, so that the classification success rate is drastically improved. To be specific, consider one sample $\vec{x}(i_1)$ of W_1, initially attributed to the group with center $\vec{c}_{w,1}$ corresponding to the 1st parasite family. However, according to the expert's classification of the Training Set samples, sample $\vec{x}(i_1)$ should have been attributed to the 4th parasite family. To deal with this discrepancy, we first consider the centers of all groups belonging to family 4 and we choose the center that has minimum distance from $\vec{x}(i_1)$ with vector $\vec{c}_{r,1}$. Now, we revaluate centers $\vec{c}_{w,1}$, $\vec{c}_{r,1}$ and the corresponding weighting factors $S_{r,1}(N)$, $S_{w,1}(N)$, as follows:

$$\vec{c}_{r,1}\leftarrow\frac{S_{r,1}(N)\vec{c}_{r,1}(1)+\delta\beta(i_1)\vec{x}(i_1)}{S_{r,1}(N)+\delta\beta(i_1)},$$

$$\vec{c}_{w,1}\leftarrow\frac{S_{w,1}(N)\vec{c}_{w,1}(n)-\delta\beta(i_1)\vec{x}(i_1)}{S_{w,1}(N)-\delta\beta(i_1)}$$

$$S_{r,1}(N)\leftarrow S_{r,1}(N)+\delta\beta(i_1),$$
$$S_{w,1}(N)\leftarrow S_{w,1}(N)-\delta\beta(i_1)$$

where

$$\delta\beta(i_1)=\beta_{w,1}(i_1)-\beta_{r,1}(i_1),$$
$$\beta_{w,1}(i_1)=\exp\left(-A\cdot d\left(\vec{c}_{w,1},\vec{x}(i_1)\right)^2\right),$$

$$\beta_{r,1}(i_1) = \exp\left(-A \cdot d\left(\vec{c}_{r,1}, \vec{x}(i_1)\right)^2\right)$$

Subsequently, we consider another sample of W_1 and we repeat the process until all W_1 individuals are exhausted.

At this point, we repeat the classification of all samples of the Training Set to a group and the corresponding family, by employing the newly estimated groups' centers values. We compare this classification with the one furnished by the expert for the Training Set parasites and suppose that the ensemble of erroneously identified individuals is W_2. Using the above procedure we reevaluate the group centers, this time employing the characteristics vectors of W_2.

In general, suppose that the $(\nu-1)^{th}$ iteration of this process has been completed and that the comparison of the obtained classification with the one the expert furnished, generates a set W_ν of erroneous identifications. Using an arbitrary sample of W_ν with characteristic vector $\vec{x}(i_\nu)$ we recompute the centers of the corresponding right and wrong groups, $\vec{c}_{r,\nu}$, $\vec{c}_{w,\nu}$, via formulas:

$$\vec{c}_{r,\nu} \leftarrow \frac{S_{r,\nu}(N)\vec{c}_{r,\nu}(1) + \delta\beta(i_\nu)\vec{x}(i_\nu)}{S_{r,\nu}(N) + \delta\beta(i_\nu)},$$

$$\vec{c}_{w,\nu} \leftarrow \frac{S_{w,\nu}(N)\vec{c}_{w,\nu}(1) + \delta\beta(i_\nu)\vec{x}(i_\nu)}{S_{w,\nu}(N) + \delta\beta(i_\nu)}$$

$$S_{r,\nu}(N) \leftarrow S_{r,\nu}(N) + \delta\beta(i_\nu),$$
$$S_{w\nu}(N) \leftarrow S_{w,\nu}(N) - \delta\beta(i_\nu)$$

where

$$\delta\beta(i_\nu) = \beta_{w,\nu}(i_\nu) - \beta_{r\nu}(i_\nu),$$

$$\beta_{w,\nu}(i_\nu) = \exp\left(-A \cdot d\left(\vec{c}_{w,\nu}, \vec{x}(i_\nu)\right)^2\right),$$

$$\beta_{r,\nu}(i_\nu) = \exp\left(-A \cdot d\left(\vec{c}_{r,\nu}, \vec{x}(i_\nu)\right)^2\right)$$

The aforementioned procedure stops when one of the following conditions hold: 1) W_ν is empty, i.e. the algorithm has classified the Training Set samples with 100% success rate or 2) the success rate has "stagnated" for a considerable number of iterations. We note that in practice condition 1) almost always occurs and that if condition 2) holds, then the success rate is very high.

In each iteration, the repositioning of the groups' centers performed in the above procedure, reduces the distance between the vectors of the center of the right group and a sample that has erroneously classified:

$$\left\|\vec{c}_{r,\nu+1}(n+1) - \vec{x}(i_\nu)\right\| = \frac{S_{r,\nu}(N)}{S_{r,\nu}(N) + \delta\beta(i_\nu)}\left\|\vec{c}_{r,\nu} - \vec{x}(i_\nu)\right\| < \left\|\vec{c}_{r,\nu} - \vec{x}(i_\nu)\right\|$$

At the same time, the distance between the center of the group to which this sample has been erroneously assigned and the sample's characteristic vector, increases:

$$\left\|\vec{c}_{w,\nu+1} - \vec{x}(i_\nu)\right\| = \frac{S_{w,\nu}(N)}{S_{w,\nu}(N) - \delta\beta(i_n)}\left\|\vec{c}_{w,\nu} - \vec{x}(i_\nu)\right\| > \left\|\vec{c}_{w,\nu} - \vec{x}(i_\nu)\right\|$$

In the end of this step one has performed Nw iterations and obtained a sequence of centers, namely $\{\vec{c}_{j,Nw}\}$, $j = 1...M(Nw)$, in practice optimally placed as far as classification of the Training Set parasites is concerned.

Step 5: Next, we will perform automatic identification of the Test Set parasites, by exploitation of the groups centers evaluated in Step4 and their distance from the characteristics vector of each test sample. Specifically, if $\vec{x}_i^{TEST}$ is the vector of characteristics of the *i*-th element of the Test Set, we compute each distance from the sequence of group centers $d\left(\vec{c}_{j,Nw}, \vec{x}_i^{TEST}\right)$, $j = 1...M(Nw)$ and we attribute $\vec{x}_i^{TEST}$ to the group with minimum distance with center $\vec{c}_{j^*,Nw}$. Hence we identify the family of the $\vec{x}_i^{TEST}$ parasite as the one to which group with center $\vec{c}_{j^*,Nw}$ belongs.

Table 2. Results of the automatic identification process of the parasites.

Parasite Genus	Number of individuals	Percentage of Classifications with 0 erroneous identifications	Percentage of Classifications with 1 erroneous identification	Percentage of Classifications with 2 erroneous identifications
1) *Cooperia*	17	57%	34%	9%
2) *Oesophagostomum*	24	31%	48%	21%
3) *Ostertagia*	16	100%	0%	0%
4) *Trichostrongylus*	31	33%	45%	22%

Application of the Method and Results

The entire set of data consisted of 193 parasite images that were shot at an arbitrary deformation instance. We randomly divided this set into 100 pairs of Training and Test Sets almost equal in number. For each Training Set we applied the procedure described in Steps 1-4, thus classifying all its members into groups, which in turn belong to one of the 4 families.

Next, we considered all samples of the corresponding Test Set and we applied Step 5 to identify the proper family to which the sample belongs. We repeated the aforementioned process for all 100 pairs of Training and Test Sets and we kept record of the correct and erroneous test classifications in each case. The related results are summarized in Table 2.

FUTURE TRENDS

The analysis presented in this chapter is quite general and it can be easily extended to take into account the determination of the mechano-elastic properties of various objects on the basis of their deformed images. Thus, for example, one may apply a similar methodology in the case of images of molecules, DNA, red blood cells, as well as of other cells, which are obtained via microscope.

Consequently, one may employ the knowledge of the elastic properties in order to obtain straightened versions of the deformed bodies and finally one can perform automatic identification of the straightened objects. Clearly this approach is also applicable in the case of non microscopic images. Moreover, the introduced clustering method described in the Section entitled "Description of the introduced classification algorithm" can be applied in radically different projects such as grouping of curves in an image and/or painting, in writer identification, etc.

Finally, it is reasonable to expect that exploitation of the color content of the parasite body image will offer parasite automatic classification near to perfection. Therefore, research in all these topics should take place in the future.

CONCLUSION

The performed experiments verify the validity of the aforementioned hypotheses and of the related analysis. In particular, the unwrapped versions of the contours of different deformed instances of the same parasite manifest strong similarity. Hence, the straightened contours seem to be reliable representations of the undeformed parasites and they can be employed in an automatic parasite classification system. Also, the assumptions on the elastic properties of parasite bodies seem to be confirmed by the obtained results. The authors used a new classification method, which succeeds in classifying the deformed parasites to proper groups and four families with more than 95% success rate.

REFERENCES

Chandrasekharaiah, D. S., & Debnath, L. (1st Ed.). (1994). *Continuum Mechanics*. Boston, MA: Academic Press.

Craig, D. (1999). Fitting Curves and Surfaces With Constrained Implicit Polynomials. *IEEE Transactions on PAMI, 21*(1), 31-41.

Sudipto G., Rajeev, R., & Kyuseok, S. (1998). CURE: An efficient clustering algorithm for large databases. *In Proc. of 1998 ACM-SIGMOD Int. Conf. on Management of Data.*

Gillian, A., Xiaoyi, P. J., Horst, D. B., Kevin, D. W., & Andrew, R. B. (1996). *An Experimental Comparison of Range Image Segmentation Algorithms, IEEE Transactions on PAMI, 18*(7), 673-689.

Guha, S., Rastogi, R., & Shim, K. (1999). ROCK: A robust clustering algorithm for categorical attributes. *Proc. of the 15th Int'l Conf. on Data Eng.*

Jain, A. K., & Dubes, R. C. (1988). *Algorithms for Clustering Data.* Prentice Hall.

Karypis, G., Han, E. H., & Kumar, V. (n.d.). CHAMELEON: A Hierarchical Clustering Algorithm Using Dynamic Modelling. *IEEE Computer: Special Issue and Data Analysis and Mining.*

Kaufman, L., & Rousseeuw, P. J. (1990). *Finding Groups in Data: an Introduction to Cluster Analysis.* JohnWiley & Sons.

Kohonen, T. (1984). *Self-Organization and Associative Memory.* Berlin - Springer Verlag.

Lee, D., Baek, S., & Sung, K. (1997). Modified k-means Algorithm for Vector Quantizer Design. *IEEE Signal Processing Letters,* 4(1), 2-4.

Malvern, L. E. (1969). *Introduction to the Mechanics of a Continuous Medium.* Englewood Cliffs, NJ: Prentice-Hall.

Manduca, A., Dutt, V., Borup, D. T., Muthupillai, R., Ehman, R. L., & Greenleaf, J. F. (1998). *Reconstruction of Elasticity and Attenuation Maps in Shear Wave Imaging: An Inverse Approach, Medical Image Computing and Computer-Assisted Interventation—MICCAI'98, 1496,* Lecture Notes in Computer Science, Springer Berlin / Heidelberg, (pp. 606-613).

McMurtry, L. W., Donaghy, M. J., Vlassoff, A., & Douch, P. G. C. (2000). Distinguishing morphological features of the third larval stage of ovine Trichostrongylus. *Veterinary Parasitology, 90*(1-2), 73-81.

Nelder, J. A., & Mead, R. (1965). A Simplex Method for Function Minimization. *Computer Journal, 7,* 308-313.

Ng, R., & Han, J. (1994). Efficient and effective clustering method for spatial data mining. *In Proc. of the 20th VLDB Conference,* (pp.144–155), Santiago, Chile.

Panagopoulos, Th., Papaodysseus, C., Exarhos, M., Triantafillou, C., Roussopoulos, G., & Roussopoulos, P. (2004). Prehistoric Wall-Paintings Reconstruction Using Image Pattern Analysis And Curve Fitting. *IEEE Systems Man and Cybernetics, 1,* 108-113.

Papaodysseus, C., Exarhos, M., Panagopoulos, P., Roussopoulos, P., Triantafillou, C., & Panagopoulos, Th. (2008). Identification of Geometrical Shapes in Paintings and its Application to Demonstrate the Foundations of Geometry in 1650 BC. *IEEE Transactions on Image Processing, 14*(7).

Papaodysseus, C., Exarhos, M., Panagopoulos, Th., Triantafillou, C., Roussopoulos, G., Pantazi, Af., Loumos, V., Fragoulis, D., & Doumas, C. (2005). Identification of Geometrical Shapes in Paintings and its Application to Demonstrate the Foundations of Geometry in 1650 BC. *IEEE Transactions on Image Processing, 14*(7).

Román-Roldán R., Gómez-Lopera J. F., Atae-Allah C., Martínez-Aroza J., & & Luque-Escamilla, P. L. (2001). A measure of quality for evaluating methods of segmentation and edge detection. *Pattern Recognition, 34*, 969-980.

Theodoropoulos, G., Loumos, V., Anagnostopoulos, C., Kayafas, E., & Martinez-Gonzales, B. (2000). A digital image analysis and neural network based system for identification of third-stage parasitic strongyle larvae from domestic animals. *Computer Methods and Programs in Biomedicine*, *62*(2), 69-76.

Washington, C. W., & Miga, M. I. (2004). Modality Independent Elastography (MIE): A New Approach to Elasticity Imaging. *IEEE Transactions on Medical Imaging, 23*(9), 1117-1128.

KEY TERMS

Automatic Curve Classification: A process which automatically classifies curves into different groups according to their similarity.

Curve Fitting Methods: Techniques that optimally fit a curve of desired functional form into a set of pixels or data points.

Elastic Deformation Invariants: Quantities, shapes or characteristics of a body, e.g. a parasite, which remain invariant during its elastic deformation.

Image Operations: Actions performed on an image that change the colour content of its pixels usually to detect or bring out some image characteristics.

Parasite Image Segmentation: The automated procedure that isolates parasite body in its microscopic image and perhaps locates the various parasite body regions.

Parasite Mechano-Elastic Properties: The quantities and properties that characterize the body of a parasite, from the point of view of Mechanics and Elasticity Theory.

Pattern Classification Techniques: A set of methods that classify the members of a data set in different groups according to a number of group-characteristic patterns.

Chapter XXIV
Nonlinear Ultrasound Radiation-Force Elastography

Alexia Giannoula
University of Toronto, Canada

Richard S. C. Cobbold
University of Toronto, Canada

ABSTRACT

"Elastography" or "elasticity imaging" can be defined as the science and methodology of estimating the mechanical properties of a medium (including soft tissue). In this chapter, an overview of elastography and its relation to tissue pathology will be presented. The basic principles of the static and dynamic methods will be described with special emphasis on the dynamic methods that rely on the acoustic radiation force of ultrasound. Of interest are the low-frequency narrowband shear waves that can be generated by a modulated radiation force produced by the interference of two continuous-wave (CW) ultrasound beams of slightly different frequencies. The advantages of using narrowband shear waves to estimate the viscoelastic properties of tissue will be discussed. Furthermore, an implementation of the inverse-problem approach will be presented and it will be shown how harmonic maps of the local shear modulus and viscosity can be reconstructed based on both the fundamental and higher-harmonic components of the propagated narrowband shear waves.

INTRODUCTION

The elasticity of soft tissues depends, to a large extent, on their molecular building blocks (fat, collagen, etc.), and on the microscopic and macroscopic structural organization of these blocks (Fung, 1981). Pathological changes are generally correlated with local changes in tissue stiffness (Figure 1). Many cancers, such as scirrhous carcinoma of the breast, liver metastases, prostatic carcinoma, and thyroid cancer, appear as extremely hard nodules (Anderson, 1984).

Other types of breast cancers (e.g. intraductal and papillary carcinoma) are soft (Ariel, 1987). Other diseases involve fatty and/or collagenous deposits, which increase or decrease tissue elasticity. The standard medical practice of soft tissue palpation is based on qualitative assessment of the low-frequency stiffness of tissue and has been used for centuries by physicians to distinguish between normal and diseased tissues. Palpation is sometimes used to assess organs such as the liver, and it is not uncommon for surgeons at the time of laparotomy to palpate tumors that were not detected preoperatively using conventional imaging methods, such as Ultrasound, Computer Tomography (CT), or Magnetic Resonance Imaging (MRI), since none of these modalities currently provides the type of information elicited by palpation.

In many cases, despite the difference in stiffness, the small size of a pathological lesion and/or its location deep in the body, preclude its detection and evaluation by palpation. In general, the lesion may or may not possess acoustic backscatter properties, which would make it detectable using ultrasound. For example, tumors of the prostate or the breast could be invisible or barely visible

Figure 1. (a) Sonogram and (b) elastogram of an in-vivo benign breast tumour (fibroadenoma) and (c) sonogram and (d) elastogram of an in-vivo malignant breast tumour (invasive ductal carcinoma). Note that black indicates stiff and white indicates soft tissue. Adapted version, reprinted from Ultrasonics, 38, Konofagou (2000), pp. 400-404, ©2000, with permission from Elsevier.

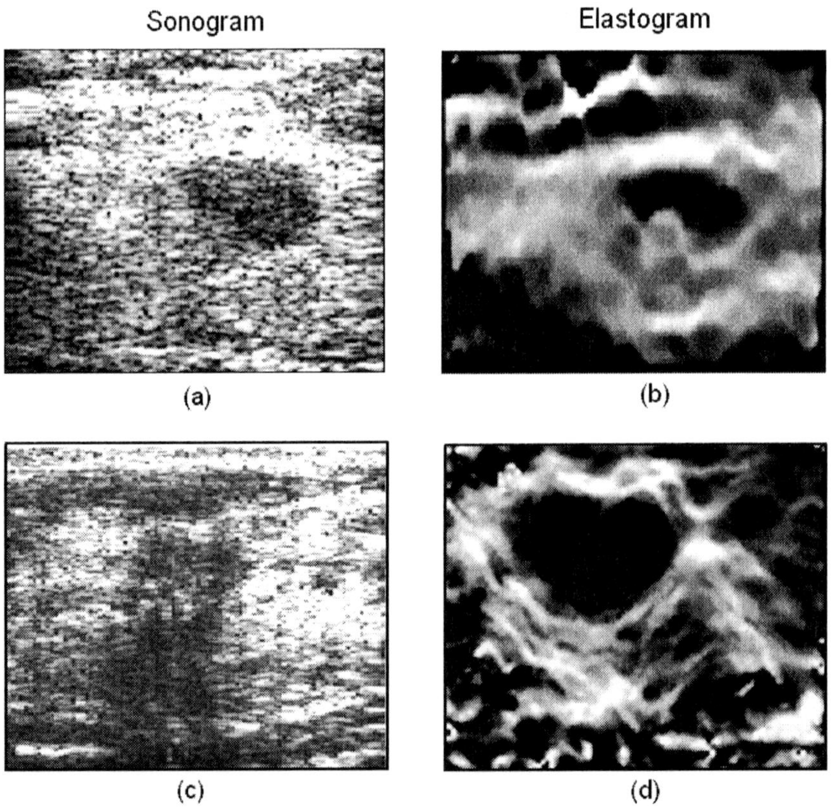

in standard ultrasound examinations, yet be much harder than the embedding tissue. Furthermore, diffuse diseases (e.g. cirrhosis of the liver) are known to significantly increase the stiffness of the liver tissue as a whole (Anderson, 1984). However, they may appear normal in conventional B-mode ultrasound examination. Based on the simple concept of palpation and the observation that echogenicity and the stiffness of tissue are generally uncorrelated (Garra, 1997; Ophir, 2001), *tissue elastography* or *elasticity imaging* (Ophir, 1991) seeks to provide non-invasive quantitative systems that can measure or image the local mechanical properties of tissue. Such systems could provide new information related to tissue structure and/or pathology (see Figure 1) and could significantly enhance the accuracy of diagnosis, even at early stages of disease.

In conventional (B-mode) ultrasound imaging, the ability to differentiate between various tissues within the body depends on changes in the acoustic properties, which in turn, depend primarily on the *bulk (elastic) modulus* (Cobbold, 2007). The range of variation of the bulk modulus is very small, i.e., significantly less than an order of magnitude. On the other hand, the shear modulus μ_l (known as the *second Lamé constant*), which is defined as the ratio of shear stress to shear strain that is involved in the passage of a transverse wave, may change by many orders of magnitude, depending on the tissue (Cobbold, 2007). This suggests that by imaging one or more characteristics of shear wave propagation, improved sensitivity to localized changes in elastic properties could be achieved, thereby, providing useful diagnostic information (Sarvazyan, 1998).

Low-frequency shear waves are known to travel within tissue with a propagation speed that is several orders of magnitude less than that of compressional waves[1]. An effective way in which localized low-frequency shear waves can be remotely generated within tissue, is by the dynamic radiation force resulting from the interference of two confocal quasi-CW ultrasound beams of slightly different frequencies. In contrast to most radiation force-based methods presented previously, the aforementioned dual-beam source can generate *narrowband* low-frequency shear waves. Such waves suffer less from the effects of dispersion, enabling the frequency-dependent shear speed and attenuation to be estimated at a specific frequency. This can be achieved by tracking the shear-wave phase delay and change in amplitude over a specific distance. Measurements at different frequencies can then be fitted to a viscoelastic model (e.g. the Voigt model, see following sections), enabling the tissue elasticity and viscosity to be extracted (Giannoula, 2008b).

In this chapter, the modulated acoustic radiation force will be modeled, based on the confocal dual-beam configuration. In order to increase the shear detection Signal-to-Noise-Ratio (SNR), higher-source pressure conditions may be needed, and thus, the presence of higher harmonics generated by nonlinear effects must be accounted for. Subsequently, the generation and propagation of short-duration shear waves at both the fundamental and harmonic modulation frequencies will be described, based on the approximate Green's functions for viscoelastic media, as derived by Bercoff (2004b). Furthermore, an implementation of the inverse-problem approach will be presented and it will be shown how harmonic maps of the local shear modulus and viscosity estimates can be obtained, based on both the fundamental and higher-harmonic components of the shear-wave spectrum. Future trends will be also discussed and conclusions will be finally drawn.

BACKGROUND

During the past two decades, various methods have been proposed for measuring or estimating the tissue elasticity. Elastography methods generally use a source of mechanical motion to produce a stress-field distribution on the probed tissue (tissue excitation). The applied stress, then, causes minute displacements within the tissue, which can be measured using magnetic resonance (MR) (Bishop, 1998; Muthupillai, 1995; Kruse, 2000), ultrasound (Ophir, 1991; Konofagou, 2000; Sugimoto, 1990) or optical techniques (Sarvazyan, 1998). The use of ultrasound has several significant advantages, including real-time imaging capabilities, very high resolution in motion estimation (~1 μm), simplicity, non-invasiveness, and relatively low cost. Overviews of elastography methods can be found in (Wilson, 2000) and (Parker, 2005).

Static vs. Dynamic Elastography

Elastography methods fall into two general categories, according to the temporal characteristics of the applied excitation: static (or quasi-static) and dynamic methods.

In *static* elastography (Ophir, 1991; Konofagou, 2000), tissue is compressed slowly and the distribution of its displacement is measured (using ultrasound, MR, etc.). The measured distribution of strain is related to the predicted distribution of stress and the resulting parameters of moduli are deduced through elasticity equations. Ophir (1991) used an external compressor to form strain images. It should be noted, that a strain image is generally formed by applying one or two-dimensional cross-correlation techniques to pairs of RF echo fields (e.g. A-lines), acquired before and after the tissue deformation (compression). Often in static methods, the strain alone is used as a surrogate for stiffness; that is, low strain means high stiffness and high strain results from softer, or low-stiffness regions (see Figure 1).

Konofagou (2000) managed to estimate shear strains from high-precision axial and lateral strain components and showed how these estimates can serve as a direct measure of tissue mobility, and thus, as a potential criterion of tissue characterization. For example, low shear strain can be generally interpreted as lack of mobility (e.g., firm binding of a tumour to its surroundings) and thereby, it may indicate a potential malignancy.

The difficulty with the static methods is that they require knowledge of boundary conditions outside of the region under investigation. An alternative means to investigate tissue elastic properties is to generate transient acoustic waves within the body and measure the associated transient motion in the spatiotemporal domain. These are known as *dynamic* elastography methods (Catheline, 1999; Fatemi, 1998; Nightingale, 2002; Lerner, 1988; Sandrin, 2004; Sarvazyan, 1998; Sugimoto, 1990; Yamakoshi, 1990) and have the advantage of potentially revealing the dynamic properties of the interrogated medium (such as viscosity). At the same time, they overcome boundary problems linked to the static methods.

Dynamic Elastography Methods

It is possible to create stress in a dynamic method by using external mechanical vibration (Catheline, 1999; Krouskop, 1987; Lerner, 1988; Sandrin, 1999; Yamakoshi, 2000) or by using an acoustic radiation force generated by a focused ultrasound beam (Bercoff, 2004a; Catheline, 2004; Fatemi, 1998; Konofagou, 2003; Nightingale, 2002; Nightingale, 2003; Sarvazyan, 1998; Sugimoto, 1990). An overview of these two classes of elastography methods will be presented in the following two subsections.

Stress Generation Using External Mechanical Vibration

Krouskop (1987) proposed a method to measure non-invasively the elastic modulus in soft tissue *in vivo*, by exciting a specific tissue region with an external vibrator (operating at approximately 10 Hz) and measuring the resulting tissue motion using pulsed Doppler ultrasound.

Lerner (1988) proposed an ultrasonic imaging modality called *sonoelasticity imaging*, which measured and imaged tissue displacement in response to externally applied low-frequency monochromatic mechanical vibration (10-100

Hz) using color Doppler ultrasound. An advantage of sonoelasticity imaging was its ease of implementation on modern ultrasound scanners, its low computation requirements, and its ability for real-time implementation.

Yamakoshi (1990) applied low-frequency (less than 200 Hz) sinusoidal vibration at the surface of the interrogated medium and the resulting motion (both amplitude and phase) was measured from the Doppler frequency shift of the reflected ultrasound waves. The vibration phase image was used to determine the shear wave propagation velocity.

Catheline (1999) proposed an ultrasound-based technique, which they called *transient elastography*, to deal with artifacts induced by diffraction in sonoelastography (e.g. wave reflection or standing waves). This method used a low-frequency (40–250 Hz) pulsed excitation to create displacements in tissue, which were then detected using pulse-echo ultrasound. The numerical values of elasticity and viscosity were deduced from the wave propagation (using cross-correlation techniques). This technique was effective, but required frame rates exceeding those available in ultrasound scanners at that time.

The work of Catheline (1999) was extended by Sandrin (1999) with the study of two-dimensional (2-D) shear wave propagation. Specifically, with a method entitled *time-resolved 2-D pulsed elastography* (Sandrin, 1999), a low-frequency (50-200 Hz) pulsed shear wave was generated using an external vibrating device, while an ultra-fast ultrasonic imaging system, specifically designed for this application, acquired 2-D frames at a very high frame rate (up to 10,000 frames/s). The tissue displacement that was induced by the slowly propagating shear wave was measured using standard cross-correlation techniques. A single low-frequency pulsed excitation was necessary to acquire the full data set. Thus, acquisition times were considerably reduced compared to MRI or Doppler detection methods. Furthermore, the proposed technique could be applied in the presence of tissue movement.

Stress Generation Using Acoustic Radiation Force

The elasticity imaging methods described previously are characterized by the application of stress throughout the entire interrogated object. However, it is possible to create a localized stress field within tissue with the acoustic radiation force of ultrasound, the principles of which will be presented in the following subsection. The concept of assessing the mechanical properties of tissue by monitoring its response to the acoustic radiation force, was first proposed by Sugimoto (1990), who attempted to quantify tissue hardness by applying a minute deformation in the tissue using the radiation force of a focused ultrasound beam and measuring the induced deformation with a pulse-echo method as a function of time.

A technique known as *shear wave elasticity imaging* (*SWEI*) was introduced by Survazyan (1998). In this method, localized shear waves (1 kHz) were remotely generated in tissue by the radiation force of a focused ultrasound beam using a short modulating pulse. The propagation of the induced shear waves was detected using a laser-based optical system and a magnetic resonance imaging (MRI) system and the local shear modulus parameter was estimated.

Nightingale (2002) proposed the acoustic radiation force impulse (*ARFI*) method. It used a short-duration (< 1 ms) acoustic radiation force to generate localized displacements in a 2-D region-of-interest (ROI) in tissue and the tissue response was determined using ultrasound correlation-based techniques. It was reported that the system was capable of measuring displacements down to the limits projected by the Cramer-Rao lower bound (Kay, 1993), i.e., about 0.2 μm. Nightingale (2003) applied also the above process to visualize the propagation of the induced transient shear waves and used direct inversion methods to estimate the shear elastic modulus parameter.

The *supersonic shear imaging* (*SSI*) technique, described Bercoff (2004a), provided a new ultrasound method for real-time (less than 30 ms) quantitative mapping of the viscoelastic properties of soft tissue. By successively focusing the "pushing" beam (~100-µs pulse) at different depths at a supersonic speed, two quasi-plane shear waves of stronger amplitude can be created that propagate in opposite directions, by the constructive interference of all the resulting shear waves from each "push". These were imaged by an ultrafast ultrasound scanner (6000 frames/s).

Fatemi (1998) proposed a technique known as *ultrasound-stimulated-vibro-acoustography* (*USVA*), in which two quasi-CW ultrasound beams of slightly different frequencies are used to remotely generate a localized dynamic (oscillatory) radiation force at the difference frequency, typically in the low kHz range. In fact, this method forms the basis of the method described below (Giannoula, 2008b). Fatemi (1998) created a modulated field in the intersection zone which caused tissue in the focal region to vibrate at the beat frequency. In response, the region emitted low-frequency longitudinal waves (known as *acoustic emission*), which could be detected externally by a hydrophone and depended on the radiation force and the elastic properties of the medium (Fatemi, 1998; Fatemi, 2000). It should be noted, that in the above work, lossless media and linear ultrasound propagation were assumed. Under these assumptions, the presence of an obstacle (scatterer) was required for the generation of the modulated radiation-force and the acoustic-emission fields. By ignoring the shear-wave generation and propagation, the authors obtained high-resolution, but qualitative only, maps of the local mechanical properties of tissue.

By using a similar dual-beam setup, Konofagou (2003) proposed a technique named *harmonic motion imaging* (*HMI*), for estimating the local Young's modulus from the oscillatory (harmonic) tissue motion induced by a dynamic (harmonically-varying) radiation force. Similarly to USVA, this method estimates tissue motion *during* and not *after* the application of the force (the latter applies to most shear-based methods, such as these presented above). This could potentially provide a better estimate of the mechanical properties of the excited lesion or tumour and would be less affected by the surrounding tissue.

Principles of the Acoustic Radiation Force

All elastography methods descried in the previous subsection relied on the use of the acoustic radiation force of ultrasound for the generation of stress within the excited medium. It should be noted, that understanding the acoustic radiation force dates back to 1902, when Rayleigh (1902) described a theory of the acoustic radiation pressure as an acoustic counterpart of the radiation pressure produced by electromagnetic waves. Since then, several theories have been proposed in order to further explain the underlying physics and controversy has arisen from improperly posed problems, confusion over definitions and the difficulties associated with nonlinear phenomena (Biquard, 1932; Beyer, 1978; Lee, 1993; Torr, 1984).

When ultrasound is incident on an obstacle whose properties differ from that of the propagation medium, a force will be exerted and this consists of two components: the first is an oscillatory component with a time-average of zero, arising from the time-varying acoustic pressure acting on the body. The second is a steady component that is known as the radiation pressure. Its presence is an inherent property of the nonlinear relation between pressure and density in the propagation media (Cobbold, 2007). Thus, in a fluid it seems reasonable to express the total radiation pressure by:

Radiation Pressure = pressure due to nonlinearity + pressure due to attenuation which asserts that provided attenuation is present, a radiation pressure will exist even when the propagation medium is perfectly linear.

In the absence of any obstacle, a finite-amplitude acoustic wave propagating in a lossless medium, whose density is nonlinearly related to the pressure, will result in a transfer of momentum from the wave to the medium. If the medium is also viscous, additional momentum will be transferred (Westervelt, 1951). Both forms of momentum transfer, i.e., those resulting from nonlinearity and absorption, contribute to the radiation pressure acting in the propagation direction. In comparison to the effects of tissue nonlinearity, the effects of attenuation in soft tissue, at frequencies in the MHz frequency range, can be expected to be dominant, as assumed in this chapter.

HARMONIC ULTRASOUND RADIATION-FORCE IMAGING

The radiation force exerted in an infinite isotropic, homogeneous, and attenuating medium is considered here. In addition, because the pressure in the focal zone region may be large, it is necessary to account for the presence of harmonics generated by nonlinear effects (Giannoula, 2007; Giannoula, 2008b).

Description of the Proposed Dual-Beam System Model

For a finite-amplitude ultrasound beam propagating in an attenuating medium, it can be shown that the force per unit volume, generated at location **r**, is given by (Nyborg, 1998):

Figure 2. (a) Illustrating the principles of a simple confocal radiation force imaging system used to generate low-frequency shear waves. (b) Transducer A (inner) is a confocal circular disk of aperture radius a_1=1.3 cm and transducer B (outer) is a confocal annular disk with inner and outer radii a_{21}=1.4 cm and a_{22}=2.1 cm, respectively (see also Section 2.2). The dynamic radiation force produced by the interference of the two beams is also shown at the common focal point (at a distance of 7.0 cm from the transducers).

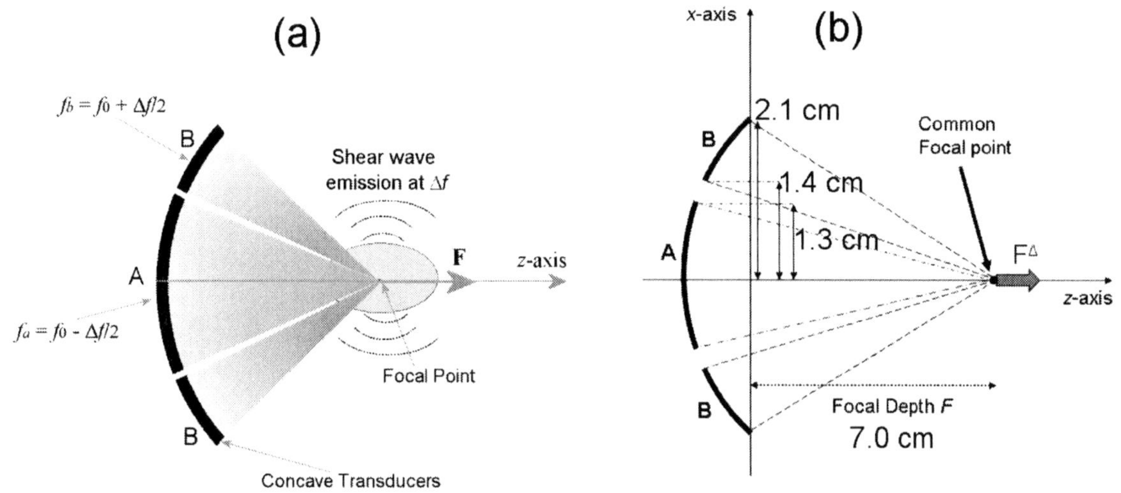

$$\mathbf{F}_n(\mathbf{r},t)=\frac{2\alpha_n \mathbf{I}_n(\mathbf{r},t)}{c}, \quad n=1,2,\ldots \qquad (1)$$

where c is the propagation speed, the subscript n denotes the n'th harmonic of the fundamental frequency f_0 and $\mathbf{I}_n(\mathbf{r},t)$ is the acoustic intensity vector. Moreover, if the attenuation coefficient is assumed to have a power-law frequency dependance, then the attenuation can be written as $\alpha_n(f)=\alpha_0 f^{\gamma}$, where γ is typically close to unity in most soft tissues. For a focused acoustic beam, the force is applied throughout the focal region of the beam and for absorbing media (such as tissue), it is assumed to be in the direction of the wave propagation, i.e. the z-axis.

With reference to Figure 2, we consider two coaxial confocal quasi-CW[2] ultrasound beams A and B excited at the angular frequencies $\omega_a=\omega_0-\Delta\omega/2$ and $\omega_b=\omega_0+\Delta\omega/2$, where ω_0 and $\Delta\omega$ are the center and difference frequencies, respectively, such that $\Delta\omega \ll \omega_0$. If the beams propagate in the z-direction with a common focal point at $(0, 0, z_0)$ then, in the region of intersection, the resulting pressure can be written as:

$$p_n(\mathbf{r},t)=p_{n,a}(\mathbf{r})e^{jn\omega_a t}+p_{n,b}(\mathbf{r})e^{jn\omega_b t}, \quad n=1,2,\ldots \qquad (2)$$

where $p_{n,a}(\mathbf{r})$ and $p_{n,b}(\mathbf{r})$ are the complex amplitude functions of the ultrasonic beams at the n'th harmonic. The resultant intensity field at the region of interference will contain two high-frequency static (time-invariant) components and a low-frequency (dynamic) components at $n\Delta\omega=n(\omega_b-\omega_a)$ (Nyborg, 1998). All high-frequency terms can be neglected, since they do not fall within the low acoustic frequency range.

Based on (1), the modulated (time-varying) radiation force corresponding to the n'th harmonic is therefore given by (Giannoula, 2008b):

$$\mathbf{F}_n^{\Delta}(\mathbf{r},t)=\frac{2\alpha_0 n^{\gamma}(f_a^{\gamma}+f_b^{\gamma})}{c}\times \frac{Re\{[p_{n,b}(\mathbf{r})\mathbf{v}_{n,a}^{*}(\mathbf{r})+p_{n,a}(\mathbf{r})\mathbf{v}_{n,b}^{*}(\mathbf{r})]e^{j(n\Delta\omega t+\Delta\phi_n(\mathbf{r}))}\}}{2}, \quad n=1,2,\ldots \qquad (3)$$

where $\mathbf{v}_{n,a}(\mathbf{r})$ and $\mathbf{v}_{n,b}(\mathbf{r})$ denote the particle velocities, $*$ denotes the complex conjugate, $\Delta\varphi_n(\mathbf{r})$ is the phase difference at which the corresponding n'th harmonics of the two beams arrive at point $\mathbf{r}$ and for convenience, we have chosen the time $t=0$ to correspond to the time at which the 'tone bursts' from the two sources reach the geometric focus. Details of the above derivation can be also found in (Giannoula, 2008a).

For our simulations, which were written in Matlab (The MathWorks, Inc., Natick, MA), a confocal source consisting of two simple coaxial concave radiation sources with a common geometric focal depth of 7.0 cm was assumed. As shown in Figure 2(b), the outer aperture radius was 1.3 cm for beam-A, while for beam-B the inner and outer aperture radii were 1.4 cm, 2.1 cm, respectively. The source pressure amplitude was taken to be 372 kPa (Zemp, 2003) at excitation frequencies of 2.0 MHz ± 250 Hz. The medium was assumed to have a propagation speed of $c=1550$ m/s, a density of 1050 g/m^3, a nonlinearity coefficient[3] of $\beta=5.0$, an attenuation characterized by $\gamma=1.1$ and $\alpha_0=0.3$ dB/(cm MHz$^{1.1}$).

To calculate the fields generated by the transducers for $n=1,2,\ldots$, we made use of a modified version of the 2nd-order operator splitting nonlinear model of Zemp (2003), that enabled the harmonic field distribution to be calculated for $n=1$-4 with reasonable accuracy. The axial pressure amplitudes of the first four harmonics for beam-A and beam-B are shown in Figure 3. Fifty propagation planes were used to capture the axial variations of the harmonics. Close to the transducer, the approximations used in the nonlinear propagation algorithm caused errors in the calculated pressure profiles, but over the region of the last maxima and beyond, the accuracy is quite sufficient. In the region of the geometric focus, a dynamic component of the radiation force will be present at the fundamental modulation frequency of 500 Hz, as well as at the harmonic frequencies of $n\Delta f$ (i.e., at 1000 Hz, 1500 Hz, etc, for $n = 2,3, \ldots$). The corresponding spatial force-field patterns on the geometric focal plane at $t = 0$, 2.0 ms, etc, are shown in Figure 4 for $n = 1$-4. The forces per unit volume have been normalized with respect to the maximum fundamental force at focus.

As illustrated in Figure 2, the radiation force described in (3), causes media in the focal zone to vibrate at the difference frequency. As a result, low-frequency longitudinal and shear waves will be generated that propagate away from this zone. In contrast to most shear wave-based elasticity imaging methods previously described, it will be shown that these tone-burst generated shear waves can have a relatively narrow bandwidth.

Shear-Wave Propagation Induced by the Modulated Radiation Force

To predict the manner in which shear waves are generated and propagate in an elastic medium due to the creation of a localized force field it is necessary to use the Navier-Stokes equation (Cobbold, 2007). Aki (2002) derived analytical expressions of the displacement field for purely elastic media, known as the Green's functions $\mathbf{G}(\mathbf{r},t)$. Bercoff (2004b) extended this model to account for viscous effects and obtained approximate expressions of the Green's functions based on the Voigt model for a viscoelastic medium. In both cases, it was found that the displacement field $\mathbf{u}(\mathbf{r}, t)$ could be written as the sum of three types of waves: a pure compressional wave $\mathbf{u}^c(\mathbf{r},t)$ propagating at a speed c, a pure shear wave $\mathbf{u}^s(\mathbf{r},t)$ that propagates at a much smaller speed c_s and a coupling term $\mathbf{u}^{cs}(\mathbf{r},t)$, that contains both types of waves.

Now the i'th component (i = x, y, z) of the total shear displacement field due to the fundamental component of the radiation force $\mathbf{F}^{\Delta}(\mathbf{r},t)$ acting in the j-direction can be expressed as (Bercoff, 2004b):

$$u_i(\mathbf{r},t) \approx F_j^{\Delta}(\mathbf{r},t) ** [G_{ij}^{s}(\mathbf{r},t) + G_{ij}^{cs}(\mathbf{r},t)] = u_i^{s}(\mathbf{r},t) + u_i^{cs}(\mathbf{r},t), \quad (4)$$

where the approximation applies to soft-tissue[4] media and $**$ denotes a four-dimensional (4-D) spatiotemporal convolution. The approximate expression of the viscoelastic Green's function for the pure shear term as derived by Bercoff (2004b) based on the Voigt model, is given by

Figure 3. Axial pressure amplitude of the n'th harmonic component (n=1...4) for (a) beam A (confocal circular disk) and (b) beam B (confocal annular ring).

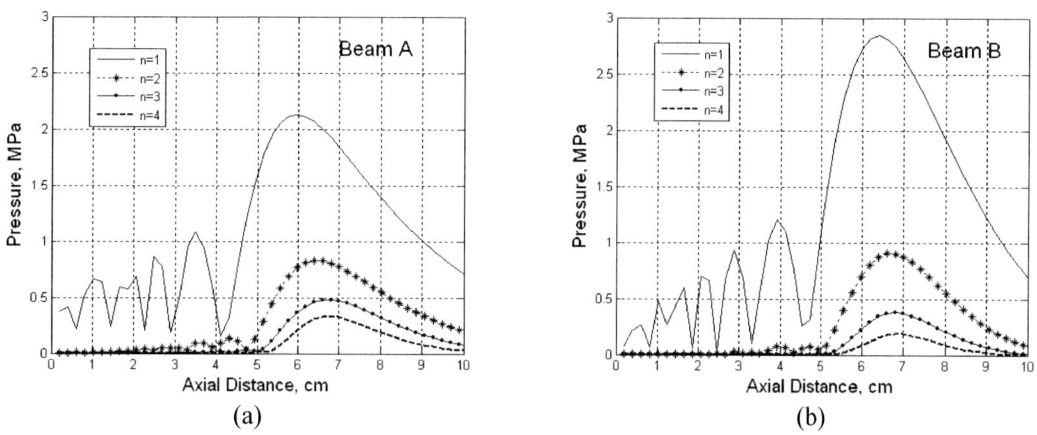

Figure 4. Normalized radiation force per unit volume on the geometric focal plane (7.0 cm) for: (a) the fundamental (500 Hz), (b) the second harmonic (1000 Hz), (c) the third harmonic (1500 Hz) and (d) the fourth harmonic (2000 Hz).

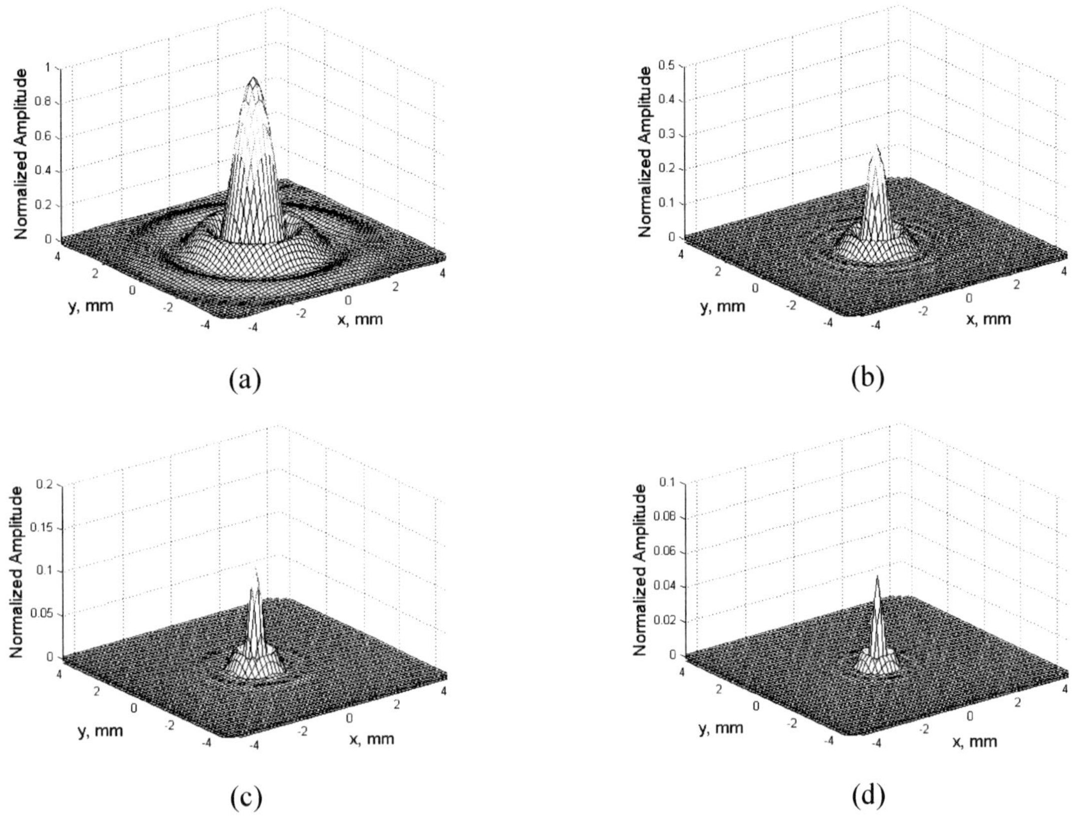

$$G_{ij}^{s}(\mathbf{r},t) = \frac{1}{4\pi\rho c_s} \times$$

$$\frac{1}{\sqrt{2\pi v_s t}} \frac{(\delta_{ij} - \gamma_i \gamma_j)}{r} \exp\left[-\frac{(t - r/c_s)^2 c_s^2}{2 v_s t}\right], \quad (5)$$

where $i = x, y, z, r = |\mathbf{r}|, \gamma_i = \partial r / \partial i$, ρ is the density of the medium and δ_{ij} is the Krönecker δ-function with $\delta_{ij} = 1$ if $i = j$ and 0 otherwise. In addition, $v_c = (\eta_c + 2\eta_s)/\rho$, $v_s = \eta_s/\rho$ denote the kinematic bulk and kinematic shear viscosity, respectively, where η_c and η_s are the bulk and shear viscosities. The coupling term, containing both longitudinal and shear wave components, can be written in a similar manner (Bercoff, 2004b). The coupling term has a r^{-3} dependence (see (23) in Bercoff (2004b)), which causes both components to rapidly reduce with distance (near-field term, (Sandrin, 2004)), as compared to the pure shear term expressed by (5), which varies as r^{-1} (far-field term).

In the immediate region surrounding the geometric focus, the primary component of the force is along the z-axis and in the following analysis, this is assumed to be the only component of significance, i.e., $i = j = z$. The origin of our coordinate system is taken to be at the geometric focus ($z = 7.0$ cm).

First, we consider the modulated n'th-harmonic radiation force to be a spatial impulse at the origin (point force) that varies sinusoidally in time at the beat frequency $n\Delta f$, such that each harmonic modulation waveform consists of a short cosine wave of duration D starting at t=0. It should be noted that as the duration is increased, the bandwidth of the shear waves will decrease, making it possible to determine the wave propagation characteristics at a specific frequency. However, for many periods of the modulation frequency, depending on the peak pressure, there will be an associated temperature rise. For in vivo use, the maximum temperature change is limited by regulatory specifications of the thermal index (TI), which increases with the modulation waveform duration (Abbott, 1999). We shall limit our discussion to values of D that correspond to periods of a few cycles, thereby limiting the TI while still maintaining a reasonably narrow bandwidth.

With the help of (3), the n'th harmonic component of the radiation force in the z-direction is described by

$$F_n^{\Delta}(0,t) = \delta(\mathbf{r}) \times$$

$$\frac{2\alpha_0 n^{\gamma}(f_a^{\gamma} + f_b^{\gamma})p_{n,a}(0)p_{n,b}(0)}{\rho c^2} H(t)H(D-t) \times$$

$$\cos[n \cdot 2\pi\Delta f \cdot t + \Delta\phi_n(0)],\ n = 1,2,... \qquad (6)$$

where H(.) denotes a Heaviside step functions. If N_h harmonics are considered for each beam, then the modulated finite-amplitude radiation force generated by the interference of these beams, can be written as $F^{\Delta}(0,t) = \sum_{n=1}^{N_h} F_n^{\Delta}(0,t)$, where $F_n^{\Delta}(0,t)$ is given by (6).

The finite-amplitude shear component can be written as a time convolution between the total radiation force and the shear Green's function, i.e.

$$u_z^s(\mathbf{r},t) = \frac{2\alpha_0}{\rho c^2}\int_0^D G_{zz}^s(\mathbf{r},\tau) \times$$

$$\left[\sum_{n=1}^{N_h} n^{\gamma}(f_a^{\gamma} + f_b^{\gamma})p_{n,a}(0)p_{n,b}(0)\cos[n\Delta\omega(t-\tau) + \Delta\phi_n(0)]\right]d\tau$$

$$(7)$$

where the shear waveform has been taken to consist of a short modulated wave of duration D starting at $t = 0$ and $G_{zz}^s(r,t)$ is the shear component of the viscoelastic Green's function (given by (5) for $i = j = z$).

The influence of several parameters on the spatiotemporal profile of the fundamental component of the shear displacement field was described in (Giannoula, 2008a; Giannoula, 2008b). The manner in which the characteristics of the viscoelastic propagation medium, i.e., the shear viscosity and speed, affect the evolution of the fundamental shear-wave component was analyzed.

Reconstructing Harmonic Maps of the Local Shear Modulus and Viscosity

From measurements of the shear displacement on an imaging plane as a function of time, it is possible to derive maps of the local shear modulus and viscosity of the medium, based on inverse algorithms (Bercoff, 2004a; Catheline, 2004).

The inverse problem approach in elastography is based on the shear-wave propagation equation. This can be written in the frequency domain, for a viscoelastic, isotropic, piece-wise homogeneous solid, as follows (Aki, 2002; Bercoff, 2004a):

$$\Im_t\left[\frac{\partial^2 u(x,z,t)}{\partial t^2}\right] - \frac{1}{\rho}(\mu_l + j\eta_s\omega) \times$$

$$\Im_t[\Delta u(x,z,t)] = 0 \qquad (8)$$

where $u(\mathbf{r},t)$ is the total shear displacement, $\Im_t$[.] denotes its Fourier transform (with respect to time), μ_l and η_s are the shear modulus and viscosity, respectively, and $\Delta = \frac{\partial^2}{\partial x^2} + \frac{\partial^2}{\partial y^2} + \frac{\partial^2}{\partial z^2}$ denotes the 3-D Laplacian operator. If the imaging area is specified to be the (x, z) plane, then only two of the above three second-order spatial derivatives can be experimentally measured. Therefore, a strong assumption, that the out-of-plane spatial derivative $\left(\frac{\partial^2 u}{\partial y^2}\right)$ is negligible, needs to be made (Catheline, 2004), i.e., $\Delta \approx \frac{\partial^2}{\partial x^2}+\frac{\partial^2}{\partial z^2}$.

As a result, it can be shown that (8) yields the following expressions for the local shear modulus and viscosity:

$$\mu_l(x,z:\omega)=\rho\ \mathrm{Re}\left\{\frac{\Im_t\left[\partial^2 u(x,z,t)/\partial t^2\right]_\omega}{\Im_t\left[\Delta u(x,z,t)\right]_\omega}\right\}$$

$$\eta_s(x,z:\omega)=\frac{\rho}{\omega}\mathrm{Im}\left\{\frac{\Im_t\left[\partial^2 u(x,z,t)/\partial t^2\right]_\omega}{\Im_t\left[\Delta u(x,z,t)\right]_\omega}\right\} \quad (9)$$

where Re{.} and Im{.} denote the real and imaginary parts. The above equations can be averaged over a range of frequencies around the excitation frequency (i.e., in our case, around the harmonic modulation frequency $n\Delta f$) and have the potential to provide quantitative estimates of the local shear modulus and shear viscosity based on either the fundamental or the higher-harmonic shear components.

In the forward problem, a circular inclusion of negligible thickness with a radius of 6.0 mm, centered at (x=15.0 mm, y=15.0 mm) was assumed to have a shear modulus and viscosity 6.0 kPa and 5.0 Pa·s, respectively. The corresponding shear modulus and viscosity of the background medium were taken 2.0 kPa and 0.1 Pa·s. A finite-amplitude modulated force at Δf=100 Hz was assumed to have duration 20.0 ms (two cycles). Furthermore, the source pressure, center frequency and attenuation coefficient were taken to be 450 kPa, 2.5 MHz and 0.35 dB/(cm·MHz$^{1.1}$), respectively. The approximate viscoelastic Green's functions (including the coupling term) were used. The displacement field was sampled throughout a 30×30 mm^2 field in order to determine $\Delta u(x,z,t)$ and $\partial^2 u(x,z,t)/\partial t^2$. Examples of the reconstructed maps of the local shear modulus and viscosity on the (x,z) plane are shown in Figure 5, based on the fundamental and second-harmonic component of the calculated displacement fields. Except within the immediate focal zone (Bercoff, 2004a), the reconstruction results are a reasonable approximation to the assumed distribution for both the fundamental and the second harmonic.

In Figure 6, reconstructed maps are shown under noisy conditions, based on the first four harmonic components and the average of the first three harmonic components, for a modulation frequency of 100 Hz. Specifically, Gaussian noise of zero mean and (normalized) variance 0.2 was added to the calculated total shear displacement field (corresponding to SNR values of approximately 60 dB) and the inverse equations described by (9) were next applied. The shear viscosity within the circular inclusion region was assumed 2.0 Pa·s. Good estimation results have been obtained especially from the fundamental and second-harmonic component. For the higher harmonics ($n=3,4$), noise amplification is observed especially at larger distances from the source and this is probably attributed to the derivatives involved in the inverse algorithm, known as highpass operations which tend to amplify noise. However, taking the average of the first three reconstructed maps gives better reconstruction results, through the smoothing effect on outliers.

Discussion

As discussed earlier in this chapter, the class of dynamic elastography methods that use the acoustic radiation force of ultrasound to generate transient motion within tissue, has been recently receiving growing interest. Such methods have shown great promise to provide quantitative stiffness estimates in a locally excited region of interest within the interrogated medium in a non-invasive manner.

Figure 5. Maps of the estimated local (a), (c) shear modulus and (b), (d) shear viscosity from (a)-(b) the fundamental and (c)-(d) the second-harmonic shear displacement on the (x,z) plane. A modulation frequency of 100 Hz was assumed, along with an emission duration of 20.0 ms.

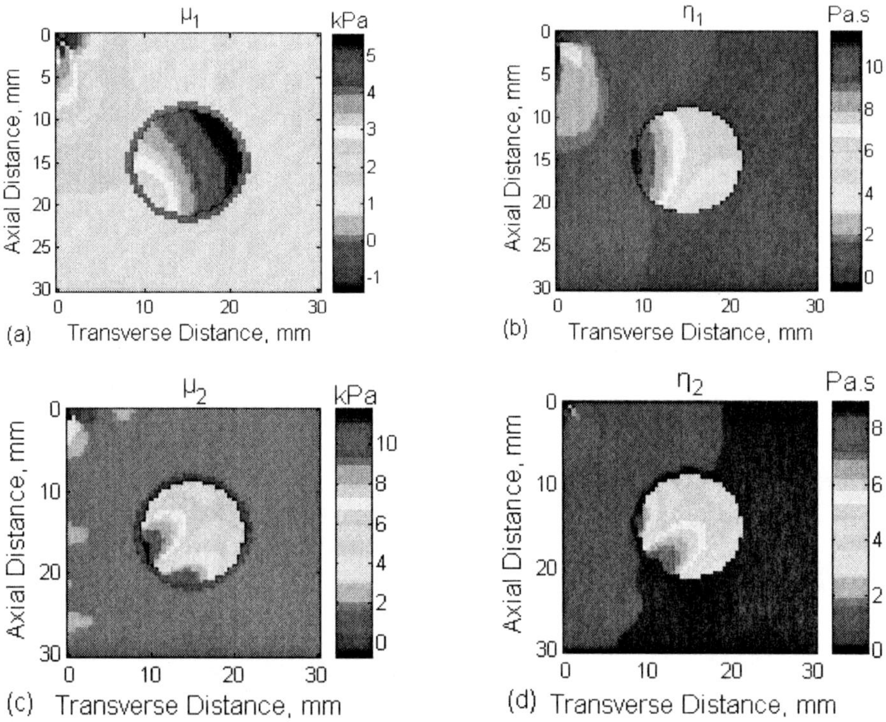

A specific methodology for remotely generating low-frequency shear waves within a medium was proposed in this section, based on narrow-band radiation-force excitations resulting from two intersecting confocal quasi-CW ultrasound beams of slightly different frequencies. In this way, a highly-localized modulated force field can be created at an easily controllable modulation frequency. In contrast to most elastography methods presented so far, which make use of a broadband excitation (short pulse), an important advantage of the above modulated source is that the spectrum of the generated low-frequency (<1 kHz) shear waves will not be significantly distorted as they propagate through tissue by different frequency-dependent effects (Giannoula, 2008b) and as a result, the viscoelastic parameters can be more accurately determined at a specific frequency.

The proposed dual-beam source should be capable of producing sufficiently accurate 2-D maps of the local shear modulus and viscosity of a locally excited region of tissue at both the fundamental and multiples of the modulation frequency, by using conventional ultrasound equipment for tissue excitation. For detecting the associated tissue motion (i.e., acquisition of 2-D images of the induced tissue displacement), a B-mode ultrasound scanning system would be needed, operating at a high frame, i.e., > 3000 frames per second. Such ultrafast scanners can nowadays be constructed (Catheline, 2004).

Figure 6. Maps of the estimated local (left column) shear modulus and (right column) shear viscosity from (a)-(b) the fundamental, (c)-(d) the second-harmonic, (e)-(f) the third-harmonic, (g)-(h) the forth-harmonic and (i)-(j) the mean average of the first three harmonic components on the (r,z) plane. The modulation frequency was assumed 100 Hz and the emission duration 20.0 ms.

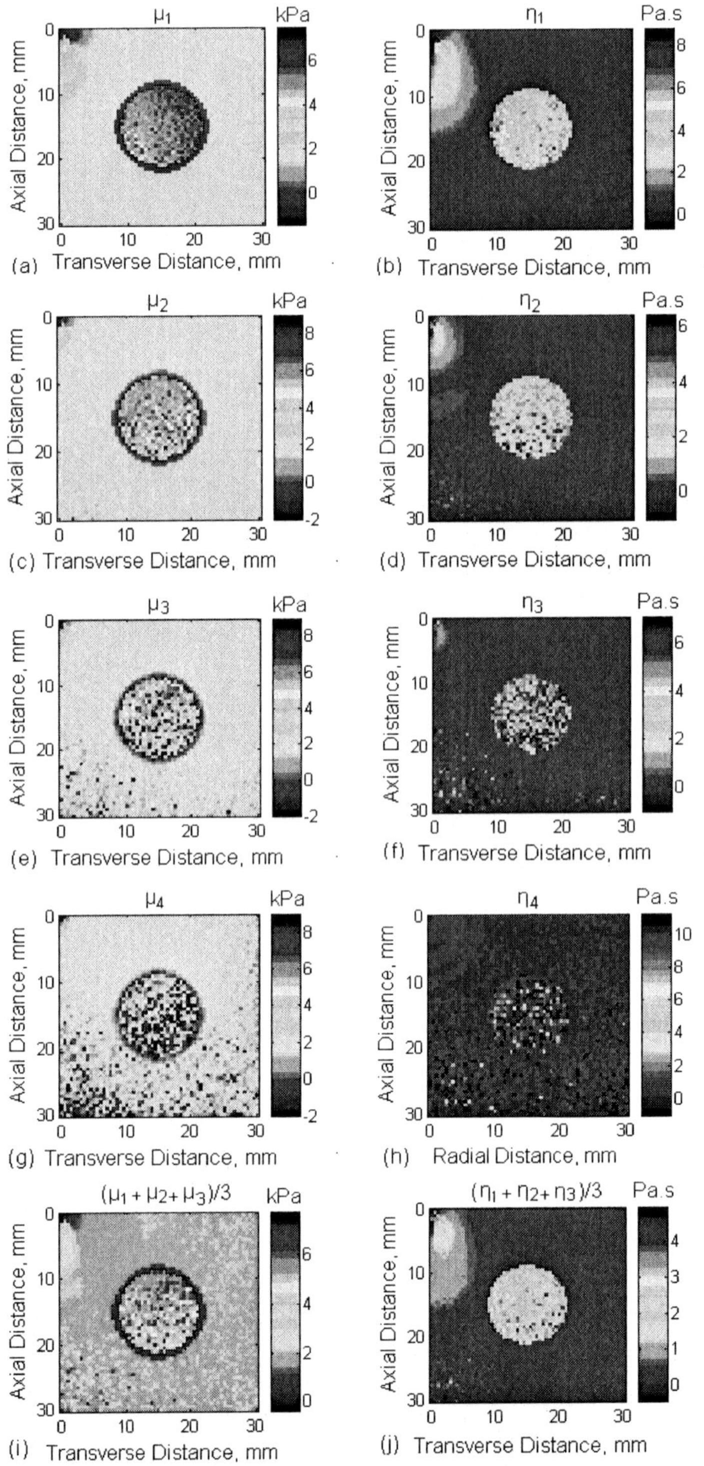

FUTURE TRENDS

For the *in-vivo* application of the proposed method, several challenges should be addressed and more realistic clinical conditions should be considered. Specifically, the method should be experimentally validated in real biological soft tissues, which are known to exhibit inhomogeneous and/or anisotropic behaviour. Another challenge often encountered *in-vivo*, is the physiological motion that many organs experience due to the respiration and/or the cardiac cycle. The effects of such motion on the proposed model and possible ways of compensating for it need also to be examined.

The above challenges appear to be significant future avenues that should be explored in order for the field of tissue elastography to provide valuable diagnostic information. In fact, several studies have been recently presented toward these trends, i.e., under more practical clinical situations (Bai, 2006; Genisson, 2003; Fahey, 2006).

Particularly for the proposed methodology, work is also being carried out in order to assess the performance of the generated local viscoelastic maps, based on image quality metrics that are commonly used in elastography. Such metrics involve the observed contrast, the contrast transfer efficiency (CTE), contrast-to-noise-ratio (CNR) (Ponnekanti, 1995) and also, the SNR and resolution. Furthermore, fusion algorithms for combining efficiently the generated local maps from several spectral components (e.g. from the fundamental and the higher-harmonic components) are also sought, in order to generate elastogram images of improved quality (e.g. increased CTE and SNR).

CONCLUSION

An overview of elastography and its major categories was provided in this chapter, with special emphasis on the dynamic elastography methods that use the acoustic radiation force of ultrasound. Furthermore, a specific methodology was proposed for remotely generating low-frequency narrowband shear waves by using the modulated radiation force resulting from two intersecting CW beams of slightly different frequencies. The advantages of using narrowband shear waves to estimate the viscoelastic properties of tissue were discussed. Nonlinear ultrasound propagation was also assumed in this chapter, so that a high-intensity force field is created in the focal zone, leading in turn, to the generation of shear waves of sufficient energy that can propagate and be detected at several wavelengths away from the source. Subsequently, an implementation of the inverse-problem approach was presented and two-dimensional (2-D) spatial maps of the local shear modulus and viscosity were derived, based on the fundamental and higher-harmonic components of the shear-wave spectrum, for both noise-free and noisy conditions.

ACKNOWLEDGMENT

We are grateful to the National Science and Engineering Research Council of Canada and the Canada Institute of Health Research, for providing partial financial support of this work.

REFERENCES

Abbott, J. G. (1999). Rationale and derivation of *MI* and *TI* – a review. *Ultrasound Med. Biol.*, *25*, 431-441.

Aki, K., & Richards, P. G. (2002). *Quantitative Seismology*. Sausalito, California: University Science Books.

Anderson, W. A. D. (1984). *Pathology* (8'th ed.). Saint Louis, Mo, USA: CW Mosby Co.

Ariel, I. M., & Cleary J. B. (1987). *Breast cancer diagnosis and treatment*. New York, USA: McGraw-Hill.

Bai, P., Wan, M., Wang, S., Zhang, D., & Dang, J. (2006). A novel method for evaluating tissue inhomogeneity in elastography. *Progress in Natural Science*, *16*(5), 474-479.

Bercoff, J., Tanter, N., & Fink, M. (2004a). Supersonic shear imaging: a new technique for soft tissue elasticity mapping. *IEEE Trans. Ultrason., Ferroelect. Freq. Contr.*, *51*, 396-409.

Bercoff, J., Tanter, M., Muller, M., & Fink, M. (2004b). The role of viscosity in the impulse diffraction field of elastic waves induced by the acoustic radiation force. *IEEE Trans. Ultrason., Ferroelect. Freq. Contr.*, *51*, 1523-1536.

Beyer, R. T. (1978). Radiation pressure – the history of a mislabeled tensor. *J. Acoust. Soc. Am.*, *63*, 1025-1030.

Biquard, P. (1932). Les ondes ultra-sonores. *Rev. d'Acoust.*, *1*, 93-109.

Bishop, J., Poole, G., Leitch, M., & Plewes, D. B. (1998). Magnetic resonance imaging of shear wave propagation in excised tissue. *J. Magn. Reson. Imaging*, *8*, 1257–1265.

Catheline, S., Wu, F., & Fink, M. (1999) A solution to diffraction biases in sonoelasticity: The acoustic impulse technique. *J. Acoust. Soc. Am.*, *105*, 2941–2950.

Catheline, S., Gennisson, J. L., Delon, G., Fink, M., Sinkus, R., & Abouelkaram, S. (2004). Measurement of viscoelastic properties of homogeneous soft solid using transient elastography: An inverse problem approach. *J. Acoust. Soc. Am.*, *116*, 3734-3741.

Cobbold, R. S. C. (2007). *Foundations of Biomedical Ultrasound*. New York: Oxford Univ. Press.

Fahey, B. J., Hsu, S. J., Wolf, P. D., Nelson, R. C., & Trahey, G. E. (2006). Liver ablation guidance with acoustic radiation force impulse imaging: challenges and opportunities. *Physics in Med. Biol.*, *51*, 3785-3808.

Fatemi, M., & Greenleaf J. (1998). Ultrasound-stimulated vibro-acoustic spectrography. *Science*, *280*, 82-85.

Fatemi, M., & Greenleaf, J. (2000). Probing the dynamics of tissue at low frequencies with the radiation force of ultrasound. *Phys. Med. Biol.*, *45*, 1449-1464.

Fung, Y. C. (1981). Ch. 4 in *Biomechanical properties of living tissues*, New York, USA: Springer Verlag.

Garra, B. S., Céspedes, E. I., Ophir, J., Spratt, R. S., Zuurbier, R. A., Magnant, C. M., & Pennanen, M. F. (1997). Elastography of breast lesions: Initial clinical results. *Radiology*, *202*, 79-86.

Gennisson, J. L., Catheline, S., Chaffai, S., & Fink, M. (2003). Transient elastography in anisotropic medium: application to the measurement of slow and fast shear wave speeds in muscles. *J. Acoust. Soc. Am.*, *114*(1), 536-541.

Giannoula, A., & Cobbold, R. S. C. (2007). Propagation of narrowband shear waves induced by a finite-amplitude radiation force. *Proc. IEEE Ultrason. Symp.*, (pp. 2267-2270).

Giannoula, A. (2008a). *Propagation of shear waves generated by a finite-amplitude ultrasound radiation force in a viscoelastic medium.* PhD dissertation, University of Toronto, Canada.

Giannoula, A., & Cobbold, R. S. C. (2008b). Narrowband shear wave generation by a finite-amplitude radiation force: the fundamental component. *IEEE Trans. Ultrason., Ferroelect. Freq. Contr.*, *55*(2), 343-358.

Kay, S. M. (1993). Fundamentals of Statistical Signal Processing, Volume I: Estimation Theory. N. J., USA: Prentice Hall.

Konofagou, E., Hannigan, T., & Ophir, J. (2000). Shear strain estimation and lesion mobility assessment in elastography. *Ultrasonics, 38*, 400-404.

Konofagou, E., & Hynynen, K. (2003). Localized Harmonic Motion Imaging: Theory, Simulations and Experiments. *Ultrasound Med. Biol., 29*, 1405-13.

Krouskop, T. A., Dougherty, D. R., & Vinson, F. S. (1987). A pulsed Doppler ultrasonic system for making noninvasive measurements of the mechanical properties of soft tissue. *J. Rehabil. Res. Dev., 24*(2), 1-8.

Kruse, S. A., Smith, J. A., Lawrence, A. J., Dresner, M. A., Manduca, A., Greenleaf, J. F., & Ehman, R. L. (2000). Tissue characterization using magnetic resonance elastography: preliminary results. *Phys. Med. Biol., 45*, 1579-1590.

Lee, C. P., & Wang, T. G. (1993). Acoustic radiation pressure. *J. Acoust. Soc. Am., 94*, 1099-1109.

Lerner, R. M., Parker, K. J., Holen, J., Gramiak, R., & Waag, R. C. (1988). Sono-elasticity: medical elasticity images derived from ultrasound signals in mechanically vibrated targets. In L.W. Kessler (Ed.), *Acoustical Imaging* (pp. 317-327). Plenum Press, New York.

Muthupillai, R., Lomas, D. J., Rossman, P. J., Greenleaf, J. F., Manduca, A., & Ehman, R. L. (1995). Magnetic resonance elastography by direct visualization of propagating acoustic strain waves. *Science, 269*, 1854-57.

Nightingale, K., Soo, M. S., Nightingale, R., & Trahey, G. (2002). Acoustic radiation force impulse imaging (ARFI): In vivo demonstration of clinical feasibility. *Ultrasound Med. Biol., 28*(2), 227-235.

Nightingale, K., McAleavey, S., & Trahey, G. (2003). Shear-wave generation using acoustic radiation force: In vivo and ex vivo results. *Ultrasound Med. Biol., 29*, 1715-1723.

Nyborg, W. L. (1998). Acoustic streaming. In M.F. Hamilton & D.T. Blackstock (Eds.), *Nonlinear Acoustics* (pp. 207-231). New York: Academic Press.

Ophir, J., Cespedes, I., Ponnekanti, H., Yazdi, Y., & Li, X. (1991). Elastography: a quantitative method for imaging the elasticity of biological tissues. *Ultrasonic Imaging, 13*, 111-134.

Ophir, J., Kallel, F., Varghese, T., Konofagou, E., Alama, S. K., Krouskop, T., Garra, B., & Righetti, R. (2001). Imagerie acoustique et optique des milieux biologiques - Optical and acoustical imaging of biological media: Elastography. *Comptes Rendus de l Académie des Sciences – Series IV - Physics, 2*(8), 1193–1212.

Parker, K. J., Taylor, L. S., & Gracewski, S. (2005). A unified view of imaging the elastic properties of tissue. *J. Acoust. Soc. Am., 117*, 2705-2712.

Ponnekanti, H., Ophir, J., Huang, Y., & Cespedes, I. (1995). Fundamental mechanical limitations on the visualization of elasticity contrast in elastography. *Ultrasound Med. Biol., 21*, 533-543.

Rayleigh, L. (1902). On the pressure of vibrations. *Phil. Mag., 3*, 338-346.

Sandrin, L., Catheline, S., Hennequin, X., & Fink, M. (1999). Time-resolved 2-D pulsed elastography. *Ultrasonic Imaging, 21*, 259-272.

Sandrin, L., Cassereau, D., & Fink, M. (2004). The role of the coupling term in transient elastography. *J. Acoust. Soc. Am., 115*, 73-83.

Sarvazyan, A. P., Rudenko, O. V., Scott, D., Swanson, J., Fowlkes, B., & Emelianov, S. Y. (1998). Shear wave elasticity imaging: a new ultrasonic technology of medical diagnostics. *Ultrasound Med. Biol., 24*(9), 1419-1435.

Sugimoto, T., Ueha, S., & Itoh, K. (1990). Tissue hardness measurement using the radiation force of focused ultrasound. *Proc. IEEE Ultrason. Symp.*, (pp. 1377-1380).

Torr, G. R. (1984). The acoustic radiation force. *Am. J. Phys., 52*, 402-408.

Westervelt, P. J. (1951). The theory of steady forces caused by sound waves. *J. Acoust. Soc. Am., 23*, 312-315.

Wilson, L. S., Robinson, D. E., & Dadd, M. J. (2000). Elastography- the movement begins. *Phys. Med. Biol., 45*, 1409-1421.

Yamakoshi, Y., Sato, J., & Sato, T. (2000). Ultrasonic imaging of internal vibration of soft tissue under forced vibration. *IEEE Trans. Ultrason., Ferroelect. Freq. Contr., 37*, 45-53.

Zemp, R. J., Tavakkoli, J., & Cobbold, R. S. C. (2003). Modeling of nonlinear ultrasound propagation in tissue from array transducers. *J. Acoust. Soc. Am., 113*, 139-152.

KEY TERMS

Acoustic Radiation Force: The force that is exerted when an ultrasound wave hits an obstacle that absorbs, scatters, or reflects energy. This force is in the direction of propagation and is also known as the *time-averaged (Langevin) radiation pressure*.

Elastography (or Elasticity Imaging): The general class of quantitative methods, which aim at measuring or imaging the mechanical properties of a medium, including soft tissue.

Finite-Amplitude Acoustic Wave: Propagation of an acoustic wave within a medium under conditions where the pressure and density are nonlinearly related. The *small-signal* approximation that is involved in the linear propagation theory is no longer valid. The pressure is considered sufficiently high that nonlinear effects arise, which cause the generation of higher harmonics.

Inverse-Problem: It involves the mathematical processes where the values of some parameters, characterizing a system under investigation, must be inferred from the observed (measured) data.

Narrowband Spectrum: It describes a signal whose frequency spectrum occupies a narrow range of frequencies (as opposed to broadband).

Shear Modulus: The ratio of the shear stress to the shear strain (or angular deformation), that is related to the passage of a transverse wave (where a shearing motion is involved). It is also known as the *second Lamé constant*.

Shear Viscosity: A coefficient that characterizes the viscous properties of a fluid and is related to the absorption (loss) of energy (or else, damping) due to the presence of velocity gradients in the fluid. This means that adjacent layers move at differing speeds and as a result, there is a frictional drag force that causes energy to be dissipated.

Shear (or Transverse) Wave: Form of wave propagation in a solid medium where the particle movement is at right angles to the direction of propagation.

ENDNOTES

1. Kruse (2000) measured the low-frequency shear speed (in the range 75-300 Hz) to be around 1.5-2.5 m/s in porcine liver and 1-2.2 m/s in porcine kidney. Typical values of the compressional speed of sound have been reported around 1550-1600 m/s in liver and 1560-1570 m/s in kidney (see Figure 1.11 in (Cobbold, 2007)).
2. The ultrasound beams are characterized as *quasi*-CW, since the transmitted waveforms are of finite duration, although they are made long enough to appear continuous.
3. The *coefficient of nonlinearity* β is a dimensionless parameter characterizing the

nonlinearity of a medium, which can be expressed by the amount of distortion imposed in a sinusoidal waveform, causing it to become more like a sawtooth. In terms of frequency content, this is equivalent to harmonic generation at integer multiples of the original frequency (Cobbold, 2007).

4 As noted by Sandrin (2004), for soft tissue-like media, the bulk modulus λ_l is much greater than the shear modulus μ_l, so that the effects of the longitudinal term are negligible compared to the shear and coupling terms.

Chapter XXV
Dynamic Contrast Enhancement:
Analysis's Models and Methodologies

Valentina Russo
University La Sapienza, Italy

Roberto Setola
University CAMPUS Bio-Medico, Italy

ABSTRACT

The aim of this chapter is to provide an overview about models and methodologies used for the Dynamic Contrast Enhancement (DCE) analysis. DCE is a non-invasive methodology aimed to diagnostic the nature of a lesion on the base of the perfusion's dynamic of specific contrast agents. The idea at the base of DCE is that, in several pathological tissues, including tumors and inflammatory diseases, the angiogenic process is abnormal, hence the characterization of vascularisation structure may be used to support the diagnosis. In this chapter, we will describe the basic DCE procedures and introduce some of its most innovative evolution based on the pharmacokinetic analysis technique (PK), and the empirical model (EM). Even if DCE is still a medical research topic, there is large interest for this type of approach in biomedical applications as witnessed by the availability of specific tools in the last generation top-class US, CT and MR machines.

INTRODUCTION

Normal and pathological tissues rely on the presence of the blood for an adequate supply of nutrients and for removal of waste metabolic materials. As tissues develop, a proper structured vascular network is "developed" at the same time. This process is known as angiogenesis (Padhani and Husband, 2001).

In pathological tissues, including tumors and inflammatory diseases, the angiogenic process is often abnormal, leading to the development of vascular beds, characterized by an excessive proportion of blood vessels with peculiar morphological and dynamic properties. Hence the characterization of vascularisation structure may be used to support non-invasive diagnoses of several pathologies. This analysis is generally performed using the Dynamic Contrast-Enhancement (DCE) procedure (Jackson, 2003; Jackson, 2004). This method aims to determine the degree of morbidity of a disease on the base of the local vessel morphology analyzing how a specific contrast media perfuse into the tissues. This type of approach may be included into those field of Biomedical Image researches that are moving from the analysis of a single image (or a spatial sequence) to the temporal examination of images' sequence, in order to emphasize physio-pathologic information strictly relates with the dynamic properties of the observed process. This passage imposes to provide physicians with sophisticated analysis tools, allowing huge quantities of raw data to be processed and analyzed. As for this purpose, development in imaging processing, computer vision and artificial intelligence in medical image interpretation have shown that software tools can pursue the objective of detecting, extracting and measuring useful features of the dynamic process under investigation, thus supporting the diagnosis process.

In addition to diagnostic issue, the kinetic of dynamic contrast enhancement may be used in clinical practice as a pharmacodynamic indicator of biological activity (i.e. for antivascular cancer drugs): it can define the biologically active dose and foresee the efficacy of a pharmacological treatment.

In this chapter, we will describe the basic DCE procedure and introduce some of its most innovative evolution based on the pharmacokinetic analysis technique (PK), and the empirical model (EM).

BACKGROUND

Quantitative characterization of microvascular structure using DCE is a powerful tool, able to provide valuable information for clinical purposes and/or for therapeutic trials. One goal of DCE is to characterize tissue regions, since some of their features (blood flow, vascular characteristics, or tissue integrity) are expected to vary in pathological tissue with respect to normal one.

In a typical DCE study, the dynamic information shows the rate at which tissue "enhances", and subsequently the rate at which Contrast Agent (CA) washes out. The enhancement is thought to be the result of the CA arriving via the system blood flown and diffusing into the interstitial space around these vessels (which is known as the extravascular extracellular space - EES). The rate and the amplitude of enhancement depend on the density and permeability of the microvasculature and on the relative size of the EES. The degree of enhancement is, therefore, related to the distribution and concentration of the CA in the vessels and in the ESS; hence the shape of the enhancement curve, then, reflects blood flow, vascular volume, extravascular volume and vessel permeability (Srikanchana et al., 2004).

The CA is used generally as an intravascular marker while the leakage into the interstitial space is generally ignored. In practice the kinetics of CA distribution are more complex and additional data can be obtained from explicit modelling of the contrast (enhancement) leakage process. In the presence of leaky capillary endothelial membranes, intravascular CA will pass into the ESS, causing enhancement. The leakage rate depends on the surface area of leaky endothelium, on the permeability of the endothelium itself and on the concentration gradient of the CA across the vessel wall. It has become apparent that quantification of contrast leakage may be a powerful indicator of the state of neo-vascular angiogenesis in pathologies, such as tumors and inflammatory processes. As for cancer research, this is very appealing, since the inhibition of angiogenesis presents new therapeutic chances of targeting of newly formed vessels, with the final aim at inhibiting their onset and growth.

Quantification of the CA enhancement effect can be performed using a variety of techniques ranging from simple measurements of the rate of enhancement (Florie et al., 2006) to complex algorithmic analysis, applying pharmacokinetic models to the imaging data, in order to measure the transfer constant (K^{trans}) of the contrast agent between the blood stream and the EES (Brix et al., 1999).

DCE analysis can be performed by non-compartmental (model-independent) or compartmental methods. Non-compartmental methods estimate the exposure to a CA by estimating the area under the curve of a concentration-time graph and is highly dependent on estimation of total CA exposure. Total CA exposure is most often estimated by Area Under the Curve (AUC) methods. Compartmental methods estimate the concentration-time graph using Pharmacokinetic (PK) models to describe and predict the concentration-time curve. Pharmacokinetic (PK) models are hypothetical structures that are used to describe the fate of a drug (in our case the CA) in a biological system, after its administration. PK compartmental models are often similar to kinetic models used in other scientific disciplines, such as chemical reactor engineering and rely on the definition of the compartment, that is a portion of space characterized by an uniform distribution of system properties (components concentration, temperature, pressure, pH).

Compartmental model are generally distinguished in terms of number of compartments that are needed for a complete description of the target systems (Padhani and Husband, 2001):

- **One compartemental model:** Following CA administration, the body is depicted as a kinetically homogeneous unit (see Figure 1.a); this configuration assumes that the CA achieves instantaneously an uniform distribution throughout the body and that the CA equilibrates instantaneously between tissues. Thus the CA concentration–time profile shows a mono-phasic response (i.e. it is mono-exponential). Notice that this does not imply that the CA concentration in plasma equals the concentration in the tissues; however, changes in the plasma concentration quantitatively reflect changes in the tissues.
- **Two compartemental model:** The two-compartment model resolves the body into a central compartment and a peripheral compartment (see Figure 1.b). Although these compartments have no physiological or anatomical meaning, it is assumed that the central compartment comprises tissues that are highly perfused, while the peripheral compartment refers to less perfused tissues. A two-compartment model assumes that, after the CA administration into the central compartment, CA transfers between that compartment and the peripheral compartment. Notice that the CA does not achieve instantaneous distribution, (i.e. equilibration), between the two compartments;
- **Multicompartmental model:** In this model the CA distributes into more than two

Figure 1. (a) One compartmental model; (b) Two compartmental model

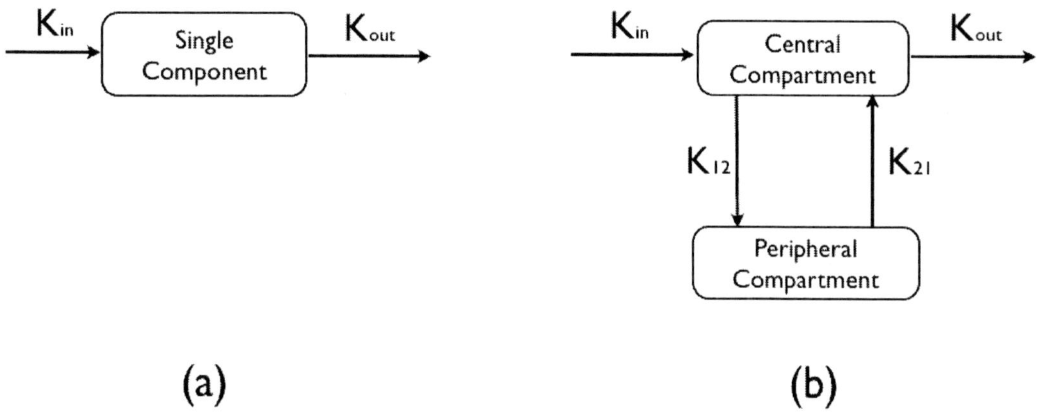

compartments and the concentration–time profile is described by several exponential terms; at least one exponential term for each assumed compartment.

The advantage of compartmental with respect to non-compartmental analysis is the ability to predict the concentration at any time. The disadvantage is the difficulty in developing and validating the proper model.

Dynamic Contrast Enhancement

Classic DCE

Dynamic Contrast Enhancement (DCE) is an approach, used in radiological framework, to evaluate the vascularisation of suspected or anomalous tissue. This non-invasive method determines the type of the local vascularisation analyzing the perfusion's dynamic of specific CA insight the tissues (Florie et al., 2006). Specifically, from the knowledge of the time evolution of the backscatter signal intensity corresponding to each ROI (Region Of Interest), one can identify a set of parameters useful for diagnose, such as: contrast wash-in and wash-out time (speed), contrast concentration (intensity) and in which way the contrast media perfuses into the lesion (uniformity) (Horsfield et al., 2004; Kier et al., 2005; Florie et al., 2006). To evaluate these parameters, the fundamental hypothesis is that the change of the intensity in the image corresponds to augment local concentration.

The DCE procedure is generally arranged as follows: the specific CA is injected and several acquisitions of images are performed at intervals, over a time period ranging from 30 seconds to several minutes, giving as result a sequence of images. DCE can be performed, with substantially the same conceptual framework, on images produced via US (Ultra Sound), CT (Computer Tomography) and MR (Magnetic Resonance) exams, where specific contrast media are used.

Even if DCE is still a medical research topic, there is large interest for this type of approach in clinical applications. Indeed, the last generation top-class US, CT and MR machines have dedicated tools to perform DCE analysis. Unfortunately, these tools are largely vendor oriented, devoted to support diagnoses for specific anatomical districts (e.g., evaluation of a lymph node, discrimination of adnexal masses, etc.) and limited to a single type of source (e.g., US or CT or MR). Recently some projects are on going to overcome these drawbacks, providing to radiologist a user-friendly framework to correctly perform the analysis (Russo et al., 2007).

Notice that, while usual CT and MR analysis are performed on spatial sequences, DCE is done on a temporal sequence: different scans are performed on the same anatomical region, at different times. Then, the images are suitable arranged, as illustrated in Figure 2, in order to create the temporal sequence.

Substantially, basic DCE analysis can be reduced to the evaluation of the Contrast-Enhancement (CE) curve illustrated schematically in Figure 3 (Horsfield et al., 2004; Marret et al. 2004; Kier et al., 2005; Florie et al., 2006; Russo et al., 2007).

CE is defined, for each pixel and with respect to any image into the sequence, as:

$$I(T_k, x, y) = \left[i(T_k, x, y) - i_0(x, y)\right] \quad (1)$$

where $I(T_k,x,y)$ is the intensity at the abscissa (x,y) at sample time T_k, $i_0(x,y)$ is the basal value (i.e. the mean value of intensity registered before the perfusion of the Contrast Media and assumed as background noise). Sometimes, to reduce the effect of noise and artifacts due to patient's motion, Eq. (1) is evaluated with respect to a sub-ROI averaging the data associated with all the pixels inside the region.

By inspecting the CE Curve (see Figure 3), it is possible to evaluate the relevant parameters (Kier et al., 2005; Marret et al., 2004) for diagnoses and, specifically:

Figure 2. Logical process to create a temporal sequence from N spatial sequence

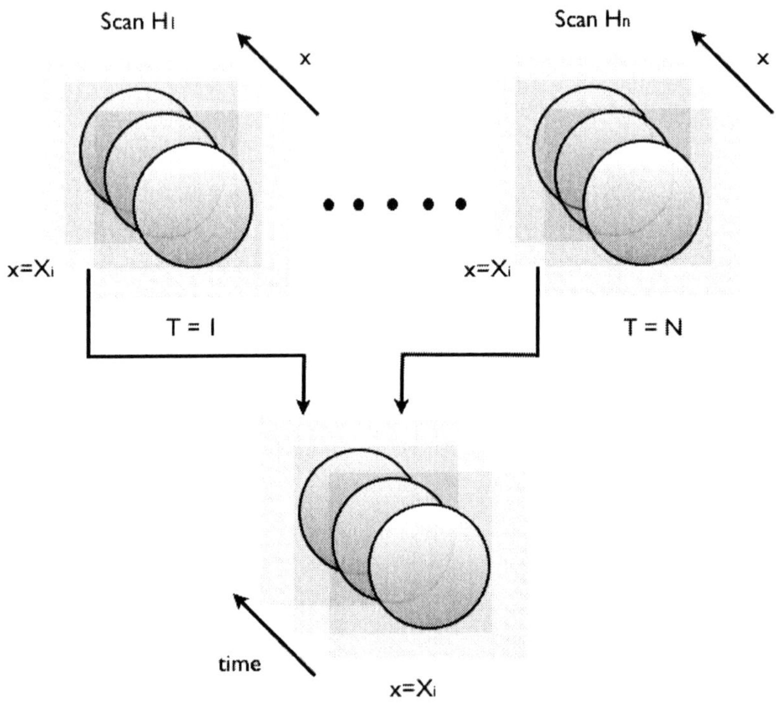

Figure 3. Contrast enhancement curve, with the definition of some of the relevant parameters: AUC, LPI, TTP and SLOPE

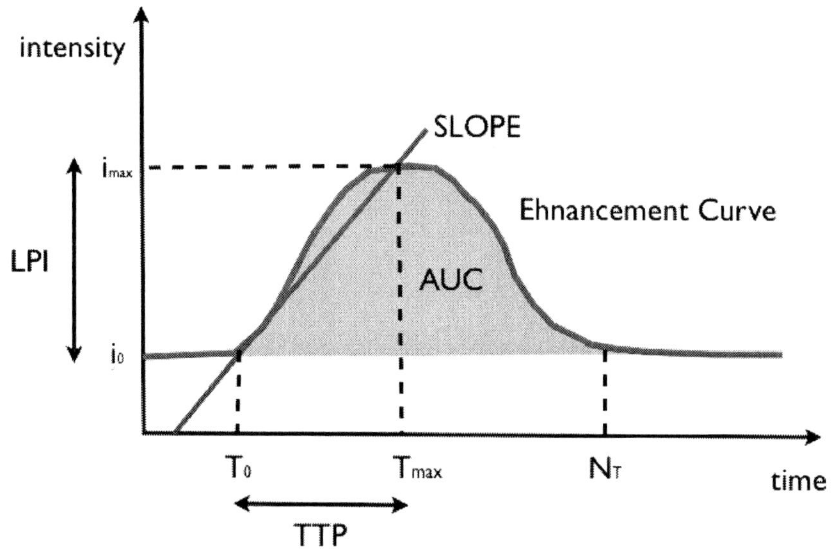

- **Area under curve (AUC):** Represents the area under the CE Curve; it measures the quantity of CA absorbed by the region investigated, hence it yields an estimation of blood flow that diffuses into the region:

$$AUC(A) = \sum_{k=1}^{M}\left\{(T_k - T_{k-1})\frac{1}{N}\sum_{(x,y)\in A}\left[i(T_k,x,y)-i_0(x,y)\right]\right\} \quad (2)$$

all the quantities are referred, for generality purpose, to the sub-ROI A that includes N pixel, and with respect to a time sequence composed by M frames, not necessarily timely equispaced.

- **Local peak intensity (LPI):** Is the maximum increment of the intensity with respect to the baseline intensity i_0 (the pure tissue answer without any CA response). The intensity variation depends exclusively on the local presence of CA, hence this quantity gives an estimation of the maximal quantity of blood that, at a given time instant, comes to the region:

$$LPI(A) = \max_{k} \max_{(x,y)\in A} \left[i(T_k,x,y)-i_0(x,y)\right] \quad (3)$$

where the max operator is evaluated with respect to all the frames into the sequence and for all pixels inside the sub-ROI.

- **Time to peak (TTP):** It is the time when the intensity reaches its maximum value. It gives an indication about whether this region is directly supplied with blood or through revascularization:

Figure 4. AUC (Area Under Curve) colour map with the corresponding values; Enhancement Curve of whole ROI, in the upper figure; Enhancement Curve of the select portion of M-SM layer (green) and Ms-M layer (red), in the lower figure.

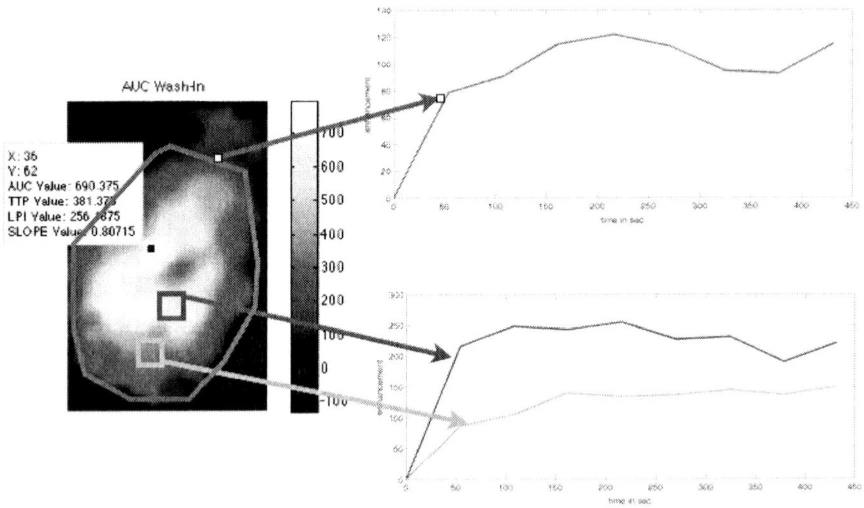

$$TTP(A) = T_k :=$$

$$\left[i\left(T_k, x, y\right) - i_0(x, y) \right] \equiv LPI(A) \quad (4)$$

some authors suggest the use of *T90* quantities, which is the time taken to reach 90% of the maximum enhancement value instead of TTP.

- **Average Rising (SLOPE):** It is a measurement of the slope of the curve between the started rising point and the peak; it is related to the average blood flow perfusion to the tissues and joins temporal and intensity aspects into a single parameter:

$$SLOPE(A) = \frac{LPI(A)}{TTP(A)} \quad (5)$$

These parameters are generally represented via specific colour maps, in order to provide an immediate overview of the ROI as illustrated in Figure 4 where we report the AUC, and the related parameters, associated with a bowel wall affected by Crohn's inflammation.

Some software tools, as DyCoH (Russo, Setola et al. 2007), allow the user to inspect quickly the different colour maps associated with the parameters (2) – (5) to read the values assumed in each specific location in order to identify the most relevant areas and to compare the CE in different sub-ROI (Figure 4).

Pharmacokinetic Model Analysis

DCE studies produce time series images that enable pixel-by-pixel analysis of contrast kinetic within a disease. These time-signal curves can be analysed with descriptive "heuristic" such as initial slope, time to peak, or rate of wash-out. These methods are valuable and easy to apply; however, they provide no insight into the underlying physiology. Moreover, they are highly dependent on the imaging protocol and scanner. Pharmacokinetic (PK) models instead provide a means of summarizing contrast enhancement data in terms of parameters directly related with underlying vascular anatomy and physiology (Choyke et al., 2003). The use of PK models leads to the derivation of those parameters which are independent of the scanning acquisition protocol or any features associated with it. Each of the PK analysis approaches uses curve fitting techniques to characterize the Arterial Input Factor (AIF) and tissue contrast concentration curve.

Commonly used PK models assume that the CA resides and exchanges between two compartments in the disease: the vascular space and the ESS. CA reaches the lesion through the vascular space by perfusion and diffuses between the vascular space and the EES; the rate of diffusion from the vascular space to the EES determined by the concentration in plasma and EES, and the permeability of the capillary-EES interface. As clarified by Tofts el al. (1999) and by Srikanchana et al. (2004) the essential features of a variety of models are covered by the Generalized Kinetic Model (GKM). Other modelling approaches are designed to separate the contribution of blood volume, flow and permeability to signal changes seen during DCE. These approaches may well represent the future of this but are currently too demanding in terms of imaging speed, image reproducibility and over all time consuming for routine clinical use. The Brix model (Srikanchana et al. 2004), which will be described in the follow, is one of several models that deal with the situation in which the arterial concentration is not directly assessed.

General Kinetic Model

The physiological processes of GKM are described in Figure 5, where the GKM simplifies the anatomy into two functional components, the vascular space and the EES. A CA, when introduced into the vascular space, will leak into the EES at a characteristic rate and then will leak back into

Figure 5. Block diagram of the general kinetic model (GMK)

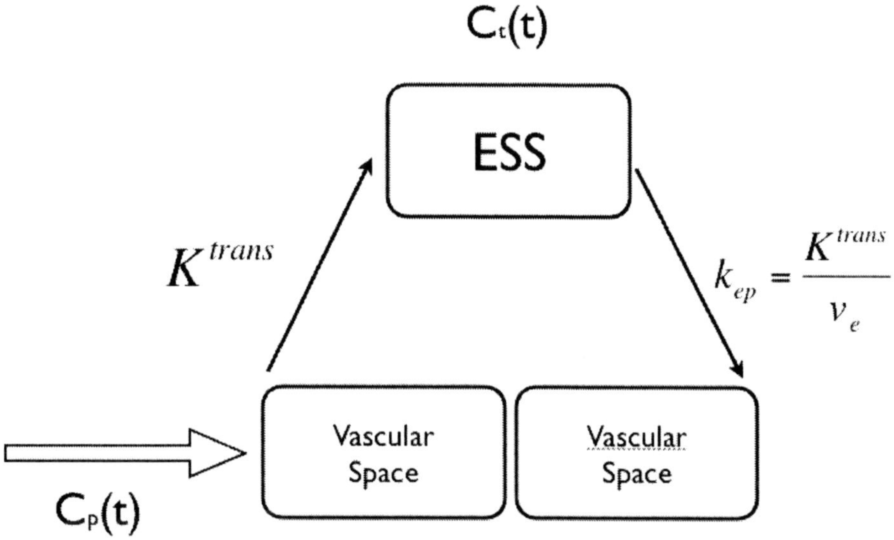

the vessel at another rate. Thus the net change in concentration can be described as:

$$\frac{dC_t}{dt} = K^{trans}\left(C_p - \frac{C_t}{v_e}\right) \quad (6)$$

where v_e is the ESS fractional volume index and K^{trans} is the transfer constant related to "wash in". Moreover the transfer constant k_{ep}, defined as:

$$k_{ep} = \frac{K^{trans}}{v_e} \quad (7)$$

characterizes the "wash-out" dynamic of CA from the tissue. C_p is the concentration of CA in the blood plasma, while C_t is the concentration of CA in the tissue under investigation (i.e., tumour or inflammatory tissue). Hence, the concentration of CA within the tumour or inflammatory tissue is determined by the blood plasma concentration curve and the two parameters K^{trans} and v_e (Choyke et al., 2003). Furthermore, these parameters can be numerically evaluate on the base of a variable concentration input function. Solving the above is convolution integral:

$$C_t(t) = K^{trans}\left[C_p(t) \otimes e^{k_{ep}t}\right] \quad (8)$$

To evaluate K^{trans} and k_{ep} a numerical solution for the GKM via a non-linear fitting algorithm is allowed. The constant k_{ep} is formally the flux rate constant between the ESS and blood plasma and can be derived from the shape of the CA with respect to the volume, whereas the transfer constant and the ESS require absolute values of CA concentration (Choyke et al., 2003).

On the basis of data of dynamic MRI - CE (Choyke et al., 2003), show that K^{trans} controls the height of the C_t curve, while $k_{ep}=K^{trans}/v_e$ determines the shape of the curve: smaller k_{ep}, more delayed the enhancement. K^{trans} is a function of flow (perfusion) and permeability; larger the flow and the permeability, larger is K^{trans} (Choyke et al., 2003). The transfer constant K^{trans}, formally called "volume transfer constant", has several physiologic interpretations, depending on the balance between capillary permeability and blood flow in the tissue of interest. In high permeability situations (as in the Kety Model, see below) the transfer constant equals the blood plasma flow per unit volume tissue (see Eq. 10); in the opposite case of low permeability (PS-Limited Model, see below) the transfer constant corresponds to the product of blood vessel permeability and the corresponding surface area in the unit volume of tissue (see Eq. 12).

Several authors have proposed different specification of K^{trans} (Tofts et al., 1999) in order to emphasize some specific agents and to improve parameters set up.

One of these is the *Flow-Limited Model (High Permeability)* provided by Kety (Tofts et al., 1999; Choyke et al., 2003). This model is based on two assumptions: first, the arterial and venous blood have well-defined concentrations, supplying and draining the tissue under study. Second, permeability is high, venous blood leaves the tissue with a CA concentration that is all times in equilibrium with the tissue itself. Thus, soon after injection of the CA, the arterial concentration is high and the venous concentration is low, then the most of the CA is being removed from the blood as it passes through the tissue. For an extracellular tracer, the Kety model can be extended by setting the venous concentration equal to that of the ESS. In this case the following differential equation relates tissue concentration C_t to arterial plasma concentration C_p:

$$\frac{dC_t}{dt} = F\rho\left(1 - Hct\right)\left(C_p - \frac{C_t}{v_e}\right) \quad (9)$$

with K^{trans} given by:

$$K^{trans} = F\rho\left(1 - Hct\right) \quad (10)$$

where F is the perfusion (or flow) of whole blood per volume unit, ρ is the density of tissue and Hct is the Hematocrit.

A different model is the *PS-Limited Model (Low Permeability)* (Tofts et al., 1999; Choyke et al., 2003). This model assumes that there is a high flow, hence the blood plasma can be considered as a single pool, with equal arterial and venous concentration. The transport of CA out of the vasculature is slow enough to deplete the intravascular concentration. The rate of uptake is determined by the permeability surface area product of the capillary wall and the concentration difference between the blood plasma and the ESS. If the contribution of the tracer in the intravascular space is ignored the transport equation is:

$$\frac{dC_t}{dt} = PS\rho\left(C_p - \frac{C_t}{v_e}\right) K^{trans} = PS\rho \quad (11)$$

with K^{trans} given by:

$$K^{trans} = PS\rho \quad (12)$$

where PS is the permeability surface area product per unit of volume.

The previous two models can be integrated into the *Mixed Flow and PS-Limited Model* (Tofts et al., 1999; Choyke et al., 2003). This model assumes that the CA uptake may be limited by both blood flow and permeability. In this case the transport equation is:

$$\frac{dC_t}{dt} = EF\rho\left(1 - Hct\right)\left(C_p - \frac{C_t}{v_e}\right) \quad (13)$$

where E, the *extraction ratio,* is the fractional reduction in capillary blood concentration as it passes through the tissue

$$E = \frac{C_a - C_t}{C_a} \quad (14)$$

Immediately after CA injection, when there is no back flow from ESS to blood plasma, E is a constant and it can be considered as an appropriate index to characterize the specific tissue and CA. Notice that, after a while, as the tissue concentration grows up after injection, backflow increases and the extraction ratio decreases, inducing a variation of E that becomes a time varying function.

Brix Model

The Brix model (Brix et al., 1999; Srikanchana et al., 2004) is also a two compartment model in which the AIF is assumed to be the result of a prolonged constant infusion that takes the shape of square wave, i.e. the CA instantly reaches a plateau, remains constant for a while and then instantly is over. The input function K_{in}, the elimination constant k_{el}, and the rate constants K_{12} and K_{21} describe the transfer of CA respectively to and from the peripheral compartment. Figure 6, shows the block diagram of a Brix model. The mathematical expression of the temporal response of $C_t(t)$ is:

$$C_t(t) = 1 + A\left[v\left(e^{k_{el}t'} - 1\right)e^{k_{el}t} - u\left(e^{k_{21}t'} - 1\right)e^{k_{21}t}\right] \quad (15)$$

where A is a fitting parameter depending on the properties of the tissue, on the type of sequence and on the infusion rate (K_{in}).

Brix noted that the Tofts approximation (see below) yields good results only in the brain, but it was not able to fit the kinetic of other organs. Hence Brix proposed a more complete mathematical description, including a term referring to an adjustable AIF parameter, in order to realize a larger accordance with clinical data.

Tofts Model

The Tofts model takes a different approach with respect to the arterial input function (AIF), but retains the fundamental assumptions of the GKM (Tofts and Kermode, 1991; Tofts et al. 1999). Whereas all the previous models were based on two exponential function (that reflecs the behaviour of the two compartmental model), Tofts developed a new model based on three exponential function. In this model the input function is assumed to be the result of a pulse bolus injected into a two compartment system. This system of compartments modifies the pulse bolus into a bi-exponential arterial input function. This was then used in the solution of the GKM leading to three exponential solutions as:

$$C(t) = D\left[b_1 e^{(-m_1 t)} + b_2 e^{(-m_2 t)} + b_3 e^{(-m_3 t)}\right] \quad (16)$$

where $m_3 = k/v_p$, $b_1 = ka_1/(m_3 - m_1)$, $b_2 = ka_2/(m_3 - m_2)$, $b_3 = -(b_1 + b_2)$, and a_1, a_2, m_1, m_2 have been determined empirically from plasma curve. Notice that, the exponential parameters are usually

Figure 6. Block diagram of Brix model

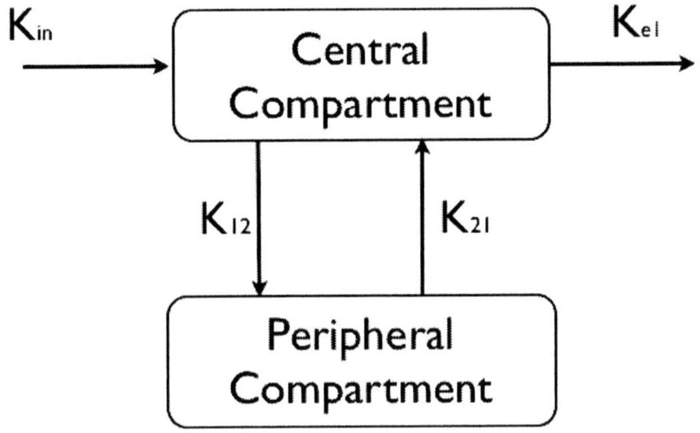

Figure 7. Block diagram of Tofts model

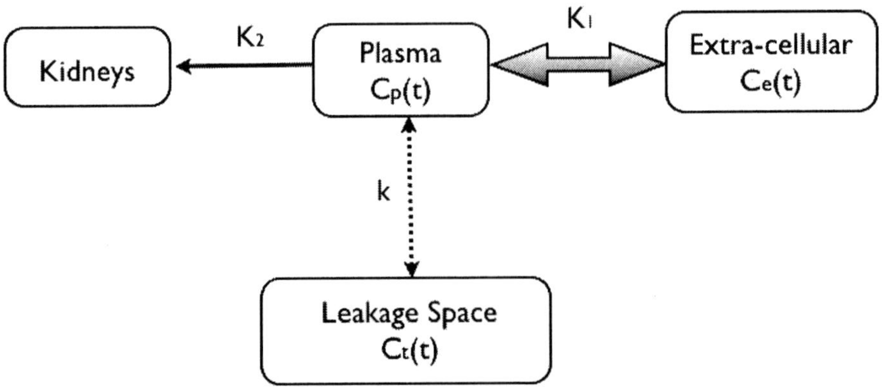

estimated from other "pooled" measurements of the AIF, so it is not measured each time.

Empirical Model

A DCE image sequence is typically composed by a small number of images, generally six to ten, spaced a minute or more apart. Hence, the time evolution of each pixel can be extremely affected by noise, thus making ambitious to attempt to fit a multi-exponential model, especially with a wide number of parameters.

Indeed, it can be shown that the error in the fit, *Err*, is given by:

$$Err = \sqrt{\sum_{i=1}^{M} \frac{C_i^2 - c_i^2}{M - P}} \tag{17}$$

where M is the number of time points, P is the number of free parameters in the model, C_i is the concentration of CA, and c_i is the model estimate of the concentration of CA. Consequently for a fixed number of parameters, the fewer the number of data points, the larger the error. In practice, it is not possible to increase the number of time points without sacrificing spatial resolution, or reducing the field of view to a part of the volume.

On the other hand, it is possible to lower the error by reducing the number of parameters. For instance, one tries to measure a parameter experimentally, rather than to try estimate it. On the other way, this method introduces measurement errors into the model.

A different solution is to adopt a black-box modelling approach. In this framework we assume a general model without any specific physical meaning and try to estimate those parameters that better fit the empirical data. In this way we can largely reduce the number of free parameters to be evaluated through fit, but unfortunately we lost large part of the physical meaning of them.

Then instead of derive the model from PK equations, it is chosen empirically to seek a parsimonious fit to the time series data. This can be obtained considering a voxel-wise tissue signal intensity over time of the form:

$$f(t) = a \cdot t \cdot e^{-\frac{t^c}{b}} \tag{18}$$

where t is the elapsed time since the injection of the CA; and a, b and c are positive real adjustable parameters. Hence, this model, requiring only three parameters, is more robust with respect to experimental errors and pre-measurement of physiological properties, because (i) it does not rely on measured parameters or constants relating to the type or density of the tissue, and (ii) it does not assume any particular relationship between the observed change in signal intensity and the concentration of contrast agent. The model is defined in terms of just one exponential function and the range of its parameters can be restricted to a relatively narrow set of values. To perform data fitting thorugh this model, a nonlinear fitting algorithm is needed. The minimization problem, in the least squares sense, is not a convex one and thus a global best fit is not guaranteed. It has been experienced that the estimated values for the model parameters lie within a relatively narrow range: e.g. Gal et al. (2007) based on clinical data sets observed that a∈(0,200), b∈(0,100) and c∈(0,3).

FUTURE TRENDS

Even though DCE is still a research field, there is a growing interest in its use in clinical applications. This is largely due to its non-invasive nature, supporting diagnoses with (relatively) easy, fast and patient comfortable tests. This interest is also witnessed by the increase of literature dealing with this topic, and, moreover, by the introduction in the market of new generation top-class US, CT and MR machine specific software tools.

Substantially, DCE studies produce time series images that enable pixel-by-pixel analysis of contrast agent kinetic within a lesion. These time-signal curve can be analysed with descriptive "heuristic" parameters, such as initial slope, time to peak, or rate of wash-out. These methods are valuable and easy to apply; however, they provide no insight into the underlying physiology and they are highly dependent on the imaging protocol and scanner. To overcome these limits, Pharmacokinetic (PK) models were developed, in order to interpret contrast enhancement data in terms of parameters directly related to vascular anatomy and physiology; with this final aim, several models are under development. They differ for the assumptions done on flow rate of the plasma and permeability characteristics of blood vessels. Moreover, the most sophisticated model are moving from one compartmental model to model with two or multiple compartments, in order to take into account more complex phenomena.

Unfortunately, because DCE sequences are typically composed by few images, the fitting of experimental data is an hard task, especially in the presence of a large number of parameters. Then, some authors have proposed empirical models, which can be considered as a trade-off between the computational simplicity of the heuristic approach and the powerful synthesis of the PK one. The major disadvantage of this empirical approach is that the extracted parameters lack of any physical meaning.

Apart from the studies about the most suitable way to extract relevant information from DCE sequences, there is the need to improve registration procedures and to make the tools more user-friendly, with the final goal of developing decision systems to support physicians in the categorization, classification and diagnose of the different lesions.

CONCLUSION

In this paper we have illustrated the basic principles and the most innovative approaches developed within the Dynamic Contrast Enhancement (DCE) framework. DCE is an interesting methodology able to exploit the improvement in bio-medical imaging processing to support no-invasive diagnoses. It is based on the assumption that vascularisation in pathological tissues is largely different from that in the healthy ones, and peculiar for the specific type of pathology. Hence a contrast agent (CA) can be used to emphasise the vascularisation bed associated with the different pathologic tissue, thus resulting in a useful diagnostic tool.

Notice that in the DCE approach the diagnostic information is strictly related with the time-dynamic of the CA perfusion. This imposes to focus on an image temporal sequence referring to a given anatomic region; generally DCE is performed on a sequence of 6 to 10 images, collected in an overall elapsed time interval ranging from 30 seconds to some minutes. Unfortunately, moving from the analysis of a single image to that of a sequence, there is an exponential increase of raw data to be consider; the quantity of information become so huge to exceed the human capability. In this contest, it appears mandatory to develop a suitable Computer Aid Diagnoses (CAD), supporting the evaluation of the most relevant aspects and information contained within biomedical images.

ACKNOWLEDGMENT

The authors would thank for their capital contribution and support Dr. Riccardo Del Vescovo, Dr. Luisa Di Paola, Dr. Francesco Rosario Grasso, and Prof. Bruno Beomonte Zobel.

REFERENCES

Brix, G., M. Bahner, L., Hoffmann, U., Horvath, A., & Schreiber, W. (1999). Regional Blood Flow, Capillary Permeability and Compartmental Volumes: Measurement with Dynamic CT-Initial Experience. *Radiology, 210*, 269.276.

Choyke, P. L., Dewer, A. J., & Knopp, M. V. (2003). Functional Tumor Imaging with Dynamic Constrast-Enhanced Magnetic Resonance Imaging. *Journal of Magnetic Resonance Imaging, 17*, 509-520.

Dhillon, S., & Gill, K. (November 2005). *Clinical Pharmacokinetic. Textbook.*

Florie, J., Wasser, M. N. J. M., Arts-Cieslik, K., Akkerman, E. K., Siersema, P. D., & Stoker J. (May 2006). Dynamic Contrast Enhanced MRI of the bowel wall for assessment of disease activity in Crohn's disease. *American Journal of Roentgenology, 186*, 1384-1392.

Gal, Y., Mehnert, A., Bradley, A., McMahon, K., & Croizer, S. (2007). An evaluation of four parametric models od contrast enhancement for dynamic magnetic resonance imaging of the breast. *29th Annual International Conference of the IEEE Engineering in Medicine and Biology Society.*

Horsfield, M. A., & Morgan, B. M. A. (2004). Algorithms for Calculation of Kinetic Parameters From T1-Weighted Dynamic Contrast-Enhanced Magnetic Resonance Imaging. *Journal of Magnetic Resonance Imaging, 20*, 723-729.

Jackson, A. (April, 2003). Quantitative characterization of tumor micro vasculature using dynamic contrast enhanced MRI. *Medica Mundi 47/1.*

Jackson, A. (2004). Analysis of Dynamic Contrast Enhanced MRI. *British Journal of Radiology,* 77(suppl 2), 5154-5166.

Kier, C., Toth, D., Meyer-Wiethe, K., Schindler, A., Cangür, H., Seidel, G., & Aach, T. (February 2005). *Cerebral perfusion imaging with bolus harmonic imaging.*

Marret, H., Sauget, S., Giraudeau, B., Brewer, M., Ranger-Moore, J., Body, G., & Tranquart, F. (2004). Contrast-Enhanced Sonography helps in discrimination of benign from malignant adnexal masses. *J Ultrasound Med.*

Metzler, V., Seidel, G., Wiesmann, M., Meyer-Wiethe, K., & Aach, T. (2004). *Perfusion Harmonic Imaging of the Human Brain.*

Padhani, A. R., & Husband, J. E. (2001). Dynamic Contrast-Enhanced MRI Studies in oncology with an emphasis on quantification, validation and human studies. *Clinical Radiology, 56,* 607-620.

Patlak, C., Blasberg, R., & Fenstermacher, J. (1983). Grafical evaluation of blood flow-to-brain Barrier transfer constant form multiple time uptake data. *J.Cereb. Blood Flow Metab, 3,* 1-7.

Russo, V., Setola, R., Del Vescovo, R., Grasso, R. F., & Zobel, B. B. (2007). DyCoH: an innovative tool to Dynamic Contrast Enhancement analysis. *29th Annual International Conference of the IEEE Engineering in Medicine and Biology Society.*

Srikanchana, R., Thomasson, D., Choyke, P., & Dwyer, A. (2004). A Comparison of Pharmacokinetic Models of Dynamic Contrast Enhanced MRI. *17th IEEE Symposium on Computer-Based Medical System.*

Tofts, P. S., Brix, G., Buckley, D. L., Evelhoch, J. L., Henderson, E., Knopp, M. V, Larsson, H. B. W., Lee, T-Y., Mayer, A. A., Parker, G. J. M., Port, R. E., Taylor, J., & Wiesskoff, R. M. (1999). Estimating Kinetic Parameters From Dynamic Contrast Enhanced T1-Weighted MRI of a Diffusable Tracer: Standardized Quantities and Symbols. *Journal of Magnetic Resonance Imaging, 10*, 223-232.

Tofts, P. S., & Kermode, A. G., (1991). Measurement of Blood-Brain Barrier Permeability and Leakage Space using Dynamic MR Imaging. Fundamental concepts. *Magnetic Resonance in Medicine, 17*, 357-367.

KEY TERMS

Arterial Input Factor (AIF): Is the Input Function and it measures the Plasma Contrast Concentration (of a Contrast Agent)

Area Under Curve (AUC): Represents the area under the CE Curve; it measures the quantity of CA absorbed by the tissue, hence it yields an estimation of blood flow that diffuses into the specific region

Contrast Agent (CA): Contrast Media perfuses into the tissue

Contrast Enhancement (CE): Tissue Contrast Concentration: the shape of an Enhancement Curve reflects blood flow, vascular volume, extravascular volume and vessel permeability

Dynamic Contrast Enhancement (DCE): The perfusion's dynamic of specific Contrast Agent insight the tissues;

Extravascular Extracelllar Space (EES): Interstitial space (around vessels)

Transfer Constant (K^{trans}): Formally called volume transfer constant is the transfer constant related to "wash in" of the CA into the tissue

Transfer Constant (k_{ep}): Is the transfer constant related with the "wash-out" of the CA from the tissue; formally is the flux rate constant between the ESS and blood plasma and can be derived from the shape of the tracer concentration vs volume data

Pharmacokinetics (PK): It is referred to the evalutation of chemical compounds distribution in body over time.

General Kinetic Model (GKM): Is the basic model often used to simplifies the human anatomy into two functional components (two compartments).

Chapter XXVI
Automatic Correspondence Methods towards Point-Based Medical Image Registration:
An Evaluation Study

George K. Matsopoulos
National Technical University of Athens, Greece

ABSTRACT

The accurate estimation of point correspondences is often required in a wide variety of medical image processing applications including image registration. Numerous point correspondence methods have been proposed, each exhibiting its own characteristics, strengths and weaknesses. This chapter presents a comparative study of four automatic point correspondence methods. The four featured methods are the Automatic Extraction of Corresponding Points approach, the Trimmed Iterated Closest Points scheme, the Correspondence by Sensitivity to Movement technique and the Self-Organizing Maps network. All methods are presented, mainly focusing on their distinct characteristics. An extensive set of dental images, subject to unknown transformations, was employed for the qualitative and quantitative evaluation of the four methods, which was performed in terms of registration accuracy. After assessing all methods, it was deduced that the Self-Organizing Maps approach outperformed in most cases the other three methods in comparison.

INTRODUCTION

In this chapter, a comprehensive evaluative study of various automatic correspondence methods is presented towards point-based two-dimensional (2D) medical image registration. Four methods for automatic correspondence have been selected after literature search. Analytically, the Automatic Extraction of Corresponding Points technique (Likar & Pernus, 1999), which is a modification of the template matching technique (referred over 17x), the Trimmed Iterative Closest Point algorithm (Chetverikov, Svirko & Stepanov, 2002), which is a modification of the Iterative Closest Point algorithm (the ICP algorithm is referred over 1650x), the Correspondence by Sensitivity to Movement approach (Guest, Berry, Baldock, Fidrich & Smith, 2001), as a improvement of the template matching technique (referred over 24x) and a Self Organizing Maps network (Matsopoulos, Asvestas, Mouravliansky & Delibasis, 2004), developed by the authors (referred over 5x) are initially reviewed and their performance is compared both qualitatively and quantitatively. In the evaluation process, all presented methods are applied to dental image pairs subject to unknown transformations. Hence no a priori knowledge of actual correspondences could be assumed and therefore the performance of the four featured point correspondence methods was evaluated both visually and quantitatively in terms of registration quality, using the Root Mean Square Difference.

BACKGROUND

There are numerous applications in medical imaging where geometrical registration is performed including the alignment of data between two modalities with anatomical information (CT-CT or CT-MRI), between anatomical atlases and dynamic studies (CT-PET, CT-SPECT, MRI-PET) or between images of the same modality acquired at different times (Maintz & Viergever, 1998).

Several image features may be exploited for the matching process, depending on the modalities used, the specific application and the implementation of the transformation utilized. There are numerous comprehensive surveys of medical image registration (Hajnal, Hill & Hawkes, 2001; Zitova & Flusser 2003), in terms of imaging modalities and employed techniques. The medical image registration methods can be classified into two main categories: image similarity-based methods and point-based methods. In image similarity-based methods, the registration of different images involves the optimization of a quantity measuring the similarity between the images, under constraints imposed by the preferred transformation model (Johnson & Christensen, 2003; Pluim, Maintz & Viergever, 2003). On the other hand, in point-based methods, registration involves the determination of the coordinates of corresponding features/points in different images such as landmark points, ridges or surfaces, and the estimation of a geometrical transformation using these corresponding features (Bookstein, 1997; Pitiot, Thompson & Toga, 2002; Pizer, Fritsch, Yushkevich, Johnson & Chaney, 1996). The corresponding features can be determined either manually or automatically.

In the literature, numerous automatic correspondence methods have been devised (Cao, Pan, Li, Balachandran, Fitzpatrick, Chapman & Dawant, 2004; Chetverikov, Svirko & Stepanov, 2002). According to the general methodology, a correspondence method incorporates two main steps; namely, detection and matching. The detection step aims at extracting salient anatomical points of the visible anatomy and/or geometrical interest points located at the locus of the optimum of some geometric property, such as L-shaped corners, T-shaped junctions and Y-shaped junctions (Laliberte, Gagnon & Sheng, 2003; Likar & Pernus, 1999). After the detection of these interest points, the correspondence between them can be established by the matching step.

DATA ACQUISITION

The four correspondence methods featured in this chapter were evaluated on 96 dental image pairs, subject to unknown transformations. The following semi-controlled geometry protocol was employed: a dry mandible was mounted on a device which permitted the object and the film to be rotated vertically and horizontally relative to the central part of the X-ray beam. The focus of the object and the object-to-film distance were kept constant at 40 cm and 0.5 cm, respectively. The radiographs were digitized with a flatscanner (Agfa Arcus II) producing 8-bit gray scale image files. The reference radiograph was taken with the central ray of the X-ray beam perpendicular to the long axes of the teeth as judged subjectively and with no resulting overlaps of adjacent tooth surfaces. Corresponding images were then obtained by moving the object either vertically or horizontally relative to the X-ray beam at 0°, 3° and 6°, respectively. This corresponds to motion about the x- and y- axis in three-dimensional space. Four dry mandibles were used in order to produce a total of 96 *in vitro* dental pairs grouped into four sets of 24 image pairs each (Sets I-IV). In each set, the same acquisition parameters were kept; thus brightness and/or contrast correction was not priory required. Furthermore, the acquired images, however, included white background representing regions outside the film limits and had to be preprocessed by suitably cropping them; thus excluding the undesired parts. The size of the cropped *in vitro* radiographs used in the study was 428×310 pixels.

METHODOLOGY

In general, all point correspondence methods are based on the same principal: Given a pair of 2D images (reference image and corresponding image) of the same anatomical scene and a set of interest points (control points) in the reference image, I_R, the automatic correspondence algorithm detects a set of homologous points (corresponding points) in the corresponding image, I_C. The homologous points may be drawn from a predefined pool of candidate points or simply estimated from scratch. Once the corresponding points are detected, they are utilized together with their respective control points to define a global transformation, which in turn is used to register the corresponding images. In our case the control points were extracted using the general purpose method adopted by Likar et al. (1999) for obtaining points around edges and ridges on dental images. The rest of this section is concerned with presenting the methodology adopted in order to evaluate the four point correspondence methods featured in this chapter. Moreover, a brief description of each method is presented, focusing on the distinct characteristics of each scheme.

The Automatic Extraction of Corresponding Points Method

The Automatic Extraction of Corresponding Points (AECP) method employs a template matching scheme to obtain correspondences (Di Stefano, Mattocia & Tombari, 2004). In order to determine the correspondence of a point (x, y), a circular area of radius r from the reference image is propagated over a circular area of radius R from the corresponding image, which is centered at (x, y). As the template circulates over the designated area of the corresponding image, the differences between the template and the area underneath are recorded. Therefore, for each pixel (x, y) of the reference image, its neighborhood of radius r is compared to the equally sized neighborhood of each pixel lying on a radius R around (x, y) on the corresponding image. This means that the digital circle of radius r around (x, y) is compared to all digital circles of radius r centered at $(x+k, y+l)$ on the corresponding image with $k^2 + l^2 < R^2$. In order to compare the neighborhoods in question, the mean absolute difference of intensities is used as a similarity measure (Likar & Pernus, 1999). Thus, for each pixel of the reference image and for $k^2 + l^2 < R^2$:

$$Sim((x,y),(x+k,y+l)) = \frac{1}{N} \sum_{\substack{\forall i,j \\ i^2+j^2<r^2}} \left| I_R(x+i,y+j) - I_C(x+k+i,y+l+j) \right| \quad (1)$$

where N is the number of pixels in the neighborhood of radius r.

The area which gives an average intensity value that minimizes Equation (1) is assumed to be the neighborhood of the corresponding point. Hence, the center of that area is considered to be the corresponding point of (x, y) in the corresponding image. This particular technique prerequisites that $R \geq r$. In fact, for small R values, the search area is reduced and hence the likelihood of an erroneous corresponding point is increased. On the other hand, if R is very large, the search area is broadened, increasing the computational cost. In this study, the values $R = 25$ and $r = 5$ were used. The effect of varying the two radii is discussed later.

The Trimmed Iterative Closest Point Algorithm

The Iterated Closest Point (ICP) algorithm (Besl & McKay, 1992) is broadly used for allocating corresponding points, due to its robustness, simplicity and fast execution time. Numerous variants of the ICP have been devised over the years. We are particularly interested in the Trimmed Iterated Closest Point (TICP) algorithm variant (Chetverikov, Svirko & Stepanov, 2002), which has the capability to maximize the efficiency of the original ICP scheme. TICP requires the extraction of a suitable pool of candidate points from the corresponding image as well as the definition of control points on the reference image. Those two point sets are utilized by TICP as the scheme tries to minimize the average distance between the two sets by finding the closest point from the reference set to the corresponding set, in an iterative manner.

The innovation of this approach lies with the fact that it only considers a predefined number of points that have the minimum distances, instead of working with the entire sets. The parameters of the point transformations are calculated over a minimal set of points, thus increasing the robustness of the algorithm. In our case the similitude transformation was adopted to estimate the corresponding points and the average Euclidean distance between the point sets was considered as our measure of match. Moreover, the number of points extracted from the corresponding image may differ from that of the reference image. This asymmetry widens the search area for the correspondences and hence lessens the possibility of finding spurious corresponding points. The TICP algorithm eventually converges to an optimal set of corresponding points, provided that proper points of interest were selected on both the reference and the corresponding image.

The Correspondence by Sensitivity to Movement Technique

The Correspondence by Sensitivity to Movement (CSM) algorithm is an advanced variant of the Template Matching scheme for allocating point correspondences. As with AECP, Template Matching estimates corresponding points by matching a region from the reference image to a region from the corresponding image (one-to-one match) and hence a unique correspondence is calculated per control point. On the other hand, CSM considers several candidate corresponding points for each control point, using a weighting scheme (Guest, Berry, Baldock, Fidrich, Smith & 2001).

The algorithm comprises of three distinct stages. Firstly, a number of candidate corresponding points, called "tentative points", are calculated for each control point. The tentative points are bound to a specific region on the corresponding image. A similarity measure is then calculated for each tentative point. In our case a simple correlation scheme was employed to realize those similarity measures. The tentative points together with their similarity measures form the match-map. During the second stage of the algorithm the control points on the reference image are slightly displaced towards all directions and a new match-map is estimated in each case. Each new tentative point is calculated by summing over the match-map, while taking distances from the control point to each point in the match-map into account. Tentative corresponding points $\underline{q_i}$ are calculated using Equation (2) shown below.

$$\underline{q_i} = \frac{\sum K_i \underline{x_i}}{\sum K_i} \qquad (2)$$

where $\underline{x_i}$ is the vector from the control point to point i in the match-map. K_i is a constant defined by $K_i = \frac{m_i}{1+\left|\underline{x_i}\right|^2}$, where m_i is the similarity value for point i. The sums involved in Equation (2) are calculated over the entire match-map. Using Equation (2), a cloud of tentative corresponding points is estimated for each minor movement of a control point. The final stage of CSM involves analyzing the distribution of those tentative points for each control point. If the tentative points are scattered along a line, the point closest to the line is considered as the corresponding point, otherwise the centroid of the scatter is selected.

In effect, the particular approach calculates several candidate corresponding points and then selects the optimal point by running a simple reliability test. By moving each control point over a specified area of the reference image, several scattered candidate points are estimated. In general, if those points are scattered over a relatively small area on the corresponding image, the candidate points are considered to be reliable. On the contrary, wildly scattered candidate points indicate an erroneous estimation process or an unreliable control point.

The Self-Organizing Maps Network

The Self Organizing Maps (SOMs) is a neural network algorithm, which is able to train itself in an unsupervised manner, through an iterative process (Matsopoulos, Asvestas, Mouravliansky & Delibasis, 2004). The SOMs model was introduced by Kohonen (1990) and comprises of a layer of m neurons arranged in a one-dimensional or two-dimensional grid. In our case, a neuron j *is* placed at each control point $\mathbf{P}_j$ from the reference image. A weight vector $\mathbf{w}_j$, which holds the parameters of a local transformation, is then associated with each neuron. The local transformation preferred in this study is a typical similitude transformation, involving a rotation, a scaling and two translation parameters. The network is firstly initialized by setting the weight vector $\mathbf{w}_j$ of every neuron j to the parameters of the identity similitude transformation. After the network is properly initialized the training iterations begin. At each iteration n, a random signal $\mathbf{s}(n)$, is generated and presented to the network. The random signal generator is similar to the one used in simulated annealing (Matsopoulos, Asvestas, Mouravliansky & Delibasis, 2004). The components of the random signal are random numbers within a predefined range and correspond to the parameters of a local similitude transformation. The generated random signal is then applied to all network neurons. The neuron j with weight vector $\mathbf{w}_j$ is declared as the winning neuron, according to the rule below:

$$j = \arg\max_i \left\{ MoM\left(\mu_{A_i}\left(I_R\right) \mu_{T_{\mathbf{s}(\mathbf{n})}(A_i)}\left(I_C\right) \right) \right\} \qquad (3)$$

where A_i is a square region centered around $\mathbf{P}_i$, $T_{s(n)}(A_i)$ is a geometric transformation of the region A_i with parameter vector $\mathbf{s}(n)$, $\mu_{A_i}(I)$ denotes the restriction of an image I to the region A_i and *MoM* is the preferred measure of match, which in our case is gradient correlation (Gonzalez & Woods, 1992).

This practically means that the wining neuron is the one that achieves the maximum measure of match subsequent to the application of signal **s**(n). After the winning neuron j is found, the neuron itself as well as its neighboring neurons i have their weight vectors modified according to the following equation:

$$\mathbf{w}_i(n+1) = \mathbf{w}_i(n) + h_{ij}(n)\left[s(n) - \mathbf{w}_i(n)\right] \quad (4)$$

where h_{ij} is a Gaussian type function which depends on the distance between the winning neuron and its neighboring neurons and n. At this point, a single iteration is complete; hence a new random signal is presented to the network and the process described above is repeated. The training of the network terminates after a fixed number of iterations is reached (for example n = 5,000). After the training is completed, the weight vectors of the neurons contain the optimal local transformation parameters. The control points obtained from the reference image are then transformed according to those parameters in order to produce their estimated corresponding points.

Comparison Implementation

The point correspondence methods previously described were applied on all 96 acquired medical dental image pairs. Given a reference image and an initial set of points, the four methods in comparison calculated a set of estimated homologous points on the corresponding images. Those estimated points were used to determine a global transformation towards image registration. A typical affine transformation was used for this purpose, which is defined by the following equation:

$$\begin{pmatrix} x' \\ y' \\ 1 \end{pmatrix} = \begin{pmatrix} a_1 & a_2 & dx \\ a_3 & a_4 & dy \\ 0 & 0 & 1 \end{pmatrix} \times \begin{pmatrix} x \\ y \\ 1 \end{pmatrix} \quad (5)$$

where a total of six (6) parameters are required to define the affine transformation.

Therefore, each pixel of the corresponding image with coordinates (x, y), is transformed to its new coordinates (x', y'), where $x' = a_1x + a_2y + dx$ and $y' = a_3x + a_4y + dy$. The parameters of the affine transformation were calculated using the corresponding points acquired by the four methods in comparison. For all four cases, the optimal values of the selected geometrical transformation parameters were obtained by a Least Squares approach in conjunction with Singular Value Decomposition (SVD) (Press, Teukolsky, Vetterling & Flannery, 1992). Having fully defined the transformations, in each case, they were applied on the corresponding images in order to suitably register them.

The produced registered images were utilized to qualitatively and quantitatively assess the four methods. The performance of each featured point correspondence scheme depends on a number of parameters. The optimal parameters were selected after a series of trials on several image pairs from all available sets, in order to enhance the validity of the study. Those parameters are summarized in Table 1. As can be seen in Table 1, identical parameters were used for common properties of the four methods, in order to conduct a meaningful and fair comparison. The major parameters affecting each scheme are further discussed later.

RESULTS

As mentioned, four data sets were used to qualitatively and quantitatively evaluate the four automatic point-based correspondence methods in comparison. All four sets comprise of image pairs obtained using semi-controlled geometry protocols. The performance of the four point correspondence methods was evaluated in terms of registration accuracy.

Table 1. Parameters used for the qualitative and quantitative evaluation of AECP, TICP, CSM and SOMs

Parameter	*AECP*	*TICP*	*CSM*	*SOMs*
Measure of Match	Absolute Intensity Difference	Euclidean Distance	Correlation	Gradient Correlation
Transformation	-	Similitude		
Maximum Displacement	80 pixels			
Maximum Rotation	25 degrees			
Maximum Scaling	10 %			
Stopping Number of Iterations	-	500	-	5,000
Inner Search Radius	5 pixels	-	-	-
Outer Search Radius	25 pixels	-	-	-
Match-Map Size	-	-	15×15 pixels	-

Qualitative Evaluation

The registration quality of the four methods in comparison was visually assessed by superimposing the edges of the reference image on the aligned corresponding image. The edges were detected by applying a 3×3 Sobel gradient filter (Gonzalez & Woods, 1992). An example is shown in Figure 1 featuring an image from Set III (shown in Figure 1(a)).

As can be seen in Figure 1, the registered image produced using the corresponding points estimated through the SOMs method (Figure 1(e)) is more accurate than the other three methods in comparison (Figure 1(b)-(d)). The white outline of the edges in Figure 1**Error! Reference source not found.**(e) fits the aligned corresponding image more accurately than the images obtained using AECP (Figure 1(b)), TICP (Figure 1**Error! Reference source not found.**(c)) and CSM (Figure 1(d)). This may also be verified by calculating the absolute difference of the reference image with respect to its registered counterpart. This case is illustrated in Figure 2.

The images shown there were obtained by evaluating the absolute difference between the intensity of the reference image and the intensity of the transformed corresponding image, on a pixel by pixel basis. In this case the darker the resulting difference the higher the registration quality. Yet again, SOMs (Figure 2(e)) performs better than all other three methods in comparison, in terms of registration quality. However, in both Figure 1 and Figure 2, it can be seen that although AECP (Figure 1(b) and Figure 2(b)) and CSM (Figure 1(d) and Figure 2(d)) perform generally worse than SOMs, they clearly outperform TICP (Figure 1(c) and Figure 2(c)) for the particular example.

Quantitative Evaluation

Quantitative evaluation of the four methods was performed using the Root Mean Square Difference (RMSD) between the reference and the finally aligned corresponding image (Zacharaki, Matsopoulos, Asvestas & Gröndahl, 2004). The RMSD is calculated as follows:

$$RMSD = \sqrt{\frac{\sum_{i=1}^{N}\left(I_R(\vec{r}_i) - I_{GTR}(\vec{r}_i)\right)^2}{N}} \qquad (6)$$

Figure 1. Visual Assessment of the Four Point Correspondence Methods, in Terms of Registration Accuracy. (a) Reference Dental Image Drawn From Set III. Registered Corresponding Image with the Edges of the Reference Image Superimposed for (b) AECP, (c) TICP, (d) CSM and (e) SOMs.

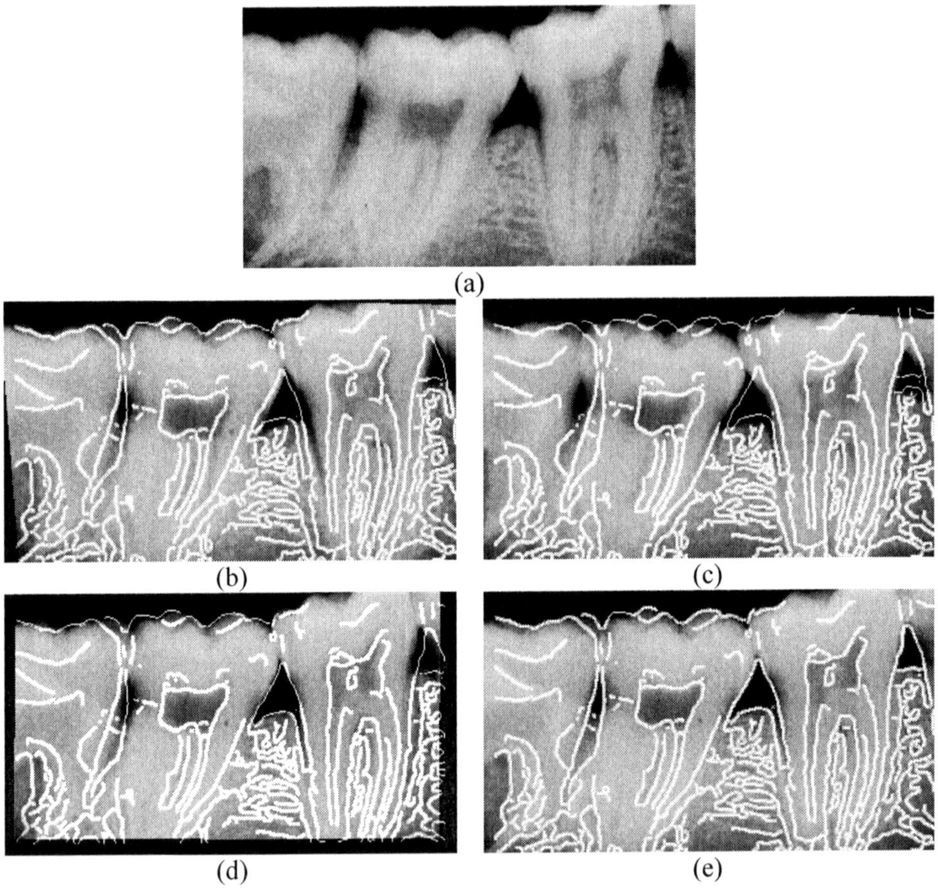

where the sum is calculated only over the N pixels belonging to the region of overlap of the reference (I_R) and the finally aligned image, using the geometrical transformation (I_{GTR}). Generally, a small value of RMSD corresponds to a small average intensity difference between homologous pixels in the reference and the registered corresponding image. This, in turn, suggests that the smaller the value of RMSD obtained, the higher the quality of the intensity-based image registration.

The results for a sample of 24 image-pairs from Set III are presented in Table 2 using the affine transform. From Table 2, it is evident that SOMs outperforms the other three methods for the vast majority of the radiographic pairs in terms of the RMSD metric. In particular, in 14 out of the 24 sample pairs, the SOMs network achieved better than all three methods in comparison. Moreover, the mean RMSD over the entire sample of 24 dental pairs is greatly improved using the SOMs algorithm (6.689) against AECP (9.561), TICP (9.563) and CSM (11.576). Finally, the robustness of SOMs is verified by its relatively low standard deviation of the RMSD (1.146) against the three

Figure 2. Visual Assessment of the Four Point Correspondence Methods, in Terms of Registration Accuracy. (a) Reference Dental Image Drawn from Set III. Absolute Difference Between the Reference Image and the Registered Corresponding Image with the Edges of the Reference Image Superimposed for (b) AECP, (c) TICP, (d) CSM and (e) SOMs.

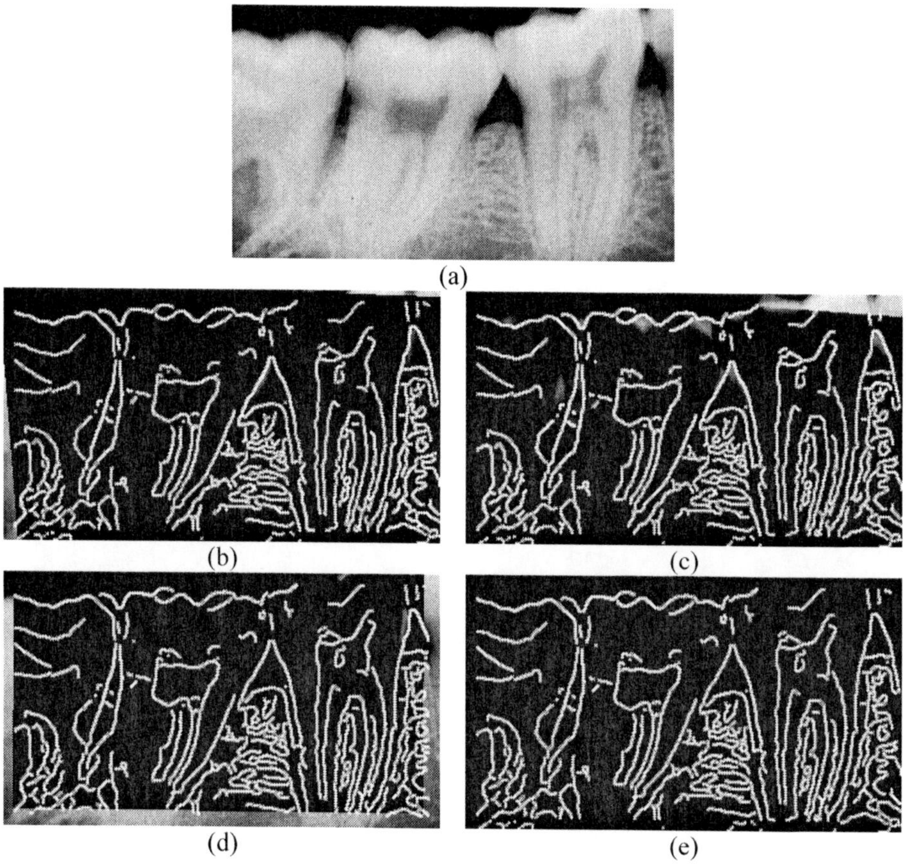

compared methods (1.895, 4.745 and 2.929, respectively), as revealed in Table 2.

The results for a sample of 24 image-pairs from Set III are presented in Table 2 using the affine transform. From Table 2, it is evident that SOMs outperforms the other three methods for the vast majority of the radiographic pairs in terms of the RMSD metric. In particular, in 14 out of the 24 sample pairs, the SOMs network achieved better than all three methods in comparison. Moreover, the mean RMSD over the entire sample of 24 dental pairs is greatly improved using the SOMs algorithm (6.689) against AECP (9.561), TICP (9.563) and CSM (11.576). Finally, the robustness of SOMs is verified by its relatively low standard deviation of the RMSD (1.146) against the three compared methods (1.895, 4.745 and 2.929, respectively), as revealed in Table 2.

Quantitative analysis over the all four sets of 96 total dental image pairs has shown that the Self-Organizing Maps approach performs better than the other three point correspondence methods on average. Those considerations are illustrated in Table 3. There, SOMs exhibits a

Table 2. Performance of the four automatic correspondence methods in terms of registration accuracy using the RMSD for the entire Set III.

Dental Image Pairs	*AECP*	*TICP*	*CSM*	*SOMs*
Pair-1	9.874	6.170	20.930	6.743
Pair-2	10.951	6.548	9.515	6.684
Pair-3	9.514	6.454	8.652	7.956
Pair-4	10.730	7.181	10.242	6.644
Pair-5	8.892	17.902	9.266	8.105
Pair-6	10.608	5.730	11.883	6.509
Pair-7	11.200	7.591	12.657	7.370
Pair-8	4.503	3.702	6.760	5.502
Pair-9	6.821	8.854	12.350	5.506
Pair-10	11.502	12.239	12.680	6.916
Pair-11	9.747	14.993	13.192	7.847
Pair-12	10.320	4.130	7.165	4.219
Pair-13	10.478	6.544	9.810	5.706
Pair-14	11.857	7.962	13.773	6.344
Pair-15	7.175	13.375	11.782	5.708
Pair-16	8.799	4.976	10.182	6.523
Pair-17	6.084	8.753	12.606	6.133
Pair-18	10.459	6.748	12.559	6.355
Pair-19	12.463	16.980	13.528	7.501
Pair-20	9.802	7.846	14.649	9.057
Pair-21	9.427	15.800	10.888	6.689
Pair-22	7.874	11.088	9.012	5.321
Pair-23	10.398	21.002	9.729	6.272
Pair-24	9.991	6.950	14.015	8.919
RMSD Mean ± Std.dev.	**9.561 ± *1.895***	**9.563 ± *4.745***	**11.576 ± *2.929***	**6.689 ± *1.146***

Table 3. Performance of the four automatic correspondence methods in terms of registration accuracy using the RMSD for all Sets (Average Values over Sets I-IV).

Data Sets	*AECP*	*TICP*	*CSM*	*SOMs*
Semi-Controlled Geometry Set I (24 pairs)	6.252 ± *1.113*	7.357 ± *1.858*	13.412 ± 2.192	7.253 ± *1.234*
Semi-Controlled Geometry Set II (24 pairs)	16.545 ± *3.767*	16.738 ± *3.500*	21.233 ± 6.351	14.038 ± *3.208*
Semi-Controlled Geometry Set III (24 pairs)	9.561 ± *1.895*	9.563 ± *4.745*	11.576 ± 2.929	6.689 ± *1.146*
Semi-Controlled Geometry Set IV (24 pairs)	18.612 ± *10.796*	20.805 ± *9.778*	17.258 ± 4.248	9.618 ± *2.339*

much lower average RMSD over AECP, TICP and CSM for Sets II-IV. Especially for Set IV, SOMs achieved acceptable correspondences, while the other three methods failed for most image pairs in the particular set. In addition, the much lower standard deviation measurements obtained for SOMs in most cases, suggests that the technique is quite robust as it exhibits consistent performance.

DISCUSSION

In this study, four methods for estimating point correspondences were considered: the Automatic Extraction of Corresponding Points (AECP) technique, the Trimmed Iterated Closest Points (TICP) approach, the Correspondence by Sensitivity to Movement (CSM) algorithm and the Self Organizing Maps (SOMs) network. The four methods were evaluated using a large variety of dental radiographs, obtained by a semi-controlled geometry protocol. After quite an extensive qualitative and quantitative analysis, it was concluded that the SOMs approach outperformed in most cases AECP, TICP as well as CSM in terms of registration quality, based on the RMSD measurement.

All four methods in comparison depend on several parameters which control key aspects of their algorithms. The preferred values for the parameters used to evaluate all methods are quoted in Table 1. When possible the same values were employed for common properties of the four methods, throughout the study. Nevertheless, the values shown in Table 1 were obtained after several trials using images from all featured sets, in order to ensure the best possible performance out of each method. Furthermore, as can be seen in Table 1, there are numerous parameters unique to each method. The effect of varying those parameters has to be examined comprehensively to assess the results obtained previously. For this purpose, the same image pair (from Set III) was used for all methods in order to obtain comparable results. In addition, each method exhibits its own strengths and weaknesses, which are reviewed in some further detail throughout this section.

As mentioned earlier, the Automatic Extraction of Corresponding Points (AECP) technique is based on Template Matching. The method improves the efficiency of the original Template Matching scheme, by employing circular templates and hence limiting the search area on the corresponding image (Likar & Pernus, 1999). AECP allocates correspondences by propagating a circular template of radius r (inner radius) from the reference image over a designated circular area of radius R (outer radius) on the corresponding image. Therefore, the size of the two circular areas, defined by their radii, is of particular importance for the AECP scheme. A dental pair from Set III was employed to examine the behavior of AECP when varying those two radii. The results are demonstrated in Figure 3. Figures 3(a) and (b) show how the RMSD and the execution time of the method respond to adjusting the inner radius r. Equally, Figures (c) and (d) demonstrate the effects of varying the outer radius R. As illustrated in Figure 3, the optimal values for the two radii are $r = 5$ and $R = 25$, which are used throughout the study. The execution time of the particular approach increases almost exponentially when increasing the value of the radii, especially when raising the value of the inner radius (Figure 3(b)); thus using any value $r \geq 9$ and $R \geq 100$ would be impractical.

AECP greatly improves the efficiency of the original Template Matching scheme. In general, AECP exhibits execution times reduced as much as 50% compared to its descendant method, without affecting the accuracy of the produced corresponding points. There are some cases, nevertheless, where the particular approach suffers from an increased number of false correspondences. This mainly occurs in corresponding images which are transformed by large rotations or translations. As AECP does not search the corresponding image in a strictly exhaustive manner, the algorithm may be confused and consider an erroneous search

Figure 3. Performance of the Automatic Extraction of Corresponding Points method in Terms of the RMSD and Execution time for Varying Values of the Two Radii. The Method was Applied to a Dental Image from Set III. Effects on Varying the Inner Radius from 3 to 15 Pixels, on (a) the RMSD Between the Reference and the Registered Corresponding Image and (b) the Execution Time. Effects of Varying the Outer Radius from 5 to 125 Pixels, on (c) the RMSD and (d) the Execution Time.

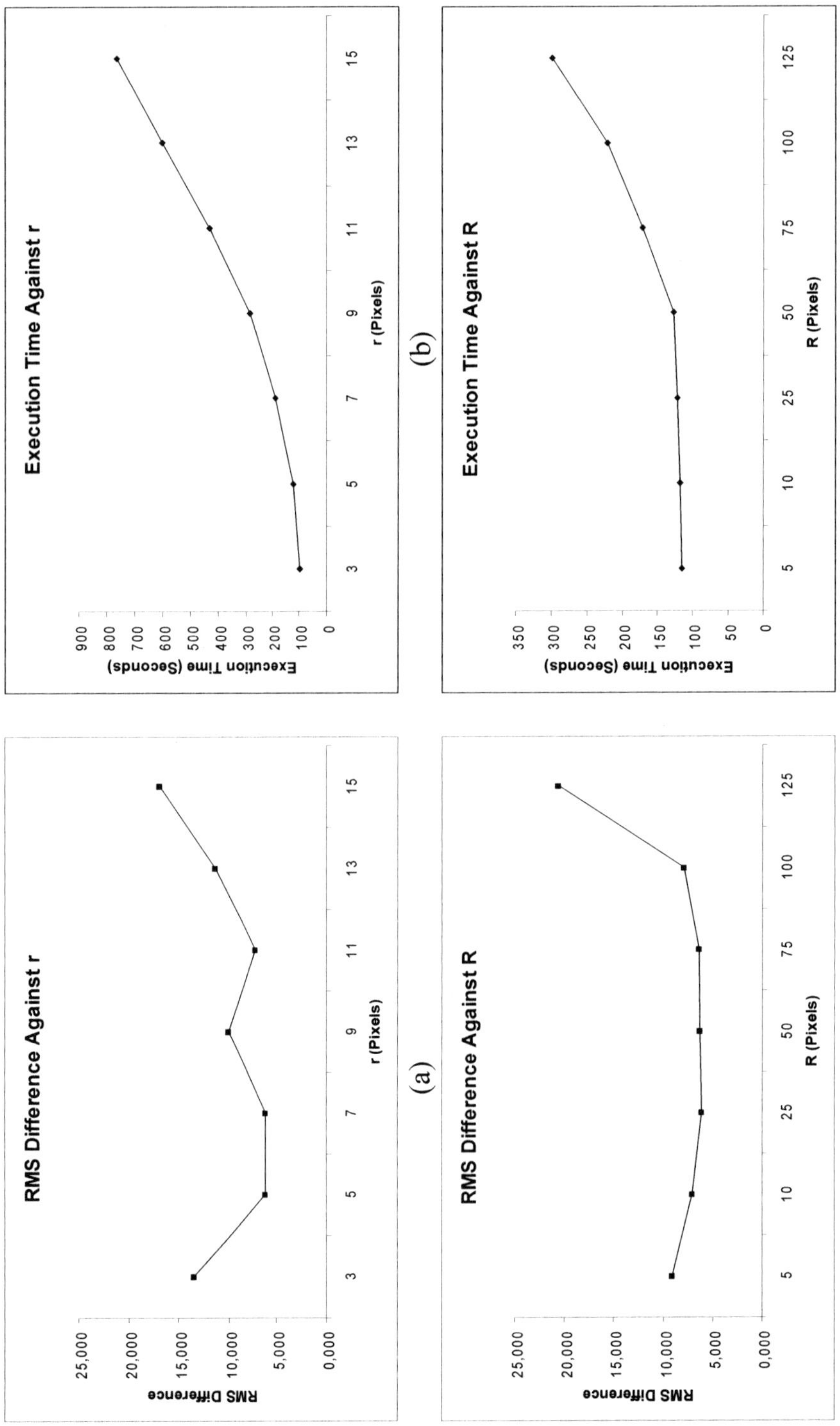

area, which in turn will give rise to a spurious corresponding point. Furthermore, AECP is a complete solution for extracting points of interest and estimating their correspondences. Since the particular study is only concerned with point correspondence, the feature extraction part of the algorithm was deliberately excluded from the evaluation process.

The Trimmed Iterated Closest Point algorithm used throughout the chapter is an improved version of ICP (Besl & McKay, 1990). The basic idea of TICP is to calculate correspondences between two or more point clouds. In our case, the first point cloud is considered to be the set of initial points on the reference image, while the second one is a set of candidate points on the corresponding image. Therefore, the particular approach requires points of interest to be extracted from both the reference and the corresponding image. TICP then tries to match those two sets of points

Figure 4. Performance of the Trimmed ICP Method for Varying the Number of Trials (Iterations). A Dental Image from Set III was Used and the Method was Applied with the Number of Trials Ranging from 50 to 1,000. The Effects on Performance were Recorded in Terms of (a) the RMSD and (b) the Execution Time.

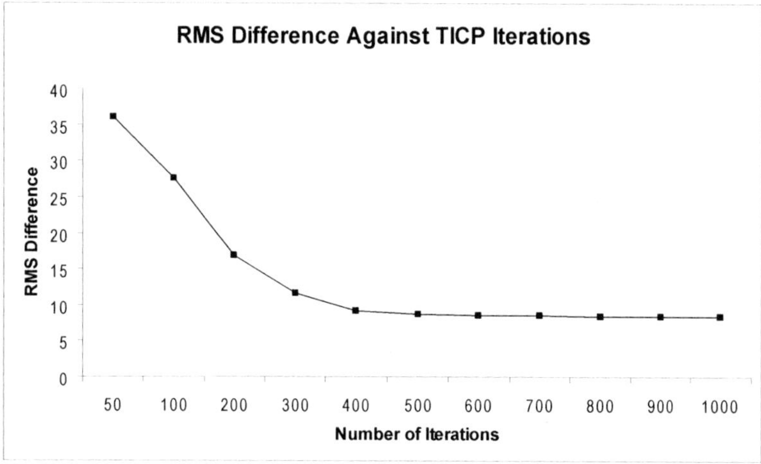

(a)

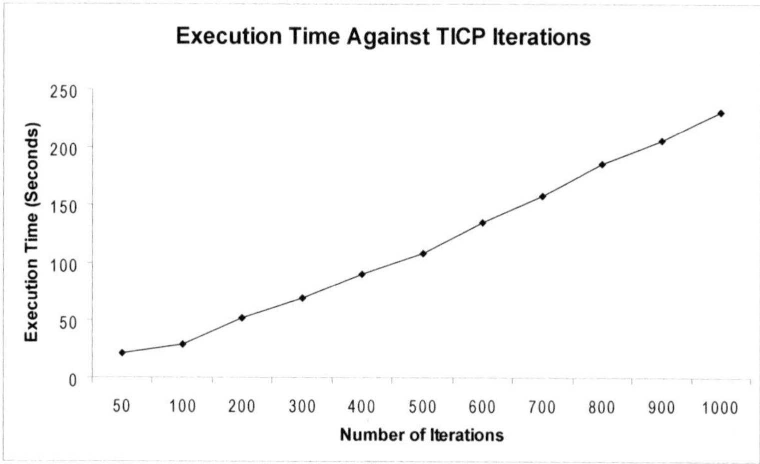

(b)

in an iterative manner as described earlier. All ICP variants adopt a trial-and-error approach to allocate correspondences. As a result the accuracy of the estimated corresponding points should improve after each iteration (trial). Obviously the more iterations are completed the more accurate the results obtained. However, there is a certain number of iterations beyond which minimal accuracy improvements are recorded. Since an increased number of trials negatively impacts on the efficiency of TICP, the preferred number of trials is usually selected such that accuracy and execution time are balanced.

An example is shown in Figure 4, where an image pair from Set III is considered. TICP was applied to the particular image pair for a varying number of iterations, ranging from 50 to 1,000. As can be seen in Figure 4(a), no significant performance gain is observed after 500 iterations, in terms of the RMSD. Since convergence time increases steadily with the number of trials (Figure 4(b)), the particular value was considered to be sufficient and therefore was selected for evaluating TICP throughout the study.

Although the TICP method can be highly efficient and fast, it is heavily dependent upon the performance of the preferred point extraction method. The reason for this is that the algorithm itself is not able to calculate the point correspondences but it merely links points from one set to another. Therefore, ICP variants are generally not suitable for allocating point correspondences unless there is a predefined set of candidate corresponding points on the corresponding image. Those points may be either defined automatically or manually.

Another method based on Template Matching is the Correspondence by Sensitivity to Movement (CSM) technique (Guest, Berry, Baldock, Fidrich & Smith, 2001). As mentioned, CSM firstly performs minor movements to the control points on the reference image thus producing a candidate (or tentative) corresponding point for each such movement. The set of tentative points associated with a control point define its match-map. The size of the match-map refers to the area within which acceptable tentative corresponding points are considered. The size of the match-map, usually expressed by a cubic area, is of particular importance for CSM, as only candidate points within the match-map are estimated. In order to assess the optimal size of the match-map, several trials were conducted featuring varying sizes ranging from 3×3 to 33×33 pixels. The performance of CSM in each case was evaluated in terms of the RMSD between the reference and the registered corresponding image, using a dental image from Set III.

The results shown in Figure 5(a) indicate that the optimal match-map size is 15×15 pixels, which was adopted as the preferred value throughout the study. As can be seen in Figure 5(a), either excessively small or large match-maps hinder the efficiency of the CSM algorithm. The reason for this is that small match-maps simply do not provide sufficient space for candidate correspondences, while large ones may well confuse the algorithm by producing spurious candidates, thus scattering the tentative corresponding points over a large area, as with the AECP approach. On the other hand, the size of the match-map does not have an immense effect in the execution time of the algorithm. This is illustrated in Figure 5(b). Although the execution time for CSM does rise as the match-map size increases, the effect is minimal compared to AECP, which also features a similar template scheme.

By examining the distribution of candidate corresponding points over minor displacements of the control points, CSM ensures that the estimated corresponding points are as reliable as possible. In effect, the particular method initially performs a Template Matching scheme for defining the match-maps and then it examines the reliability of the estimated correspondences by assessing their sensitivity to the movement of their respective control point. In that way only reliable corresponding points may be extracted. Therefore, CSM favours robustness over execution time, as

Figure 5. Performance of the Correspondence by Sensitivity to Movement Algorithm for Varying the Size of the Match-Map. The Match-Map was Varied from 3 to 33 Pixels Wide and the Tests were Performed on a Dental Image from Set III. The Performance was Assessed in Terms of (a) the RMSD and (b) the Execution Time.

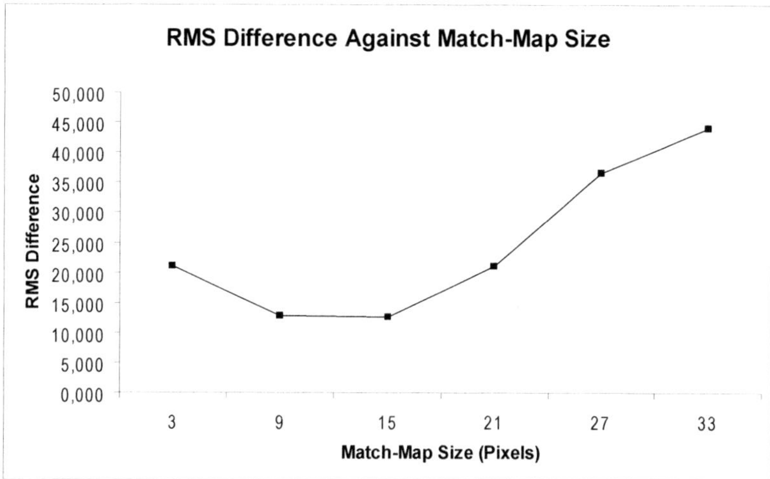

(a)

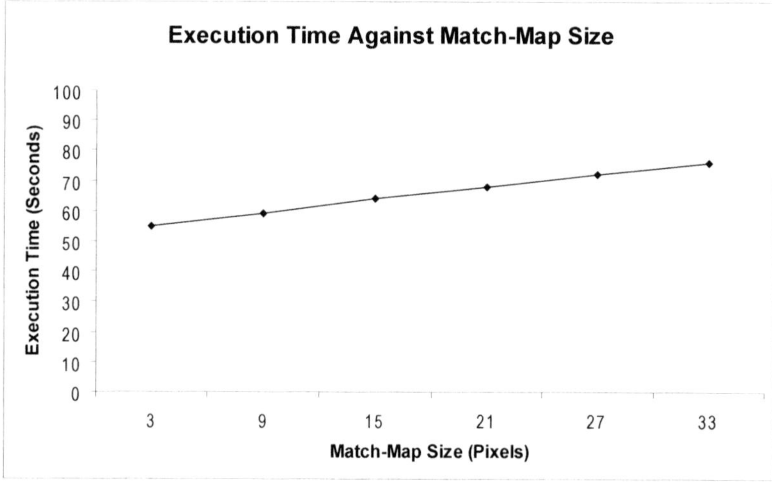

(b)

it is generally slower than AECP and TICP. On the other hand, although CSM is an improvement over the original Template Matching scheme, it does not always guarantee superior performance over its descendant method. In fact, there are cases where the efficiency of CSM degrades due to the characteristics of the featured image pair. Poor quality blurred images are especially unfavourable for CSM.

As with any other iterative method, the Self Organizing Maps approach is greatly affected by the number of iterations executed. Again, the more

Figure 6. Performance of the Self Organizing Maps Methods for a Varying Number of Iterations. A Dental Image from Set III was Used and the Method was Applied with a Varying Number of Stopping Iterations Ranging from 500 to 15,000. The Effects on the Performance were Recorded in Terms of (a) the RMSD and (b) the Execution Time.

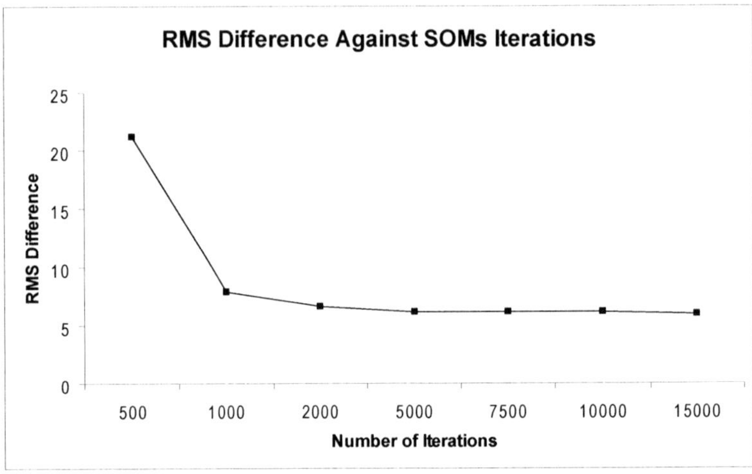

(a)

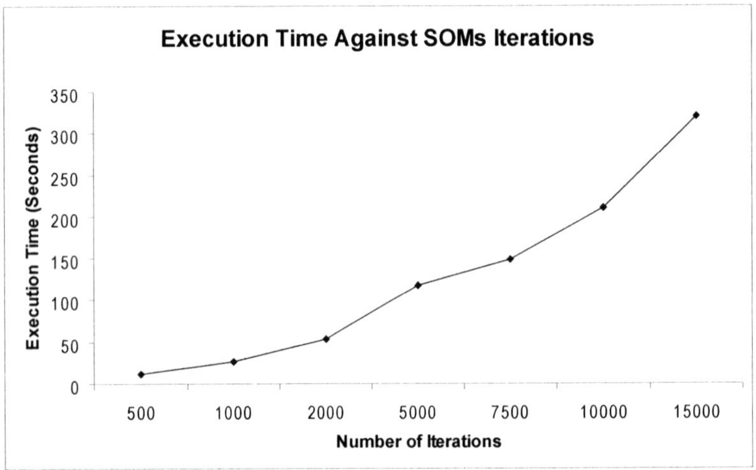

(b)

iterations performed, the better the accuracy of the corresponding points, up to a certain number where no further noticeable improvement can be accounted. For the particular image pairs included in this study, it was observed that SOMs did not improve point accuracy noticeably for more than 5,000 iterations. In some instances (especially in small images) performance was saturated for even less iterations, but the value of 5,000 was universally adopted to suffice all cases.

As can be seen in Figure 6, the SOMs algorithm was tested on a dental image pair from Set III using a fluctuating number of iterations (from 500 to 15,000). There, it is quite clear that employing more than 5,000 iterations does not improve the accuracy noticeably (Figure 6(a)).

Moreover, the fact that the convergence time of the particular approach raises dramatically as the number of trials increases (Figure 6(b)), using a larger number of iterations would hinder the efficiency of the method, as the execution time of the algorithm increases without any performance gain.

After qualitative and quantitative evaluation of all four methods over all four dental image sets, it was concluded that SOMs outperformed AECP, TICP and CSM on average. However, the superiority of SOMs comes at a cost to convergence time. In general SOMs was the slowest method of all four methods examined. It took about 4 minutes to calculate the point correspondences of 50 control points. For the same images and number of control points, AECP and CSM estimated the correspondences in approximately 3 minutes, while TICP in about 2 minutes. All tests featured in this study were performed on a typical desktop workstation (AMD Opteron 165, 1800 MHz processor with 2 GB of RAM).

FUTURE TRENDS

The presented comparative study involves the evaluation of four automatic correspondence methods and the evaluation of their performance in 2D dental radiographs. The study could be extended either to incorporate more methods to define automatic correspondence on the same image data or the application of these methods to define correspondence on 2D unimodal image pairs from other modalities. Finally, a future step may include the evaluation of the performance of various automatic correspondence methods applied to three-dimensional (3D) unimodal or multimodal image data such as CT or MRI data, towards automatic point-based registration.

CONCLUSION

This chapter presented a comprehensive evaluative study comparing four commonly used methods for obtaining point correspondences towards image-based registration. The Automatic Extraction of Corresponding Points (AECP), the Trimmed ICP (TICP), The Correspondences by Sensitivity to Movement (CSM) and the Self Organizing Maps (SOMs) techniques were all assessed both visually and quantitatively. The four methods were applied individually on 96 dental image pairs subject to unknown transformations. In general, the SOMs approach outperformed in most cases the other three methods in comparison in terms of the average RMSD between the reference image and the registered corresponding image. On the other hand, AECP and TICP performed evenly in most cases.

REFERENCES

Besl, P. J., & McKay, N. D. (1992). A method of registration of 3-D shapes. *IEEE Transactions in Pattern Analysis and Machine Intelligence, 14*(2), 239-256.

Bookstein, F. (1997). Shape and the information in medical images: a decade of the morphometric synthesis. *Computer Vision and Imaging Understanding, 66*, 97–118.

Cao, Z., Pan, S., Li, R., Balachandran, R., Fitzpatrick, M. J., Chapman, W. C., & Dawant, B. M. (2004). Registration of medical images using an interpolated closest point transform: method and validation. *Medical Image Analysis, 8*, 421-427.

Chetverikov, D., Svirko, D., & Stepanov, D. (2002). The trimmed iterative closest point algorithm. *International Conference of Pattern Recognition, 3*, 545-548.

Di Stefano, L., Mattocia, S., & Tombari, F. (2004). An algorithm for efficient and exhaustive template matching. *Image Analysis and Recognition, 3211*, 408-415.

Gonzalez, R., & Woods, R. (1992). *Digital image processing.* Addison Wesley.

Guest, E., Berry, E., Baldock, R. A., Fidrich, M., & Smith, M. A. (2001). Robust point correspondence applied to two- and three-dimensional image registration. *IEEE Transactions in Pattern Analysis and Machine Intelligence, 23*(2), 165-179.

Hajnal, J. V., Hill, D. L. G., & Hawkes, D. J. (2001). *Medical image registration.* CRC Press.

Johnson, H., & Christensen, G. (2002). Consistent landmark and intensity-based image registration. *IEEE Transactions in Medical Imaging, 21*, 450-461.

Kohonen, T. (1990). The self-organizing map. *Proceedings of the IEEE, 78*(9), 1464-1480.

Laliberte, F., Gagnon, L., & Sheng, Y. (2003). Registration and fusion of retinal images: an evaluation study. *IEEE Transactions in Medical Imaging, 22*(5). 404-418.

Likar, B., & Pernus, F. (1999). Automatic extraction of corresponding points for the registration of medical images. *Medical Physics, 26*, 1678–1686.

Maintz, J. B. A., & Viergever, M. A. (1998). A survey of medical image registration. *Medical Image Analysis, 2*(1), 1-36.

Matsopoulos, G. K., Asvestas, P. A., Mouravliansky, N. A., & Delibasis, K. K. (2004). Multimodal registration of retinal images using self organizing maps. *IEEE Transactions in Medical Imaging, 23*, 1557-1563.

Pitiot, A., Thompson, P. & Toga, A. (2002). Adaptive elastic segmentation of brain MRI via shape model guided evolutionary programming. *IEEE Transactions in Medical Imaging, 21*, 910–923.

Pizer, S., Fritsch, D., Yushkevich, P., Johnson, V., & Chaney, E. (1996). Segmentation, registration, and measurement of shape variation via image object shape. *IEEE Transactions in Medical Imaging, 18*, 851–865.

Pluim, J. P. W., Maintz, J. B., & Viergever, M. A. (2003). Mutual information based registration of medical images: a survey. *IEEE Transactions in Medical Imaging, 22*, 986-1004.

Press, W. H., Teukolsky, S. A., Vetterling, W. T., & Flannery, B. P. (1992). *Numerical recipes in C: the art of scientific computing.*

Zacharaki, E. I., Matsopoulos, G. K., Asvestas, P. A., Gröndahl, K., & Gröndahl, H. G. (2004). A digital subtraction radiography scheme based on automatic multiresolution registration. *Dentomaxillofacial Radiology, 33*, 1-14.

Zitova, B., & Flusser, J. (2003). Image registration methods: a survey. *Image and Vision Computing, 21*, 977–1000.

KEY TERMS

Automatic Point Correspondence: The automatic process of estimating the homologous points on the corresponding image of a set of initial points from the reference image.

Dental Imaging: The representation of dental elements on a film, acquired through specific radiographic protocols

Image Registration: The process of matching a corresponding image to a reference image, using suitable transformations

Iterated Closest Points: Automatic point correspondence method which works by minimizing the average distance from a set of points on the reference image to a set of points on the corresponding image

Point Extraction: The automatic or manual process of extracting points of interest from an image

Self Organizing Maps: Automatic iterative method for allocating point correspondences, based on Kohonen's neural network

Template Matching: Automatic point correspondence method based on matching regions from the reference image to transformed regions of the corresponding image

Chapter XXVII
Anomaly Detection in Medical Image Analysis

Alberto Taboada-Crispi
Universidad Central de Las Villas, Cuba

Hichem Sahli
Vrije Universiteit Brussel, Belgium

Maykel Orozco-Monteagudo
Universidad Central de Las Villas, Cuba

Denis Hernández-Pacheco
Universidad Central de Las Villas, Cuba

Alexander Falcón-Ruiz
Universidad Central de Las Villas, Cuba

ABSTRACT

Various approaches have been taken to detect anomalies, with certain particularities in the medical image scenario, linked to other terms: content-based image retrieval, pattern recognition, classification, segmentation, outlier detection, image mining, as well as computer-assisted diagnosis, and computer-aided surgery. This chapter presents, a review of anomaly detection (AD) techniques and assessment methodologies, which have been applied to medical images, emphasizing their peculiarities, limitations and future perspectives. Moreover, a contribution to the field of AD in brain computed tomography images is also given, illustrated and assessed.

INTRODUCTION

In general terms, anomaly detection (AD) can be considered as the process of detecting a small fraction of the data that differs, in some sense, from the global trend or pattern defined by the data set. The goal of an anomaly detector can be thought as the identification of the most unusual samples in a data set, without having any *a priori* information about their properties, other than they are rare and have a low probability of occurrence.

By their nature, anomalies do not permit a positive definition of their properties, making difficult a general formulation of the AD problem. Most of the approaches to detect anomalies use, instead, a negative definition: anomalies are data samples that do not conform to the rule or model of normalcy. This led to a broad group of anomaly detectors that are based on some type of a mathematical model, or description, characterizing the data under interest. Data fitting this description is considered as normal; those not fitting the model are considered anomalous. The general taxonomy for AD in image analysis can be thought to be composed of: (1) Observation field definition, (2) Background model estimation and (3) Detection.

This chapter discusses the particularities of the AD techniques in the context of medical images, their current status and perspectives. The Chapter is organized as follows: the next section presents the AD problem in pathology, gives an overview of the state-of-art in AD, and discusses AD algorithms assessment, where we propose a new evaluation measure. Then, we propose an AD algorithm for brain computed tomography (CT) images. In the last sections we analyze future trends in the domain and give some conclusions.

BACKGROUND

Most AD algorithms for medical image analysis are profoundly influenced by the specific image datasets used and by the medical or biological task. *Figure 1* shows this diversity at a glance. Most reported studies have dealt with detection of tumors in digital mammography (Huang, 2004; Selvi, 2005; Wei, 2005; Peng, 2006; Chiracharit, 2007; Ikedo, 2007; Karnan, 2007), lung CT images (Minhas, 2005; Sluimer, 2006), and brain magnetic resonance (MR) images (Gering, 2003; Prastawa, 2004; Lee, 2005; Benamrane, 2006; Menze, 2006; Shinkareva, 2006; Bouix, 2007; Ekin, 2007), but many others can be mentioned.

Since the foundational work of Sklansky and Ballard (1973) on automatic location of tumors in radiographs using pattern-recognition-related methods, there have been several approaches focused in the detection of anomalies represented in medical images. Among others, one can cite the detection of different kind of tumors (Krivacic, 2004; Iyatomi, 2006; Strzelecki, 2006; Xu, 2006; Kelm, 2007; Montgomery, 2007), hemorrhages, multiple sclerosis, malformations and more (Bertelli, 2006; Shinkareva, 2006; Stoitsis, 2006). Any lesion (characterizing a disease, as Alzheimer's (Ashton, 2006), or due to an accident) that is structurally and compositionally distinct from surrounding healthy tissue could be highlighted by an appropriate imaging modality and therefore could be detected by an AD approach.

Most AD works in the medical scenario are focused on studying organs more prone to develop certain types of cancers: breast, lungs, and brain. Variety of studies comprises AD techniques applied to images of cells (Krivacic, 2004; Spinosa, 2005), as well as to whole body scans (Ashton, 2006; Huang, 2007). In addition, image analysis of some other organs have benefited from AD procedures, e.g. the prostate (Kelm, 2007), the carotid artery (Stoitsis, 2006), the heart (Bertelli, 2006;

Figure 1. Medical images used for AD

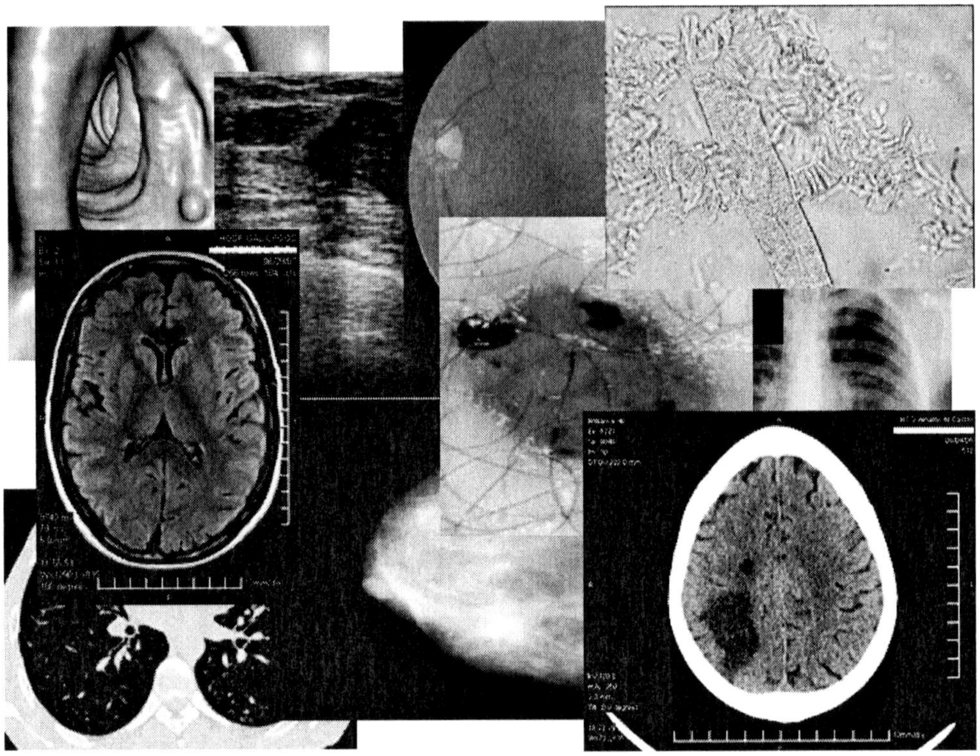

Strzelecki, 2006), the nasopharyngeal structure, the tympanic membrane (Xie, 2006), the retina (Xiaoxue, 2004), and the skin (Iyatomi, 2006).

To deal with AD, several imaging modalities have been used:

- Photography: conventionally taken (Iyatomi, 2006), or specially derived with M-modes (Bertelli, 2006), or obtained with the extension of an endoscope, or a microscope (Krivacic, 2004; Xie, 2006; Goode, 2007).
- Electrical impedance tomography (Minhas, 2005).
- Ultrasound-based systems (Huang, 2004; Stoitsis, 2006; Strzelecki, 2006; Ikedo, 2007).
- X rays (Sklansky, 1973; Müller, 2005).
- Computed tomography (CT) (Messmer, 2006; Sluimer, 2006).
- Magnetic resonance imaging (MRI) (Gering, 2003; Prastawa, 2004; Lee, 2005; Benamrane, 2006; Bouix, 2007; Ekin, 2007; Vovk, 2007).
- Functional magnetic resonance imaging (fMRI) (Shinkareva, 2006).
- Magnetic resonance spectroscopy imaging (MRSI) (Menze, 2006; Kelm, 2007).
- Single photon emission computed tomography (SPECT) and positron emission tomography (PET) (Montgomery, 2007).

Environmental and genetic changes cause great variability in the anatomical structures from one individual to another, which make the AD over medical images procedure very difficult. This variability is even higher in the condition of disease or abnormality. However, current medical imaging systems, with proper calibration and exploitation, assure certain standardized conditions. For instance, as shown in *Figure 2*, modern CT systems provide 4096 gray-level images, representing different density levels (given in Hounsfield Units, HU), arbitrarily established at 0 HU for water and -1000 HU for air. *Figure 2* shows default settings for CT (0 ± 2000/2 HU, on top) and re-scaled window/level adjustments for brain matter (35 ± 70/2 HU, right) and bone analysis (800 ± 2000/2 HU, left) in the multi-slice CT scanner, Philips 'Brilliance 40' (64-channel thin-slice).

As illustrated in *Table 1*, even those imaging modalities that look very close in appearance, as X ray/CT and MR images, may have different gray-levels to represent a given normal or abnormal tissue. Bright X ray/CT images are associated to high density tissues (i.e. high attenuation of X rays), and dark X ray/CT images are associated to low density tissues (Müller, 2005; Messmer, 2006; Sluimer, 2006). For MR, on the other hand, brighter regions are related to higher signal intensities.

Overview of AD Approaches

AD has its own foundations, based on statistics (Markou, 2003a), neural networks (Markou, 2003b), machine learning, and image mining (Hodge, 2004), however, in some cases the AD strategy is not applied directly but associated to other image analysis techniques such as classification, segmentation, image mining and content-based image retrieval.

Special Cases

AD in medical images can be seen as a special case of:

- Classification approach using generally two classes: normal and anomaly (Pokrajac, 2005; Selvi, 2005; Spinosa, 2005; Menze, 2006; Shinkareva, 2006; Strzelecki, 2006; Bouix, 2007). It should be highlighted that

Figure 2. Density levels in a 12 bit DICOM image and window/level adjustments

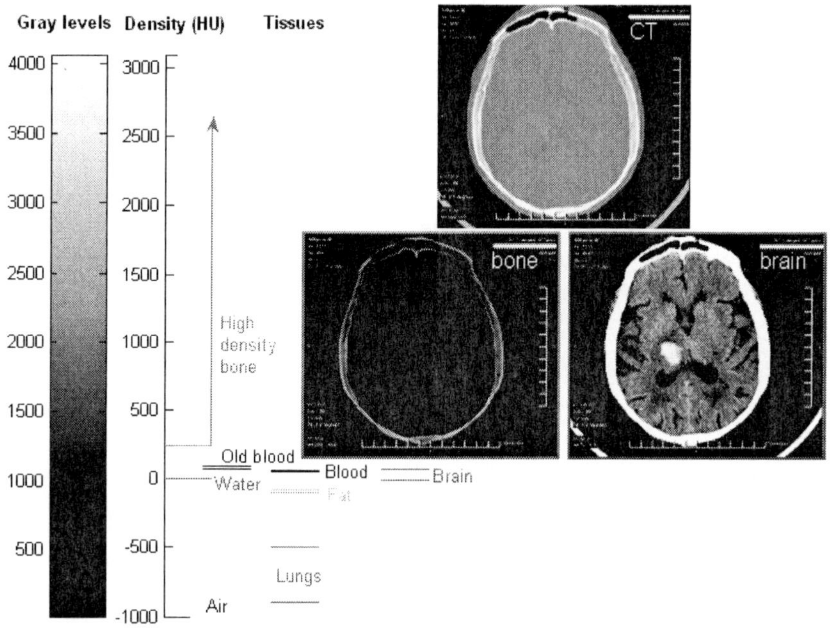

Table 1. Normal and abnormal tissues vs. imaging modalities

Structure			Image acquisition modality		
Normal/ anomaly	Tissue	Approximate Density (HU)	X ray/CT	T1 MR	T2 MR
Normal	Air	-1000	Very dark	Very dark	Very dark
	High density bone	> 250	Very bright	Very dark	Very dark
	Fat	-90 ± 10	Dark	Bright	Bright
	Water	0 ± 5	Dark	Dark	Bright
	Brain matter	35 ± 35	Intermediate	Intermediate	Intermediate
Anomaly	Bleeding or hemorrhage	55 ± 5 (fresh) 80 ± 10 (old)	Bright	Bright	Bright
	Infarction		Dark	Dark	Bright
	Tumors		Dark (if no calcified)	Dark	Bright

typical classification algorithms are not suited to deal with the critical data imbalance (normal class is much more abundant than the infrequent anomaly class) of most AD problems, but it could assist in some stage to pre-classify the normal tissues. AD application itself requires the classifier to act as a detector rather than as a classifier.

- Segmentation technique allowing the segmentation of abnormal regions in an image, combining detection and delineation (Gering, 2003; Huang, 2004; Prastawa, 2004; Lee, 2005; Ségonne, 2005; Bertelli, 2006; Strzelecki, 2006; Bouix, 2007; Huang, 2007; Montgomery, 2007).
- Content-based image retrieval to extract anomaly images from a database and indicate the anomaly within the retrieved image (Lehmann, 2005; Hersh, 2006; Xu, 2006). In case of databases containing normal (non-pathologic) cases, dissimilarity retrieval is applied.
- Medical image mining (Lehmann, 2005; Peng, 2006), as well as outlier detection (Prastawa, 2004; Rousseeuw, 2006) can be applied to detect anomalies.

Statistical Methods

Statistical methods comprise parametric and non-parametric techniques. Parametric methods assume that data distributions are Gaussian in nature, characterized by their mean and covariance, and exploit probabilistic/Gaussian mixture modeling, hidden Markov models, Markov random fields (MRF) (Gering, 2003; Selvi, 2005), conditional random fields (Lee, 2005) and hypothesis testing, by using robust statistics: minimum volume estimation, convex peeling, principal component analysis (PCA), and expectation maximization (EM) plus deterministic annealing (Markou, 2003a; Hodge, 2004; Rousseeuw, 2006; Daszykowski, 2007; Ekin, 2007). Non-parametric methods, as histogram analysis, include density estimation based on the *k*-nearest neighbors algorithm with Euclidean or Mahalanobis distance (Markou, 2003a), local kernel models or Parzen windowing (Hodge, 2004; Prastawa, 2004), and features matching (between training and test data) using some dissimilarity measures. In this context, the work of Pokrajac *et al.* (2005) proposed a method using measures of dissimilarity (Mahalanobis distance and the Kullback-Leibler divergence) to compute the difference between spatial probability distributions of regions of interest (such as lesions, tumors, areas of brain activity, etc.) in an image of a new subject and each of the considered classes represented by historical data.

Neural Networks

Both, supervised (as multi-layer perceptrons) (Strzelecki, 2006) and unsupervised (as self-organizing maps, SOM) (Huang, 2004) neural networks can be useful for AD in medical imaging. Radial basis functions (Minhas, 2005), learning vector quantization, probabilistic neural networks, Hopfield networks, support vector machines (SVM) (Lee, 2005; Wei, 2005; Menze, 2006; Xu, 2006; Chiracharit, 2007), synchronized oscillator network (Strzelecki, 2006), and adaptive resonance theory can be used.

Gering (2003) recognizes deviations from normalcy by using a contextual dependency network that incorporates context (immediate and broad) to detect tumors in MR images. All training is performed on healthy tissue, and it extends EM-based segmentation with region-level properties to derive a multi-level MRF approach. Classification of every voxel considers: the voxel itself, the surrounding neighborhood (Markov) of the voxel, the region where the voxel belongs (entire connected region), the global setting (position of the voxel's region relative to other regions), and user guidance.

Huang & Chen (2004) integrate SOM and watershed segmentation (Pratikakis, 2005) for textural analysis to extract contours of breast tumors from ultrasound images. Menze *et al.* (2006) applied linear and nonlinear feature extraction, including independent component analysis, PCA, and wavelet transformations, combined with classifiers such as linear discriminant analysis or Fisher's linear discriminant, chemometric methods (Rousseeuw, 2006), SVM (Kelm, 2007), and ensemble methods to classify echo time *in vivo* MRSI and detect recurrent brain tumors.

Machine Learning and Data Mining

Unlike the statistical and neural network methods, the machine learning approaches can deal with multi-type vectors and symbolic attributes. These approaches can use rule-based systems and decision trees, e.g. C4.5. In the AD scenario, we are interested in rules describing infrequent out-of-the-norm cases, while association rule mining algorithms may generate certain redundant rules. Based on the normal regions, data mining techniques can generate models of normality to recognize deviations from them, considered as anomalies.

Xiaoxue *et al.* (2004) used a multiple-instance learning mining approach to detect hard exudates in retinal images from diabetic patients. In general, the training images only have vague class labels, but no other information. Therefore, a mining approach is adequate to the problem of learning the characteristics of anomalies. They extracted relevant image features, discover anomalies and deal with errors in the training data.

Wei *et al.* (2005) propose the use of relevance vector machine (RVM), as a classifier, to detect micro-calcifications in digital mammograms as a supervised-learning problem. RVM is a machine-learning procedure based on Bayesian estimation theory, with a sparse decision function defined by a very small number of relevance vectors. RVM is not only accurate but also computationally efficient.

Goode *et al.* (2007) propose an automated, online approach to AD in high-content screening assays for pharmaceutical research based on machine learning approach as well.

Hybrid Systems

More recently, statistical, neural networks or machine learning methods have been combined in hybrid systems to obtain better performance. However, combining AD algorithms is different than combining classifier ensembles because, in the latter, classification algorithms deal with combining discrete class labels (e.g. using some voting technique), while in AD, the anomaly scores or rankings of the algorithms are combined instead.

Hybrid systems proliferate in recent works on AD in the medical image context. For instance, a genetic algorithm to search for bright spots in mammograms has been combined with a knowledge-discovery mechanism to improve its performance (Peng, 2006).

Neural networks, fuzzy logic and genetic algorithms have been combined in a hybrid system to detect anomalies present in brain MR images and to specify their nature (malign or benign tumors) (Benamrane, 2006). A neural network classifier, a Bayesian classifier, and a classifier based on hidden Markov chains were joined by a behavior knowledge space fusion rule for a semi-automatic classification process (Bertelli, 2006).

Assessment of AD Algorithms

To evaluate the performance of AD systems, one requires a suitable ground truth, and appropriate similarity measures. The same procedure can be used to fine-tune the parameters of the AD systems (operation point), deciding the threshold value which represents an intolerant deviation from normalcy, to recognize lesions from healthy surroundings. However, obtaining an acceptable ground truth is a very difficult task, and standard performance evaluation measures such as the misclassification rate are irrelevant in the AD context.

Ground Truth

The most common approach to evaluate the results of an AD technique is to compare them with those of a group of experts (segmented by hand) for a set of images. Human experts have excellent recognition capabilities due to prior global knowledge; however, their delineation ability is poor. The intra-expert coefficients of variation have been reported around 6.5%, and the inter-expert coefficients of variation is in the order of 22.1% according to (Ashton, 2006), or around 15% in both intra and inter-operator coefficients in accordance with (Gering, 2003), coinciding with our experience. Phantoms (synthetic images (Gering, 2003; Pokrajac, 2005) or known physical objects) could be used as well to evaluate the AD algorithms, at least in a preliminary stage, but this is not a trivial task.

Unlike the hundreds of datasets of medical images available for some other image analysis tasks, particular annotated datasets for AD algorithm assessment are very uncommon. This lack of gold standards for validating AD algorithms, forced Bouix *et al.* (2007) to focus their attention on a common agreement principle to assess algorithms for brain tissue classification without a ground truth. They found this technique suitable for AD, but not sufficient for a precise performance evaluation of brain tissue classifiers.

Performance Measures

Having a suitable ground truth (showing anomaly regions) for the considered AD problem, the assessment of the AD algorithm requires the definition of similarity measures to compare the reference data with the AD system output. Several measures have been used, from differences in size of the detected anomalies (Strzelecki, 2006) to numerous distances between boundaries of segmented anomalies, using e.g. the Hausdorff distance (Prastawa, 2004), or measures of spatial overlap (Bouix, 2007).

In this context, a ground truth can be seen as a binary image, X, showing 0 (black) in the normal regions and 1 (white) in the anomaly regions. In the same way, the AD results could be represented as a binary image, Y, with similar assignation of values. Both, X and Y, are defined over the same finite grid of N spatial sites (see example of *Figure 8*). *Figure 3* depicts a schematic reasoning, based on information theory, to compute popular measures of similarity between Y and X. The following notations are considered:

- a = number of occurrences of x_i = 1 and y_i = 1 (anomalies detected as anomalies), known as true positives.
- b = number of occurrences of x_i = 0 and y_i = 1 (non-anomalies detected as anomalies), known as false positives.
- c = number of occurrences of x_i = 1 and y_i = 0 (anomalies detected as non-anomalies), known as false negatives.
- d = number of occurrences of x_i = 0 and y_i = 0 (non-anomalies detected as non-anomalies), known as true negatives.

Several similarity (and corresponding dissimilarity) coefficients can be computed as simple measures for evaluation. In general, the most popular measures (represented in the bottom right corner of *Figure 3*) are:

- S_e = sensitivity, detection rate, or recall, which is the probability of detecting anomalies correctly, defined as

$$S_e = \text{Recall} = p(Y=1 \mid X=1)$$
$$=1-p(Y=0 \mid X=1)=\frac{a}{a+c}=1-\frac{c}{a+c} \quad (1)$$

- S_p = specificity, which is the probability of detecting normalcy correctly[1], computed as

$$S_p = p(Y=0 \mid X=0)$$
$$=1-p(Y=1 \mid X=0)=\frac{d}{b+d}=1-\frac{b}{b+d} \quad (2)$$

- P_p = positive predictive value, precision, or Bayesian detection rate, which is the probability of having positives correctly detected, that is

$$P_p = \text{Precision} = p(X=1 \mid Y=1)$$
$$=1-p(X=0 \mid Y=1)=\frac{a}{a+b}=1-\frac{b}{a+b} \quad (3)$$

Figure 3. Information theory-based similarity between two sets

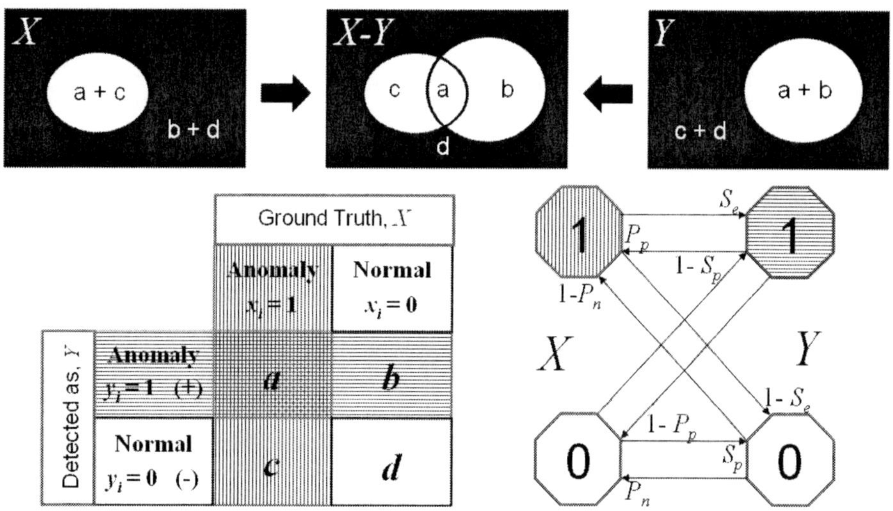

- P_n = negative predictive value, or Bayesian negative rate, which is the probability of having negatives correctly detected, according to

$$P_n = p(X=0 \mid Y=0) = 1 - p(X=1 \mid Y=0) = \frac{d}{c+d} = 1 - \frac{c}{c+d} \quad (4)$$

- R_C = classification rate, accuracy, or simple matching coefficient[2], which is the rate of correct classifications, computed as

$$R_C = D_{sm} = p(X=Y) = 1 - p(X \neq Y) = \frac{a+d}{a+b+c+d} = 1 - \frac{b+c}{a+b+c+d} \quad (5)$$

Due to the large number of zeros (black areas) in the binary images X and Y (($d+b$) >> ($a+c$)), the above measures are usually biased in the AD context. Remember that anomalies are very uncommon events, much more infrequent in a massive screening program[3]. To have a better idea of this imbalance in the data, we can use the *base rate* (rate of anomalies), R_B, which is normally <<1 in most AD scenarios, and corresponds to the prior probability of anomaly,

$$R_B = p(X=1) = 1 - p(X=0) = \frac{a+c}{a+b+c+d} = 1 - \frac{b+d}{a+b+c+d} \quad (6)$$

To deal with this critical imbalance of the data, some authors have used the following coefficients instead:

- D_T = Tanimoto distance, or Rogers distance, which is similar to the classification rate but it gives double weight to ($b+c$) in the denominator

$$D_T = \frac{a+d}{a+d+2(b+c)} \quad (7)$$

- D_R = distance of Russel and Rao, which does not involve the term d in the numerator,

$$D_R = \frac{a}{a+b+c+d} \quad (8)$$

- D_J = distance of Jaccard (Bouix, 2007), which discards completely the term d,

$$D_J = \frac{a}{a+b+c} \quad (9)$$

- D_C = distance of Czekanowski, Dice, Sorensen or F-measure, which is similar to the distance of Jaccard, but giving double weight to a,

$$D_C = F_{measure} = \frac{2S_eP_p}{S_e+P_p} = \frac{2a}{2a+b+c} \quad (10)$$

In this paper, we propose to adapt a measure for intrusion detection introduced by Gu *et al.* (2006), to fine-tune and assess AD algorithms in the medical image analysis scenario. The proposed measure, referred to as *the AD rate* or *capability*, R_{AD}, can be seen as the ratio of the mutual information, $I(X;Y)$, between the ground truth, X, and the AD output image, Y, and the entropy of the ground truth, $H(X)$,

$$R_{AD} = \frac{I(X;Y)}{H(X)} = \frac{H(X) - H(X \mid Y)}{H(X)} = 1 - \frac{-\sum_x \sum_y p(x)p(y \mid x)\log\frac{p(x)p(y \mid x)}{p(y)}}{-\sum_x p(x)\log p(x)} \quad (11)$$

where, (equation 12)

$$H(X) = -R_B \log R_B - (1-R_B)\log(1-R_B) \quad (13)$$

$$H(X\,|\,Y) = -R_B S_e \log\frac{R_B S_e}{R_B S_e + (1-R_B)(1-S_p)} - R_B(1-S_e)\log\frac{R_B(1-S_e)}{R_B(1-S_e)+S_p(1-R_B)} - (1-R_B)S_p \log\frac{(1-R_B)S_p}{(1-R_B)S_p + R_B(1-S_e)} - (1-R_B)(1-S_p)\log\frac{(1-R_B)(1-S_p)}{(1-R_B)(1-S_p)+S_e R_B} \quad (12)$$

Therefore, $R_{AD}\,(0 \le R_{AD} \le 1)$ takes into account all the important aspects of detection capability, according to

$$R_{AD} = 1 - \frac{a\log P_p + b\log(1-P_p) + c\log(1-P_n) + d\log P_n}{(a+c)\log R_B + (b+d)\log(1-R_B)} \quad (14)$$

The proposed *AD rate* provides an intrinsic measure of AD capability and it is sensitive to operation parameters (Gu, 2006) of the AD system. We have verified all these advantages over the more traditional measures.

PROPOSED AD ALGORITHM FOR BRAIN CT IMAGING

Unlike the abundant works on AD in brain MR imaging, there is no much work on AD in brain CT scanning. In this section, we propose an AD algorithm for brain CT imaging. CT is cheaper and more widely available than MR imaging systems. Therefore, efforts to detect anomalies (lesions) from brain CT images are plenty justified.

In general, MR outperforms CT to detect brain tumors, but CT is better for the detection of calcification, hemorrhages and bony details. CT is very useful for diagnosing cerebrovascular accidents, intracranial hemorrhage, and for evaluating skull fractures. CT scanning may be used, as well, replacing MR, in the presence of patients semiconscious, unable to remain motionless, suffering of claustrophobia, or carrying metallic implants.

Materials and Methods

Data Collection and Preliminary Stage

Data of 27 brain CT studies, have been collected, at the University Hospital "Arnaldo Milián Castro", Santa Clara, Cuba, using a multi-slice CT scanner, model Philips 'Brilliance 40' (64-channel thin-slice). In total, 890 slices of size 512×512 voxels and resolution of 12 bits, i.e. 4096 gray-levels, have been used for this study.

Compared to most of the published works on medical AD, where a statistical model of common background tissues is first determined, and then anomalies are determined (Ashton, 2006), the proposed approach uses a combination of feature-based and histogram-based classification scheme. In order to assess our method, we selected, with the help of radiologists and neurologists, a set of regions representing the following normal classes (*Figure 4*): air/background (BG), cerebrospinal fluid (CSF), white and gray matter (WM and GM, respectively), and skull high density bone (HDB). From these regions, we extracted patches of 16×16 voxels. Each patch corresponds to an area of 8mm × 8mm at the given resolution. For each of the extracted patches, the histogram, and feature vector consisting of two elements: the gray-level median and the threshold-entropy, have been estimated for the classification, as described in the following sub-sections.

Feature-Based Classification

To pre-classify CSF and BM (WM+GM) regions, we did try 40 different features, which has been

Figure 4. Patches of 16×16 voxels taken from normal class regions in a brain CT image (left) and its normalized average histograms (right)

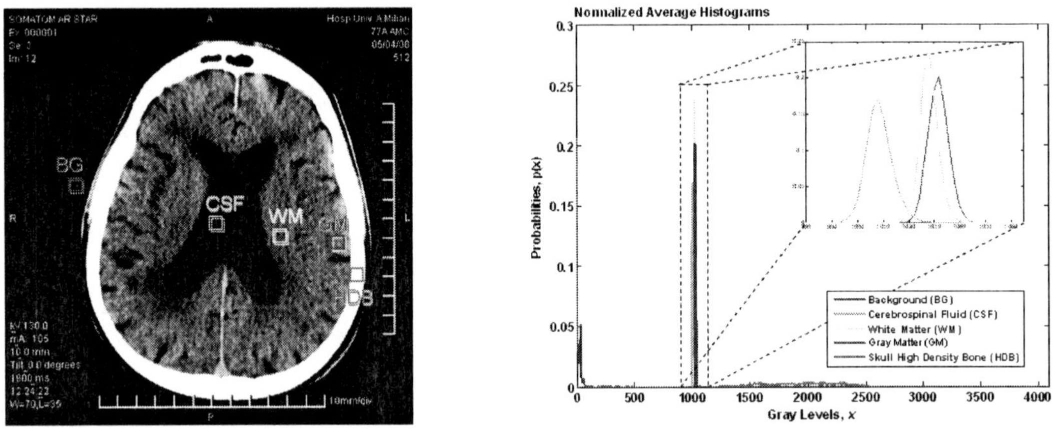

Figure 5. Behavior of best ranked features at (pre)classifying CSF and BM normal patches

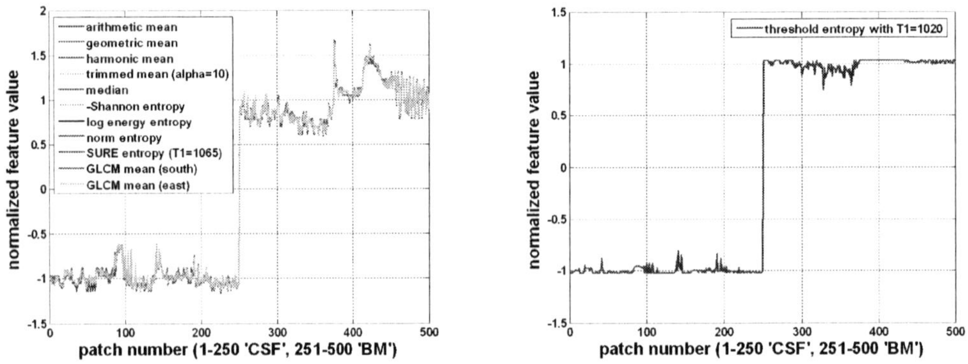

used in numerous works (Huang, 2004; Lehmann, 2005; Müller, 2005; Pokrajac, 2005; Radke, 2005; Benamrane, 2006; Peng, 2006; Sluimer, 2006; Stoitsis, 2006; Strzelecki, 2006; Xu, 2006; Taboada, 2007). Namely:

- **Entropy-based measurements:** Shannon entropy, p-norm entropy, log energy entropy, threshold-entropy, and SURE entropy.
- **Central tendency of the gray-level values:** Arithmetic mean, Trimmed mean, Median, Harmonic mean and Geometric mean.
- **Dispersion of the gray-level values:** Range, Inter quartile range, Standard deviation, Variance, and Median absolute deviation based on means and on medians.
- **Shape of the probability distribution:** Skewness and Kurtosis.
- **Gray-level co-occurrence matrix (GLCM)-based texture measurements:** (Xie, 2006). Contrast, dissimilarity, similarity, homogeneity, angular second moment, energy, maximum probability, entropy,

mean, variance, standard deviation, and correlation. For these GLCM features, we used east and south orientations, and a distance of one, reducing the number of gray-levels to 20 (985-1065, width = 4).

For every labeled patch, we computed the 40 features and we ranked them according to their *classification relevance* by using the FSV (Feature selection via concave minimization and support vector) function in Spider, a Machine Learning Toolbox for MATLAB (http://www.kyb.tuebingen.mpg.de/bs/people/spider/index.html).

According to this ranking, the best performing features, to recognize brain areas in CT images, are the entropy-based features, followed by those representing the central tendency. The dispersion parameters and the shape of the probability distributions perform poorly, as it can be expected from *Figure 4*. Surprisingly, none of the GLCM features was ranked amongst the first 8 best features.

In order to assess the 12 best ranked features (median and arithmetic, geometric, harmonic, and trimmed at 10% means; Shannon's, log energy, 2-norm, SURE, and threshold entropies; and GLCM means in the south and east directions), we selected a set of patches from the CSF and BM classes. Every feature has been normalized according to the mean (μ) and the standard deviation (σ) (estimated over the set of patches).

$$x_n(i) = \frac{x_i - \mu}{\sigma} \quad (15)$$

Figure 5 depicts the plots of the normalized feature values (x_n), for the selected set of 250 CSF patches (patches numbered 1 to 250 in *Figure 5*), and 250 BM patches (patches numbered 251-375 from WM; and patches 376-500 from GM). As it can be seen, all the considered 12 features can distinguish CSF (patches 1-250, corresponding to normalized feature values around -1) from BM (patches 251-500, around +1). However, within BM, the subclasses WM (patches 251-375) and GM (patches 376-500) can not be differentiated. From the 12 considered features, only the threshold entropy H_{thr} (16), with threshold $T_1 = 1020$ (*Figure 5* right) being the gray-level intersection between the CSF and BM prototype histograms, performs slightly different.

$$H_{thr} = \#\{i, \quad x_i > T_1\} \quad (16)$$

As 11 of these features behave similarly, we decided to use a feature vector consisting of two elements: (i) the gray-level median m_{50} (because it is the best suited feature in the presence of artifacts) and (ii) the threshold entropy H_{thr} to (pre)classify the patches under test. Therefore, the feature-based classification will use two prototype vectors (each of two elements, m_{50} and H_{thr}), V_{CSF} and V_{BM} for the classes CSF and BM, respectively. The classes will be characterized by their means (m_{CSF} and m_{BM}, for the CSF and the BM classes, respectively) and covariance matrices (C_{CSF} and C_{BM}).

For the classification, the Mahalanobis-inspired distance (Rousseeuw, 2006; Daszykowski, 2007; Taboada, 2007), D_M, between the feature vector of the *i*-th patch, V_i, and the prototype feature vectors, V_{CSF} and V_{BM}, are computed:

$$D_M(V_i, V_{CSF}) = \sqrt{(V_i - m_{CSF})^T C_{CSF}^{-1} (V_i - m_{CSF})}$$
$$D_M(V_i, V_{BM}) = \sqrt{(V_i - m_{BM})^T C_{BM}^{-1} (V_i - m_{BM})} \quad (17)$$

The *i*-th patch is (pre)assigned to the class for which the distance D_M has a minimum value, as the nearest neighbor pattern matching in (Gering, 2003).

Histogram-Based Classification

Despite their simplicity, histogram-based techniques have proved their worth as a low-cost, low-level approach. Therefore, to complement the feature-based classification, we propose a histogram-based scheme with variable-bin-size histograms.

The variable-bin-size histograms are based on the traditional window/level adjustments used to visually analyze CT images of BM and skull (*Figure 2*). More precisely, we forced a first bin to include gray-level values below 985, BG class, and a last bin over 1250, matching the HDB. The rest of the bins are adjusted as in the brain window/level adjustment (985-1065, width=4). Finally we obtain 23 bins: 0, 985, 989, …, 1061, 1065, 1250, and 4095.

After computing the variable-bin-size histogram of every patch, we estimated an average (prototype) normalized histogram for the CSF and BM classes, respectively. Let, h_{CSF} and h_{BM} be such reference histograms. Then, we evaluated several histogram-based distances, D_h, reported in the literature (Lehmann, 2005; Rousseeuw, 2006; Stoitsis, 2006; Taboada, 2007). Namely, the L1, L2 and L∞ norms, Matusita distance, Bhattacharyya distance, and χ^2 distance, Histogram intersection, Kullback-Leibler divergence, Harmonic mean of Kullback-Leibler (symmetric), and the Earth Mover's distance.

In order to measure the ability of the considered distances for the separation between classes, we propose the use of a *separation measure*, *S*, subtracting the two histogram-based distances. For instance, if the expected class is BM, then S_i is computed for the *i*-th patch (with histogram h_i) by using D_h as

$$S_i = D_h(h_i,h_{CSF}) - D_h(h_i,h_{BM}). \quad (18)$$

The analysis of the ranking of the 10 distances, with respect to the classification rate and the separation measure, showed that the best results are obtained using the χ^2 distance ($D_{h1}=D\chi^2$) and L∞ norm ($D_{h2}=D_{L\infty}$).

$$D_{\chi^2}(x,y) = \sum_{i=1}^{n}\frac{(x_i - y_i)^2}{x_i + y_i}, \quad (19)$$

$$D_{L\infty}(x,y) = \max_{1\le i\le n}|x_i - y_i|. \quad (20)$$

Classification Stage

The block diagram of the classification stage is shown in *Figure 6*. After loading the image slice or the whole set of slices (of size 512×512 each) from a CT study, a sliding window of 16×16 voxels generates a set of patches with 50% of overlapping (in total, 3969 patches per slice) (Taboada, 2007). An important part of these patches (N_e) can be immediately pre-classified as BG, or HDB. The rest of the patches (N_r = 3969 – N_e) will be classified using the following procedure.

For the feature-based classification, we get:

$$minD_M(i) = \min(D_M(V_i,V_{CSF}), D_M(V_i,V_{BM})),\ 1<i<N_r,$$

$$\text{if } minD_M(i) = D_M(V_i,V_{CSF}), \text{ then } Mclass(i) = \text{CSF},\ 1<i<N_r,$$

$$\text{if } minD_M(i) = D_M(V_i,V_{BM}), \text{ then } Mclass(i) = \text{BM},\ 1<i<N_r. \quad (21)$$

For the histogram-based classification, the nearest neighbor pattern matching approach is applied, using the first best ranked distances D_{h1} and D_{h2}:

$$minD_h(i) = \min(D_{h1}(h_i,h_{CSF}), D_{h1}(h_i,h_{BM})),\ 1<i<N_r,$$

$$\text{if } minD_h(i) = D_{h1}(h_i,h_{CSF}), \text{ then } hclass(i) = \text{CSF},\ 1<i<N_r,$$

$$\text{if } minD_h(i) = D_{h1}(h_i,h_{BM}), \text{ then } hclass(i) = \text{BM},\ 1<i<N_r. \quad (22)$$

$$minD_{h2}(i) = \min(D_{h2}(h_i,h_{CSF}), D_{h2}(h_i,h_{BM})),\ 1<i<N_r,$$

if $minD_{h2}(i) = D_{h2}(h_i, h_{CSF})$, then $h2class(i) =$ CSF, $1<i<N_r$,

if $minD_{h2}(i) = D_{h2}(h_i, h_{BM})$, then $h2class(i) =$ BM, $1<i<N_r$. (23)

As there are only two possible normal classes, the final classification is as follows:

if $hclass(i) = Mclass(i)$, then $class(i) = hclass(i)$, else $class(i) = h2class(i)$. (24)

After these stages, it may happen that some anomalies had been inadvertently pre-classified as pertaining to a normal class (CSF or BM), i.e. there may be some false negatives. To improve the AD performance, we computed the robust distance (Rousseeuw, 2006), D_{rob}, among all the feature vectors (V) characterizing the patches pre-classified in the same class,

$$D_{rob}(V) = \sqrt{(V - m_{rob})^T S_{rob}^{-1} (V - m_{rob})}. \quad (25)$$

We can detect anomaly patches by their large values of D_{rob}. The robust distance D_{rob} is very similar to D_M in (17), but unlike the classical centre (mean), a robust method uses a minimum covariance determinant (MCD), m_{rob}, as a multivariate location estimate. In addition, D_{rob} uses a scatter matrix, S_{rob}, instead of the covariance matrix in (17) and it is not affected by the masking effect. We use the MCD method (Rousseeuw, 2006), implemented in the MATLAB function FAST-MCD (available at http://www.agoras.ua.ac.be).

Figure 6. Proposed AD system: Block diagram of the classification stage

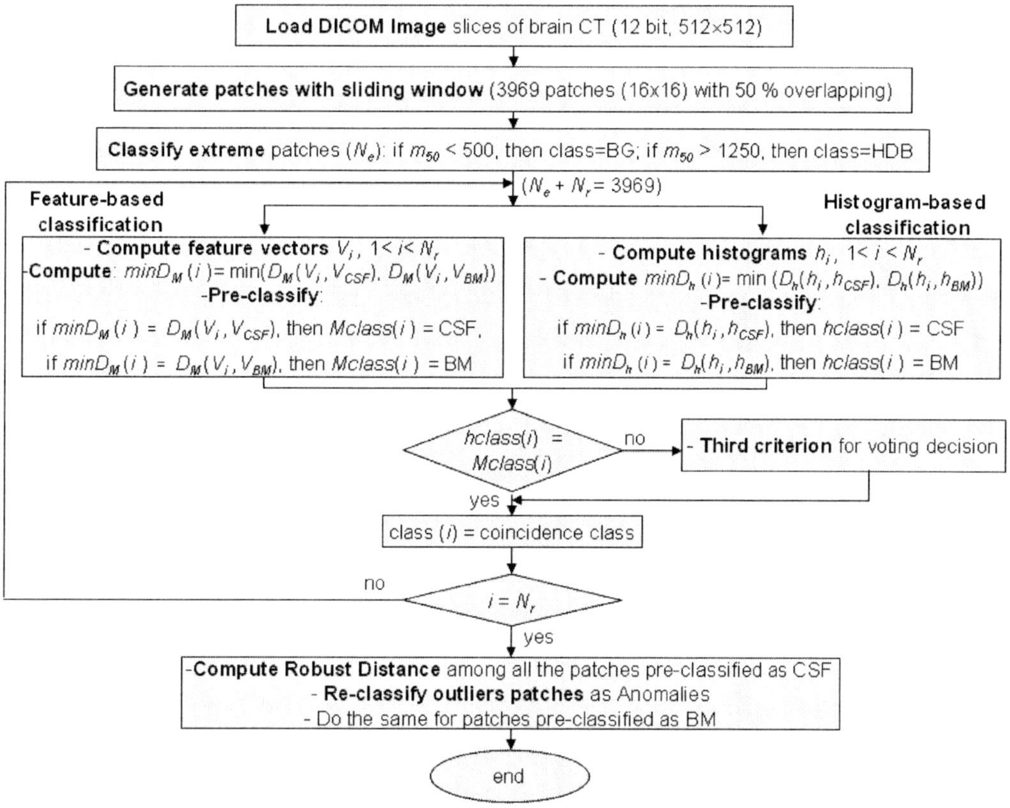

Results and Discussion

Pre-Classification Stage

Combining both best 'gross classifier' approaches: feature-based using the vector (m_{50}, H_{thr}), and histogram-based with χ^2 and $L\infty$ norm distances as D_{h1} and D_{h2}, respectively, the obtained rate of classification was 100%.

Note that the performed pre-classification (BM or CSF) is just an intermediate stage to deal with the variable 'background' (normal tissues) where the anomalies can appear in disguise. The final purpose is to detect the anomalies or lesions represented in the CT images.

For all the patches, pre-classified as normalcy, in a particular class (BM or CSF), the robust distance is computed as in (25) to reclassify those patches with associated D_{rob} over a threshold computed with the FASTMCD function.

We should note that, applying (25) with the mean and the covariance matrix estimated in the training stage (m_{CSF} and C_{CSF} for CSF class, or m_{BM} and C_{BM} for BM class), where only normal patches were used (no outliers or anomalies), one may obtain similar results. Despite the higher computational burden, we propose the robust distance with the MCD estimate because this robust approach circumvents any slight calibration or performance issue biasing the data under assessment (or those used for training) by re-adjusting the characteristics of the mean and covariance matrix.

Classification Stage

We performed some evaluation of the AD algorithm of *Figure 6* for the classification stage by using 10 slices, containing various representative lesions: tumors, hemorrhages and infarctions areas (*Figure 7* shows four of them). Observe that some are hyper-dense (brighter than the surrounding tissue) and some are hypo-dense (darker than surroundings).

The hyper-dense lesions have been detected almost always, i.e. bleeding, hemorrhage, calcifications, or calcified tumors, as in the example of *Figure 8*, although sometimes they could be

Figure 7. Examples of lesions to detect with the AD system here implemented

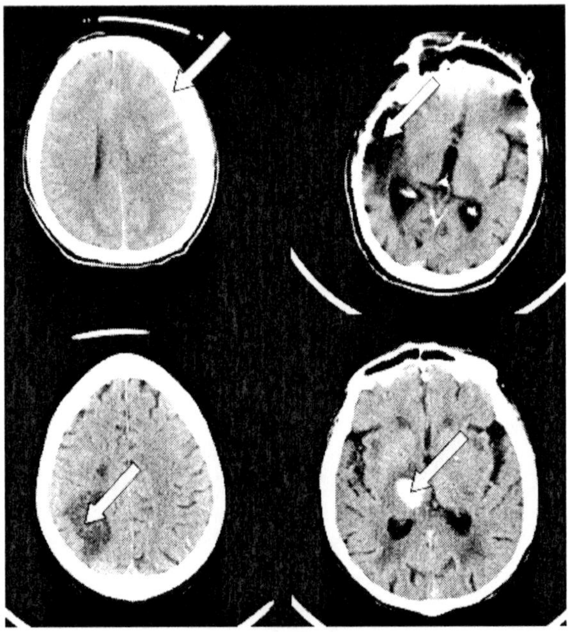

confused with GM, which is part of the BM normal class.

In the obtained AD results for the 10 slices (images), we observe an overall sensitivity of 74.2%, specificity of 99.8%, and positive predictive value of 84.1%. The Jaccard distance (65%) has a similar behavior as the proposed *AD rate* (60%), but the latter is even more sensitive to any variation of performance.

The proposed AD algorithm can not identify hypo-dense lesions with gray-level values between those of normal classes, BM and CSF, and sometimes totally overlapped with the latter. Hence, we will need to incorporate in future work other criteria to correctly discriminate these classes. A good candidate should take into account position and region properties such as area, elongation, compactness, etc.

FUTURE TRENDS

The universe of applications of AD algorithms for medical image analysis will consolidate and advance in the near future. Automatic annotations of anomalies in medical images by AD systems will help teaching and research, along with several clinical applications, including region-based compression algorithms for telemedicine. Definitively, more AD algorithms will succeed in clinical practice in the near future because it will be a market for them; they will be faster and easier to use, more reliable, and interactively correctable if needed. Recently, certain AD systems have evolved from simple detection to interpretation, characterization and follow-up (Sluimer, 2006; Stoitsis, 2006); that will be the future.

Unfortunately, appropriate medical image databases carefully annotated for AD algorithm benchmarking are not currently available. Al-

Figure 8. Example of performance evaluation of AD system

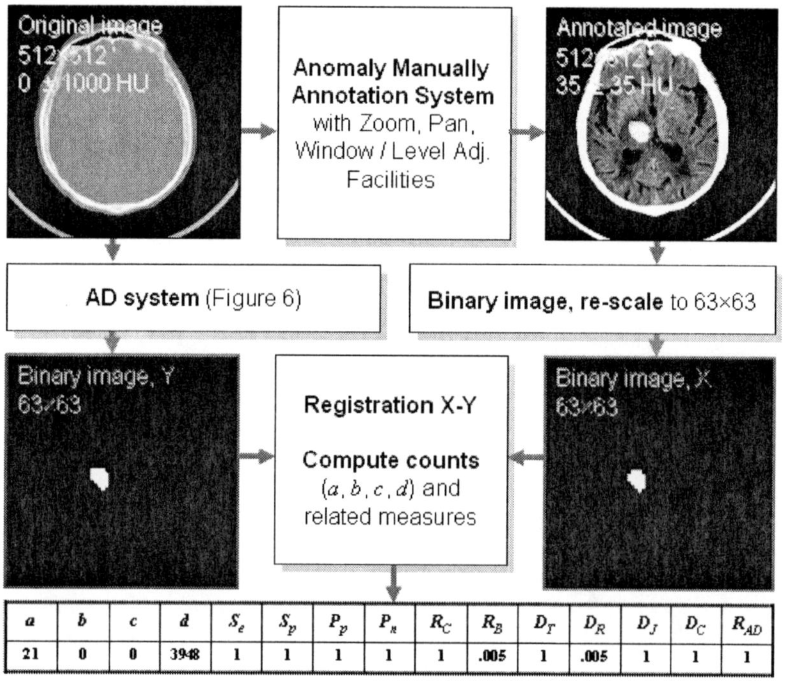

a	b	c	d	S_e	S_p	P_p	P_n	R_C	R_B	D_T	D_R	D_J	D_C	R_{AD}
21	0	0	3948	1	1	1	1	1	.005	1	.005	1	1	1

though, in certain areas, this necessity has been recognized and first steps are being undertaken (Sluimer, 2006; Messmer, 2006), more efforts should be focused in this direction to allow objective comparison of particular AD algorithms.

For certain applications, such as surgical planning, surgical guidance (DiMaio, 2007), volumetric analysis (Ashton, 2006), time series analysis (Radke, 2005; Huang, 2007), and computer aided diagnosis (Iyatomi, 2006; Peng, 2006; Sluimer, 2006), images should be annotated. However, manual annotation is a subjective and very expensive task. In these applications, automatic segmentation of anomalies by using AD algorithms can save much of the time required for sketching contours, with very high stability. AD systems will take care increasingly of this annotation process, or at least be considered as a starting point or as a second opinion reading in a screening program.

More and more AD algorithms will be incorporated into the medical imaging equipment, as well as in computer-assisted diagnosis and computer-aided surgery systems, to help and complement doctors' interpretations. As AD algorithms will be part of the imaging systems, to reduce their effective computational time, some processing stages should be performed from the time the data are acquired.

Bioinformatics, pharmaceutical research, nanomedicine and neurosciences are currently some of the most prolific research fields, which should benefit to a great extent from medical imaging AD systems. Online distributed approaches for AD will become more available in applications such as high content screening with immediate corrective action, early termination, and redesign of assays (Goode, 2007). Opportunities may arise where AD at the organ level images will benefit from findings at the molecular, cellular, and atomic levels. On the other hand, results at the organ level imaging and microscopy combined, merging macro and micro worlds, may help researches on physiological functions. We believe that AD systems will evolve from simple detection to interpretation, characterization and follow-up.

CONCLUSION

AD in medical image analysis is a complex field associated to several imaging modalities to study lesions, structurally and compositionally distinct from surrounding healthy tissue, in certain organs. There have been numerous works on AD systems for digital mammography, lung CT, and brain MR imaging. Other areas have started to obtain encouraging results, and new applications are devised these days.

To evaluate the performance of AD systems, annotated datasets (ground truth) and some adequate assessment measures as gold standards should be defined. In this work, we did propose the AD rate or capability, R_{AD}, a very complete measure for this purpose.

AD associated to brain CT images, although not undertaken before in the literature, presents a group of challenging problems. Histogram-based and feature-based measurements were combined with a nearest neighbor pattern matching approach to obtain a pre-classification of image patches decomposed with a sliding window. Later, robust distance computation inside every normal class decides if there is any outlier (anomaly) or not. Better results could be obtained by using machine learning approaches to produce useful rules, such as age of the patient, as well as region-based measures. According to these rules, part of the 'normal regions' may be re-classified as anomalies, improving final results.

REFERENCES

Ashton, E. (2006). *Method and system for automatic identification and quantification of abnormal anatomical structures in medical images.* United States Patent 7,103,224.

Benamrane, N. *et al.* (2006). Fuzzy Neural Networks and Genetic Algorithms for Medical Images Interpretation. *Proc. Geometric Modeling and Imaging— New Trends, IEEE Computer Society.*

Bertelli, L. *et al.* (2006). A semi-automatic system for segmentation of cardiac M-mode images. *Pattern Analysis and Applications*, *9*(4), 293-306.

Bouix, S. *et al.* (2007). On evaluating brain tissue classifiers without a ground truth. *NeuroImage*, *36*, 1207–1224.

Chiracharit, W. *et al.* (2007). Normal mammogram detection based on local probability difference transforms and support vector machines. *IEICE Transactions on Information and Systems, E90-D*(1), 258-270.

Daszykowski, M. *et al.* (2007). Robust statistics in data analysis — A review of Basic concepts. *Chemometrics and Intelligent Laboratory Systems*, *85*, 203–219

DiMaio, S. *et al.* (2007). Challenges in image-guided therapy system design. *NeuroImage*, *37*, 144–151.

Ekin, A. *et al.* (2007). Improving information quality of MR brain images by fully automatic and robust image analysis methods. *Journal of the Society for Information Display*, *15*(6), 367-376.

Gering, D. T. (2003). *Recognizing deviations from normalcy for brain tumor segmentation*. PhD Thesis. Department of Electrical Engineering and Computer Science. Massachusetts Institute of Technology.

Goode, A. *et al.* (2007). *Distributed Online Anomaly Detection in High-Content Screening.* CMU-CS-07-177, School of Computer Science, Carnegie Mellon University.

Gu, G. *et al.* (2006). *An Information-Theoretic Measure of Intrusion Detection Capability.* ASIACCS'06 , March 21-24, Taipei, Taiwan, 90-101.

Hersh, W. (2006). Medical Image Retrieval Protocol. *ImageCLEFmed 2006*, available at http://www.clef-campaign.org/, last updated - 14 June 2006.

Hodge, V. J., & Austin, J. (2004). A Survey of Outlier Detection Methodologies. *Artificial Intelligence Review*, *22*, 85–126.

Huang, Y. L., & Chen, D. R. (2004). Watershed Segmentation For Breast Tumor In 2-D Sonography. *Ultrasound in Med. & Biol.*, *30*(5), 625–632.

Huang, X. *et al.* (2007). *System and Method for Whole Body Landmark Detection, Segmentation and Change Quantification in Digital Images.* Patent WO2007044508.

Ikedo, Y. *et al.* (2007). Development of a fully automatic scheme for detection of masses in whole breast ultrasound images. *Medical Physics*, *34*(11), 4378-4388.

Iyatomi, H. *et al.* (2006). Quantitative assessment of tumor extraction from dermoscopy images and evaluation of computer-based extraction methods for an automatic melanoma diagnostic system. *Melanoma Research*, *16*(2), 183-190.

Karnan, M., & Thangavel, K. (2007). Automatic detection of the breast border and nipple position on digital mammograms using genetic algorithm for asymmetry approach to detection of microcalcifications. *Computer Methods and Programs in Biomedicine*, *87*(1), 12-20.

Kelm, B. M. *et al.* (2007). Automated Estimation of Tumor Probability in Prostate Magnetic Resonance Spectroscopic Imaging: Pattern Recognition vs. Quantification. *Magnetic Resonance in Medicine*, *57*, 150–159.

Krivacic, R. T. *et al.* (2004). A rare-cell detector for cancer. *Proc. of the National Academy of Sciences of the United States of America, Clinical Cancer Research, 101*(29), 10501 – 10504.

Lee, C.-H. *et al.* (2005). Segmenting Brain Tumors with Conditional Random Fields and Support Vector Machines. *Lecture Notes in Computer Science, 3765*, 469-478.

Lehmann, T. M. *et al.* (2005). Automatic categorization of medical images for content-based retrieval and data mining. *Computerized Medical Imaging and Graphics, 29*, 143–155.

Markou, M., & Singh, S. (2003a). Novelty Detection: A Review, Part 1: Statistical Approaches. *Signal Processing, 83*, 2499–2521.

Markou, M., & Singh, S. (2003b). Novelty Detection: A Review, Part 2: Neural network-based approaches. *Signal Processing, 83*, 2481–2497.

Menze, B. H. *et al.* (2006). *Optimal Classification of Long Echo Time In Vivo Magnetic Resonance Spectra in the Detection of Recurrent Brain Tumors.* Multidimensional Image Processing, IWR, University of Heidelberg.

Messmer, P. *et al.* (2006). A CT Database for Research, Development and Education: Concept and Potential. *Journal of Digital Imaging, 0*(0), 1-6, Online publication 07 August 2006.

Minhas, A. S., & Reddy, M. R. (2005). Neural network-based approach for AD in the lungs region by electrical impedance tomography. *Physiol. Meas., 26*, 489–502

Montgomery, D. W. G. *et al.* (2007). Fully automated segmentation of oncological PET volumes using a combined multiscale and statistical model. *Medical Physics, 34*(2), 722-736.

Müller, H. *et al.* (2005). Benefits of Content-based Visual Data Access in Radiology. *RadioGraphics, 25*, 849-858.

Peng, Y. *et al.* (2006). Knowledge-discovery incorporated evolutionary search for microcalcification detection in breast cancer diagnosis. *Artificial Intelligence in Medicine, 37*(1), 43-53.

Pokrajac, D. *et al.*, (2005). Applying spatial distribution analysis techniques to classification of 3D medical images. *Artificial Intelligence in Medicine, 33*, 261-280.

Prastawa, M. *et al.* (2004). A brain tumor segmentation framework based on outlier detection. *Medical Image Analysis, 26*(8), 275–283.

Pratikakis, I. *et al.*, (2005). Three-Dimensional Multiscale watershed segmentation of MR images, in *Medical Image Analysis Methods,* Editor. Lena Costaridou, CRS - Taylor & Francis, 271—314.

Radke, R. J. *et al.* (2005). Image Change Detection Algorithms: A Systematic Survey. *IEEE Transactions on Image Processing, 14*(3), 294-307.

Rousseeuw, P. J. *et al.* (2006). Robustness and Outlier Detection in Chemometrics. *Critical Reviews in Analytical Chemistry, 36*, 221–242.

Ségonne, F. (2005). *Segmentation of Medical Images under Topological Constraints.* PhD Thesis. Department of Electrical Engineering and Computer Science. Massachusetts Institute of Technology.

Selvi, S. T. *et al.* (2005). *Breast Cancer Detection Using MMRF.* Proceedings of the International Conference on Information and Automation, December 15-18, Colombo, Sri Lanka, 127-132.

Shinkareva, S. V. *et al.* (2006). Classification of functional brain images with a spatio-temporal dissimilarity map. *NeuroImage, 33*, 63–71.

Sklansky, J., & Ballard, D. (1973). Tumor Detection in Radiographs. *Computers and Biomedical Research, 6*(4), 299-321.

Sluimer, I. *et al.* (2006). Computer Analysis of Computed Tomography Scans of the Lung: A Survey. *IEEE Trans. on Medical Imaging, 25*(4), 385-405.

Spinosa, E. J., & de Carvalho, A. (2005). Support vector machines for novel class detection in Bioinformatics. *Genet. Mol. Res., 4*(3), 608-615.

Stoitsis, J. *et al.* (2006). A Modular Software System to Assist Interpretation of Medical Images—Application to Vascular Ultrasound Images. *IEEE Transactions on Instrumentation and Measurement, 55*(6), 1944-1952.

Strzelecki, M. *et al.* (2006). Classification and segmentation of intracardiac masses in cardiac tumor echocardiograms. *Computerized Medical Imaging and Graphics*, *30*, 95–107.

Taboada-Crispi, A., & Sahli, H. (2007). Experimental System for Image Anomaly Detection Based on Features and Distances. *Ingeniería Electrónica, Automática y Comunicaciones*, *28*(2), 8-13.

Vovk, U. *et al.* (2007). A Review of Methods for Correction of Intensity Inhomogeneity in MRI. *IEEE Transactions on Medical Imaging, 26*(3), 405-421.

Wei, L. *et al.* (2005). Relevance vector machine for automatic detection of clustered microcalcifications. *IEEE Transactions on Medical Imaging, 24*(10), 1278-1285.

Xiaoxue, Y. *et al.* (2004). *Abnormality detection in retinal images*. Technical Report MIT-3845, MIT, Massachusetts Institute of Technology.

Xie, X. (2006). *Defect Detection in Random Colour Textures*. PhD Thesis. Faculty of Engineering. Department of Computer Science. University of Bristol.

Xu, R. *et al.*, (2006). Target Detection with Improved Image Texture Feature Coding Method and Support Vector Machine. *International Journal of Intelligent Technology*, *1*(1), 47-56.

KEY TERMS

Anomaly: Deviation or departure from the normal or common order, form or rule; one that is peculiar, irregular, abnormal or difficult to classify. In image analysis, anomalies are unknown targets, which are relatively small and with low probability of occurrence. Tumors, micro-calcifications, and vascular irregularities are examples of anomalies in the medical image analysis framework.

Anomaly Detection (AD) Systems: Systems used to detect anomalies. They can be developed with no prior knowledge of the data, or modeling both normality and anomalies, or modeling only normality. In the medical imaging context, the third approach is the best suited. AD systems can be based on statistical methods, neural networks, or machine learning.

Imaging Modalities: Different physical principles involved in the acquisition of an image. In the medical imaging context, we can mention: photography, endoscope, microscopy, electrical impedance tomography, ultrasound-based systems, X rays, CT, MRI and fMRI, MRSI, SPECT, PET and PET/CT.

Content-Based Image Retrieval: Process of retrieving images from databases based on its real visual contents (features of texture, shape, and color) by using signal processing, pattern recognition and computer vision methods.

Segmentation: The partitioning of digital images into different regions, which group elements (pixels or voxels) with similar feature values.

Ground Truth: The image gold standard for assessing detection/classification algorithms. This term was originally used to designate the true information gathered in ground to evaluate remote sensing techniques like aerial photographs or satellite imagery, but it has been generalized to other scenarios.

Measures of Performance: Measures used to evaluate the performance of AD algorithms, by using images with available ground truths. Most of them are based on the coincidences (true positives and true negatives) and not coincidences (false positives and false negatives) between regions detected/classified by algorithms under assessment and the corresponding regions in the ground truth.

Window/Level Adjustment: Mapping of portions of the image dynamic range to the dynamic range of the display monitor. For instance, a 12 bit CT image should be re-scaled for brain matter analysis with a window/level adjustment around 35 ± 35 Hounsfield Units (i.e. gray-levels between 1000 and 1070). This is the base of the variable-bin-size histogram approach in this work.

ENDNOTES

1. Its complementary dissimilarity measure, $(1-S_p)$, is known as the false alarm rate.
2. Its complementary dissimilarity measure, $(1-R_C)$, is known as the misclassification rate and it is proportional to the square of the Euclidean distance, which is the Hamming distance in communications.
3. In a context where all the patients are expected to have certain degree of lesions or anomalies, e.g. a follow up program or a confirmation study, the imbalance is not that critical, but still $(d+b) >> (a+c)$.

Chapter XXVIII
Evaluation of Medical Image Compression

C. Delgorge-Rosenberger
Université d'Orléans, France

C. Rosenberger
GREYC – ENSICAEN – Université Caen Basse Normandie – CNRS, France

ABSTRACT

The authors present in this chapter an overview on evaluation of medical image compression. The different methodologies used in the literature are presented. Subjective evaluation uses some a priori knowledge such as the judgment of experts or the ability to realize a correct diagnosis. Objective evaluation generally takes into account the value of metrics: the PSNR is an example of such a criterion. The goal of hybrid evaluation is to realize a reliable judgment while having a simple computation. The authors discuss on the benefits and drawbacks of these approaches. The European Project called OTELO in which they were involved, gives feedback on ultrasound image compression.

INTRODUCTION

Medical imaging is an important and a powerful technique whose goal is to facilitate the expert diagnosis. Many image processing algorithms can be used within this context such as: image filtering, compression, segmentation, interpretation or retrieval... One important issue concerns the evaluation of different image processing results for the medical expert: as for example, image filtering can improve the image quality but can disturb the ability of a medical expert to make a diagnosis.

The proposed chapter deals with the particular field of the evaluation of medical image compression. Image compression for medical applications is an important topic as many image acquisitions are transmitted and stored for a further analysis. In this context, we want to minimize the size of the compressed image while keeping a sufficient quality for the diagnosis. Several evaluation methods have been proposed in the state of the art. We propose in this chapter to make an overview of these approaches. We present different evaluation techniques for either an expert in image processing or for a medical expert. We discuss the advantages and drawbacks of each method. The European OTELO project (Delgorge *et al.*, 2005) in which we have been involved, provides a good experience feedback in the evaluation of medical image compression.

The main objective of the European OTELO project (mObile Tele-Echography with an ultra Light rObot) was to develop a robotic tele-echographic system. A light weight robot holds and moves a real probe on a distant patient according to the expert gesture and permits an image acquisition using a standard ultrasound device (see Figure 1). Ultrasound images constitute the only feedback information available to the medical expert to remotely control the distant robotized system. The expert controls the remote probe holder robot by using a dedicated input device and based on the quality of the received information. The diagnosis made by the specialist strongly depends on the quality of these images. An important task also concerns the evaluation of the quality of the compressed images. Many experimental results are presented in this chapter in order to illustrate the behaviors of the different evaluation methods.

We can distinguish three types of evaluation methods in the state of the art. The first one concerns the subjective evaluation. The quality of a compression result, for any medical types of images, is traditionally evaluated by considering a visual test where many experts examine a large

Figure 1. the OTELO tele-echographic system

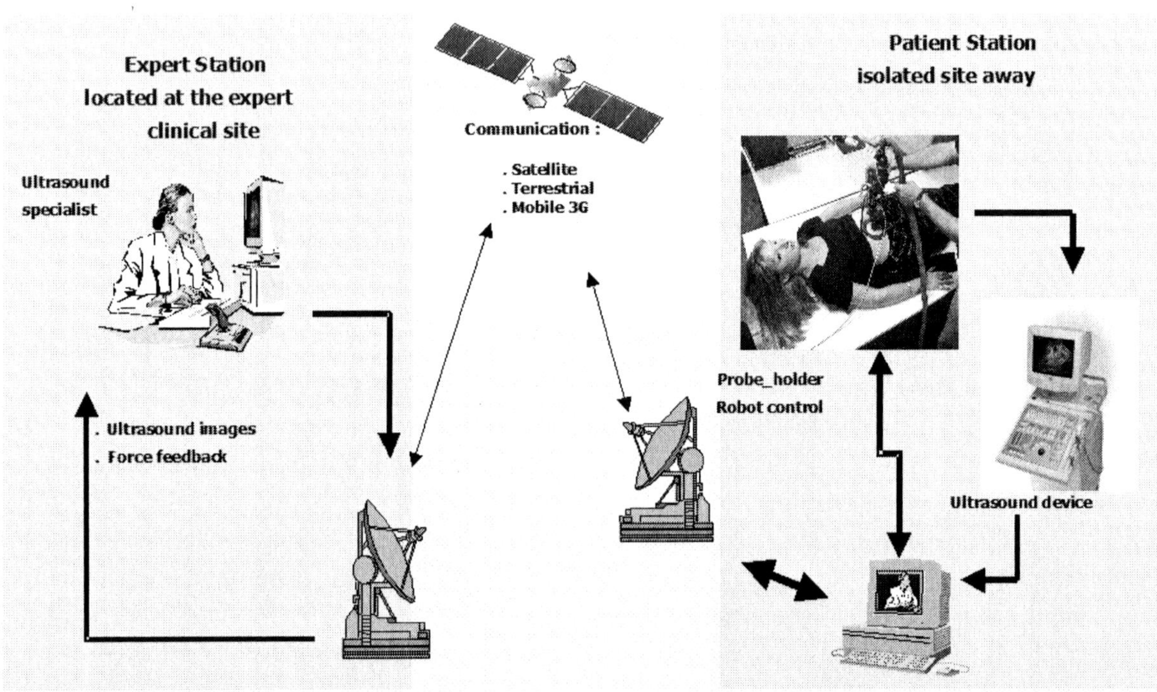

set of images and score each one based on their quality or the ability to make a correct diagnosis. Second, we present the objective evaluation methods. Many statistical criteria have been proposed in the literature to automatically evaluate different compression results of a single image. We propose to compare many of them and discuss their efficiency. Subjective and objective evaluation methods have many advantages and drawbacks. These two approaches are complementary. That is why many works propose an hybrid approach. These methods are presented in the main trust of this article. The goal of these methods is to make a reliable judgment (similar to a medical expert) while using some statistical criteria to make the evaluation of a large set of compression results possible. The future trends in the domain are then proposed and a conclusion is given.

BACKGROUND

Image compression is an important issue in medical imaging as the distant visualization of medical images is now possible through high bandwidth networks for different applications (discussion between experts on a difficult case, storage of medical images of a patient...) and as telemedecine becomes an emergent technology nowadays (Delgorge et al., 2005).

Image compression is an image processing algorithm whose objective is to decrease the size of storage of the image while preserving as much as possible its visual quality (see Figure 2). Even if this definition is quite simple, the main problem is to evaluate the quality of a compression result. As for example, the result given in Figure 2 is clearly not very good but it is difficult to say if this quality would be satisfactory for a medical expert to make a diagnosis.

We present in the following sections two classical approaches for the evaluation of medical image compression results.

Subjective Evaluation

The evaluation of image processing results can be realized in a subjective way. It can be done through different approaches:

- The quality of a result can be visually appreciated by an user on a benchmark image. The well known « Lena » image is an example. All researchers in image processing can rather easily compare the results they

Figure 2. Example of a JPEG compression result (ratio 5%) of an ultrasound image

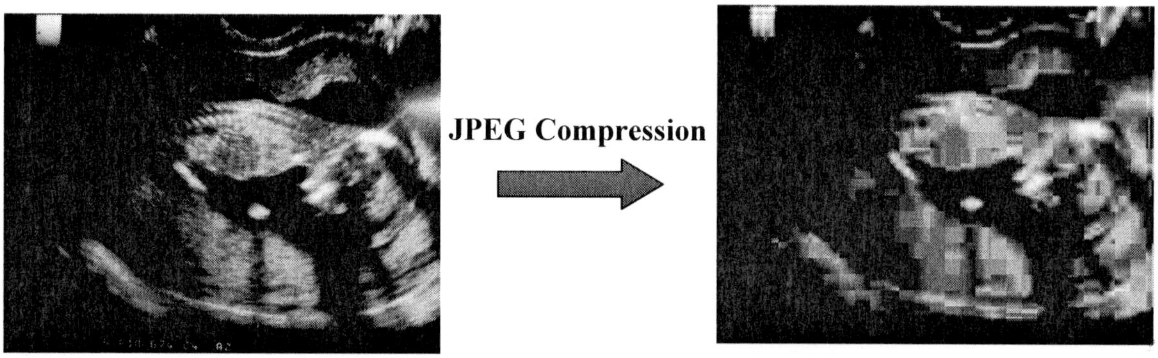

obtain using their own algorithm with some from the state of the art;

- It is also possible to use a synthetic ground truth in order to compare the results of different algorithms. As for example, synthetic images can be used in order to evaluate the quality of a medical image segmentation result;
- The use of a phantom (synthetic material) also permits to evaluate some image processing results while keeping all acquisitions artifacts;
- Another solution consists in asking as many experts as possible to quantify the quality of the obtained results. For medical applications, many approaches were defined in the literature such as the simple visualization of results, the visual comparison of results or the performance quantification in term of ability to realize a correct medical diagnosis.

Nowadays, the two first methods are rarely used because the achieved evaluation reliability is poor. The two last methods are more and more used with many alternatives. We present in this section, the possible solutions and some associated feedbacks.

In the multimedia world, the quantification of the subjective quality perceived by an observer remains the only reference as regards to the quality of images (Klein, 1993). The International Consultative Committee of Radio communication (CCIR) defined multiple standardized evaluation methods to define the image quality. The principle of a subjective test is contingent upon a standardized structure, which consists of an observers group, a quantification method for the appreciation of the visual quality (i.e. a subjective scale of quality notation), a set of test images, a display material, a test room and a protocol defining the notation process of the images as well as the experimental conditions.

The three most current tests are the following (International Telecommunication Union, 2002):

- **Method with one stimulus:** It makes it possible to evaluate many imagery systems. A set of images degraded by various treatments is presented in a random order. The appreciation of the image quality is given by the expert without any reference image. The scale of notation can be defined or built by the observer itself as the test advances. Figure 3 shows an example of such a subjective evaluation with 5 possible scores (from unacceptable to very good). The main problem of this approach is that it requires a certain number of images for an observer in order to stabilize the scale of scores. Note also that the original image is not given, that is not very comfortable for the observer.
- **Method with double stimulus:** Images are evaluated per pair: an original image (the reference) and a compression result. The observer must score this result according to the preset scale. In general, two categories of scales are proposed: the first translates the feeling of the visual quality of the image (that can be considered as a criterion of "nice image"), the second translates the degree of degradation (that is a criterion of "good image" for the application).
- **Comparative method:** Different images representing the multiple treatments we want to compare are presented at the observer. The comparison is realized considering the different compression results. The observer must sort all of them considering the alteration associated to the original image. Figure 4 gives an example where an expert is asked to sort 5 compression results given the original image.

Figure 3. Example of an evaluation using only one stimulus

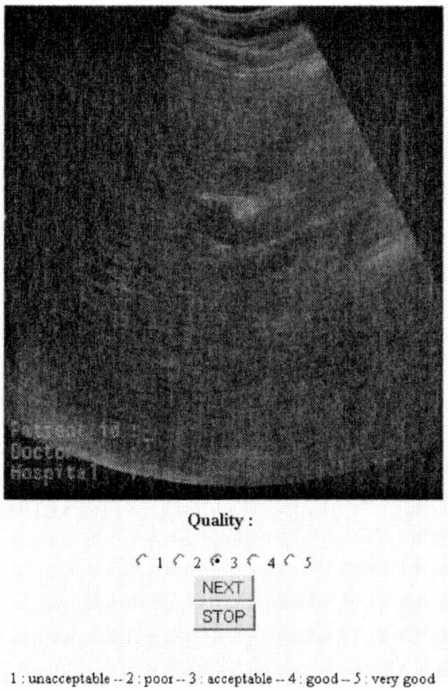

A large quantity of recommendations is published (International Telecommunication Union, 2002). They relate mainly to:

- the environment of the test: displaying conditions, the visualization material, distance of the expert to the screen,
- the resolution and contrast of the screen,
- the image database used for the test,
- observers (or experts): they must be at least 15, their vision must be measured and corrected if necessary, their experiment must be raised (specialty, age),
- the protocol of the test: it must be precisely explained to the observers,
- the duration of test: it must last at least 30 minutes,
- the analysis and the presentation of the results.

This kind of tests implies that all the experts follow a very rigorous protocol. This approach requires important human and financial fundings. This is why, it is not rare to find in the literature some studies taking as a starting point these recommendations but not following them all completely (Naegele-Jackson *et al.*, 2002; Azpiroz-Leehan *et al.*, 2004). Moreover, such qualitative and subjective evaluations depend of

Figure 4. Example of an evaluation using the comparative approach

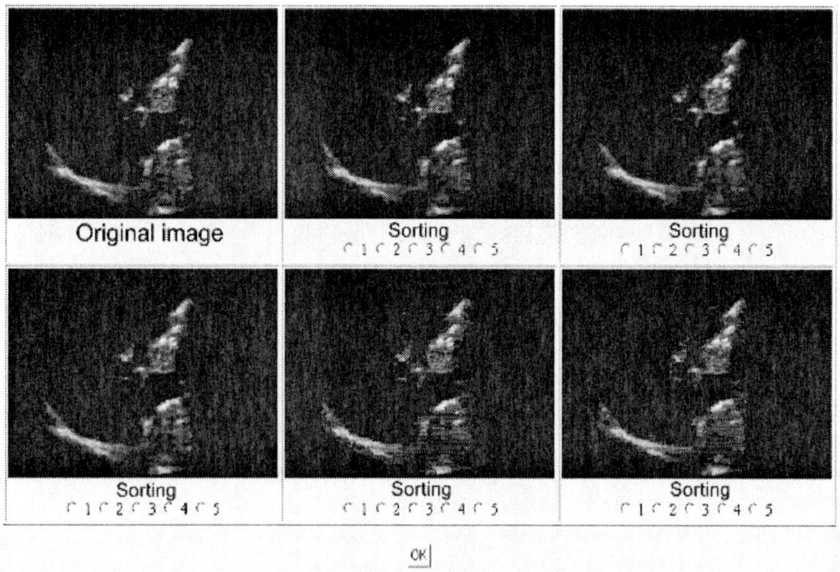

the medical specialty of the expert, its motivation, its availability, its tiredness or its interest in such tests.

Receiver Operating Characteristic (ROC) curves provide many tools to analyze the behavior of models, algorithms or human judgments. It can be used to compare different compression methods by considering the medical application (Weatherburn *et al.*, 2003). In order to choose a compression method or a parameter, we can evaluate the number of cases corresponding to a correct diagnosis. Figure 5 shows an example of ROC curves. We look for a compression method that maximizes the correct positive rate while minimizing the false positive rate. In this case, the Test A has to be preferred than the other one.

Objective Evaluation

A subjective evaluation permits to take into account the medical expertise. The main drawback of this approach is that these tests are very time and manpower consuming. In the literature, many statistical criteria are available and offer a simple tool to evaluate the quality of a compression result according to the original one.

Statistical Criteria

There are several methods to evaluate an image quality. The quality of a compression result can be represented thanks to the ***pixel distance*** between the compression result and the original image. The most known distance is the Minkowski one. From this measure, we obtain many distances: the Euclidean distance, the Manhattan distance, the Chebychev distance and the mean square error (MSE). These measures can be calculated considering the neighborhood of a pixel and not only with one pixel (Tamtaoui *et al.*, 1999). In the image processing literature, the most frequently used measures are the mean square error (MSE) and the peak signal to noise ratio (PSNR) (Yang, 2005; Zhong, 2005).

The similarity between two images can be translated thanks to ***correlation measures***. Several criteria have been proposed in (Linfoot, 1958) and are based on the power spectral density: in particular, the fidelity, the structural content and the normalized cross correlation. The Czekanowski coefficient (Andreautos *et al.*, 1998) measures the correlation between two images considering parameters extracted from both of them.

Figure 5. Example of ROC curves

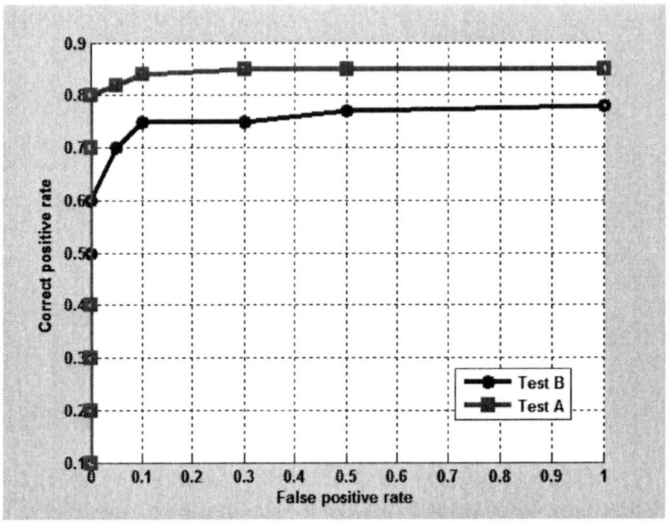

Figure 6. Comparison of two compression results with same PSNR

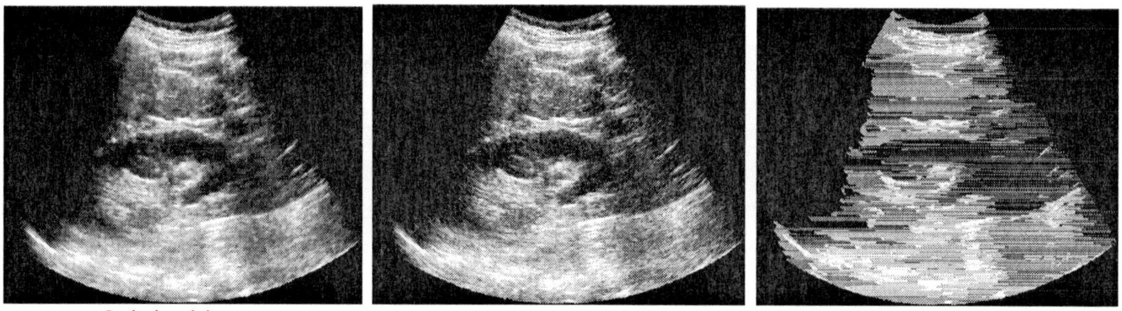

Original image Jpeg-LS result Jpeg result

The above mentioned distances can be calculated in the ***spectral*** field. The goal is also to isolate the image distortion on particular frequency bands or to separate the distortions due to the spectral phase or magnitude (Avcibas *et al.*, 2002).

T-J Chen proposed in (Chen 2003) a new quality measure based on the Moran ***statistics***. The Moran I coefficient translates the studied area clearness, it measures a structural distortion and not a gray level pixel variation. The compressed image statistical properties are used in (Turaga *et al.*, 2004) to evaluate the distortion due to the compression.

Some ***graphical criteria***, based on the histograms of images, have been proposed. The graphical distance also measures the dissimilarity between two histograms or uses the difference image histogram to represent a fidelity measure between the original image and the compression result (Sundersingh, 2000).

Discussion

The main advantage of objective criteria is the simplicity of computation. It is then possible to automatize the evaluation of a large set of compression results. The important drawback of all these statistical criteria is the fact that they do not always correspond to the human visual system (HVS) – representing the observer's visual perception.

The definition of the distance measures depends on the kind of degradations introduced in the image by the compression algorithm. The problem of a graphical measure based on the histogram is the fact that the histogram is not a single function: the same histogram can represent two completely different images.

Moreover, the MSE and PSNR distance measures are very popular due to their simplicity of mathematical definition, even if many studies showed that these criteria are not enough relevant. As for example, Figure 6 shows the bad reliability of the PSNR measure. Two different compression methods (obtained by using the Jpeg-LS and Jpeg algorithms) give two compression results with different compression rate but a similar PSNR value (PSNR=32.5dB). We can clearly see that the Jpeg result quality is visually worst than the Jpeg-LS one, whereas the PSNR evaluates as equal their quality. In this example, we understand that the PSNR is not an efficient criterion for a medical application.

In the OTELO project framework, we studied some statistical criteria and compared them with respect to the results of an expert evaluation. We selected several criteria of different types according to some previous works in the literature (Avcibas *et al.*, 2002): distance mea-

Table 1. Statistical criteria chosen for the OTELO study

D1	Minkowski distance - Mean absolute error
D2	Minkowski distance - Mean square error
D3	Minkowski distance - Modified infinity norm
D4	Neighborhood error - 8 neighbors
D5	Neighborhood error - 24 neighbors
D6	Multi-resolution error
C1	Normalized cross correlation
C2	Image fidelity
C3	Czekonowski correlation
S1	Spectral phase error
S2	Spectral phase-magnitude error
S3	Block spectral magnitude error
S4	Block spectral phase error
S5	Block spectral phase-magnitude error
S6	Block spectral error
P1	Peak signal to noise ratio

sures, denoted *Dx* ; correlation measures *Cx*; spectral measures *Sx* ; PSNR measure *P1* (see Table 1). The three best criteria are D5, S2 and S1, reaching for D5 a maximal value of 65.3%. This means that this criterion is able to reproduce the ability of a medical expert to compare two compression results in **65.3%** of the cases. One can notice that the PSNR criterion, often used for the comparison of compression results, ranks only at the ninth place.

MAIN FOCUS OF THE CHAPTER

We focus in this section on the hybrid evaluation approach. This methodology has for objective to realize a reliable judgment while keeping a simple computation (see Figure 7).

Human Visual System (HVS) Based Criteria

The objective of these criteria is to give some evaluation results close to those we would obtain with a subjective evaluation while having the same calculation simplicity as the objective criteria. Since 1950, many models have been proposed with the goal to simulate the human visual system (HVS), representing the visual perception. The first HVS models were based on an approach called single channel. In this case, the HVS is considered as a simple space filter

Figure 7. Hybrid evaluation

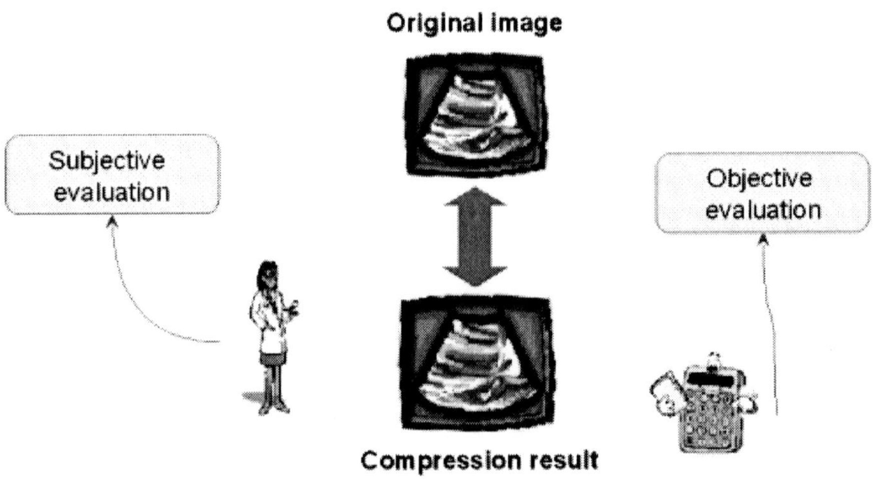

whose characteristics are defined by a function of sensitivity to contrast.

Le Callet and Barba (Le Callet & Barba, 2001) proposed on this principle, a criterion for the evaluation of a compression result. It carries out the combination of perceptual errors between the original image and the compression result to obtain a quality score. The performances of the criterion (evaluated using a subjective evaluation) allow a benefit of about 30% of effectiveness (measured by the coefficient correlation factor) compared to the PSNR. Mathematical models of observers were also developed for the nuclear medicine (Pommert & Höhne 2002). The compression result, the error image or a simple statistical criterion are then balanced by one of these models. The definition of artificial models of observers concerns a rather long and expensive procedure and is dependent on the type of tested images.

Some studies model the HVS and then define some criteria from this model (Carnec, 2004). One can also find in the literature many criteria proposing to combine statistical metrics and some characteristics of the HVS. In the following study (Miyaji *et al.*, 2000), the SNR is balanced by local factors reflecting visual perception (the effect of mask, frequential characteristics). When some specificities of the image are taken into account, one can note that the correlation of the criterion with subjective quality increases (compared to the only use of statistical metrics). The error of evaluation noted by this HVS based criterion decreases about 30% compared to the PSNR.

For the OTELO project, we studied also some HVS based criteria: human visual system based measures H*x* ; contrast measure T*1* (see Table 2). The T1 and H1 criteria gave good results, obtaining respectively the second and fifth place considering the results of all the statistical and HVS based criteria. The T1 criterion is able to reproduce the ability of a medical expert to compare two compression results in **65.3%** of the cases.

Fusion of Evaluation Criteria

The models proposed in the literature to represent the HVS are either too simple or too complex: they do not represent in an efficient way the HVS and they are too complex to obtain a criterion easily usable. In order to mitigate these various disadvantages, some works propose to combine several statistical measures (Cane, 1997) and bring them closer to the HVS (see Figure 8). One can find some works on combinations of criteria by linear regression, analysis of the variance and construction of a Kohonen chart (Avcibas *et al.*, 2002) or with a genetic algorithm (Olivès, 1998; Delgorge *et al.*, 2006).

A possible method for the fusion of evaluation criteria consists in combining linearly the best ones. A combined criterion can be written as follows:

$$C_{FUSION} = \sum_{i=1}^{N} a_i . C_i \qquad (1)$$

Where a_i are coefficients that permit to define the importance of the criterion C_i in the computation of C_{FUSION} and to take into account its variation interval. These coefficients have to be determined by optimization by considering some evaluation examples given by experts. The value N corresponding to the number of criteria to fuse and can be set by the user. The choice of criteria to fuse can be done according to their efficiency (used alone) or by selecting them in the optimization process (Delgorge et al. ; 2006).

Table 2. HVS based criteria chosen for the OTELO study

H1	Absolute norm Human Visual System
H2	L2 norm Human Visual System
H3	Similarity
H4	DCTune error
T1	Contrast measure

Figure 8. Fusion of evaluation criteria

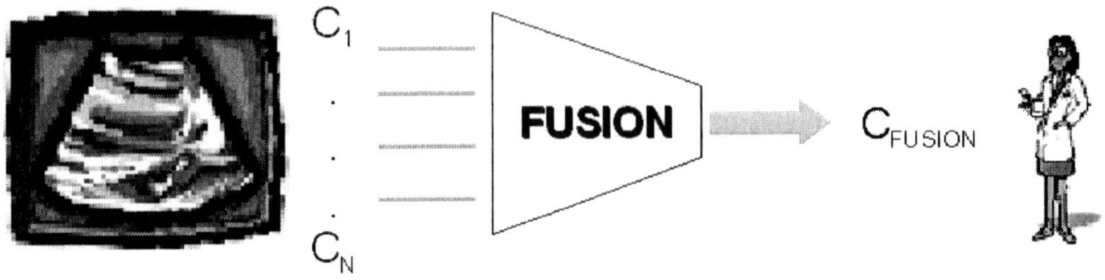

Figure 9. One solution to learn the medical expertise

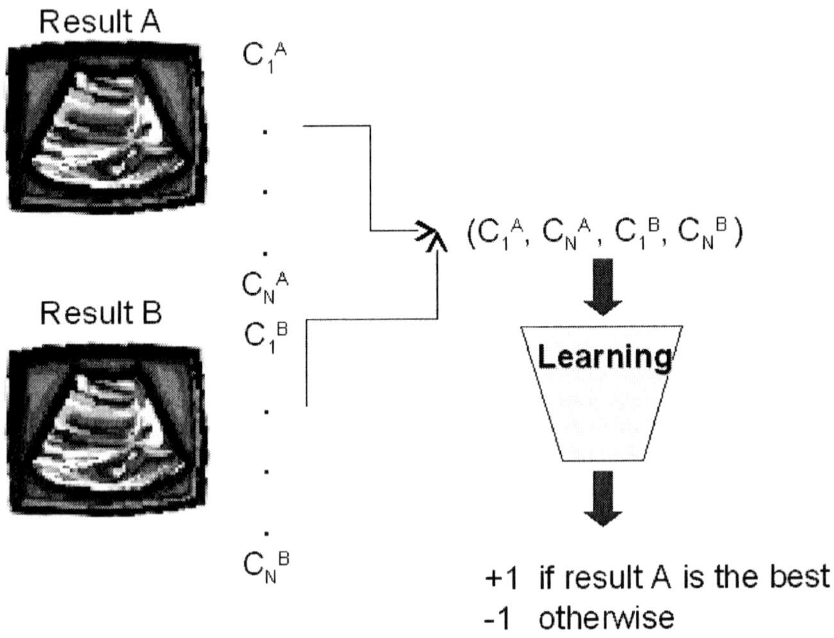

The optimization method can be a classical linear method (such as simplex) without selection of criteria to fuse. In the other case, a genetic algorithm can be used.

This last approach has been applied in the OTELO project, in order to improve the evaluation of compression results quality and to perform better than the statistical criteria. We combined the minimal number of statistical criteria while obtaining an evaluation as close as possible to the medical judgment. The highest similarity rate of correct comparison obtained is **75.3%** for the fusion of 9 selected criteria. The selection process of criteria to fuse permits also to determine complementary ones.

Medical Expertise Learning

The fusion of statistical criteria can be done according to another approach: the learning of the medical assessment data. In this case, the objective is to define an algorithm that is able to compare two compression results similarly as a medical expert. In the previous section, the decision function for the comparison of two compression results was set (as for example, induced by the choice of a linear combination). With this new approach, the decision function is estimated thanks to a learning algorithm (see Figure 9). The support vector machine (SVM) has been proposed as the learning algorithm for the OTELO application (Delgorge *et al.*, 2006).

Suppose we have two compression results A and B we want to compare. We compute on each compression result N different evaluation criteria (that can be selected previously). As for example, for the compression result A, we have a vector $c_1^A, \ldots, c_N^A$ where c_i^A is the value of the criterion number i. We have so two vectors for each compression result we can merge in a single one denoted $COMP = c_1^A, \ldots, c_N^A, c_1^B, \ldots, c_N^B$. This pattern represents the comparison of the compression results A and B. We can use some judgments given by experts on the comparison of different compression results as reference. Given this reference, if the result A is better judged than the result B by experts, the COMP vector must lead to a an exit of the comparison algorithm equals to 1.

In the OTELO project experiments, when 95% of the whole data set is used in the learning database, the system obtains a successful recognition rate of **92.8%**, for the fusion of 5 criteria computed for each of the two compression results to compare.

Discussion

As for us, hybrid evaluation is nowadays the best approach to quantify the performance and the quality of an image processing result. The definition of a single evaluation tool for any medical applications is impossible. It is so necessary to take into account the particular context of the application and also different evaluation approaches. This is also the case for different domains such as paper reviewing. The evaluation of a paper is based on different criteria (clarity, adequacy to the literature review, contribution...) that are taken into account by the evaluator based on its experience and expertise.

We presented three possible methods in the medical image compression. Table 3 sums up the results we obtained in the context of the OTELO project. Note that the best objective evaluation criterion gave a performance equals to 65,3% based on medical experts judgment. The medical expertise learning shows clearly its benefit.

FUTURE TRENDS

Image processing is now a mature technology. The evaluation of a processing result is an important task especially in medical imaging. Different approaches have been proposed in the literature. Nevertheless, few techniques are used for the validation of a new algorithm. Generally, the PSNR is used to compare multiple compression results even if different studies showed that this evaluation criterion does not give a reliable judgment.

We think that two main future trends have to be considered.

The first one concerns the analysis of evaluation methodologies. Even if some new criteria are proposed in the literature, none validation are generally provided. The systematic comparison of evaluation criteria is necessary to increase the reliability of the judgment that is realized. It will have also an impact on the progress in defining new image compression methods.

Table 3. Hybrid evaluation results

Approaches	Performance
Human Visual System criterion	65,3%
Fusion of criteria	75,3%
Medical expertise learning	**92,8%**

The second issue concerns the proposition of new hybrid evaluation criteria. They combine the advantages of objective and subjective evaluation methods. An hybrid evaluation criterion, through integrating some visual perception considerations, is an elegant and interesting solution. The expertise learning is another solution which is similar to a medical expert training. New criteria can be developed integrating many aspects such as the medical application, the type of image or the type of displaying tool.

CONCLUSION

Evaluation of medical image compression is a great challenge as this processing is more and more used for storage and telemedecine applications. The difficulty for the medical application is that a medical expert does not see the same thing than a non expert. The main interest of a medical expert is to quantify in which measure the processing will facilitate its diagnosis. A non expert will appreciate the quality of an image considering the alterations of the compression result. Many studies have to be done in order to define a metric that embeds this kind of information.

ACKNOWLEDGMENT

This work was funded by the European Commission under OTELO project (IST 2001-32516).

REFERENCES

Andreutos, D., Plataniotis, K. N., & Venetsanopoulos, A. N. (1998). Distances Measures for Color Image Retrieval. *IEEE ICIP International Conference on Image Processing.*

Avcibas, I., Sankur, B., & Sayood, K. (2002). Statistical evaluation of image quality measures. *Journal of Electronic imaging, 11*(2), 206-223.

Azpiroz-Leehan, J., Leder, R., & Lerallut, J.-F. (2004). Quantitative and qualitative evaluation of filter characteristics for wavelet packet compression of MR images. *In 26th Annual International Conference of the Engineering in Medicine and Biology Society*, (pp. 1537-1540).

Cane, B. Mc (1997). On the Evaluation of Image Segmentation Algorithms. *DICTA'97* and *IVCN'Z'97*, (pp. 455-459).

Carnec, M. (2004). *Critères de qualité d'images couleur avec référence réduite perceptuelle générique*. Phd Thesis de l'Ecole Polytechnique de l'Université de Nantes.

Chen, T.-J., Chuang, K.-S., Wu, J., Chan, S. C., Hwang, I.-M., & Jan, M.-L. (2003). A novel image quality index using Moran I statistics. *Physics in Medicine and Biology, 48*, 131-137.

Delgorge, C., Courreges, F., Al Bassit, L., Novales, C., Rosenberger, C., Smith-Guerin, N., Bru, C., Gilabert, R., Vannoni, M., Poisson, G., & Vieyres, P. (2005). A tele-operated mobile ultrasound scanner using a light weight robot. *IEEE Transactions on Information Technology in BioMedicine, special issue mHealth, 9*(1).

Delgorge, C., Rosenberger, C., Poisson, G., & Vieyres, P. (2006). Towards a new tool for the evaluation of the quality of ultrasound compressed images. *IEEE Transactions on Medical Imaging, 25*, 1502 – 1509.

International Telecommunication Union (2002). ITU-R-BT.500-11 Methodology for the subjective assessment of the quality of television pictures. *Recommendation on Broadcasting Service.*

Klein, S. A. (1993) Image quality and image compression: a psychophysicist's viewpoint. *Digital and human vision*, (pp. 73–88).

Le Callet, P., & Barba, D. (2001) Critère de qualité visuelle d'images couleur - application à l'évaluation réaliste de codeurs d'images. *Colloque GRETSI.*

Linfoot, E. H. (1958). Quality Evaluation of Optical Systems. *Optica Acta, 5*(1-2), 1-13.

Miyaji, S., Hamada, T., & Matsumoto, S. (2000). Development of a Digital Compressed Picture Quality Assessment System Considering Human Visual Perception. *Systems and Computers in Japan, 5*, 97–109.

Naegele-Jackson, S., Holleczek, P., Rabenstein, T., Maiss, J., & Sackmann, M. (2002). Influence of compression and network impairments on the picture quality of video transmissions in telemedicine. *In Proceedings of the 35th Annual Hawaii International Conference on System Sciences,* (pp. 2060–2068).

Olivès, J.-L. (1998). *Optimisation globale d'un système imageur à l'aide de critères de qualité visuelle.* PhD thesis de l'Ecole Nationale Supérieure de l'Aéronautique et de l'Espace ENSAE.

Pommert, A., & Höhne, K.H. (2002). Evaluation of Image Quality in Medical Volume Visualization: The State of Art. *Lecture Notes in Computer Science, 2489*, 598–605.

Sundersingh, B. J. (2000). *Qualitative Evaluation of Data Compression in Real-Time Ultrasound Imaging.* PhD Thesis University of Tennessee, Memphis.

Tamtaoui, A., Ribagnac, M., & Aboutajdine, D. (1999). Elaboration de criteres de mesure de qualité objective pour la qualité subjective. *Colloque GRETSI*, (pp. 845-848)

Turaga, D. S., Chen, Y. & Caviedes, J. (2004). No reference PSNR estimation for compressed pictures. *Signal Processing Image Communication, 19*, 173-184.

Weatherburn, G. C., Ridout, D., Strickalnd, N. H., Robins, P., Glastonbury, C. M., Curati, W., Harvey, C., & Shadbolt, C. (2003). A comparison of conventional film, CR hard copy and PACS soft copy images of the chest: Analyses of ROC curves and inter-observer agreement. *European Journal of Radiology, 47*, 206-214.

Yang S.-B. (2005). Smooth side-match weighted vector quantizer with variable block size for image coding. *IEEE Proceedings Vision and Image and Signal Processing, 152*, 763-770.

Zhong, J., & Ning, R. (2005). Image Denoising based on wavelets and multifractals for singularity detection. *IEEE Transactions on Image Processing, 14*, 1435-1447.

KEY TERMS

Fusion: Combination of different data in order to improve decision making.

Hybrid Evaluation: The goal of this approach is to obtain a judgment as reliable as the subjective one while having an easy computation.

Human Visual System (HVS): It refers to the visual perception of humans that is simulated by researchers in evaluation.

Objective Evaluation: It is a quantitative evaluation generally based on statistical criteria. None *a priori* knowledge is used for the evaluation.

Peak Signal-to-Noise Ratio (PSNR): The PSNR is most commonly used as a measure of quality of reconstruction in image compression.

Receiver Operating Characteristic (ROC): ROC curves provides tools to analysis the behavior of models, algorithms or human judgments.

Subjective Evaluation: It is a quantitative or a qualitative evaluation involving experts or some *a priori* knowledge.

Chapter XXIX
Advanced ROI Coding Techniques for Medical Imaging

Charalampos Doukas
University of the Aegean, Samos, Greece

Ilias Maglogiannis
University of Central Greece, Lamia, Greece

ABSTRACT

Medical images are often characterized by high complexity and consist of high resolution image files, introducing thus several issues regarding their handling. Current compression schemes produce high compression rates, sacrificing however the image quality and leading this way to unenviable examination. Region of Interest (ROI) coding has been introduced as an efficient technique for addressing such issues, by performing advanced image compression and preserving quality in diagnostically critical regions. This chapter discusses the basic ROI approaches and provides an overview of state of the art ROI coding techniques for medical images along with corresponding results.

BACKGROUND

Medical imaging has a great impact on medicine, especially in the fields of diagnosis and surgical planning. Proper assessment requires high image quality, which is translated into higher requirements for storage capacity and transmission bandwidth in applications like electronic health records and telemedicine applications. Medical image compression can reduce redundancy of the image data in order to be able to store or transmit data in an efficient form. Compression can be lossy or lossless; Lossy compression methods, especially when used at low bit rates, achieve higher compression ratio and size/rate reduction but also introduce compression artifacts. Lossless compression methods may also be preferred for high value content, such as medical imagery or image scans made for archival purposes. The tradeoff between lossy and lossless image compression can be addressed by introducing the Region of Interest (ROI) coding; for most medical images, the diagnostically significant information is localized over relatively small regions of interest. In this case, region-based coding offers better utilization of the available bit rate since the high quality should be maintained only for the aforementioned diagnostically significant regions and the rest of the image can be encoded at a lower bit rate.

INTRODUCING BASIC CONCEPTS OF ROI CODING

The functionality of Region of Interest (ROI) is important in medical applications where certain parts of the image are of higher diagnostic importance than others. In such a case, these regions need to be encoded at higher quality than the background. During image transmission for telemedicine purposes, these regions are required to be transmitted first or at a higher priority. In transformation-based ROI coding methods, the coefficients associated with the ROI are transferred ahead of those associated with the background. Therefore, when an image is coded with an emphasis of ROI, it is necessary to identify the coefficients required for the reconstruction of the ROI. Thus, a ROI mask is introduced to indicate which coefficients have to be transmitted exactly in order for the receiver to reconstruct the ROI. Usually, the wavelet transform (Burrus et. al., 1998; I. Daubechies, 1998) is applied to the image at the encoder side and the resulting coefficients not associated with the ROI are scaled down (shifted down) so that the ROI associated bits are placed in higher bit planes The mask in wavelet domain is a map pointing out all the related coefficients for the reconstruction of the ROI. The corresponding locations of the coefficients in next scale are calculated from the current scale. An example calculation of the ROI mask is as follows (Liu et. al. 2004):

Let R^n the wavelet domain of an image and $\Omega \in R^n$ the Region of Interest. The characteristic function $\chi_\Omega(x)$ is defined as:

$$\chi_\Omega(x) = \begin{cases} 1, & \text{if } x \in \Omega \\ 0, & \text{if else} \end{cases} \qquad (1)$$

Then the ROI mask will be generated according to:

$$g_i(x) = \left(\tilde{W}_i \circ x_\Omega\right)(x) + \tilde{I}_i x_\Omega(x) \qquad i \in \Lambda \qquad (2)$$

where $\tilde{W}_i$ stands for the wavelet operator for the ith subband, Λ is the index set of all subbands and $\tilde{I}_i$ is identity operator equipped with down-sampling operation respectively.

ROI coding has been applied on different types of medical images. For instance, MAXSHIFT of JPEG2000 (ISO/IEC JTC 1/SC 29/WG 1 (ITU-T SG8), JPEG 2000 Part II Final Committee Draft, 2000), set partitioning in hierarchical trees (SPIHT) (A. Said and W.A. Pearlman, 1996), embedded block coding with optimized truncation (EBCOT) (Taubman, 2000), adaptive integer wavelet transforms (IWTs) (Minami et. al. 2001) and region-based discrete wavelet transform (RB-DWT) (S. Li and W. Li, 2000) are the most common transformations utilized for region coding on still medical images. Variations of the aforementioned algorithms have been proposed for application on volumetric (i.e. three dimensional) images (e.g., 3D SPHIT (Xiong et. al., 1998)). Additional techniques allow the implementation of multiple and arbitrary ROI coding as well as dynamic coding for scalable medical image compression. Regarding medical video compression, similar techniques allow the annotation of regions with higher diagnostic importance within the video sequence (Liu et. al., 2004). Figure 1 presents two medical image samples and a medical video image compressed using ROI coding.

Figure 1. Image samples compressed with Region of Interest (ROI) coding: (a) skin lesion image, (b) MRI image, and (c) medical video image (snapshot); (d) – (f) same images with background compressed at higher factor than the ROI.

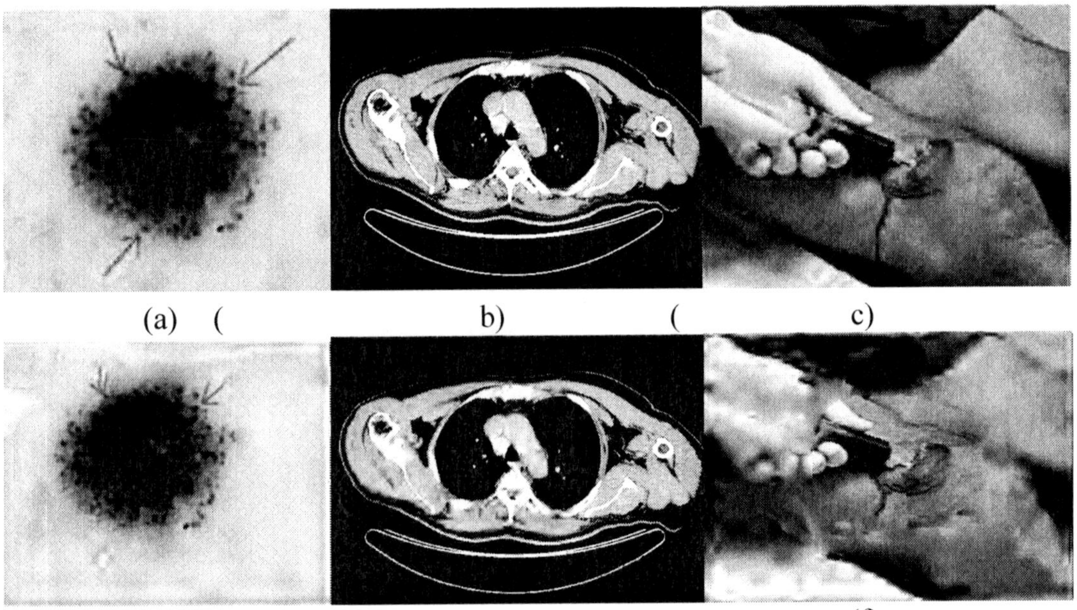

(a) (b) (c)

(d) (e) (f)

ROI CODING TECHNIQUES FOR 2-D MEDICAL IMAGES

This section provides ROI coding techniques applied on still 2-D medical images. The principle of the general-scaling method (also defined in Part II of the JPEG2000 Imaging Standard (ISO/IEC JTC 1/SC 29/WG 1 (ITU-T SG8) JPEG 2000 Part II Final Committee Draft, 2000)) is to scale (shift) coefficients so that the bits associated with the ROI are placed in higher bit-planes than the bits associated with the background (see Figrue 2(b)). Then, during the embedded coding process, the most significant ROI bit-planes are placed in the bit-stream before any background bit-planes of the image. Depending on the scaling value, some bits of the ROI coefficients might be encoded together with non-ROI coefficients. Thus, the ROI will be decoded, or refined, before the rest of the image. Regardless of the scaling, a full decoding of the bit-stream results in a reconstruction of the whole image with the highest fidelity is available. If the bit-stream is truncated, or the encoding process is terminated before the whole image is fully encoded, the ROI will be of higher quality than the rest of the image.

According to the MAXSHIFT method, (defined in ISO/IEC JTC 1/SC 29/WG 1 (ITU-T SG8) JPEG 2000 Part I Final Committee Draft Version 1.0, Mar. 2000.), the scaling value is computed in such a way that it makes possible to have arbitrary shaped ROIs without the need for transmitting shape information to the decoder. This means also that the decoder does not have to perform ROI mask generation either. The mapping of the ROI from the spatial domain to the wavelet domain is dependent on the used wavelet filters and it is simplified for rectangular and circular regions. The encoder scans the quantized coefficients and chooses a scaling value s such that the minimum

Figure 2. Illustration of coefficient scaling in image compression: (a) Full image compression, (b) general ROI scaling-based method, (c) MAXSHIFT method.

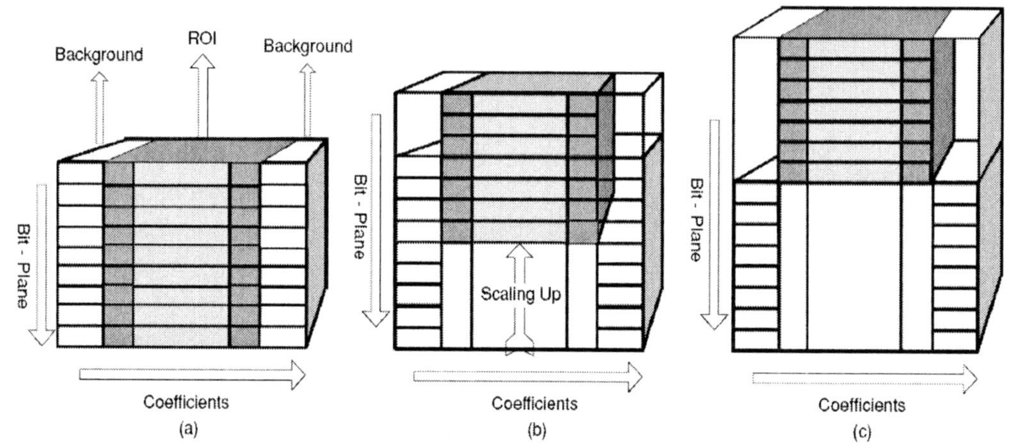

coefficient belonging to the ROI is larger than the maximum coefficient of the background (non-ROI area). As illustrated in Figure 2(c) all of the wavelet coefficients that are not part of the ROI are scaled down by (s + D), where D is a small constant. As a result all the wavelet coefficients corresponding to the background have a magnitude < 1. The decoder, after receiving the bit-stream, just scales up (by s + D) all coefficients that have a magnitude < 1; therefore no extra information about the shape of the ROI is required.

The advantages of the MAXSHIFT method, in comparison to the scaling based method, is that encoding of arbitrary shaped ROIs is possible without the requirement of shape information provision and without the need for calculating the ROI mask. The encoder is simpler, since no shape encoding is required, i.e. shape is implicit. The decoder is almost as simple as a non- ROI capable decoder, while it can still handle ROIs of arbitrary shape. The MAXSHIFT method however, results in slightly higher bit-rates, while no background information is available before the whole ROI is decoded (A. Bradley and F. Stentiford, 2002). Performance metrics of the MAXSHIFT and general scaling method in the context of medical images are provided by Anastassopoulos and Skodras (2002), proving the referred consumption regarding the superiority of the MAXSHIFT method.

The ROI coding schemes included in JPEG2000 standard, provide better image quality in critical diagnostic areas. However lossy-to-lossless compression of ROI is not supported, unless the ROI consists of the whole image. Liu et. al. (2002) propose a lossy-to-lossless ROI compression scheme. The scheme is based on Set Partitioning in Hierarchical Trees (SPIHT) (A. Said and W. A. Pearlman, 1996) and Embedded Block Coding with Optimized Truncation (EBCOT) (D. Taubman, 2000). The input images are segmented into the foreground and background respectively and a chain code-based shape coding scheme by Liu et. al. (2002) is used to code the ROI's shape information. Then, the critically sampled shape-adaptive integer wavelet transforms (Minami et. al., 2001) are performed on the foreground and background image separately to facilitate lossy-to-lossless coding. Finally, the shape coding bit-stream, the foreground bit-stream, and the background bit-stream are combined into a single bit-stream. In this algorithm extraneous coefficients outside the ROIs are not coded. Regarding the SPIHT, the multipass "zerotree" coding is adapted in order to reduce the redundancy. Using methods provided by Tasdoken and Cuhadar (2003), the spatial orientation trees in the wavelet domain are divided into categories, according to whether all or some coefficients are inside or outside the ROIs. In order to improve SPIHT's coding efficiency, the EBCOT's context model for bit-pale coding is borrowed. The latter applies the arithmetic coding on sign bits and refinement bits as well. The wavelet transform used in EBCOT is replaced again with a shape-adaptive wavelet transform (Minami et. al., 2001). A modification is also made, so that only coefficients inside ROIs are coded after performing the wavelet decomposition. Experiments conducted on chromosome images proved the efficiency of the proposed schemes both in the context of lossy and lossless image compression.

The Region-based Integer Wavelets Transform (RB-IWT) proposed by Tasdoken and Cuhadar, (2003) is another ROI coding scheme based on SPIHT. In this implementation, the integer wavelet transform (Dewitte and Cornelis, 1997) is utilized in order to obtain the representation of the partitioned image plane rather than differentiating the coefficients associated with each region. The specific approach is suggested as a low-complexity implementation based on the lifting mechanism that also enables lossless coding of image regions. The ROI is obtained through an integer wavelet decomposition of the partitioned image signal, which maps the partitioned image plane into a partitioned wavelet coefficient plane. These parse representations of the arbitrary shape regions are encoded using a modified SPIHT algorithm. Experimental results provided by the authors, proved that the proposed RB-IWT method performs better than SPIHT based ROI coding.

Penedo et al. (2003) propose a two ROI wavelet-based coding methods with application to digital mammography. In both methods, after segmenting the breast region, Region-Based Discrete Wavelet Transform (RBDWT) (S. Li and W. Li, 2000) is applied. Then in the first method an Object-Based extension of the Set Partitioning in Hierarchical Trees (OB-SPIHT) (Said and Pearlman, 1996) coding algorithm is used, while the second method utilizes an Object- Based extension of the Set Partitioned Embedded bloCK (OB-SPECK) (Islam and Pearlman, 1999) coding algorithm. Using RBDWT it is possible to efficiently perform wavelet sub-band decomposition of an arbitrary shape region, while maintaining the same number of wavelet coefficients. Both OB-SPIHT and OB-SPECK algorithms are embedded techniques, i.e. the coding method produces an embedded bit-stream which can be truncated at any point, equivalent to stopping the compression process at a desired quality. The wavelet coefficients with larger magnitude are those with larger information content. In a comparison, with full-image compression methods as SPIHT and JPEG2000, OB-SPIHT and OB-SPECK exhibit much higher quality in the breast region at the same compressed file size.

A different approach is presented by Dilmaghani et. al. (2003), where the Embedded Zerotree Wavelets (EZW) coding technique is adopted for ROI coding in Progressive Image Transmission (PIT). Using sub-band decomposition and image wavelet transform to eliminate or reduce the correlation in the sub-images at different resolutions, the whole frequency band of the original image is split into different sub-bands at different resolution. The EZW algorithm is effectively applied to wavelet coefficients to refine and encode the most significant ones. The optimum bit allocation, b_i, for any sub-band with bandwidth w_i, and average power of P_i is derived as follows:

$$bi = \frac{w_i}{W}B + \sum_{i=1}^{N}\left(\frac{w_j w_i}{W}\right)\log 2\left(\frac{P_i w_i}{P_j w_i}\right), \quad i=1,2,...N \tag{3}$$

where B and W are the given total bit-rate and the total bandwidth respectively. Equation 3 is used to assign the bit rate to each band. Due to the partially localized nature of the wavelet transform, it is possible to specify an arbitrary region to be compressed. This is performed by specifying the corresponding wavelet coefficients of the ROI in the wavelet space and then applying the EZW algorithm on these coefficients. The latter belong to different scales and thus to different resolutions in the wavelet domain. The constraint on the bit-rate is limited to the size of the ROI. In order to send the ROI, a recognizable image is firstly send to the receiver, and then the requested ROI is progressively improved.

Another ROI coding technique is based on vector quantization (VQ) (Cziho et. al., 1997; Nasrabadi and King, 1998). In VQ, the image is divided into small non-overlapping blocks. At the encoder side, each vector x_i of the image is compared to the elements of a codebook $W = \{w_0,w_1,...,w_{N-1}\}$, called the codevectors or codewords, and only the index of the nearest codevector is transmitted. In the Region-of-Interest VQ (ROI-VQ) approach a separate codebook is generated for every region (or image 'object', i.e. organ). The properties of these codebooks, (i.e. the codebook size and the block size), are chosen according to the medical importance of the given object. If an object is diagnostically important, a large codebook containing small codewords is created. Inversely, for less important regions, the block size is smaller and/or the codebook contains less codevectors. This compression algorithm has been adapted for echoendoscopic images of the esophagus wall. The ROI-VQ method succeeds in obtaining a good rate/distortion performance, and preserving the quality on the most important part, (i.e. on the esophagus wall).

Finally a wavelet based ROI coding algorithm implemented for Personal Digital Assistants (PDAs) is described by Doukas et. al. (2005). The algorithm is based on octave decomposition, which repeatedly divides the lower sub-band into 4 sub-bands. The ROI shape is given by the user as a binary mask form on the source image and the wavelet coefficients on the ROI and on the Region of None Interest (RONI) are quantized with different step sizes. For this purpose, a corresponding binary mask is obtained, on the wavelet transform domain.

ROI CODING IN VOLUMETRIC MEDICAL IMAGES

Volumetric medical images have introduced further problems regarding their handling and transmission, due to the sheer volume of data they contain. Thus, the use of a compression method enhanced with ROI coding for diagnosis in critical areas, is considered essential in this case.

Three-dimensional wavelet coding provides better performance compared to corresponding 2D methods by exploiting the inter-slice correlation that exists in such image data. An evaluation of conventional ROI coding schemes on volumetric images, called SA –DWT exists in the work by Ueno and Pearlman (2003). In this algorithm only samples within an object are transformed (S. Li and W. Li, 2000) according to the shape information additionally sent to the decoder. The length of each one-dimensional segment to be transformed varies from segment to segment. Compared with scaling-based ROI (SB-ROI), fewer samples are necessary to encode the object, so more efficient coding of the object can be expected. However flexible ROI coding such as user-driven ROI coding on interactive applications is difficult to realize. In user-driven ROI coding, the user modifies or specifies an ROI in the middle of the coding process. In SA-DWT the wavelet transform needs to be performed again when the ROI is specified /modified. This, it would cause significant increase of computational cost for efficiently using transmitted until that time code data. The object and background are faithfully reproduced without the pixel blending artifacts in the case of MAXSHIFT. With the exception of very low coding rates, SA-ROI has better compression performance than SB-ROI.

A hybrid model of lossless compression in the region of interest, with high-rate, motion-compensated, lossy compression in other regions is applied on colon CT images in Gokturk et. al. (2001). The colon wall is segmented through a sequence of 3-D morphological image processing techniques. The output of the motion compensated coding acts as an initial approximation for ROI areas. Once the ROI is segmented in each slice, a hybrid compression scheme is used for coding the images. The first slice of the volume is compressed with a lossless coder. Each slice is then coded by motion compensated coding, which also acts as a prediction filter for ROI. Finally, the difference between the real-image ROI block and the predicted-image ROI block is coded by an entropy minimizing lossless coder.

An extension to 3D-SPIHT that allows 3D ROI coding in volumetric images is presented by Agrafiotis et. al. (2003). In order to identify the coefficients that affect the ROI, a three dimensional bitmap mask is maintained at the encoder. This mask undergoes a similar to wavelet transform, where at each step the necessary coefficients for the perfect reconstruction of the ROI at the current level of decomposition are identified. In order to assign greater priority to the ROI, the coefficients of the bitmap mask are scaled up through a fixed number of left bit shifts (S). The larger the number of left shift bits, the greater the emphasis placed on the ROI and the faster the lossless reconstruction of it.

ROI CODING IN MEDICAL VIDEO SEQUENCES

The storage requirements for medical video sequences are even higher. Conventional compression methods of captured video mostly rely on a combined motion estimation–compensation strategy, followed by an often frequency-based, residual coding method. These methods may provide impressive compression ratios (100:1) with relatively small amounts of image quality degradation (Ang et. al., 1991; Bernabe et. al., 2000). Unfortunately, the compression of medical video sequences (e.g. angiogram or endoscopic video sequences) using conventional video compression methods is non-optimal (Gibson et. al., 2000), due to the particular structure of medical video data and mainly due to the unusual motion patterns and large amounts of background texture. A wavelet-based ROI encoder for compression of angiogram video sequences is presented in Gibson et. al., (2004). The specific approach is a combination of a three-dimensional (3-D) wavelet compression scheme based on the SPIHT algorithm, ROI detection and bit allocation, and a wavelet-based texture modeling approach that models the high frequency texture for some of the diagnostically unimportant background areas of an image. This allows for a larger proportion of the total bit allocation to be used within the ROI area. In terms of compression performance, the proposed method can operate at a compression ratio around 10:1 with differences between the original and compressed images assessed as being not of diagnostic significance by trained cardiologists. A pixel (x,y) is defined as a point within a ROI according to the following equation:

$$R(x,y)=\begin{cases}1, & Df(x,y)>k_A T\\ 0, & \text{otherwise}\end{cases} \qquad (4)$$

$Df(x,y)$ is a two-dimensional spatial Gaussian filter applied to the deviation of the frame difference function. $K_A T$ is an empirically chosen constant, selected based on the precautionary idea that it is preferable to include diagnostically non-significant areas into the ROI than it is to exclude significant areas for the ROI. The ROI map $R(x,y)$ is post-processed into a block-based representation—in this case, using blocks of 16x16 pixels in size. Thus in case a pixel with a given block is labeled as belonging to the ROI, then all of the pixels in that block will be labeled as being part of the ROI. Hence, the ROI is strictly expanded when described as a collection of blocks. ROI encoding is performed by representing each block by a single bit and transmitting the resultant bit stream uncompressed. Although techniques such as run length encoding would likely work well on this bit stream, the net effect on the required total bandwidth would prove negligible. Additional experiments were conducted comparing the efficiency of the proposed method against the conventional 3D-SPIHT coding algorithm. The corresponding results prove the efficiency of the proposed methods in the context of less quality distortion in ROI for different bit rates.

COMPARISON OF SURVEYED TECHNIQUES AND DISCUSSION

In this chapter several techniques enabling ROI coding image compression in distributed telemedicine systems for various types of medical image modalities are discussed. These techniques are summarized in Table 1, presenting a quick overview of their basic features.

As presented, the General Scaling, the MAXSHIFT, the EZW-based and the ROI-VQ methods require additional coefficients to decode the object, whereas in the rest of the discussed techniques both the background and the ROI are coded using the same number of coefficients as the entire image. A few methods require the ROI shape information to be incorporated into the bit-stream, whereas most of them support arbitrary ROI coding. The exact decoding of the object feasibility refers to the ability of the method to preserve the entire ROI without pixel blending artifacts. Finally, corresponding metrics (in PSNR per bits per pixel) are provided in the last column of Table 1, proving the efficiency of each method.

A CASE STUDY APPLICATION OF MEDICAL IMAGE ROI CODING

Medical image ROI coding is mostly utilized for reducing the required size and bit rate for storing, manipulating and transmitting images and maintaining quality for assessment at the same time. The application domain is thus mostly telemedicine applications using different kinds of image modalities; mammograms are coded properly in order to keep only the required visual information for more efficient storage (Penedo et. al., 2003; S. Li and W. Li, 2000; Islam and Pearlman, 1999; Dilmaghani et. al.,2003). Echoendoscopic images (Cziho et. al.,1997; Nasrabadi and King, 1998) and angiogram video sequences are transmitted more efficiently over telemedicine networks utilizing proper ROI coding respectively.

In the context of telemedicine applications and medical ROI coding, a transmission and examination application of DICOM images on mobile devices (Doukas et. al., 2005) is discussed in this section. The application enables scalable compression, retrieval and decompression of medical images on mobile devices, enhanced with ROI coding for advanced image examination of specific areas within the image. The system can be used for accessing medical images at a health care center, where the electronic medical record system resides, at a medical treatment/care center established at a sports facilities center, at a treatment center on an island, on an urban area, or even remotely on patient's site, and in an ambulance. An inherent feature of the proposed application is its support for mobility making this suitable for heterogeneous radio access network infrastructures. The application adopts the Distortion Limited Wavelet Image Codec (DLWIC) algorithm (Shapiro, 1999). In DLWIC, the image to be compressed is firstly converted to the wavelet domain using the orthonormal Daubechies wavelet transform (Daubechies, 1998). The transformed data is then coded by bit-levels and the output is coded using QM-coder (Lehtinen, 1999), an

Table 1. Overview of the discussed ROI coding techniques, presenting the related references, the applicable medical image category (2-D still images, volumetric images and video sequences), and the image type each method is applied to.

ROI coding method	**Reference**	**Medical Image category**	**Image type applied to**	**Corresponding results: (PSNR in dB) (bits per pixel**	**Comments**
General ROI-based scaling method	Anastassopoulos and Skodras (2002), ISO/IEC JTC 1/SC 29/WG 1 (ITU-T SG8) JPEG 2000 Part II Final Committee Draft (2000)	2-D still images	Nephrostogram	44.91 (0.08 bpp)	Part of JEPG2000. The image can be resolved even in case of truncated bit-stream.
MAXSHIFT	Anastassopoulos, and Skodras (2002), ISO/IEC JTC 1/SC 29/WG 1 (ITU-T SG8) JPEG 2000 Part I Final Committee Draft Version 1.0 (2000)	2-D still images	Nephrostogram	44.90 (0.08 bpp)	Simple decoding process without needing ROI mask generation.
Lossy-to-lossless ROI coding	Liu et. al. (2002), Said and Pearlman (1996), D. Taubman (2000), Liu et. al. (2002), Minami et. al. (2001)	2-D still images	Chromosome Images	44.4 (0.08 bpp)	Lossless image compression provided, ROI must be predetermined.
RB-IWT	Tasdoken and Cuhadar (2003), Said and Pearlman (1996), Anastassopoulos and Skodras (2002)	2-D still images	--	35 (0.8 bpp)	A low complexity ROI coding mechanism.
OB-SPIHT, OB-SPECK	Penedo et. al. (2003), S. Li and W. Li (2000), Islam and Pearlman (1999)	2-D still images	Mammogram	54.2 (0.8 bpp)	The bit-stream can be truncated, proved high quality compression in breast region.
EZW-based ROI	Dilmaghani et. al. (2003), Doukas et. al. (2005)	2-D still images	Mammogram, knee CT scans	N/A	The ROI is decoded progressively at the receiver.
Hybrid coder	Gokturk et. al. (2001)	Volumetric images	Colon CT scans	32.0 (0.52 bpp)	ROI must be predetermined.
ROI-VQ	Cziho et. al. (1997), Nasrabadi and King (1998)	2-D still images	Echoendoscopic images	31.58 (0.03 bpp)	Obtains good rate/distortion performance preserving ROI quality.
SA-DWT	Ueno and Pearlman (2003)	Volumetric images	MRI Chest	52.5 (0.50 bpp)	Requires more computation power than other techniques.
Extended 3D-SPIHT	Agrafiotis et. al. (2003), Gibson et. al. (2004)	Volumetric images, Medical Video sequences	MRI Head, Angiogram video sequences	38.78 (0.52 bpp)	Similar to General scaling method, quite simple and efficient, Efficient ROI coding in medical video sequences.

advanced binary arithmetic coder. The algorithm processes the bits of the wavelet transformed image data in decreasing order concerning their significance in terms of Mean Square Error (MSE). This produces a progressive output stream enabling the algorithm to be stopped at any phase of the coding. The already coded output can be used to construct an approximation of the original image. The proposed medical application follows a three-tier architecture, consisting of the client part, the DICOM Server and the Electronic Medical Record System - Remote Database Management System (EMR-RDBMS). Client requires a Java enabled web - browser and communicates using HyperText Transfer Protocol (HTTP) and Remote Method Invocation (RMI) protocols with the server. Figure 2 presents screenshots from the application in use. Conducted experiments evaluating the performance of the transmission of medical images over wireless networks have proved that wavelet compression and ROI coding can reduce transmission time over 50% in cases of slow networks (e.g., GRPS).

CONCLUSION

ROI coding preserves image quality in diagnostically critical regions by performing advanced image compression, enabling better image examination and addressing issues, regarding image handling and transmission in telemedicine systems. Therefore ROI coding is considered quite important in distributed and networked electronic healthcare. The presented coding techniques have been classified according to the image type they apply on; two-dimensional still medical images, volumetric images and medical video sequences. The ROI mask generation, the coding and the transmission process are described in the relative sections. A comparison between the referred techniques informs the reader about their feasibilities and characteristics, such as object decoding, user-driven ROI selection and shape information transmission. Corresponding results are also provided indicating the efficiency of each method.

FUTURE TRENDS

The results presented so far, from the research community are promising for the future. It is now necessary to adapt the existing algorithms in order to decrease complexity. This will enable their use in portable and mobile devices, which have limited computing power allowing the support of moving and commuting physicians. Current and future

Figure 3. Application screenshots: (a) for a Tablet PC, (b) for a PDA, (c) for ROI support on lossy compressed image.

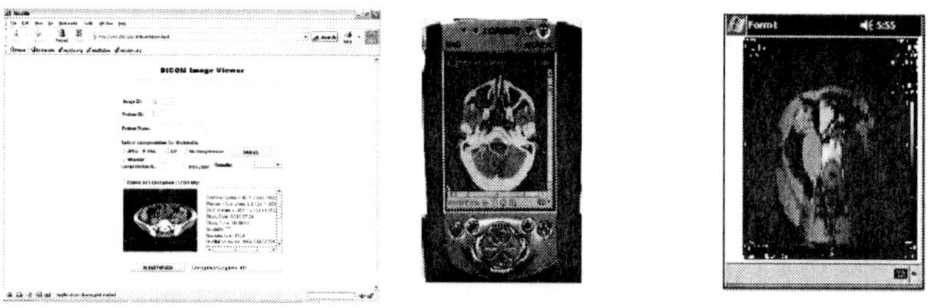

(a) (b) (c)

research trends in the discussed context should also focus in addressing ROI coding issues like complexity in large medical datasets (Schelkens et. al., 2003), improved coding of volumetric images (Kontos and Megaloikonomou 2004) and the automatic selection of diagnostically important areas before coding (Nguyen et. al., 2005).

REFERENCES

Agrafiotis, D., Bull, D. R., & Canagarajah, N. (2003). ROI coding of volumetric medical images with application to visualization. *3rd International Symposium on Image and Signal Processing and Analysis*, (p. 217).

Anastassopoulos, G., & Skodras, A. (2002). JPEG2000 ROI coding in Medical Imaging Applications. *2nd IASTED Int. Conf. on Visualisation, Imaging and Image Processing*, VIIP2002.

Ang, P. H., Ruetz, P. A., & Auld, D. (1991). Video compression makes big gains, *IEEE Spectrum, 28*, 16 – 19.

Bernabe, G., Gonzalez, J., Garcia, J. M., & Duato, J. (2000). A new lossy 3-D wavelet transform for high-quality compression of medical video. *IEEE EMBS International Conference on Information Technology Applications in Biomedicine*, (p. 226).

Bradley, A., & Stentiford, F. (2002). JPEG2000 and Region of Interest Coding. *Presented at DICTA2002.*

Burrus, C. S., Gopinath, R. A., & Guo, H. (1998). Introduction to Wavelets and the Wavelet Transform: A Primer. Englewood Cliffs, NJ: Prentice-Hall

Burrus, C. S., Gopinath, R. A., & Guo, H. (1993). Introduction to Wavelets and the Wavelet Transform—A Primer. *ICASSP 93.*

Cziho, A., Cazuguel, G., Solaiman, B., & Roux, C. (1998). Medical image compression using region-of-interest vector quantization. *20th Annual International Conference of the IEEE Engineering in Medicine and Biology Society.* (pp. 1277).

Daubechies, I. (1998). Orthonormal bases of compactly supported wavelets. *Commun. Pure Applied Math. 41*, 909–996.

Dewitte, S., & Cornelis, J. (1997). Lossless integer wavelet transform. *IEEE Signal Processing Letters, 4*, 158 – 160.

Dilmaghani, R., Ahmadian, A., Ghavami, M., Oghabian, M., & Aghvami, H. (2003). Multi rate/resolution control in progressive medical image transmission for the Region of Interest (ROI) using EZW. *25th Annual International Conference of the IEEE EMBS*, Mexico.

Doukas, C. N., Maglogiannis, I., & Kormentzas, G. (2005). Medical Image Compression using Wavelet Transform on Mobile Devices with ROI coding support. *27th Annual International Conference of the IEEE EMBS.*

Gibson, D., Spann, M., & Woolley, S. I. (2000). Comparative study of compression methodologies for digital angiogram video. *Presented at the ISPACS 2000*, Honolulu.

Gibson, D., Spann, M., & Woolley, S. I. (2004). A wavelet-based region of interest encoder for the compression of angiogram video sequences. *IEEE Transactions on Information Technology in Biomedicine, 8*, 103 – 113.

Gokturk, S. B., Tomasi, C., Girod, B., & Beaulieu, C. (2001). Medical image compression based on region of interest, with application to colon CT images. *23rd Annual International Conference of the IEEE Engineering in Medicine and Biology Society*, (p.2453).

Islam, A., & Pearlman, W. A. (1999). An embedded and efficient low-complexity hierarchical image coder. *SPIE Visual Comm. and Image Processing*, (pp. 294).

Kontos, D., & Megalooikonomou, V. (2004). Fast and effective characterization of 3D Region of Interest in medical image data. Medical Imaging 2004: Image *Processing, edited by J. Michael Fitzpatrick, Milan Sonka, Proceedings of SPIE Vol. 5370* (SPIE, Bellingham, WA, 2004) (pp. 1324-1331)

Lehtinen, J. (1999). Distortion of a Wavelet Image Codec. *Acta Cyberntica, 14*, 342-356.

Li, S., & Li, W. (2000). Shape-adaptive discrete wavelet transform for arbitrary shaped visual object coding. *IEEE Trans. Circuits Syst. Video Technol., 10*, 725–743.

Liu, C., Xia, T., & Li, H. (2004). ROI and FOI algorithms for wavelet-based video compression. *5th Pacific Rim Conf. Multimedia*, Tokyo, (pp. 241).

Liu, Z., Ha, J., Xiong, Z., Wu, Q., & Castleman, K. (2002). Lossy-to-lossless ROI coding of chromosome images using modified SPIHT and EBCOT. *IEEE International Symposium on Biomedical Imaging*, (pp.317).

Liu, Z., Ha, J., Xiong, Z., Wu, Q., & Castleman, K. (2002). Cascaded Differential and Wavelet Compression of Chromosome Images. *IEEE Trans. on Biomedical Engineering, 49*, 323-283.

Menegaz, G., & Grewe L. (2002). 3D/2D object-based coding of head MRI data. *2002 International Conference on Image Processing*, (1), 181-184.

Minami, G., Xiong, Z., Wang, A., & Mehrotra, S. (2001). 3-D wavelet coding of video with arbitrary regions of support. *IEEE Trans. Circuits Syst. Video Technol., 11*, 1063–1068.

Nasrabadi, N. M., & King, R. A. (1998). Image coding using vector quantization: a review. *IEEE Trans.Com., 36*, 957-971.

Nguyen, T. D., Kim, S. H., & Kim, N. C. (2005). An Automatic Body ROI Determination for 3D Visualization of a Fetal Ultrasound Volume. R. Khosla et al. (Eds.): *KES 2005, LNAI 3682*, (pp. 145–153).

Penedo, M., Pearlman, W. A., Tahoces, P. G., Souto, M., & Vidal, J. J. (2003). Region-based wavelet coding methods for digital mammography. *IEEE Transactions on Medical Imaging, 22*, 1288 – 1296.

Said, A., & Pearlman, W. A. (1996). A new, fast and efficient image codec based on set partitioning in hierarchical trees. *IEEE Trans. Circuits Syst. Video Technol., 6*, 243–250.

Schelkens, P., Munteanu, A., Barbarien, J., Galca, M., Giro-Nieto, X., & Cornelis J., (2003). Wavelet Coding of Volumetric Medical Datasets, *IEEE Transactions On Medical Imaging, 22*(3), 441-458.

Shapiro, J. M. (1999). Embedded image coding using zerotrees of wavelet coefficients. *IEEE Trans. Signal Processing, 31*(12), 3445-3462.

Tasdoken, S., & Cuhadar, A. (2003). ROI Coding with Integer Wavelet Transforms and Unbalanced Spatial Orientation Trees. *25th Annual International Conference of the IEEE-EMBS.*

Taubman, D. (2000). High performance scalable image compression with EBCOT, *IEEE Trans. Image Processing, 9*, 1158–1170.

Ueno, I., & Pearlman, W. (2003). Region of Interest coding in volumetric images with shape-adaptive wavelet transform. *SPIE/IS&T Electronic Imaging 2003.*

Xiong, Z., Wu, X., & Yun, D. Y. (1998). Progressive coding of medical volumetric data using three-dimensional integer wavelet packet transform. *IEEE Multimedia Signal Processing*, (pp. 553-558).

KEY TERMS

Distributed Telemedicine: Store-and-forward telemedicine involves acquiring medical data (like medical images, biosignals etc) and then transmitting this data to a doctor or medical specialist at a convenient time for assessment offline. Dermatology, radiology, and pathology are common specialties that are conducive to asynchronous telemedicine.

Medical Image Coding: Refers to image compression as the application of data compression on digital images. In effect, the objective is to reduce redundancy of the image data in order to be able to store or transmit data in an efficient form. Image compression can be lossy or lossless. Lossy compression methods, especially when used at low bit rates, introduce compression artifacts. Lossless compression methods may also be preferred for high value content, such as medical imagery or image scans made for archival purposes.

ROI Coding: The Region Of Interest (ROI) coding it is a function that enables a non-uniform distribution of the image quality between a selected region (the ROI) and the rest of the image (background). ROI coding of medical images allows the compression of diagnostically important regions at better quality without affecting the visual assessment procedure, whereas areas like the background can be coded at lower quality in order to decrease image size and improve storage and/or transmission procedures.

Volumetric Medical Image: A typical 3D data set is a group of 2D slice images acquired by a CT or MRI scanner. Usually these are acquired in a regular pattern (e.g., one slice every millimeter) and usually have a regular number of image pixels in a regular pattern. This is an example of a regular volumetric grid, with each volume element, or voxel represented by a single value that is obtained by sampling the immediate area surrounding the voxel.

Wavelet: A one-dimensional pulse, usually the basic response from a single reflector. Its key attributes are its amplitude, frequency and phase. The wavelet originates as a packet of energy from the source point, having a specific origin in time, and is returned to the receivers as a series of events distributed in time and energy. The distribution is a function of velocity and density changes in the subsurface and the relative position of the source and receiver.

Wavelet Coding: Wavelet coding or compression is a form of data compression well suited for image compression (sometimes also video compression and audio compression). Wavelet compression can be either perfect (lossless) or lossy, where a certain loss of quality is accepted. Using a wavelet transform, the wavelet compression methods are adequate for representing transients, such as percussion sounds in audio, or high-frequency components in two-dimensional images, for example an image of stars on a night sky. This means that the transient elements of a data signal can be represented by a smaller amount of information than would be the case if some other transform, such as the more widespread discrete cosine transform, had been used.

Chapter XXX
Segmentation Methods in Ultrasound Images

Farhang Sahba
Medical Imaging Analyst, Canada

ABSTRACT

Ultrasound imaging now has widespread clinical use. It involves exposing a part of the body to high-frequency sound waves in order to generate images of the inside of the body. Because it is a real-time procedure, the ultrasound images show the movement of the body's internal structure as well. It is usually a painless medical test and its procedures seem to be safe. Despite recent improvement in the quality of information from an ultrasound device, these images are still a challenging case for segmentation. Thus, there is much interest in understanding how to apply an image segmentation task to ultrasound data and any improvements in this regard are desirable. Many methods have been introduced in existing literature to facilitate more accurate automatic or semi-automatic segmentation of ultrasound images. This chapter is a basic review of the works on ultrasound image segmentation classified by application areas, including segmentation of prostate transrectal ultrasound (TRUS), breast ultrasound, and intra-vascular ultrasound (IVUS) images.

INTRODUCTION

Among different image modalities, ultrasound imaging is one of the most widely used technologies for the diagnosis and treatment of diseases such as breast and prostate cancer. Ultrasound equipment is less expensive to purchase and maintain than many other imaging systems such as X-ray, computed tomography (CT), or magnetic resonance imaging (MRI). These images are the result of reflection, refraction, and deflection of ultrasound beams from different types of tissue with different acoustic impedances. The detection of the object boundaries in such images is crucial for diagnostic and classification purposes.

However, attenuation, speckle, shadows, and signal dropout can result in missing or diffused boundaries. Also the contrast between areas of interest is often low. These obstacles make segmentation of these images a challenge. Further complications arise when the quality of the image is influenced by the type and particular settings of the machine. Despite these factors, ultrasound imaging still remains an important tool for clinical applications and any effort to improve segmentation of these images is highly desirable. Thus, there is currently an interest in understanding how to apply image segmentation to ultrasound data. Figure 1 demonstrates the basic principle of an ultrasound imaging transducer. Using an ultrasound transducer, a pulse of energy is transmitted into the body along the path shown by line 1. After this beam encounters any surface, including tissue or structures within an organ, a part of the transmitted energy is backscattered along the original trajectory and received by the transducer which now acts as a receiver. These returning waves are converted to electrical signals, amplified, and finally shown. After that, the direction of the transmitted beam changes to attain the data from the next line close to the first one. The ultrasound transducer repeats the same procedure to cover 64-256 lines and makes the entire image (Webb, 2003).

This chapter contains an overview of the ideas representing the ultrasound segmentation problem in particular clinical applications.

BACKGROUND

Many methods have been introduced to facilitate more accurate segmentation of ultrasound images. The performance of these methods is generally improved through the use of expertise or prior knowledge. All segmentation methods usually require at least some user interaction to adjust critical parameters. The type of user interaction varies, depending on the amount of time and effort required from the user.

This chapter is a review of ultrasound image segmentation methods and focuses on clinical applications that have been investigated in different clinical domains. It centers on reviewing the ideas behind the incorporated knowledge of ultrasound physics such as speckle structure, as well as prior information about the intensity or shape model. We review some principal works in this area according to their applications where the major-

Figure 1. The basic principle of an ultrasound imaging transducer (© 2003 IEEE, Reprinted, with permission from IEEE Press Series in Biomedical Engineering 2003. "Introduction to Biomedical Imaging", by A. Webb).

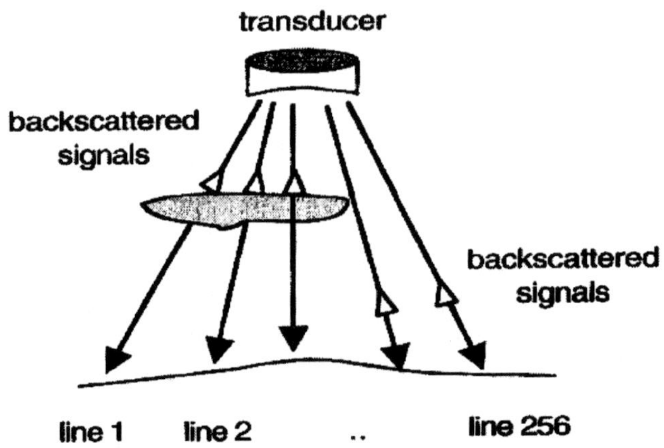

ity of efforts have been focused. These include segmentation of prostate transrectal ultrasound (TRUS), breast ultrasound, and intravascular ultrasound (IVUS) images.

ULTRASOUND IMAGE SEGMENTATION ACCORDING TO CLINICAL APPLICATIONS

Based on clinical application, ultrasound image segmentation can be categorized in various groups. In this section, we mention some important methods in each group.

Prostate Segmentation

Prostate cancer is one of the most frequently diagnosed malignancies in the adult and aging male population (Mettlin,1995). Ultrasound imaging is a widely used technology for the detection and intervention of this cancer and may help to reduce death rate if used in early stages.

As the prostate boundaries play an important role in the diagnosis and treatment of prostate cancer, it is crucial for many clinical applications to accurately detect them. These applications include the accurate placement of needles during the biopsy, accurate prostate volume measurement from multiple frames, constructing anatomical models used in treatment planning, and estimation of tumor border. These images are the result of reflection, refraction, and deflection of ultrasound beams from different types of tissues with different acoustic impedances (Insana et al., 1993).

Some factors, such as poor contrast, speckle, and weak edges, however, make the ultrasound images inherently difficult to segment. Furthermore, the quality of the image may be influenced by the type and particular settings of the machine.

Currently, the prostate boundaries are generally extracted from TRUS images (Insana et al., 1993). This kind of imaging has been a fundamental tool for prostate cancer diagnosis and treatment.

Prostate boundaries must generally be outlined in 2D TRUS image slices along the length of the prostate. But as previously mentioned, the signal-to-noise ratio in these images is very low. Therefore, traditional edge detectors fail to extract the correct boundaries.

Consequently, many methods have been developed to facilitate automatic or semi-automatic segmentation of the prostate boundaries from the ultrasound images. Figure 2 shows segmentation of some sample ultrasound images of the prostate using the method presented by Nanayakkara et al. (2006); it contains the ground truth boundaries drawn by an expert as well as contours generated by the computerized method.

Knoll et al. (1999) proposed a technique for elastic deformation of closed planar curves restricted to particular object shapes. Their method is based on a one-dimensional dyadic wavelet transform as a multi-scale contour parameterization technique to constrain the shape of the prostate model. Important edges at multiple resolutions are extracted as the first step. Then a template matching procedure is used to obtain an initial shape of the contour. The shape of the contour is constrained to predefined models during deformation. While they reported that the method provides an accurate and fully automatic segmentation of 2D objects, the dependence of the statistically derived prior model has limited its capability for segmentation of aberrant shapes.

Richard et al. (1996) presented a texture-based algorithm for prostate segmentation. This method segments a set of parallel 2D images of the prostate into prostate and non-prostate regions to form a 3D image. This algorithm is a pixel classifier which classifies each pixel of an ultrasound image using four associated texture energy measures. One of the drawbacks of this approach is that the number of clusters cannot be predicted for an image; therefore, the resulting image may be

Figure 2. Four samples for prostate boundary detection. The solid line shows the contour generated by the computerized method and the dotted line shows the corresponding manual outline (Reprinted (partially), from Physics in Medicine and Biology, 51, N.D Nanayakkara, J. Samarabandu, and A. Fenster, "Prostate segmentation by feature enhancement using domain knowledge and adaptive region based operations", pp. 1831–1848, 2006, with permission from IOP publishing Ltd).

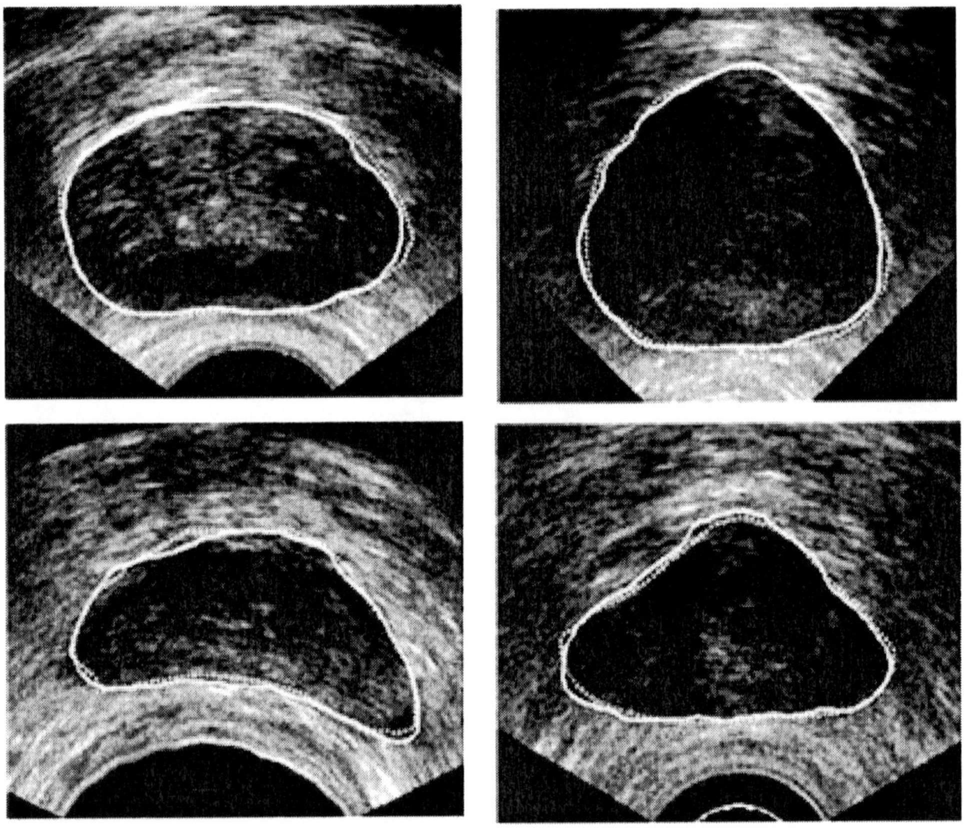

represented by a set of disconnected regions and no post-processing technique is proposed for preventing or overcoming the problem of such discontinuities.

Ladak et al. (2000) proposed a cubic spline interpolation technique for semi-automatic segmentation of the prostate. The algorithm uses an initial contour based on four points given by the user. The user selects four points around the prostate and then uses the discrete dynamic contour. A model is used to refine the boundary. Although this semi-automatic algorithm can segment a wide range of prostate images, at least four initial points must be defined accurately by the user (radiologist). In addition, it is less satisfactory when the prostate has an irregular shape and cannot be perfectly approximated by the initial points. For such cases, further human intervention is required to achieve satisfactory results.

Wang et al. (2003) presented two methods for semi-automatic three-dimensional (3D) prostate boundary segmentation using 2D ultrasound images. The segmentation process is initiated by manually placing four points on the boundary of a selected slice. Then an initial prostate boundary is determined. It is refined using the discrete dynamic contour until it fits the actual prostate boundary. The remaining slices are then segmented by iteratively propagating the results to other slices and implementing the refinement.

Hu et al. (2003) proposed an algorithm for semi-automatic segmentation of the prostate from 3D ultrasound images. In this method, the authors use model-based initialization and mesh refinement using deformable models. Six points are required to initialize the outline of the prostate using shape information. The initial outline is then automatically deformed to better fit the prostate boundary.

Chiu et al. (2004) introduced a semi-automatic segmentation algorithm based on the dyadic wavelet transform and the discrete dynamic contours. In this method, a spline interpolation is first used to determine the initial contour based on four user-defined initial points. Then the discrete dynamic contour refines the initial contour based on the approximate coefficients as well as the wavelet coefficients generated using the dyadic wavelet transform. A selection rule is also used to choose the best contour.

Abolmaesumi et al. (2004) used an interactive multi-model probabilistic data association filter to extract prostate contours from transrectal ultrasound images. As the first step, a Sticks filter is used to enhance the image. The problem is then addressed by considering several equally spaced radii from a seed point towards the boundary of the prostate. In this method, the border of the prostate is represented as the trajectory of a moving object. This motion is modeled using a set of dynamical models where their measurement points are presented as candidate edge points along each radius. As the method does not use any numerical technique, their results show that the convergence is also fast.

Pathak et al. (2000) proposed an edge-guided boundary delineation algorithm for prostate segmentation provided as a visual guide to the observer. This step is followed by manual editing. For automatic edge detection, the algorithm first uses a Sticks filter to enhance contrast and reduce speckle. Then, an anisotropic diffusion filter is applied to smooth the result of the previous stage. Finally, some basic prior knowledge such as shape and echo pattern is used to extract the most probable edges. After these stages, by using a manual linking procedure on the detected edges, the final boundary is indicated.

Shen et al. (2003) presented a statistical shape model for segmentation of the prostate in ultrasound images. A Gabor filter bank is employed in both multiple scales and multiple orientations to represent the image characteristics around the prostate boundaries. As these features give both edge directions and edge strengths, they can provide the information for deformation of the prostate model. This strategy can generate both coarse and fine image features that further allow the model to focus on particular features at different deformation steps. To make the proposed method more robust against local minima, several hierarchical deformation strategies are proposed as well. In another work, the authors have also introduced an adaptive focus deformable model, which uses the concept of an attribute vector (Shen et al., 2001).

Figure 3 shows segmentation of an ultrasound image of the prostate using the method presented in (Shen et al., 2003). This figure demonstrates the results of the algorithm in the different steps (iterations). As can be seen, the method is robust with respect to a bad initialization.

Betrounia et al. (2005) proposed a method for the automatic segmentation of trans-abdominal ultrasound images. Adaptive morphological and median filtering are employed together to detect the noisy areas and smooth them. Using this method, the contours of the prostate can be enhanced without changing the critical information in the image. An optimization algorithm is then employed to search for the contour initialized from a prostate model. The algorithm has been shown

Figure 3. Demonstration of the algorithm represented in (Shen et al., 2003). The dashed contour indicates the manually segmented prostate. The solid contours show the resulting the automatic algorithm in the different steps (iterations). The final segmentation results are shown in the right-bottom corner; a case of the bad initialization. (© 2003 IEEE, Reprinted with permission from IEEE Transaction on Medical Imaging, 2003, 22(4), pp. 539-551, "Segmentation of Prostate Boundaries from Ultrasound Images Using Statistical Shape Model", by D. Shen, Y. Zhan and C. Davatzikos).

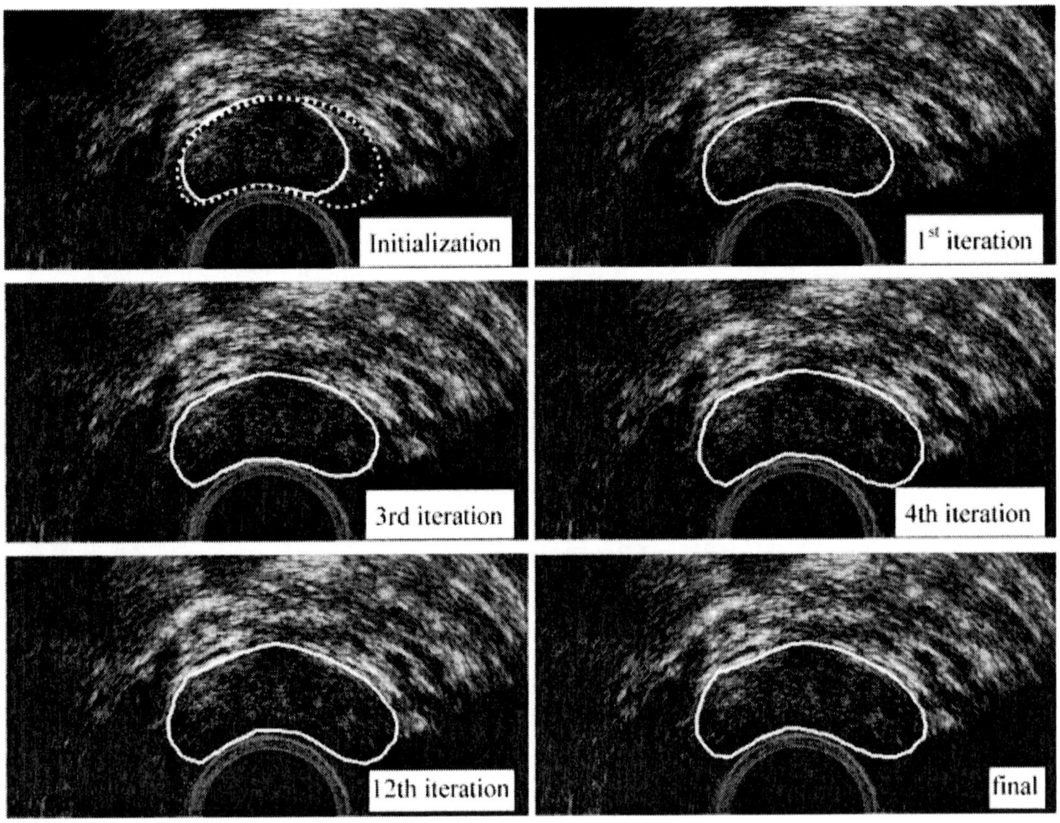

to have accurate results in terms of average distance and average coverage index in comparison to those obtained by manual segmentation.

Breast Cancer

Breast cancer is one of the leading causes of death in women. Along with digital mammography, ultrasound has been one of the most commonly used methods for early detection and diagnosis of breast cancer in the last decade. Ultrasound can help to distinguish whether a mass is benign or malignant (cancerous). Automatic segmentation of breast tumors using ultrasound imaging can assist physicians in making faster and more accurate diagnoses (Noble et al., 2006). The problem with segmenting ultrasonic breast images is mostly the variance of the lesion's shape and the fact that often the borders of the lesion are not well distinguished. Figure 4 demonstrates three different manually segmented ultrasonic breast lesions with great differences in their shapes and sizes as represented in (Madabhushi et al., 2003).

Figure 4. Three manually segmented tumors with different shapes and sizes (© 2003 IEEE, Reprinted with permission from IEEE Transaction on Medical Imaging, 2003, 22(2), pp. 155–169, "Combining low-, high-level and empirical domain knowledge for automated segmentation of ultrasonic breast lesions", by A. Madabhushi and D. N. Metaxas).

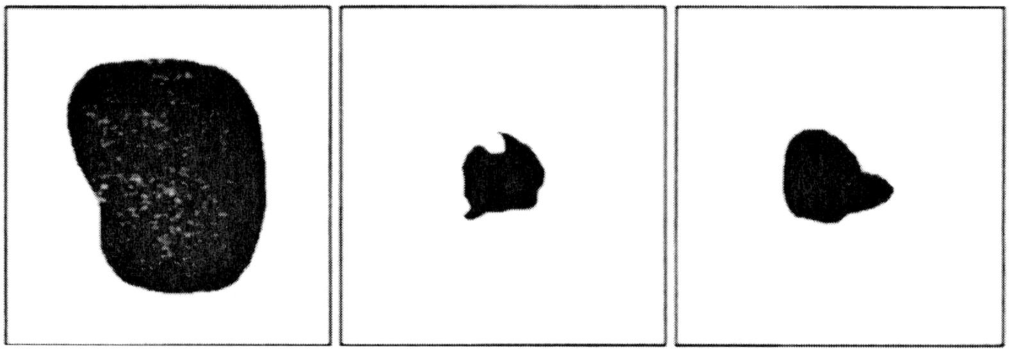

Huang et al. (2004) proposed an approach that combines a neural network classifier with a morphological watershed segmentation method to extract precise contours of a breast tumor from ultrasound images. Textural analysis is employed to generate the inputs of the neural network to classify US images. The features of the texture contain auto covariance coefficients to classify US images using a self-organizing map. After these features have been classified, an adaptive preprocessing procedure is selected by neural network output and then watershed transformation automatically determines the contours of the tumor. This method contains a preprocessing step which helps the watershed algorithm through a good selection of markers. The self-organizing map is used in order to select the appropriate preprocessing filter locally from a set of nine predefined filters. Figures 5 demonstrates two malignant and benign cases of breast ultrasound images. In this figure, the first, second, and third rows show the original magnified monochrome breast image, the contours manually sketched, and the contours determined by the proposed system in (Huang et al., 2004) , respectively.

Chen et al. (2002) presented a method based on a neural network. The aim of this method is to make the classification based on a set of input features. These features are variance contrast, autocorrelation contrast, and the distribution distortion in the wavelet coefficients. These are inputs of a multilayer perceptron neural network with one hidden layer which is trained by error backpropagation. Image texture is an important component in their method.

Xiao et al. (2002) discussed a method for simultaneous estimation of video-intensity inhomogeities and segmentation of US image tissue regions. The number of regions (classes) needs to be specified. It employs a combination of the maximum a posteriori (MAP) and Markov random field (MRF) methods to estimate the US image distortion field. The approach shows consistent segmentations under different time gain compensation (TGC) settings on the tested data.

Figure 5. Contour segmentation. The first row: Original magnified monochrome breast ultrasound images (left malignant and right benign case); the second row, manual sketch contour; and the third row, automatic sketch contour. (Reprinted from Ultrasound in Medicine & Biology, 30(5), Y. L Huang and D. R. Chen, "Watershed segmentation for breast tumor in 2-D sonography", pp. 625–632, 2004, with permission from Elsevier).

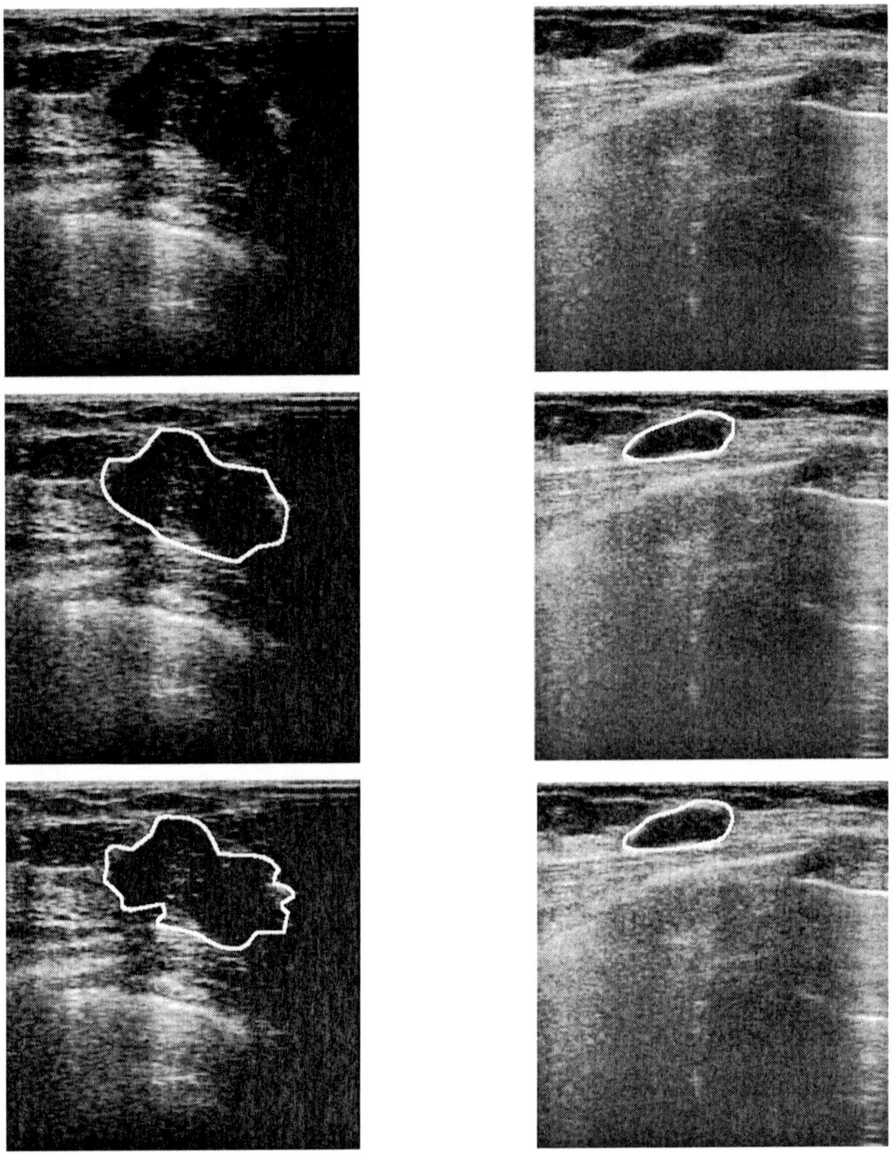

Horsch et al. (2001) introduced a segmentation technique that is based on maximizing a utility function over partition margins which are defined through gray-value thresholding of a preprocessed image that has enhanced mass structures. It requires the manually defined lesion center. The problem of shadowing is not discussed. Shape, echogeneity, margin, and posterior acoustic behavior are computed as four features to test the effectiveness when directed at distinguished malignant and benign masses. The authors have further evaluated their method in (Horsch et al., 2004) to assess the advantages of the different mentioned features using linear discriminant analysis. It is shown that the two best features are depth-to-width ratio for shape and normalized radial gradient for margin.

Sahiner et al. (2004) developed 2D and 3D intensity-gradient active contour models for automated segmentation of the mass volumes. For initialization of the active contour, texture and morphological features were automatically extracted from the segmented masses and their margins. Algorithm parameters were determined empirically. To find the segmentation result, depth to width ratio, a posterior shadowing feature measure, and texture features were computed around the boundary of each 2D slice and then linear discriminant analysis was used to classify volumes.

Madabhushi et al. (2003) proposed a method that uses the combination of intensity and texture with empirical domain-specific knowledge, along with directional gradient and a deformable shape-based model. A second-order Butterworth filter is used to remove speckle noise, and then the contrast of the tumor regions is enhanced. The image pixels are probabilistically classified based on intensity and texture information and then a region growing technique is used to obtain an initial segmentation of the lesion. The boundary points are found to supply an initial estimate to a deformable model. It attempts to limit the effects of shadowing and false positives by incorporating empirical domain-specific knowledge. The method requires a small database for training.

There are also some other methods that take into account the domain knowledge and consider the specification of ultrasound images such as speckle or artifacts.

Intravascular Ultrasound

Intravascular Ultrasound (IVUS) is a non-invasive technique which provides real-time high-resolution images with valuable anatomical information about the coronary arterial wall and plaque. IVUS consequently provides new insights into the diagnosis and therapy of coronary disease. IVUS imaging can be used as a complementary imaging tool to contrast X-ray angiography (Radeva et al., 2003), (Noble et al., 2006). Due to the ultrasound speckle, catheter artifacts, or calcification shadows, processing of IVUS image sets is a challenge. To perform an accurate quantitative analysis, a good segmentation of the lumen, the plaque, and the wall borders is required. Methods used for IVUS segmentation usually apply contour modeling (Kovalski et al., 2000; Sonka et al., 1995; Cardinal et al., 2003; Olszewski et al., 2004; Noble et al., 2006). Figure 6 shows a schematic form of a cross-sectional anatomy of a diseased coronary artery (Sonka et al., 1995).

Cardinal et al. (2003) presented a three-dimensional IVUS segmentation model based on the fast-marching method and gray level probability density functions of the vessel wall structures. A mixture of Rayleigh PDFs model the gray level distribution of the whole IVUS pullback. Using this method, the lumen, intima plus plaque structure, and media layers of the vessel wall were computed simultaneously.

The results were obtained with average point to point distances between segmented vessel wall borders and ground truth. The authors have also shown the potential of gray level PDF and fast-marching methods in 3D IVUS image processing.

Figure 6. A schematic cross-sectional anatomy of a diseased coronary vessel. (©1995 IEEE, Reprinted with permission from IEEE Transaction on Medical Imaging, 1995, 14(4), pp. 719–732, "Segmentation of intravascular ultrasound images: A knowledge-based approach", by M. Sonka, X. M. Zhang, M. Siebes, M. S. Bissing, S. C. DeJong, S. M. Collins and C. R. McKay).

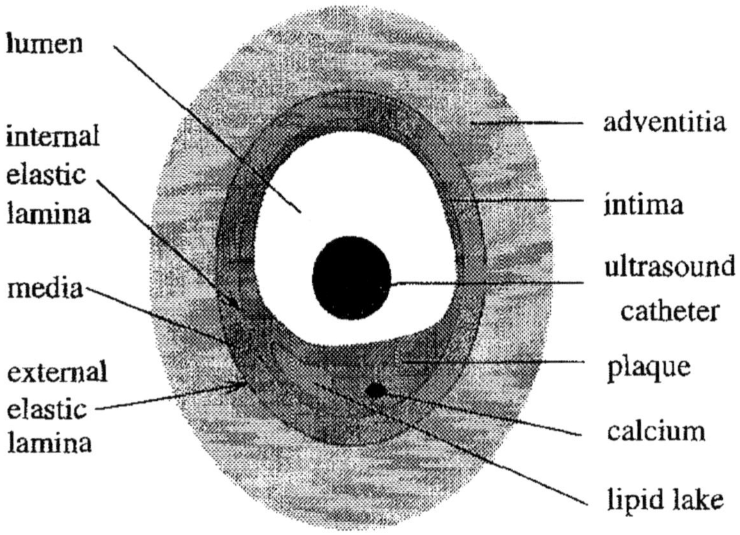

Sonka et al. (1995) introduced a semi-automatic knowledge-based method for segmentation of intravascular ultrasound images which identifies the internal and external elastic laminae and the plaque-lumen interface. This approach attempts to incorporate *a priori* knowledge about cross-sectional arterial anatomy, such as objectshape, edge direction, double echo pattern, and wall thickness. The method uses a cost function based on edge strength to find the border. However, the method does not take into account speckle statistics. To assess the performance of the method, they compared five quantitative measures of arterial anatomy derived from borders extracted by the algorithm, with measures derived from borders manually indicated by an expert.

Shekhar et al. (1999) developed a three-dimensional segmentation technique, called active surface segmentation, for semi-automatic segmentation of the lumen and adventitial borders in serial IVUS images in examinations of coronary arteries. The authors also presented a faster method, based on a fast active contours technique (a neighborhood-search method) (Klingensmith et al., 2000). Both of their works used only intensity gradient information for snakes. The technique was assessed by computing correlation coefficients and by comparing the results to the expert tracings.

Takagi et al. (2000) presented an automated contour analysis assisted by a blood noise reduction algorithm used as preprocessing step. Subtraction of two consecutive IVUS images acquired at the same position in time can increase the signal-to-noise ratio of the lumen area, i.e., obtain good contrast between the lumen and other parts in the image. As the blood echo speckles have higher temporal and spatial variations than the arterial wall, an adaptive filtering of speckle was applied based on pre-segmentation of blood and tissue areas. Their preliminary results showed that automated contour detection facilitated with a blood noise reduction algorithm appeared to be a reliable technique for area measurements in 40-MHz IVUS imaging.

Kovalski et al. (2000) developed an algorithm to identify the lumen border and the media-adventitia border (the external elastic membrane). To represent the contours in this method, a 3D balloon model is recruited by using polar coordinates. In this representation, the control points can only move along the radial direction. The reported inter-observer area variability is comparable to the result in (Klingensmith et al., 2003) except that the method in (Kovalski et al., 2000) is automatic. Figure 7 illustrates three sets of images with the lumen and media-adventitia tracings with shadowing artifacts from (Kovalski et al., 2000). The left, middle, and right columns demonstrate the original image, the manual contours, and the result of automatic procedures, respectively.

The features are extracted in three dimensions. The results for border contours obtained by this method were compared to the manually extracted results. The method suffers from some tuning of the algorithm's parameters when using different scanners.

Figure 7. The comparison between the manual and the automatic tracings of the lumen and media-adventitia for three different slices. Left: Original image; middle: Manual tracing and right: automatic detection. (Reprinted from Ultrasound in Medicine & Biology, 26(4), G. Kovalski, R. Beyar, R. Shofti, and H. Azhari, "Three-dimensional automatic quantitative analysis of intravascular ultrasound images", pp. 527–537, 2000, with permission from Elsevier).

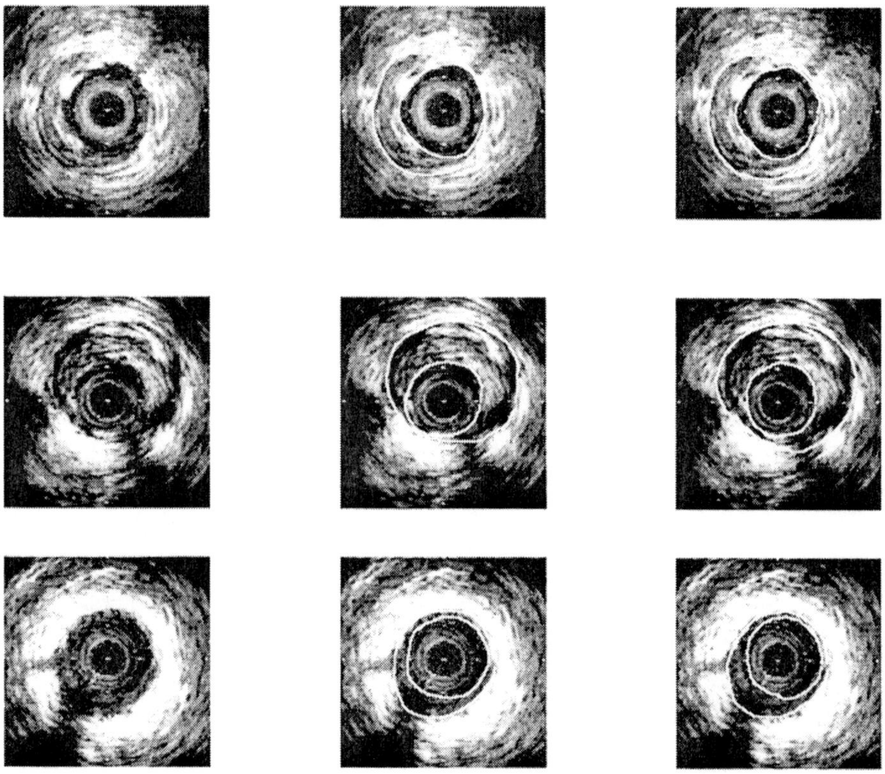

Haas et al. (2000) used an algorithm based on the optimization of a *maximum a posteriori* estimator. It implements an image generation model based on the Rayleigh distribution of the image pixels and *a priori* information about the contours. Using the property of the closed contours, they are modeled by first-order Markov random fields, expressing a strong correlation between a contour point and its two next neighbors. During the first stage, the algorithm detected the reliable points and then chose either the global or the first maximum along the radial direction depending on the contour prior energy. Dynamic programming is used to accelerate the estimation process. Additional information from the blood flow is used to initialize the segmentation in 3D image sets.

Pardo et al. (2003) proposed a statistical deformable model for 3D segmentation of anatomical organs applied to IVUS images. A bank of Gaussian derivative filters is used to generate a feature space at different orientations and scales, to locally describe each part of the object boundary. The feature space was reduced by linear discriminant analysis and a statistic discriminant snake is used in a supervised learning scheme to guide the model deformation. It is performed by minimizing the dissimilarity between the learned and found image features. The proposed approach is of particular interest for tracking temporal image sequences. Anatomical organs including IVUS are segmented and the results compared to expert tracings for validation.

As one of the approaches incorporating high-level knowledge in IVUS image segmentation, Olszewski et al. (2004) proposed a learning technique based on the human visual system. This method mimics the procedure performed by human experts for automatic detection of the luminal and the medial-adventitial borders. The approach requires no manual initialization or interaction. To verify the accuracy of the method, it is applied on a reasonable data set.

A key drawback for Intravascular Ultrasound imaging is its inability to consider the vessel curvature and the orientation of the imaging catheter (Noble et al., 2006). Therefore, the information extracted from this data is distorted, since the vessel curvature remains unconsidered. An answer for correct 3D reconstruction of the IVUS can be derived from the fusion between intravascular ultrasound images and biplane angiography (Noble et al., 2006).

FUTURE TRENDS

Ultrasonic imaging stands as one of the most important medical imaging applications of physics and engineering. There have been recent advances in transducer technology and image formation procedure which significantly improve the quality of information obtained from ultrasound devices.

There is a need for more effort in the area of segmentation validation to better evaluate the strengths and limitations of the existing methods on larger and more varied databases of images. This would be especially useful for the adoption of methods which are more appropriate in clinical applications. Future efforts for ultrasound segmentation methods should also more effectively consider imaging physics.

Basically, a 3D ultrasound image can be constructed from 2D slices which are put together. For such an application, the size and shape of the object of interest is to be extracted in each slice. This means that a fast and reliable segmentation method for individual slices is needed. Considering the correlation between the sequential frames, this can be subjected to further research.

4D ultrasound system provides a next generation for medical imaging applications which allow faster diagnosis and improve treatment success rates. A 4D ultrasound device takes multiple images in rapid succession and creates a 3D motion video, which is very valuable for diagnosis purposes. Any effort towards applying current segmentation methods in these successive frames would be desirable.

CONCLUSION

Ultrasound imaging is a non-invasive, easily portable, and relatively inexpensive image modality that has been used for clinical applications for a long time.

Ultrasound imaging can be used to visualize the anatomy of the body organs. It also has excellent temporal resolution. In this technique, by exposing a part of the body to high-frequency sound waves, we can generate images of the inside of the body.

On the other hand, segmentation is an important image processing task that partitions the image into meaningful regions. These regions are homogeneous with respect to specific characteristics or features such as gray level, texture, etc. Segmentation is an important tool in medical imaging and it is useful for many applications such as feature extraction and classification.

Although ultrasound imaging is one of the most widely used technologies for diagnosis and treatment, it is still a challenging case for segmentation tasks due to attenuation, speckle, shadows, and signal dropout. Improvements in this area of research are thus highly desirable. Many methods have been introduced in existing literature to facilitate more accurate automatic or semi-automatic segmentation of ultrasound images.

This chapter reviews the ultrasound image segmentation methods by focusing on clinical applications that contain important ideas demonstrating significant clinical usefulness.

The focus of this chapter is on reviewing the works which have incorporated prostate transrectal ultrasound (TRUS), breast ultrasound, and intravascular ultrasound (IVUS) images.

The future trend for ultrasound image segmentation can focus on improvement of the current methods such that they can be adopted for real clinical applications. Development of new and effective methods for construction of 3D images from 2D slices is also another interesting area of research.

As the next generation of ultrasound imaging devices, the 4D ultrasound system should be positioned as a top research area for image segmentation.

REFERENCES

Abolmaesumi, P., & Sirouspour, M.R. (2004). Segmentation of prostate contours from ultrasound images. *ICASSP04*, 3, 517-520.

Betrounia, N., Vermandela, M., Pasquierc, D., Maoucheb, S., & Rousseaua, J. (2005). Segmentation of abdominal ultrasound images of the prostate using a priori information and an adapted noise filter. *Computerized Medical Imaging and Graphics*, *29*, 43-51.

Cardinal, M. H. R., Meunier, J., Soulez, G., Thrasse, E., & Cloutier G. (2003). *Intravascular ultrasound image segmentation: A fastmarching method.* Medical Image Computing and Computer Assisted Intervention, Lecture Note Computer Science. Berlin: Springer-Verlag, (pp. 432–439).

Chen, D. R., Chang, R. F., Kuo, W. J., Chen, M. C., & Huang, Y. L. (2002). Diagnosis of breast tumors with sonographic texture analysis using wavelet transform and neural networks. *Ultrasound in Medicine & Biology*, *28*(10), 1301–1310.

Chiu, B., Freeman, G. H., Salama, M. M. A., & Fenster A. (2004). Prostate segmentation algorithm using dyadic wavelet transform and discrete dynamic contour. *Physics in Medicine and Biology*, *49*, 4943-4960.

Haas C., Ermert H., Holt S., Grewe P., Machraoui A., & Barmeyer J. (2000). Segmentation of 3-D intravascular ultrasonic images based on a random field model. *Ultrasound in medicine & biology, 26*(2), 297–306.

Horsch, K., Giger, M. L., Venta, L. A., & Vyborny, C. J. (2001). Automatic segmentation of breast lesions on ultrasound. *Medical Physics, 28*(8), 1652–1659.

Horsch, K., Giger, M. L., Vyborny, C. J., & Venta, L. A. (2004). Performance of computer-aided diagnosis in the interpretation of lesions on breast sonography. *Academic radiology, 11*(3), 272–280.

Hu, N., Downey, D. B., Fenster, A., & Ladak, H. M. (2003). Prostate boundary segmentation from 3D ultrasound images. *Medical Physics, 30*(7), 1648-1659.

Huang, Y. L., & Chen, D. R. (2004). Watershed segmentation for breast tumor in 2-D sonography. *Ultrasound in Medicine & Biology, 30*(5), 625–632.

Insana, M. F., & Brown, D. G. (1993). *Acoustic scattering theory applied to soft biological tissues. In Ultrasonic Scattering in biological tissues,* Boca Raton, CRC Press.

Klingensmith, J. D., Shekhar, R., & Vince, D. G. (2000). Evaluation of three dimensional segmentation algorithms for the identification of luminal and medial-adventitial borders in intravascular ultrasound images. *IEEE Transaction on Medical Imaging, 19*(10), 996–1011.

Klingensmith, J. D., Tuzcu, E. M., Nissen, S. E., & Vince, D. G. (2003). Validation of an automated system for luminal and medial-adventitial border detection in three-dimensional intravascular ultrasound. *The International Journal of Cardiovascular Imaging, 19*(1), 93–104.

Knoll, C., Alcaniz, M., Grau, V., Monserrat, C., & Juan, M.C. (1999). Outlining of the prostate using snakes with shape restrictions based on the wavelet transform. *Pattern Recognition, 32,* 1767-1781.

Kovalski, G., Beyar, R., Shofti, R., & Azhari, H. (2000). Three-dimensional automatic quantitative analysis of intravascular ultrasound images. *Ultrasound in medicine & biology, 26*(4), 527–537.

Ladak, H. M., Mao, F., Wang, Y., Downey, D. B., Steinman, D. A., & Fenster, A. (2000). Prostate boundary segmentation from 2D ultrasound images. *Medical Physics, 27,* 1777-1788.

Madabhushi, A., & Metaxas, D. N. (2003). Combining low-, high-level and empirical domain knowledge for automated segmentation of ultrasonic breast lesions. *IEEE Transaction on Medical Imaging, 22*(2), 155–169.

Mettlin, C. (1995). American society national cancer detection project. *Cancer, 75,* 1790-1794.

Nanayakkara, N. D., Samarabandu, J., & Fenster, A. (2006). Prostate segmentation by feature enhancement using domain knowledge and adaptive region based operations", *Physics in Medicine and Biology, 51,* 1831–1848

Noble, J. A., & Boukerroui, D. (2006). Ultrasound Image Segmentation: A Survey. *IEEE Transactions on Medical Imaging, 25,* 987-1010.

Olszewski, M. E., Wahle, A., Mitchell, S. C., & Sonka, M. (2004). Segmentation of intravascular ultrasound images: A machine learning approach mimicking human vision. *In International Congress Series, 1268,* 1045–1049.

Pardo, X. M., Radeva, P., & Cabello, D. (2003). Discriminant snakes for 3-D reconstruction of anatomical organs. *Medical Image Analysis, 7*(3), 293–310.

Pathak, S. D., Chalana, V., Haynor, D. R., & Kim, Y. (2000). Edge-guided boundary delineation in prostate ultrasound images. *IEEE Transactions on Medical Imaging, 19,* 1211-1219.

Radeva, P., Suri, J. S., & Laxminarayan, S. (2003). *Angiography and plaque imaging: Advanced segmentation techniques*. Boca Raton, FL: CRC Press.

Richard, W. D., & Keen, C. G. (1996). Automated texture-based segmentation of ultrasound images of the prostate. *Computerized Medical Imaging and Graphics, 20*(3), 131-140.

Sahiner, B., Chan, H. P., Roubidoux, M. A., Helvie, M. A., Hadjiiski, L. M., Ramachandran, A., Paramagul, C., LeCarpentier, G. L., Nees, A., & Blane, C. (2004). Computerized characterization of breast masses on threedimensional ultrasound volumes. *Medical Physics, 31*(4), 744–754.

Shekhar, R., Cothren, R. M., Vince, D. G., Chandra, S., Thomas, J. D., & Cornhill, J. F. (1999). Three-dimensional segmentation of luminal and adventitial borders in serial intravascular ultrasound images. *Computerized Medical Imaging and Graphics, 23*, 299–309.

Shen, D., Herskovits, E. H., & Davatzikos, C. (2001). An adaptive-focus statistical shape model for segmentation and shape modeling of 3D brain structures. *IEEE Transactions on Medical Imaging, 20*, 257-270.

Shen, D., Zhan, Y., & Davatzikos, C. (2003). Segmentation of Prostate Boundaries From Ultrasound Images Using Statistical Shape Model. *IEEE Transactions on Medical Imaging, 22*(4), 539-551.

Sonka, M., Zhang, X. M., Siebes, M., Bissing, M. S., DeJong, S. C., Collins, S. M., & McKay C. R. (1995). Segmentation of intravascular ultrasound images: A knowledge-based approach. *IEEE Transaction on Medical Imaging, 14*(4), 719–732.

Takagi, A., Hibi, K., Zhang, X., Teo, T. J., Bonneau, H. N., Yock, P. G., & Fitzgerald P. J. (2000). Automated contour detection for highfrequency intravascular ultrasound imaging: A technique with blood noise reduction for edge enhancement. *Ultrasound in medicine & biology , 26*, 1033–1041.

Wang, Y., Cardinal, H. N., Downey, D. B., & Fenster, A. (2003). Semiautomatic three-dimensional segmentation of the prostate using two dimensional ultrasound images. *Medical physics, 30*(5), 887-897.

Webb, A. (2003). *Introduction to Biomedical Imaging*. IEEE Press Series in Biomedical Engineering.

Xiao, G. F., Brady, M., Noble, J. A., & Zhang, Y. Y. (2002). Segmentation of ultrasound B-mode images with intensity inhomogeneity correction. *IEEE Transaction on Medical Imaging, 21*(1), 48–57.

KEY TERMS

Breast Ultrasound: Generation of ultrasound images from the breast for diagnostic and treatment purposes.

Image Segmentation: This is an important image processing task that partitions the image into meaningful regions.

Intravascular Ultrasound: This is an ultrasound medical imaging methodology that uses a catheter with a miniaturized ultrasound probe to visualize the inside walls of blood vessels.

Prostate Ultrasound: Generation of ultrasound images from the prostate for diagnostic and treatment purposes.

Ultrasound Imaging: This is an ultrasound-based diagnostic imaging technique used for visualizing internal organs and their structures and possible lesions.

Compilation of References

Abbott, J. G. (1999). Rationale and derivation of *MI* and *TI* – a review. *Ultrasound Med. Biol., 25*, 431-441.

Abolmaesumi, P., & Sirouspour, M.R. (2004). Segmentation of prostate contours from ultrasound images. *ICASSP04*, 3, 517-520.

AbuRahma, A. F., Kyer, P. D., Robinson, P. A., et al. (1998). The correlation of ultrasonic carotid plaque morphology and carotid plaque hemorrhage: clinical implications. *Surgery, 124*, 721-8.

Acharya, R., Wasserman, R., Stevens, J., & Hinojosa, C. (1995). Biomedical imaging modalities: a tutorial. *Computerized Medical Imaging and Graphics, 19*(1), 3-25.

Ackerman, M. (1998). The visible human project. *Proceedings of the IEEE, 86*(3), 504–511.

Adams, R., & Bischof, L. (1994). Seeded region growing. *IEEE Trans. Pattern Anal. Machine Intell., 16*, 641-647.

ADIR M-FISH Image Database. Available at: http://www.adires.com/05/Project/MFISH_DB/MFISH_DB.shtml

Adlassnig, K.-P., Combi, C., Das, A. K., Keravnou, E. T., & Pozzi, G. (2006). Temporal representation and reasoning in medicine: Research directions and challenges. *Artif Intell Med, 38*(2), 101-113.

Agam G., & Dinstein I., (1997). Geometric separation of partially overlapping nonrigid objects applied to automatic chromosome classification. *IEEE Transactions on Pattern Analysis and Machine Intelligence, 19*, 1212-1222.

Aggarwal, J. K., & Nandhakumar, N. (1988). On the computation of motion from sequences of images – A review. *Proceedings of the IEEE, 76*(8), 917-935.

Agostinelli, S. (2003). Geant4—a simulation toolkit. *Nuclear Instruments and Methods in Physics Research, A 506*, 250–303.

Agrafiotis, D., Bull, D. R., & Canagarajah, N. (2003). ROI coding of volumetric medical images with application to visualization. *3rd International Symposium on Image and Signal Processing and Analysis*, (p. 217).

Ahmed, A. A., Vias, M., Iyer, N. G., Caldas, C., & Brenton J. D. (2004). Microarray segmentation methods signifficantly influence data precision. *Nucleic Acids Research, 32*, e50.

Aki, K., & Richards, P. G. (2002). *Quantitative Seismology*. Sausalito, California: University Science Books.

Aldoori, M. I., Baird, R. N., Al-Sam, S. Z., et al. (1987). Duplex scanning and plaque histology in cerebral ischaemia. *European Journal of Vascular Surgery, 1*, 159-64.

Alexander, A. L., Tsuruda, J. S., & Parker, D. L. (1997). Estimation of eddy current artifacts in diffusion-weighted echo-planar images: the use of bipolar gradients. *Magnetic Resonance in Medicine, 38*, 1016-1021.

Alexander, D. C. (2005). Multiple-fiber reconstruction algorithms for diffusion MRI. *Annals of the New York Academy of Sciences, 1064*, 113-133.

Alexander, D. C., & Barker, G. J. (2005). Optimal imaging parameters for fiber-orientation estimation in diffusion MRI. *NeuroImage, 27*, 357-367.

Alexander, D. C., Barker, G. J., & Arridge, S. R. (2002). Detection and modeling of non-gaussian apparent diffusion coefficient profiles in human brain data. *Magnetic Resonance in Medicine, 48*, 331-340.

Allison, D. B., Cui, X., Page, G. P. (2006). Sabripour, M., Microarray Data Analysis: from Disarray to Consolidation and Consensus, *Nat. Rev. Genet. 7*, 55-65.

Alonso-Calvo, R., & Maojo, V. (2007). An Agent and Ontology-based System for integrating Public Genomic Databases. *J Biomed Inform., 40*(1), 17-29.

American Cancer Society [http://www.cancer.org]

American Society for Gastrointestinal Endoscopy [www.asge.org]

Amini, A. A., & Duncan, J. S. (1992). Bending and stretching models for LV wall motion analysis from curves and surfaces. *Image and Vision Computing, 10*(6), 418-430.

Anastassopoulos, G., & Skodras, A. (2002). JPEG2000 ROI coding in Medical Imaging Applications. *2nd IASTED Int. Conf. on Visualisation, Imaging and Image Processing*, VIIP2002.

Anbar, M. (2007). Dynamic thermal assessment. In J. D. Bronzino & N. A. Diakides (Ed.), *Medical Infrared Imaging* (pp. 8.1 – 8.23).Boca Raton, FL: CRC Press.

Anbeek, P., Vincken, K. L., van Osch, M. J., Bisschops, R. H., & van der Grond, J. (2004). Probabilistic segmentation of white matter lesions in MR imaging. *Neuroimage, 21,* 1037-1044.

Anderson, J. L., & Skare, S. (2002). A model-based method for retrospective correction of geometric distortions in diffusion-weighted EPI. *NeuroImage, 16,* 177-199.

Anderson, T., & McDicken, W. N. (1999). Measurement of tissue motion. *Proceedings of the Institution of Mechanical Engineers, 213*(3), 181-191.

Anderson, W. A. D. (1984). *Pathology* (8'th ed.). Saint Louis, Mo, USA: CW Mosby Co.

Andreassen, S., Riekehr, C., Kristensen, B., Schonheyder, H. C., & Leibovici, L. (1999). Using probabilistic and decision-theoretic methods in treatment and prognosis modeling. *Artif Intell Med, 15*(2), 121-134.

Andreutos, D., Plataniotis, K. N., & Venetsanopoulos, A. N. (1998). Distances Measures for Color Image Retrieval. *IEEE ICIP International Conference on Image Processing.*

Ang, P. H., Ruetz, P. A., & Auld, D. (1991). Video compression makes big gains, *IEEE Spectrum, 28*, 16 – 19.

Angelini, C., De Canditiis, D., Mutarelli, M., Pensky M, (2007). A Bayesian Approach to Estimation and Testing in Time-course Microarray Experiments, *Statistical Applications in Genetics and Molecular Biology*: *6*(1), 24.

Angelini, E. D., Homma, S., Pearson, G., Holmes, J. W., & Laine, A. F. (2005). Segmentation of real-time three-dimensional ultrasound for quantification of ventricular function: A clinical study on right and left ventricles. *Ultrasound in Medicine and Biology, 31*(9), 1143-1158.

Angulo, J., & Serra, J. (2003). Automatic analysis of DNA microarray images using mathematical morphology. *Bioinformatics, 19*(5), 553-562.

Arfanakis, K., Cordes, D., Haughton, V. M., Carew, J. D., & Meyerand, M. E. (2002). Independent component analysis applied to diffusion tensor MRI. *Magnetic Resonance in Medicine, 47*, 354-363.

Arfanakis, K., Haughton, V. M., Carew, J. D., Rogers, B. P., Dempsey, R. J., & Meyerand, M. E. (2002). Diffusion tensor MR imaging in diffuse axonal injury. *American Journal of Neuroradiology, 23*, 794-802.

Argyropoulos, C., Chatziioannou, A. A., Nikiforidis, G., Moustakas, A., Kollias, G., & Aidinis, V. (2006). Operational criteria for selecting a cDNA microarray data normalization algorithm. *Oncology reports,15*(4), 983-996.

Ariel, I. M., & Cleary J. B. (1987). *Breast cancer diagnosis and treatment.* New York, USA: McGraw-Hill.

Arif, M., & Rajpoot, N. M. (2007). Detection of nuclei by unsupervised manifold learning. *Proceedings of Medical Image Understanding and analysis.*

Arikidis, N., Skiadopoulos, S., Karahaliou, A., Likaki, E., Panayiotakis, G., & Costaridou, L. (2008, in press). B-spline active rays segmentation of microcalcifications in mammography. *Medical Physics.*

Armitage, P. A., & Bastin, M. E. (2001). Utilizing the diffusion-to-noise ratio to optimize magnetic resonance diffusion tensor acquisition strategies for improving measurements of diffusion anisotropy. *Magnetic Resonance in Medicine, 45,* 1056-1065.

Arnheim, R. (2004). *Visual Thinking.* Berkeley, CA: University of California Press.

Arnold, J. A. C., Modaresi, K. B., Thomas, N., et al. (1999) Carotid plaque characterization by duplex scanning. Observer error may undermine current clinical trials. *Stroke, 30,* 61-5.

Arteaga-Salas, J. M., Zuzan, H., Langdon, W. B., Upton, G. J., & Harrison, A. P. (2008). An overview of image-processing methods for Affymetrix GeneChips. *Brief Bioinform, 9*(1), 25-33.

Ashton, E. (2006). *Method and system for automatic identification and quantification of abnormal anatomical structures in medical images.* United States Patent 7,103,224.

Assaf, Y., & Basser, P. J. (2005). Composite hindered and restricted model of diffusion (CHARMED) MR imaging of the human brain. *Neuroimage, 27,* 48-58.

Assaf, Y., Freidlin, R. Z., Rohde, G. K., & Basser, P. J. (2004). A new modeling and experimental framework to characterize hindered and restricted diffusion in brain white matter. *Magnetic Resonance in Medicine, 52,* 965-978.

Asvestas, P., Matsopoulos, G. K., & Nikita, K. S. (1998). A power differentiation method of fractal dimension estimation for 2-D signals. *Journal of Visual Communication and Image Representation, 9*(4), 392-400.

Avcibas, I., Sankur, B., & Sayood, K. (2002). Statistical evaluation of image quality measures. *Journal of Electronic imaging, 11*(2), 206-223.

Azpiroz-Leehan, J., Leder, R., & Lerallut, J.-F. (2004). Quantitative and qualitative evaluation of filter characteristics for wavelet packet compression of MR images. *In 26th Annual International Conference of the Engineering in Medicine and Biology Society,* (pp. 1537-1540).

Bahrens, T. E., Johansen-Berg, H., & Woolrich, M. W. (2003). Non-invasive mapping of connection between human thalamus and cortex using diffusion imaging. *Nature Neuroscience, 6,* 750-757.

Bai, P., Wan, M., Wang, S., Zhang, D., & Dang, J. (2006). A novel method for evaluating tissue inhomogeneity in elastography. *Progress in Natural Science, 16*(5), 474-479.

Bajcsy, P., Liu, L., & Band, M. (2007). DNA microarray image processing. In G. Kamberova (Ed.), *DNA array image analysis*: Nuts & Bolts.

Bajcsy, R., & Kovacic, S. (1989). Multiresolution elastic matching. *Computer vision, graphics, and image processing, 46,* 1–21.

Bammer, R. (2003). Basic principles of diffusion-weighted imaging. *European Journal of Radiology, 45,* 169-184.

Bang, J., Dahl, T., Bruinsma, A., Kaspersen, J. H., Hernes, T. A. N., & Myhre, H. O. (2003). A new method for analysis of motion of carotid plaques from rf ultrasound images. *Ultrasound in Medicine and Biology, 29*(7), 967-976.

Bankman, I. N., Spisz, T. S., & Pavlopoulos, S. (2000). *Two-Dimensional Shape and Texture Quantification, Handbook of medical imaging.* Academic Press, Inc.

Bardies, M., Flux, G., Lassmann, M., Monsieurs, M., Savolainen, S., Strand, S. E. (2006). Quantitative imaging for clinical dosimetry. *Nuclear Instruments and Methods in Physics Research, A 569,* 467–471.

Barillot, C., Lemoine, D., Le Briquer, L., Lachmann, F., & Gibaud B. (1993). Data fusion in medical imaging: merging multimodal and multipatient images, identification of structures and 3D display aspects. *European Journal of Radiology, 17*(1), June, 22-27.

Basser, P. J., & Pierpaoli, C. (1998). A simplified method to measure the diffusion tensor from seven MR images. *Magnetic Resonance in Medicine, 39,* 928-934.

Basser, P. J., Mattiello, J., & Bihan, D. L. (1994). Estimation of the effective self-diffusion tensor from the NMR spin echo. *Journal of Magnetic Resonance, 103,* 247-254.

Basser, P. J., Mattiello, J., & Le Bihan, D. (1994). MR diffusion tensor spectroscopy and imaging. *Biophysical Journal, 66,* 259-267.

Basser, P. J., Pajevic, S., Pierpaoli, C., Duda, J., & Aldroubi, A. (2000). In vitro fiber tractography using DT-MRI data. *Magnetic Resonance in Medicine, 44,* 625-632.

Bates, D. W. (2002). The quality case for information technology in healthcare. *Medical Informatics and Decision Making,* 2(7).

Bath, P. (2003). Data mining in health and medical information. *Annual Review of Information Science and Technology, 38,* 331-369.

Bathula, D. R., Papademetris, X., & Duncan, J. S. (2007). Level set based clustering for analysis of functional MRI data. *4th IEEE International Symposium on Biomedical Imaging: From Nano to Macro,* (pp. 416-419).

Battle, A., Chechik, G., & Koller, D. (2007). Temporal and Cross-Subject Probabilistic Models for fMRI Prediction Tasks. In B. Scholkopf (Ed.), *Advances in Neural Information Processing Systems 19: Proceedings of the 2006 Conference* (pp.121-128). Cambridge: MIT Press.

Beckmann, C. F., & Smith, S. M. (2004). Probabilistic independent component analysis for functional magnetic resonance imaging. *IEEE Trans. Med. Imaging, 23*(2), 137-152.

Behrenbruch, C. P., Marias, K., Armitage, P. A., Yam, M., Moore, N. R., English, R. E., Clarke, P. J., Leong, F. J., & Brady, J. (2004). Fusion of contrast-enhanced breast MR and mammographic imaging data. *The British Journal of Radiology, 77*(2), S201-208.

Behrens, S., Laue, H., Althaus, M., Boehler, T., Kuemmerlen B., Hahn, H. K., & Peitgen, H. O. (2007). Computer assistance for MR based diagnosis of breast cancer: Present and future challenges. *Computerized Medical Imaging and Graphics, 31*(4-5), 236-247.

Bellazzi, R., & Zupan, B. (2001). Intelligent data analysis--special issue. *Methods Inf Med, 40*(5), 362-364.

Bellazzi, R., & Zupan, B. (2008). Predictive data mining in clinical medicine: Current issues and guidelines. *Int J Medical Informatics, 77*(2), 81-97.

Benamrane, N. *et al.* (2006). Fuzzy Neural Networks and Genetic Algorithms for Medical Images Interpretation. *Proc. Geometric Modeling and Imaging— New Trends, IEEE Computer Society.*

Benayoun, S., & Ayache, N. (1998). Dense non-rigid motion estimation in sequences of medical images using differential constraints. *International Journal of Computer Vision, 26*(1), 25-40.

Benjamini, Y., & Hochberg, Y. (1995). Controlling the False Discovery Rate: a Practical and Powerful Approach to Multiple Testing. *J. R. Statist. Soc., 57,* 289-300.

Bercoff, J., Tanter, M., Muller, M., & Fink, M. (2004). The role of viscosity in the impulse diffraction field of elastic waves induced by the acoustic radiation force. *IEEE Trans. Ultrason., Ferroelect. Freq. Contr., 51,* 1523-1536.

Bercoff, J., Tanter, N., & Fink, M. (2004). Supersonic shear imaging: a new technique for soft tissue elasticity mapping. *IEEE Trans. Ultrason., Ferroelect. Freq. Contr., 51,* 396-409.

Bernabe, G., Gonzalez, J., Garcia, J. M., & Duato, J. (2000). A new lossy 3-D wavelet transform for high-quality compression of medical video. *IEEE EMBS International Conference on Information Technology Applications in Biomedicine,* (p. 226).

Bertelli, L. *et al.* (2006). A semi-automatic system for segmentation of cardiac M-mode images. *Pattern Analysis and Applications, 9*(4), 293-306.

Berzin, D., & Hagiwara, I. (2002). Minimal area for surface reconstruction from crosssections, *The Visual Computer, 18*, 437–444.

Besl, P. J., & McKay, N. D. (1992). A method of registration of 3-D shapes. *IEEE Transactions in Pattern Analysis and Machine Intelligence, 14*(2), 239-256.

Betal, D., Roberts, N., & Whitehouse, G. H. (1997). Segmentation and numerical analysis of microcalcifications on mammograms using mathematical morphology. *The British Journal of Radiology, 70*(837), 903-917.

Betrounia, N., Vermandela, M., Pasquierc, D., Maoucheb, S., & Rousseaua, J. (2005). Segmentation of abdominal ultrasound images of the prostate using a priori information and an adapted noise filter. *Computerized Medical Imaging and Graphics, 29*, 43-51.

Beyer, R. T. (1978). Radiation pressure – the history of a mislabeled tensor. *J. Acoust. Soc. Am., 63*, 1025-1030.

Bezdek, J. C. (1981). Pattern Recognition with Fuzzy Objective Function Algorithms. *Plenum Press.* New York.

Bhagat, Y. A., & Beaulieu, C. (2004). Diffusion anisotropy in subcortical white matter and cortical gray matter: changes with aging and the role of CSF-suppression. *Journal of Magnetic Resonance Imaging, 20,* 216-227.

Biasi, G. M., Mingazzini, P. M., Baronio, L., Piglionica, M. R., Ferrari, S. A., Elatrozy, T. S., Nicolaides, A. N. (1998) Carotid plaque characterization using digital image processing and its potential in future studies of carotid endarterectomy and angioplasty. *Journal of Endovascular Surgery, 5(3)*, 240-6.

Bidgood W. D., & Horii, S. C. (1997). Understanding and Using DICOM, the Data Interchange Standard for Biomedical Imaging. *Journal of the American Medical Informatics Association, 4*, 199-212.

Bieniecki, W. (2004). Oversegmentation avoidance in watershed-based algorithms for color images. *In Proc. Of Modern Problems of Radio Engineering, Telecommunications and Computer Science.*

Bihan, D. L., Mangin, J., Poupon, C., Clark, C. A., Pappata, S., Molko, N., & Chabriat, H. (2001). Diffusion Tensor Imamging: Concepts and Applications. *Journal of Magnetic Resonance Imaging, 13,* 534-546.

Bilban, M., Buehler, L. K., Head, S., Desoye, G., & Quaranta, V. (2002). Normalizing DNA Microarray Data. *Curr. Issues Mol. Biol. 4*, 57-64.

Bilgili, Y., & Unal, B. (2004). Effect of region of interest on interobserver variance in apparent diffusion coefficient measures, *American Journal of Neuroradiology, 25,* 108-111.

Biquard, P. (1932). Les ondes ultra-sonores. *Rev. d'Acoust., 1*, 93-109.

Bishop, J., Poole, G., Leitch, M., & Plewes, D. B. (1998). Magnetic resonance imaging of shear wave propagation in excised tissue. *J. Magn. Reson. Imaging, 8*, 1257–1265.

Black, M. J., & Yacoob, Y. (1998). Recognising facial expressions in image sequences using local parameterised models. *Int'l J Computer Vision, 25*(1), 23-48.

Blekas, K., Galatsanos, N., Likas, A., & Lagaris, I. E. (2005). Mixture Model Analysis of DNA Microarray Images. *IEEE Transactions on Medical Imaging, 24*(7), 901-909.

Blumich, B. (2003). *NMR imaging of materials.* New York: Oxford University Press.

Bookstein, F. (1997). Shape and the information in medical images: a decade of the morphometric synthesis. *Computer Vision and Imaging Understanding, 66*, 97–118.

Borodin, P., Zachmann, G., & Klein, R. (2004). Consistent Normal Orientation for Polygonal Meshes. *Computer Graphics International 2004* (CGI), June 16–19, Crete, Greece. IEEE Computer Society Press.

Bosc, M., Heitz, F., Armspach, J. P., Namer, I., Gounot, D., & Rumbachc, L. (2003). Automatic change detection in multimodal serial MRI: application to multiple sclerosis lesion evolution. *Neuroimage 20,* 643-656.

Bouchet, L. G. Jokisch, D. W., & Bolch, W. E. (1999). A three-dimensional transport model for determining absorbed fractions of energy for electrons within trabecular bone. *J. Nucl. Med., 40,* 1947–66.

Bouix, S. *et al.* (2007). On evaluating brain tissue classifiers without a ground truth. *NeuroImage, 36,* 1207–1224.

Bouma, C., Niessen, W., Zuiderveld, K., Gussenhoven, E., & Viergever, M. (1996). Automated lumen definition from 30MHz intravascular ultrasound images. *Med Imag Analysis, 1*(4), 363-377.

Bourantas, C. V., Kalatzis, F. G., Papafaklis, M. I., Fotiadis, D. I., Tweddel A. C., Katsouras, C. S, et al (2008). ANGIOCARE: an automated system for fast three dimensional coronary reconstruction using angiographic and intracoronary ultrasound data. *Cathet Cardiovasc Interv* (in press)

Bourantas, C. V., Kourtis, I. C., Plissiti, M. E., Fotiadis, D. I., Katsouras, C. S., Papafaklis, M. I., et al. (2005). A method for 3-D reconstruction of coronary arteries using biplane angiography and intravascular ultrasound images. *Comput Med Imaging Graph, 29*(8), 597-606.

Bourantas, C. V., Plissiti, M. E., Fotiadis, D. I., Protopappas, V. C., Mpozios, G. V., Katsouras, C. S., et al. (2005). In vivo validation of a novel semi-automated method for border detection in intravascular ultrasound images. *Br J Radiol, 78*(926), 122-9.

Bozinov, D., & Rahnenführer, J. (2002). Unsupervised Technique for Robust Target Separation and Analysis of DNA Microarray Spots Through Adaptive Pixel Clustering. *Bioinformatics, 18*(5), 747-756.

Bradley, A., & Stentiford, F. (2002). JPEG2000 and Region of Interest Coding. *Presented at DICTA2002.*

Brandle, N., Bischof, L., & Lapp, H. (2003). Robust DNA microarray image analysis. *Machine Vision and Applications, 15,* 11-28.

Briesmeister, J. F. (2000). *Report LA-13709-M.* Los Alamos National Laboratory, NM.

Brix, G., M. Bahner, L., Hoffmann, U., Horvath, A., & Schreiber, W. (1999). Regional Blood Flow, Capillary Permeability and Compartmental Volumes: Measurement with Dynamic CT-Initial Experience. *Radiology, 210,* 269.276.

Brodlie, K., & Wood, J. (2001). Recent Advantages in Volume Visualization. *Computer Graphics Forum, 20*(2), 125-148.

Brody, T. A., Flores, J., French, J. B., Mello, P. A., Pandey, A., & Wong, S. S. M. (1981). Random-matrix physics: spectrum and strength fluctuations. *Rev. Mod. Phys., 53*(3), 385-479.

Bronzino, J. D. (2006). *The Biomedical Engineering Handbook.* CRC Press, 3rd ed. Boca Raton, FL: CRC Press.

Bronzino, J. D., & Diakides, N. A. (2007). *Medical Infrared Imaging.* Boca Raton, FL: CRC Press.

Brown, W. T., Wu, X., Amendola, B., Perman, M., Han, H., Fayad, F., Garcia, S., Lewin, A., Abitbol, A., de la Zerda, A., & Schwade, J. G. (2007). Treatment of early non-small cell lung cancer, stage IA, by image-guided robotic stereotactic radioablation--CyberKnife. *The Cancer Journal, 13*(2), 75-7.

Bruce, E. N. (2001). *Biomedical Signal Processing and Signal Modelling,* Wiley-Interscience, New York, NY, (pp. 13-18).

Bruining, N., von Birgelen, C., de Feyter, P. J., Ligthart, J., Li, W., Serruys, P. W., et al (1998). ECG-gated versus nongated three-dimensional intracoronary ultrasound analysis: implications for volumetric measurements. *Cathet Cardiovasc Diagn, 43*(3), 254-60.

Buchbinder, S. S., Leichter, I. S., Lederman, R., Novak, B., Bamberger, P. N., Coopersmith, H., & Fields, S. I. (2002). Can the size of microcalcifications predict malignancy of clusters at mammography? *Academic Radiology, 9*(1), 18-25.

Buck, M. J., & Lieb, J. D. (2004). ChIP-chip: considerations for the design, analysis, and application of genome-wide chromatin immunoprecipitation experiments. *Genomics, 83,* 349-360.

Buckley, M. J. (2000). Spot User's Guide. *CSIRO Mathematical and Information Sciences,* Australia,. from http://www.cmis.csiro.au/iap/Spot/spotmanual.htm

Buhler, J., Ideker, T., & Haynor D. (2000). Dapple: improved techniques for finding spots on DNA microarrays. (UWCSE Tech Rep). Washington*: UWTR Dept. of Computer Science and Eng.,* University of Washington.

Buhler, J., Ideker, T., & Haynor, D. (2000). *Improved techniques for finding spots on cDNA microarrays*: University of Washington.

Bui, A. A. (2000). *A multimedia data model with generalized stream constructs.* (Ph.D. Dissertation, University of California, Los Angeles, 2000).

Bui, A. A., Taira, R. K., El-Saden, S., Dordoni, A., & Aberle, D. R. (2004). Automated medical problem list generation: Towards a patient timeline. *Medinfo, 11*(Pt 1), 587-591.

Buonaccorsi, G., O'Connor, J. P. B., Caunce, A., Roberts, C., Cheung, S., Watson, Y., Davies, K., Hope, L., Jackson, A., Jayson, G. C., & Parker, G. J. M. (2007). Tracer Kinetic Model–Driven Registration for Dynamic Contrast-Enhanced MRI Time-Series Data. *Magnetic Resonance in Medicine, 58,* 1010–1019.

Burges, C. J. C. (1998). A Tutorial on Support Vector Machines for Pattern Recognition. *Data Mining and Knowledge Discovery, 2*(2), 121-167.

Burman, C., Kutcher, G. J., & Emami, B. (1991). Fitting of normal tissue tolerance data to an analytical function. *Int. J. Radiat. Biol. Phys., 21,* 123-35.

Burrus, C. S., Gopinath, R. A., & Guo, H. (1998). *Introduction to Wavelets and the Wavelet Transform: A Primer.* Englewood Cliffs, NJ: Prentice-Hall

Burton A., & Altman D.G. (2004). Missing covariate data within cancer prognostic studies: a review of current reporting and proposed guidelines. *British Journal of Cancer, 91,* 4–8.

Callaghan, P. H. (1991). *Principles of magnetic resonance microscopy.* Oxford, UK: Oxford University Press.

Campbell, P., & Roderick, T. (2006). Thermal imaging in surgery. In J. D. Bronzino & N. A. Diakides (Ed.), *Medical Imaging Devices and Systems, The Biomedical Engineering Handbook* (pp. 19.1 – 19.18).Boca Raton, FL: CRC Press.

Canales, R. D., Luo, Y., Willey, J. C., Austermiller, B., Barbacioru, C. C., Boysen, C., Hunkapiller, K., Jensen, R. D., Knight, C. R., Lee, K. Y., Ma, Y., Maqsodi, B., Papallo, A., Peters, E. H., Poulter, K., Ruppel, P. L., Samaha, R. R., Shi, L., Yang, W., Zhang, L., & Goodsaid, F. M. (2006). Evaluation of cDNA Microarray Results with Quantitative Gene Expression Platforms. *Nat. Biotech., 24,* 1115-1122.

Candela, G. T., Grother, P. J., Watson, C. I., Wilkinson, R. A., & Wilson, C. L. (1995). *PCASYS – a pattern-level classification automation system for fingerprints.* Technical report. NISTIR 5647: National Institute of Standards and Technology.

Cane, B. Mc (1997). On the Evaluation of Image Segmentation Algorithms. *DICTA'97* and *IVCN'Z'97,* (pp. 455-459).

Cao, Z., Pan, S., Li, R., Balachandran, R., Fitzpatrick, M. J., Chapman, W. C., & Dawant, B. M. (2004). Registration of medical images using an interpolated closest point transform: method and validation. *Medical Image Analysis, 8,* 421-427.

Cardinal, M. H. R., Meunier, J., Soulez, G., Thrasse, E., & Cloutier G. (2003). *Intravascular ultrasound image segmentation: A fastmarching method.* Medical Image Computing and Computer Assisted Intervention, Lecture Note Computer Science. Berlin: Springer-Verlag, (pp. 432–439).

Carnec, M. (2004). *Critères de qualité d'images couleur avec référence réduite perceptuelle générique*. Phd Thesis de l'Ecole Polytechnique de l'Université de Nantes.

Carters G., & Graham J. (1999). Trainable grey-level models for disentangling overlapping chromosomes. *Pattern Recognition, 32,* 1335-1349.

Carters, G., & Graham, J. (2002). Disentangling chromosome overlaps by combining trainable shape models with classification evidence. *IEEE Transactions on Signal Processing, 50*, 2080-2085.

Catarci, T., Costabile, M. F., & Matera, M. (1995). Visual metaphors for interacting with databases. *ACM SIGCHI Bulletin, 27*(2), 15-17.

Catheline, S., Gennisson, J. L., Delon, G., Fink, M., Sinkus, R., & Abouelkaram, S. (2004). Measurement of viscoelastic properties of homogeneous soft solid using transient elastography: An inverse problem approach. *J. Acoust. Soc. Am., 116*, 3734-3741.

Catheline, S., Wu, F., & Fink, M. (1999) A solution to diffraction biases in sonoelasticity: The acoustic impulse technique. *J. Acoust. Soc. Am., 105*, 2941–2950.

Celis, J. E. (2003). Integrating Proteomic and Functional Genomic Technologies in Discovery-driven Translational Breast Cancer Research. *Molecular & Cellular Proteomics*; *2*, 369-77.

Cerignani, M., Bammer, R., Sormani, M. P., Fazekas, F., & Filippi, M. (2003). Inter-sequence and inter-imaging unit variability of diffusion tensor MR imaging histogram-derived metrics of the brain in healthy volunteers. *American Journal of Neuroradiology, 24,* 638-643.

Cesaretti, J., Pennathur, A., Rosenstein, B. S., Swanson, S. J., & Fernando, H. (2008). Stereotactic Radiosurgery for Thoracic Malignancies. *The Annals of Thoracic Surgery, 85*(2), 785–791.

Chabrier, S., Emile, B., Rosenberger, C., & Laurent, H. (2006). Unsupervised performance evaluation of image segmentation. *EURASIP Journal on Applied Signal Processing*, (pp. 1-12).

Chan, H.-P., Sahiner, B., Lam, K. L., Petrick, N., Helvie, M. A., Goodsitt, M. M., & Adler, D. D. (1998). Computerized analysis of mammographic microcalcifications in morphological and texture feature spaces. *Medical Physics, 25*(10), 2007-2019.

Chan, H.-P., Sahiner, B., Petrick, N., Hadjiiski, L., & Paquerault, S. (2005). Computer-aided diagnosis of breast cancer. In: L. Costaridou (Ed.), *Medical Image Analysis Methods*, (pp. 1-49). Boca Raton: Taylor & Francis Group, CRC Press.

Chan, H.-P., Sahiner, B., Petrick, N., Helvie, M. A., Lam, K. L., Adler, D. D., & Goodsitt, M. M. (1997). Computerized classification of malignant and benign microcalcifications on mammograms: Texture analysis using an artificial neural network. *Physics in Medicine and Biology, 42*(3), 549-567.

Chan, K. L. (1993). Two approaches to motion analysis of the ultrasound image sequence of carotid atheromatous plaque. *Ultrasonics, 31*(12), 117-123.

Chandrasekharaiah, D. S., & Debnath, L. (1st Ed.). (1994). *Continuum Mechanics.* Boston, MA: Academic Press.

Chang, C., & Lin, C. (2001). LIBSVM: A Library for Support Vector Machines. Retrieved April 1, 2005, from http://www.csie.ntu.edu.tw/~cjlin/

Chang, L. C., Jones, D. K., & Pierpaoli, C. (2005). RESTORE: robust estimation of tensors by outlier rejection. *Magnetic Resonance in Medicine, 53,* 1088-1095.

Chatziioannou, A., & Moulos, P. (2007). Extending the Interpretation of Gene Profiling Microarray Experiments to Pathway Analysis Through the Use of Gene Ontology Terms. *ICCS 2007 Proceedings (22-27 July, Sheffield), QA-Gen Workshop.*

Chatziioannou, A., & Moulos, P. (2007). ANDROMEDA: A MATLAB automated cDNA microarray data analysis platform. *IFIP International Federation for Information Processing, 247*, (pp. 127-136).

Chen, D. R., Chang, R. F., Kuo, W. J., Chen, M. C., & Huang, Y. L. (2002). Diagnosis of breast tumors with sonographic texture analysis using wavelet transform and neural networks. *Ultrasound in Medicine & Biology, 28*(10), 1301–1310.

Chen, E. L., Chung, P. C., Chen, C. L., Tsa, H. M., & Chang, C. I. (1998). An automatic diagnostic system for CT liver image classification. *IEEE Transactions on Biomedical Engineering, 45*(6), 783-794.

Chen, H., Fuller, S. S., Friedman, C., & Hersh, W. (2005). *Medical Informatics: Knowledge Management and Data Mining in Biomedicine*. New York, NY: Springer.

Chen, T.-J., Chuang, K.-S., Wu, J., Chan, S. C., Hwang, I.-M., & Jan, M.-L. (2003). A novel image quality index using Moran I statistics. *Physics in Medicine and Biology, 48*, 131-137.

Chen, W., Giger, M. L., Bick, U., & Newstead, G. M. (2006). Automatic identification and classification of characteristic kinetic curves of breast lesions on DCE-MRI. *Medical Physics, 33*(8), 2878-2887.

Chen, W., Giger, M. L., Lan, L., & Bick, U. (2004). Computerized interpretation of breast MRI: Investigation of enhancement-variance dynamics. *Medical Physics, 31*(5), 1076-1082.

Chen, W., Giger, M. L., Li, H., Bick, U., & Newstead, G. M. (2007). Volumetric texture analysis of breast lesions on contrast-enhanced magnetic resonance images. *Magnetic Resonance in Medicine, 58*(3), 562-571.

Chen, Y., Dougherty, E. R., & Bittner, M. L. (1997). Ratio-Based Decisions and the Quantitative Analysis of cDNA Microarray Images. *Journal Of Biomedical Optics, 2*(4), 364–374.

Chen, Y., Kamat, V., Dougherty, E. R., Bittner, M. L., Meltzer, P. S., & Trent, J. M. (2002). Ratio statistics of gene expression levels and applications to microarray data analysis. *Bioinformatics, 18*(9), 1207-1215.

Cheng, H. D., Cai, X., Chen, X., Hu, L., & Lou, X. (2003). Computer-aided detection and classification of microcalcifications in mammograms: A survey. *Pattern Recognition, 36*(12), 2967-2991.

Chetverikov, D., Svirko, D., & Stepanov, D. (2002). The trimmed iterative closest point algorithm. *International Conference of Pattern Recognition, 3*, 545-548.

Chiracharit, W. *et al.* (2007). Normal mammogram detection based on local probability difference transforms and support vector machines. *IEICE Transactions on Information and Systems, E90-D*(1), 258-27.

Chiu, B., Freeman, G. H., Salama, M. M. A., & Fenster A. (2004). Prostate segmentation algorithm using dyadic wavelet transform and discrete dynamic contour. *Physics in Medicine and Biology, 49*, 4943-4960.

Choi, H., Castleman, K., & Bovik, A. (2004). Joint Segmentation and Classification of M-FISH Chromosome Images. In *Proc. 26th IEEE Ann. Intern. Conf (EMBS)*, San Francisco, (pp. 1636-1639).

Choyke, P. L., Dewer, A. J., & Knopp, M. V. (2003). Functional Tumor Imaging with Dynamic Constrast-Enhanced Magnetic Resonance Imaging. *Journal of Magnetic Resonance Imaging, 17*, 509-520.

Christensen, G. E., Rabbitt, R. D., & Miller, M. I. (1996). *Multiresolution elastic matching. IEEE Transaction on Image Processing, 5*, 1435–1447.

Christodoulou, C. I., Michaelides, S. C., & Pattichis, C. S. (2003). Multi-feature texture analysis for the classification of clouds in satellite imagery. *IEEE Transactions on Geoscience and Remote Sensing, 41(11)*, 2662-2668.

Christodoulou, C. I., Pattichis, C. S., Pantziaris, M., & Nicolaides, A. (2003). A Texture-based classification of atherosclerotic carotid plaques. *IEEE Transactions on Medical Imaging, 22*(7), 902 - 912.

Christodoulou, C. I., Pattichis, C. S., Pantziaris, M., Tegos, T., Nicolaides, A., Elatrozy, T., Sabetai, M., & Dhanjil, S. (1999). Multi-feature texture analysis for the classification of carotid plaques. *Presented at the Int. Joint Conf. Neural Networks IJCNN* '99 Washington DC.

Ciccarelli, O., Toosy, A. T., Parker, G. J., Wheeler-Kingshott, C. A. M., Barker, G. J., Miller, D. H., & Thompson A. J. (2003). Diffusion tractography based group mapping of major white-matter pathways in the human brain. *NeuroImage., 19*, 1545-1555.

Cimino, J. J., & Shortliffe E. H. (2006). Biomedical Informatics: Computer Applications in Health Care and Biomedicine. *Health Informatics, 3*, 120-134

Cinthio, M., Ahlgren, A. R., Bergkvist, J., Jansson, T, Persson H. W., & Lindström, K. (2006). Longitudinal movements and resulting shear strain of the arterial wall. *American Journal of Physiology – Heart and Circulatory Physiology, 291*(1), H394-H402.

Cinthio, M., Ahlgren, A. R., Jansson, J. T., Eriksson, A., Persson, H. W., & Lindström, K. (2005). Evaluation of an ultrasonic echo-tracking method for measurements of arterial wall movements in two dimensions. *IEEE Transactions on Ultrasonics, Ferroelectrics and Frequency Control, 52*(8), 1300-1311.

Clairand, I., Ricard, M., Gouriou, J., Di Paola, M., & Aubert, B. (1999). DOSE3D: EGS4 Monte Carlo code-based software for internal radionuclide dosimetry. *J. Nucl. Med., 40*, 1517–23.

Cleveland, W. S., Grosse, E., & Shyu, W. M. (1992). *Local Regression Models, Statistical Models in S*. In J. M. Chambers & T. J. Hastie (Eds.), *Practical Nonparametric Statistics* Wadsworth & Brooks/Cole Dormand, J.R. Conover, W.J., (1980)., Wiley.

Cobbold, R. S. C. (2007). *Foundations of Biomedical Ultrasound*. New York: Oxford Univ. Press.

Cohen, I., Sebe, N., Garg, A., Chen, L. S., & Huang, S. T. (2003). Facial expression recognition from video sequences: temporal and static modelling. *Computer Vision and Image Understanding, 91*, 160-187.

Cohen, R. V., Schiavon, C. A., Pinheiro, F. J. C., & Correa, J. L. (2003). *Laparoscopic Bariatric Surgery: New Technologies, Trends and Perspectives, 58*(5), I-VIII. Pubmed.

Cohen, Y., & Assaf, Y. (2002). High *b*-value *q*-space analyzed diffusion-weighted MRS and MRI in neuronal tissues- a technical review. *NMR in Biomedicine, 15*, 516-542.

Coifman, R. R., & Wickerhauser, M. V. (1992). Entropy-based algorithms for best basis selection. *IEEE Transactions on Information Theory, 38*(2), 713-719.

Coli, M., Fontanella, L., Ippoliti, L., & Merla. A. (2007). Multiresolution KLE of psycho-physiological signals. In *Proceedings of S.Co.2007, Fifth Conference on Complex Models and Computational Intensive Methods for Estimation and Prediction, Book of Short Papers*, ISBN 978-88-6129-114-0, (pp. 116-121).

Collignon, A., Maes, F., Delaere, D., Vandermeulen, D., Suetens, P., & Marchal, G. (1995). Automated multi-modality image registration based on information theory. In *Proceedings of the International Conference on Information Processing in Medical Imaging (IPMI)*, Ile de Berder, France, June 1995 (pp. 263-274). Kluwer: Yves Bizais (Ed.).

Conturo, T. E., Lori, N. F., Cull, T. S., Akbudak, E., Snyder, A. Z., Shimony, J. S., McKinstry, R. C., Burton, H., & Raichle, M. E. (1999). Tracking neuronal fiber pathways in the living human brain, *Proceedings of National Academy of Sciences USA, 96*, 10422-10427.

Conturo, T. E., McKinstry, R. C., Akbudak, E., & Robinson, B. H. (1996). Encoding of anisotropic diffusion with tetrahedral gradients: A general mathematical diffusion formalism and experimental results. *Magnetic Resonance in Medicine, 35*, 399-412.

Cootes, T. F., Edwards, G., & Taylor, C. J. (1998). Active appearance models. *Proc. European Conf. Computer Vision, 2*, 484-498.

Cootes, T. F., Taylor, C. J., Cooper, D. H. & Graham, J. (1995). Active shape models – Their training and application. *Computer Vision and Image Understanding, 61*(1), 38-59.

Cordes, D., & Nandy, R. R. (2006). Estimation of the intrinsic dimensionality of fMRI data. *Neuroimage, 29*, 145-154.

Cothren, R., Shekhar, R., Tuzcu, E., & Nissen, S. (2000). Three-dimensional reconstruction of the coronary artery wall by image fusion of intravascular ultrasound and bi-plane angiography. *Int J Card Imag, 16*, 69-85.

Craig, D. (1999). Fitting Curves and Surfaces With Constrained Implicit Polynomials. *IEEE Transactions on PAMI, 21*(1), 31-41.

Cremonesi, M., Ferrari, M., Bodei, L., Tosi, G., & Paganelli, G. (2006). Dosimetry in Peptide Radionuclide Receptor Therapy: A Review. *J Nucl Med 2006, 47*, 1467–1475.

Cristianini, N., & Shawe-Taylor, J. (2000). *Introduction to Support Vector Machines and other kernel-based learning methods*. Cambridge University Press.

Cristy, M., & Eckerman, K. (1987). Specific absorbed fractions of energy at various ages from internal photons sources *ORNL/TM-8381 V1-V7* (Oak Ridge, TN: Oak Ridge National Laboratory).

Crum, W. R., Hartkens, T., & Hill D. L. (2004). Non-rigid image registration: theory and practice. *British Journal of Radiology, 77*(2), S140-S153.

Cziho, A., Cazuguel, G., Solaiman, B., & Roux, C. (1998). Medical image compression using region-of-interest vector quantization. *20th Annual International Conference of the IEEE Engineering in Medicine and Biology Society*. (pp. 1277).

Dahl, T., Bang, J., Ushakova, A., Lydersen, S., & Myhre, H. O. (2004). Parameters describing motion in carotid artery plaques from ultrasound examination: a reproducibility study. *Ultrasound in Medicine and Biology, 30*(9), 1133-1143.

Daszykowski, M. *et al.* (2007). Robust statistics in data analysis — A review of Basic concepts. *Chemometrics and Intelligent Laboratory Systems, 85*, 203–219

Daubechies, I. (1998). Orthonormal bases of compactly supported wavelets. *Commun. Pure Applied Math. 41*, 909–996.

Daugman, J. (1980). Two-dimensional spectral analysis of cortical receptive field profiles. *Vision Research, 20*, 846-856.

Daugman, J. (1985). Uncertainty relation for resolution in space, spatial frequency and orientation optimized by two-dimensional visual cortical fields. *J Optical Society of America A, 2*(7), 1160-1171.

Davatzikos, C. (2004). Why voxel-based morphometry analysis should be used with great caution when characterizing group differences. *NeuroImage, 23*, 17-20.

Davis, M. H., Khotanzad, A., Flamig, D. P., & Harms, S. E. (1997). A Physic-Based Coordinate Transformation for 3-D Image, Matching. *IEEE Transactions on Medical Imaging, 16(3)*, 317–328.

Davis, M. H., Khotanzad, A., Flamig, D. P., & Harms, S. E. (1997). A Physic-Based Coordinate Transformation for 3-D Image, Matching. *IEEE Transactions on Medical Imaging, 16(3)*, 317–328.

Dawson, S. L., & Kaufman, J. A. (1998). The imperative for medical simulation. *Proceedings of the IEEE 8*(3), 479–483.

Delgorge, C., Courreges, F., Al Bassit, L., Novales, C., Rosenberger, C., Smith-Guerin, N., Bru, C., Gilabert, R., Vannoni, M., Poisson, G., & Vieyres, P. (2005). A tele-operated mobile ultrasound scanner using a light weight robot. *IEEE Transactions on Information Technology in BioMedicine, special issue mHealth, 9*(1).

Delgorge, C., Rosenberger, C., Poisson, G., & Vieyres, P. (2006). Towards a new tool for the evaluation of the quality of ultrasound compressed images. *IEEE Transactions on Medical Imaging, 25*, 1502 – 1509.

Dempster, A., Laird, N., & Rubin, D. (1977). Maximum likelihood from incomplete data via the EM algorithm. *Journal of the Royal Statistical Society, 39*(1), 1-38.

Denton E. R. E., Sonoda, L. I., Rueckert, D., Rankin, S. C., Hayes, C., Leach, M. O., Hill, D. L. G., & Hawkes, D. J. (1999). Comparison and Evaluation of Rigid, Affine, and Nonrigid Registration of Breast MR Images. *Journal of Computer Assisted Tomography, 23(5)*, 800-805.

Derivaux, S., Lefèvre, S., Wemmert, C., & Korczak, J. J. (2007). On machine learning in watershed segmentation. *IEEE International Workshop on Machine Learning in Signal Processing* (pp. 187-192).

Dettori, L., & Beshir, A. (2007). Texture classification of normal tissues in computed tomography using Gabor filters. In J. P. W. Pluim, J. M. Reinhardt (Ed), *SPIE Medical Imaging: Vol. 6512*, (6512Q).

Deurloo, E. E., Muller, S. H., Peterse, J. L., Besnard, A. P., & Gilhuijs, K. G. (2005). Clinically and mammographically occult breast lesions on MR images: Potential effect of computerized assessment on clinical reading. *Radiology, 234*(3), 693-701.

Dewaraja, Y. K., Wilderman, S. J., Ljungberg, M., Koral, K. F., Kenneth, Z., & Kaminiski, M. S. (2005). Accurate dosimetry in 131I radionuclide therapy using patient-specific, 3-dimensional methods for SPECT reconstruction and absorbed dose calculation. *J. Nucl. Med., 46,* 840–9.

Dewitte, S., & Cornelis, J. (1997). Lossless integer wavelet transform. *IEEE Signal Processing Letters, 4,* 158 – 160.

Dhawale, P., Rasheed, Q., Griffin, N., Wilson, D., & Hodgson, J (1993). Intracoronary Ultrasound Plaque Volume Quantification. *In: Proc Comput Cardiol, Los Alamitos (CA),* IEEE Computer Society Press (pp.121-24).

Dhawan, A. P., Chitre, Y., Kaiser-Bonasso, C., & Moskowitz, M. (1996). Analysis of mammographic microcalcifications using gray-level image structure features. *IEEE Transactions on Medical Imaging, 15*(3), 246-259.

Dhillon, S., & Gill, K. (November 2005). *Clinical Pharmacokinetic. Textbook.*

Di Romualdo, S., Merla, A., & Romani, G. L. (2007). Superimposition of thermal imaging to visual imaging using homography. In *Proceedings of the 2007 IEEE Engineering Medicine Biology Society,* (pp. 3365-8).

Di Stefano, L., Mattocia, S., & Tombari, F. (2004). An algorithm for efficient and exhaustive template matching. *Image Analysis and Recognition, 3211,* 408-415.

Diakides, N. A. (Guest Editor). (1998). Special Issue on Medical Infrared Imaging. *IEEE Engineering in Medicine and Biology,* 17, July/August.

Diakides, N. A. (Guest Editor). (2000). Special Issue on Medical Infrared Imaging. *IEEE Engineering in Medicine and Biology,* 19, May/June.

Diakides, N. A. (Guest Editor). (2002). Special Issue on Medical Infrared Imaging. *IEEE Engineering in Medicine and Biology,* 21, November/December.

Dilmaghani, R., Ahmadian, A., Ghavami, M., Oghabian, M., & Aghvami, H. (2003). Multi rate/resolution control in progressive medical image transmission for the Region of Interest (ROI) using EZW. *25th Annual International Conference of the IEEE EMBS,* Mexico.

DiMaio, S. *et al.* (2007). Challenges in image-guided therapy system design. *NeuroImage, 37,* 144–151.

Dimou, I., Manikis, G., & Zervakis, M. (2006). Classifier Fusion approaches for diagnostic cancer models, *Proceedings of the 28th IEEE, EMBS Annual International Conference,* New York City, USA, Aug 30-Sept 3, (pp. 5334-5337).

Dineley, J., Meagher, S., Poepping, T. L., McDicken, W. N., Hoskins, P. R. (2006). Design and characterisation of a wall motion phantom. *Ultrasound in Medicine and Biology, 32*(9), 1349-1357.

Dionisio, J. D., Cardenas, A. F., Taira, R. K., Aberle, D. R., Chu, W. W., McNitt-Gray, M. F., et al. (1996). A unified timeline model and user interface for multimedia medical databases. *Comput Med Imaging Graph, 20*(4), 333-346.

DiZenzo, S. (1986). A note on the gradient of a multi-image. *Comput. Vis. Graph. Image Process, 33,* 116-125.

Dodel, S., Geisel, T., & Herrmann. J. M. (2000). Comparison of temporal and spatial ICA in fMRI data analysis. *Proc. ICA 2000,* Helsinki, Finland, 543-547.

Dodel, S., Herrmann, J. M., & Geisel, T. (2002). Functional connectivity by cross-correlation clustering. *Neurocomputing,* 44-46, 1065-1070.

Donato, G., Bartlett, M. S., Hager, J. C., Ekman, P., & Senjowski, T. J. (1999). Classifying facial actions. *IEEE Trans. Pattern Analysis and Machine Intelligence, 21*(10), 974-989.

Dougherty, E. R., Astola, J. (1994). *An Introduction to Nonlinear Image Processing,* Belingham. Washington, SPIE Optical Engineering Press.

Dougherty, L, Asmuth, J. C., Blom, A. S., Axel, L., & Kumar R. (1999). Validation of an optical flow method for tag displacement estimation. *IEEE Transaction on Image Processing, 18,* 359–363.

Douglas, D. H., & Peucker, T. K. (1973). Algorithms for the Reduction of the Number of Points Required to Represent a Line or its Character. *The American Cartographer, 10*(2), 112-123.

Doukas, C. N., Maglogiannis, I., & Kormentzas, G. (2005). Medical Image Compression using Wavelet Transform on Mobile Devices with ROI coding support. *27th Annual International Conference of the IEEE EMBS.*

Draghici, S., Khatri, P., Eklund, A. C., & Szallasi, Z. (2006). Reliability and reproducibility issues in DNA microarray measurements. *Trends Genet, 22*(2), 101-109.

Drewniok, C. (1994). Multi-spectral edge detection - Some experiments on data from Landsat-TM, *Intern. J. Remote. Sens., 15*, 3743-3765.

Dreyfus, G. (2005). *Neural Networks, Methodology and Applications.* Springer.

Driver, D., & Dobbs, H. J. (2004). Improvements in radiotherapy practice: the impact of new imaging technologies. *Cancer Imaging, 4,* 142-150.

Drukker, K., Horsch, K., & Giger, M. L. (2005). Multimodality computerized diagnosis of breast lesions using mammography and sonography. *Academic Radiology, 12*(8), 970-979.

Duda, O. R., Hart, E. P., & Stork, D. G. (2001). *Pattern Classification* (pp. 259-265), Wiley.

Dudoit, S., Shaffer, J. P., & Boldrick, J. C. (2003). Multiple Hypothesis Testing in Microarray Experiments. *Statistical Science, 18*, 71-103.

Dudoit, S., Yang, Y. H., Speed, T., & Callow, M. J. (2002). Statistical Methods for Identifying Differentially Expressed Genes in Replicated cDNA Microarray Experiments. *Statistica Sinica 12*, 111-139.

Dufaux, F., & Moscheni, F. (1995). Motion estimation techniques for digital TV: a review and a new contribution. *Proceeding of the IEEE, 83*(6), 858-876.

Dunning, M. J., Smith, M. L., Ritchie, M. E., & Tavare, S. (2007). beadarray: R classes and methods for Illumina bead-based data. *Bioinformatics, 23*(16), 2183-2184.

Dupuy, A., & Simon, R. M. (2007). Critical review of published microarray studies for cancer outcome and guidelines on statistical analysis and reporting. *J Natl Cancer Inst, 99*(2), 147-157.

Eberhart, R. C., & Dobbins, R. W. (1990). Neural network performance metrics for biomedical applications, *Proceedings of Third Annual IEEE Symposium on Computer-Based Medical Systems*, (pp. 282-289).

Ebrchart, R. C, & Dobbins, R. W. (1990). *Neural Networks PC Tools A Practical Guide.* (Academic Pr., 1990).

Eckerman, K. F., Cristy, M., & Warner, G. G. (1981). Dosimetric evaluation of brain scanning agents. In E. E. Watson, A. T. Schlafke-Stelson, J. L. Coffey, & R. J. Cloutier (Eds.), *3rd Int. Radiopharmaceutical Dosimetry Symp.* (Rockville, MD: U.S. Department of Health and Human Services, Food and Drug Administration) (pp. 527–40). *HHS Publication* FDA 81-8166.

Eckerman, K., & Stabin, M. (2000). Electron absorbed fractions and dose conversion factors for marrow and bone by skeletal regions. *Health Phys., 78*, 199–214.

Edler, I., & Hertz, C. H. (1954). The use of ultrasonic reflectoscope for the continuous recording of the movements of heart walls. *Kungl Fysiografiska Sällskapets i Lund Förhandlingar, 24*(5), 1-19.

Efron, B. (1982). *The jackknife, the bootstrap, and other resampling plans*, Philadelphia, CBMS-NSF Regional Conf. Series in Applied Mathematics, Society for Industrial and Applied Mathematics (SIAM).

Eggers, G., Mühling, J., & Marmulla, R. (2006). Image-to-patient registration techniques in head surgery. *International Journal of Oral and Maxillofacial Surgery, 35*(12), 1081-95.

Eibenberger, E., Borsorf, A., Wimmer, A., & Hornegger, J. (2008). Edge-Preserving Denoising for Segmentation in CT-Images, In T. Tolxdorff, J. Braun, T. M. Deserno, H. Handels, A. Horsch, H. P. Meinzer (Ed.) *Bildverarbeitung für die Medizin 2008 - Algorithmen, Systeme, Anwendungen* (pp. 257-261). Springer-Verlag.

Eils, R., Uhrig, S., Saracoglu, K., Satzler, K., Bolzer, A., Petersen, I., Chassery, J., Ganser, M., & Speicher, M. (1998). An optimized fully automated system for fast and accurate identification of chromosomal rearrangements by multiplex-FISH (M-FISH), *Cytogenet. Cell Genet., 82*, 160-171.

Eisen, M. B. (1999). *ScanAlyse*. form http://rana.Stanford.EDU/software/

Eisen, M. B., & Brown, P. O. (1999). DNA Arrays for Analysis of Gene Expression. *Methods Enzymol, 303*, 179-205.

Ekin, A. *et al*. (2007). Improving information quality of MR brain images by fully automatic and robust image analysis methods. *Journal of the Society for Information Display, 15*(6), 367-376.

Ekman, P. (1991). *Telling Lies: Clues to deceit in the Marketplace, Politics, and Marriage*. New York, USA: W. W. Norton.

Ekman, P. (2003). Darwin, deception and facial expression. *Annals New York Academy of sciences, 100*, 205-221.

Ekman, P., & Friesen, W. V. (1971). Constants across cultures in the face and emotion. *Journal of Personality and Social Psychology, 17*(2), 124-129.

Ekman, P., & Friesen, W. V. (1978). *The Facial Action Coding System: A technique for the measurement of facial movement*. San Francisco: Consulting Psychologist Press.

Ekman, P., & Rosenberg, E. L. (2005). *What the face reveals: Basic and applied studies of spontaneous expression using the FACS*. Oxford, UK: Oxford University Press.

Elatrozy, T., Nicolaides, A., Tegos, T., et al. (1998). The objective characterisation of ultrasonic carotid plaque features. *European Journal of Vascular and Endovascular Surgery, 16*, 223-30.

El-Barghouti, N., Nicolaides, A. N., Tegos, T., et al. (1996). The relative effect of carotid plaque heterogeneity and echogenicity on ipsilateral cerebral infarction and symptoms of cerebrovascular disease. *International Angiology, 15*, 300-6.

Ergüt, E., Yardimci, Y., Mumcuoglu, E., & Konu, O. (2003). Analysis of microarray images using FCM and K-means clustering algorithm. *In IJCI 2003*, (pp. 116-121).

Errington P., & Graham J. (1993). Application of artificial neural networks to chromosome classification. *Cytometry, 14*, 627–639.

Essa, I., & Petland, A. (1997). Coding, analysis, interpretation, recognition of facial expressions. *IEEE Trans. Pattern Analysis and Machine Intelligence, 19*(7), 757-763.

Ettinger, G. J., Grimson, W. E., Lozano–Perez, T., Wells, W. M., III, White, S. J., & Kikinis, R. (1994). Automatic registration for multiple sclerosis change detection. In *Proceedings of the IEEE Workshop on Biomedical Image Analysis*, Seattle, WA, USA, 24-25 June 1994 (pp. 297-306)

Ettinger, G. J., Grimson, W. E., Lozano–Perez, T., Wells, W. M., III, White, S. J., & Kikinis, R. (1994). Automatic registration for multiple sclerosis change detection. In *Proceedings of the IEEE Workshop on Biomedical Image Analysis*, Seattle, WA, USA, 24-25 June 1994 (pp. 297-306)

European carotid plaque study group (1995). Carotid artery plaque composition - Relationship to clinical presentation and ultrasound B-mode imaging. *European Journal of Vascular and Endovascular Surgery, 10*, 23-30.

European Society for Gynaecological Endoscopy [http://www.esge.org/]

Everson, R., & Roberts, S. (2000). Inferring the eigenvalues of covariance matrices from limited, noisy data. *IEEE Trans. Signal Processing, 48*(7), 2083-2091.

Eyal, E., & Degani, H. (2007). Model-based and model-free parametric analysis of breast dynamic-contrast-enhanced MRI. *NMR in Biomedicine*.

Faerber, M., Ehrhardt, J., & Handels, H. (2007). Live-wire-based segmentation using similarities between corresponding image structures. *Computerized Medical Imaging and Graphics, 31*, 549–560.

Faerber, M., Ehrhardt, J., & Handels, H. (2005). Automatic atlas-based contour extraction of anatomical structures in medical images. *International Congress Series, 1281*, 272–277.

Fahey, B. J., Hsu, S. J., Wolf, P. D., Nelson, R. C., & Trahey, G. E. (2006). Liver ablation guidance with acoustic radiation force impulse imaging: challenges and opportunities. *Physics in Med. Biol., 51*, 3785-3808.

Falcao, A., & Udupa, J. (2000). A 3D generalization of user-steered live-wire segmentation. *Medical. Image Analysis, 4*(4) 89–402.

Falconer, J. C., & Narayana, P. A. (1997). Cerebrospinal fluid-suppressed high-resolution diffusion imaging of human brain. *Magnetic Resonance in Medicine, 37*, 119-123.

Falk, E., Shah, P. K., & Fuster, V. (1995). Coronary plaque disruption. *Circulation, 92*(3), 657-671.

Fasel, B., & Luettin, J. (2003). Automatic facial expression analysis: a survey. *Pattern Recognition, 36*, 259-275.

Fasel, I. R., Fortenberry, B., & Movellan, J. R. (2005). A generative framework for real time object detection and classification. *Int'l J Computer Vision and Image Understanding, 98*(1), 181-210.

Fatemi, M., & Greenleaf J. (1998). Ultrasound-stimulated vibro-acoustic spectrography. *Science, 280*, 82-85.

Fatemi, M., & Greenleaf, J. (2000). Probing the dynamics of tissue at low frequencies with the radiation force of ultrasound. *Phys. Med. Biol., 45*, 1449-1464.

Fayez, J. A., & Vogel, M. F. (1991). *Comparison of Different Treatment Methods of Endometriomas by Laparoscopy. Obstet. Gynecol., 78*, 660-665.

Fenton, J. J., Taplin, S. H., Carney, P. A., Abraham, L., Sickles, E. A, D'Orsi, C., Berns, E. A., Cutter, G., Hendrick, R. E., Barlow, W. E., & Elmore, J. G. (2007). Influence of computer-aided detection on performance of screening mammography. *The New England Journal of Medicine, 356*(14), 1399-1409.

Ferranti, J. M., Musser, R. C., Kawamoto, K., & Hammond, W. E. (2006). The clinical document architecture and the continuity of care record: a critical analysis. *J Am Med Inform Assoc., 13*(3), 245-52.

Finkelstein, D. B., Ewing, R., Gollub, J., Sterky, F., Somerville, S., & Cherry, J. M. (2002). *Iterative Linear Regression by Sector, Methods of Microarray Data Analysis*, S. M. Lin & K. F. Johnson (Eds.). Cambridge, MA: Kluwer Academic (pp. 57-68).

Finsterbusch, J., & Frahm, J. (2000). Diffusion tensor mapping of the human brain using single-shot line scan imaging. *Journal of Magnetic Resonance Imaging, 12*, 388-394.

Fischer, D. R. (2003). Assessments for high dose radionuclide therapy treatment planning. *Radiation Protection Dosimetry, 105*(1–4), 581–586.

Fisher, D. R. (2000). Internal dosimetry for systemic radiation therapy. *Semin. Radiat. Oncol., 10*(2), 123–132.

Fisher, R. A. (1936). The Use of Multiple Measurements in Taxonomic Problems. *Annals of Eugenics, 7*, 179-188.

Fitzpatrick, J. M., Hill, D. L. G., & Maurer, C. R. (2000). Image registration. In *Handbook of Medical Imaging, Volume 2: Medical Image Processing and Analysis* (pp. 451-507). Bellingham, WA: SPIE.

Florie, J., Wasser, M. N. J. M., Arts-Cieslik, K., Akkerman, E. K., Siersema, P. D., & Stoker J. (May 2006). Dynamic Contrast Enhanced MRI of the bowel wall for assessment of disease activity in Crohn's disease. *American Journal of Roentgenology, 186*, 1384-1392.

Flux, G., Bardies, M., Monsieurs, M., Savolainen, S., Strand, S. E., & Lassmann, M. (2006). The Impact of PET and SPECT on Dosimetry for Targeted Radionuclide Therapy. *Z. Med. Phys., 16*, 47–59.

Forbes, K. P., Pipe, J. G., Karis, J. P., & Heiserman, J. E. (2002). Improved image quality and detection of acute cerebral infarction with PROPELLER diffusion weighted MR imaging. *Radiology, 225*, 551-555.

Frakes, D. H., Dasi, L. P., Pekkan, K., Kitajima, H. D., Sundareswaran, K., Yoganathan, A. P., & Smith, M. J. T. (2008). A New Method for Registration-Based Medical Image Interpolation. *IEEE Transactions on Medical Imaging, 27*(3), 370-377.

France, L., Lenoir, J., Angelidis, A., Meseure, P., Cani, M.-P., Faure, F., & Chaillou, C. (2005). A layered model of a virtual human intestine for surgery simulation. *Medical Image Analysis,* (9).

Frangi, A. F., Niessen, W. J., & Viergever, M. A. (2001). Three-dimensional modeling for functional analysis of cardiac images: a review. *IEEE Transactions on Medical Imaging, 20*(1), 2-25.

Frank, L. R. (2001). Anisotropy in high angular resolution diffusion-weighted MRI. *Magnetic Resonance in Medicine, 45,* 935-939.

Frank, L. R. (2002). Characterization of anisotropy in high angular resolution diffusion-weighted MRI. *Magnetic Resonance in Medicine, 47,* 1083-1099.

Freeborough, P. A., & Fox, N. C. (1998). Modeling brain deformations in Alzheimer disease by fluid registration of serial 3D MR images. *Journal of Computer Assisted Tomography, 22,* 838-843.

Freitas, A., Costa-Pereira, A., & Brazdil, P. (2007). Cost-sensitive decision trees applied to medical data. *In Lecture Notes in Computer Science (including subseries Lecture Notes in Artificial Intelligence and Lecture Notes in Bioinformatics). 4654 LNCS,* 303-312.

Freudenberg, J., Schiemann, T., Tiede, U., & Hoehne, K. H. (2000). Simulation of cardiac excitation patterns in a three-dimensional anatomical heart atlas. *Computers in Biology and Medicine, 30,* 191-205.

Freund, Y., & Schapire, R. E. (1995). A decision-theoretic generalization of on-line learning and an application to boosting. *Computational Learning Theory: Eurocolt, 95,* 23–37.

Friedman, J., Hastie, T., & Tibshirani, R. (2000). Additive logistic regression: a statistical view of boosting. *The Annals of Statistics, 28*(2), 337-374.

Friedman, N., Linial, M., Nachman, I., & Pe'er, D. (2000). Using Bayesian networks to analyze expression data. *J Computational Biology, 7*(3-4), 601-620.

Friesen, W. V., & Ekman, P. (1983). *Emfacs-7: emotional facial action coding system.* Unpublished Manuscript, University of California at San Francisco

Friston, K. J., Penny, W., Phillips, C., Kiebel, S., Hinton, G., & Ashburner, J. (2002). Classical and Bayesian inference in neuroimaging: theory. *NeuroImage, 16*(2), 465–483.

Fu, L., & Medico, E. (2007). FLAME, a Novel Fuzzy Clustering Method for the Analysis of DNA Microarray Data. *BMC Bioinformatics, 8*(3).

Fuchs, H., Kedem, Z. M., & Uselton, S. P. (1977). Optimal surface reconstruction from planar contours. *Commun ACM, 20,* 693–702.

Fukunaga, K. (1990). *Statistical Pattern Recognition.* Morgan Kaufmann.

Fuller, D. B., Naitoh, J., Lee, Ch., Hardy, S., & Jin, H. (2008). Virtual HDR CyberKnife Treatment for Localized Prostatic Carcinoma: Dosimetry Comparison With HDR Brachytherapy and Preliminary Clinical Observations. *International Journal of Radiation Oncology, Biology, Physics, 70*(5), 1588-1597.

Fung, G., & Stoeckel, J. (2007). SVM feature selection for classification of SPECT images of Alzheimer's disease using spatial information. *Knowledge and Information Systems, 11*(2), 243–258.

Fung, Y. C. (1981). Ch. 4 in *Biomechanical properties of living tissues*, New York, USA: Springer Verlag.

Furhang, E. E., Sgouros, G., & Chui, C. S. (1993). Radionuclide photon dose kernels for internal emitter dosimetry. *Med. Phys., 23*(5), May 1996.

Gal, Y., Mehnert, A., Bradley, A., McMahon, K., & Croizer, S. (2007). An evaluation of four parametric models od contrast enhancement for dynamic magnetic resonance imaging of the breast. *29th Annual International Conference of the IEEE Engineering in Medicine and Biology Society.*

Galinsky, V. L. (2003). Automatic registration of microarray images. I. Rectangular grid. *Bioinformatics, 19*(14), 1824-1831.

Garbey, M., Merla, A., & Pavlidis I. (2004). Estimation of blood flow speed and vessel location from thermal video. In *Proceedings of the IEEE Computer Society*

Conference on Computer Vision and Pattern Recognition, 1, 356–363.

Garbey, M., Sun, N., Merla, A., & Pavlidis, I. (2007). Contact-free measurement of cardiac pulse based on the analysis of thermal imagery. *IEEE Transactions Biomedical Engineering, 54*(8), 1418-26.

Garra, B. S., Céspedes, E. I., Ophir, J., Spratt, R. S., Zuurbier, R. A., Magnant, C. M., & Pennanen, M. F. (1997). Elastography of breast lesions: Initial clinical results. *Radiology, 202*, 79-86.

Gavaghan, D., Garny, A., Maini, P. K., & Kohl, P. (2006). Mathematical models in physiology. *Phil. Trans. R. Soc. A 364*, 1099–1106.

Gennisson, J. L., Catheline, S., Chaffai, S., & Fink, M. (2003). Transient elastography in anisotropic medium: application to the measurement of slow and fast shear wave speeds in muscles. *J. Acoust. Soc. Am., 114*(1), 536-541.

Gérard, O., Billon, A. C., Rouet, J. M., Jacob, M., Fradkin, M., & Allouche, C. (2005). Efficient model-based quantification of left ventricular function in 3-D echocardiography. *IEEE Transactions on Medical Imaging, 21*(9), 1059-1068.

Gering, D. T. (2003). *Recognizing deviations from normalcy for brain tumor segmentation*. PhD Thesis. Department of Electrical Engineering and Computer Science. Massachusetts Institute of Technology.

Geroulakos, G., Ramaswami, G., Nicolaides, A., et al. (1993). Characterisation of symptomatic and asymptomatic carotid plaques using high-resolution real-time ultrasonography. *British Journal of Surgery, 80,* 1274-7.

Gersho, A., & Gray, R. M. (1991). *Vector Quantization and Signal Compression*. Kluwer Academic edition.

Ghosh, A. K. (2004). On the challenges of using evidence-based information: The role of clinical uncertainty. *Journal of Laboratory and Clinical Medicine, 144*(2):60-64.

Giannakeas, N., & Fotiadis, D. I. (2007). Multichannel Segmentation of cDNA Microarray Images using the Bayes Classifier. *In 29th Annual International Conference of the IEEE Engineering in Medicine and Biology Society*. Lyon, France.

Giannoglou, G. D., Chatzizisis, Y. S., Koutkias, V., Kompatsiaris, I., Papadogiorgaki, M., Mezaris, V., et al. (2007). A novel active contour model for fully automated segmentation of intravascular ultrasound images: in vivo validation in human coronary arteries. *Comput Biol Med, 37*(9), 1292-302.

Giannoni, M. F., Spezial, F., Faraglia, E., et al. (1991). Minor asymptomatic carotid stenosis contralateral to carotid endarterectomy (CEA). Our experience. *European Journal of Vascular Surgery, 5*, 237-45.

Giannoula, A. (2008). *Propagation of shear waves generated by a finite-amplitude ultrasound radiation force in a viscoelastic medium*. PhD dissertation, University of Toronto, Canada.

Giannoula, A., & Cobbold, R. S. C. (2007). Propagation of narrowband shear waves induced by a finite-amplitude radiation force. *Proc. IEEE Ultrason. Symp.*, (pp. 2267-2270).

Giannoula, A., & Cobbold, R. S. C. (2008). Narrowband shear wave generation by a finite-amplitude radiation force: the fundamental component. *IEEE Trans. Ultrason., Ferroelect. Freq. Contr., 55*(2), 343-358.

Gibbons, J. D. (1985). *Nonparametric Statistical Inference*. 2nd Ed., M. Dekker.

Gibbs, P., & Turnbull, L. W. (2003). Textural analysis of contrast-enhanced MR images of the breast. *Magnetic Resonance in Medicine, 50*(1), 92-98.

Gibson, D., Spann, M., & Woolley, S. I. (2000). Comparative study of compression methodologies for digital angiogram video. *Presented at the ISPACS 2000*, Honolulu.

Gibson, D., Spann, M., & Woolley, S. I. (2004). A wavelet-based region of interest encoder for the compression of angiogram video sequences. *IEEE Transactions on Information Technology in Biomedicine, 8*, 103 – 113.

Giger, M. L. (2004). Computer aided diagnosis in diagnostic mammography and multimodality breast imaging. *RSNA Categorical Course in Diagnostic Radiology Physics: Advances in Breast Imaging - Physics, Technology and Clinical Applications,* (pp. 205-217).

Giger, M. L., Huo, Z., Kupinski, M. A., & Vyborny, C. J. (2000). Computer-aided diagnosis in mammography. In: M. Sonka, J. M. Fitzpatrick. (Eds.) *Handbook of Medical Imaging Vol. 2, Medical Image Processing and Analysis* (pp. 915-1004). Bellingham, Washington, USA, SPIE Press.

Gilhuijs, K. G. A., Deurloo, E. E., Muller, S. H., Peterse, J. L., & Schultze-Kool, L. J. (2002). Breast MR imaging in women at increased lifetime risk of breast cancer: Clinical system for computerized assessment of breast lesions - Initial results. *Radiology, 225*(3), 907-916.

Gillian, A., Xiaoyi, P. J., Horst, D. B., Kevin, D. W., & Andrew, R. B. (1996). *An Experimental Comparison of Range Image Segmentation Algorithms, IEEE Transactions on PAMI, 18*(7), 673-689.

Glasbey, C. A., & Madria, K. V. (1998). A review of image-warping methods *Journal of Applied Statistics, 25*(2), 155–171.

Glatting, G., Landmann, M., Wunderlich, A., Kull, T., Mottaghy, F. M., Reske, S. N. (2006). Internal radionuclide therapy: Software for treatment planning using tomographic data. *Nuklearmedizin, 45*(6), 269-72.

Gletsos, M., Mougiakakou, S. G., Matsopoulos, G. K, Nikita, K. S., Nikita, A., & Kelekis, D. (2003). A computer-aided diagnostic system to characterize CT focal liver lesions: Design and optimization of a neural network classifier. *IEEE Transactions on Information Technology in Biomedicine, 7*(3), 153-162.

Glover, F., & Lagun, M. (1999). *Tabu search.* Boston, MA: Kluwer Academic Publishers.

Glynn, R. J., Schneeweiss, S., & Stürmer, T. (2006). Indications for propensity scores and review of their use in pharmacoepidemiology. *Basic Clin Pharmacol Toxicol, 98*(3), 253-259.

Gokturk, S. B., Tomasi, C., Girod, B., & Beaulieu, C. (2001). Medical image compression based on region of interest, with application to colon CT images. *23rd Annual International Conference of the IEEE Engineering in Medicine and Biology Society,* (p.2453).

Goldberg, D. (1989). *Genetic algorithms in search, optimization and machine learning.* Boston, MA. Addison-Wesley.

Golemati, S., Sassano, A., Lever, M. J., Bharath, A. A., Dhanjil, S., Nicolaides, A. N. (2003). Motion analysis of carotid atherosclerotic plaque from B-mode ultrasound. *Ultrasound in Medicine and Biology, 29*(3), 387-399.

Golemati, S., Stoitsis, J., Sifakis E. G., Balkizas, T., & Nikita K. S. (2007). Using the Hough Transform to segment ultrasound images of longitudinal and transverse sections of the carotid artery. *Ultrasound in Medicine and Biology, 33*(12), 1918-1932.

Gollub, J., Ball, C. A., Binkley, G., Demeter, K., Finkelstein, D. B., Hebert, J. M., Hernandez-Boussard, T., Jin, H., Kaplper, M., Matese, J. C., Schroeder, M., Brown, P. O., Botstein, D., & Sherlock, G. (2003). The Stanford Microarray Database: data access and quality assessment tools. *Nucleic Acids Res., 31,* 94-96.

Gonzalez, R. C., & Woods, R. E. (2002). Image Enhancement in the Spatial Domain. In *Digital image processing* (pp. 75-146). Reading, MA. Addison-Wesley.

Gonzalez, R. C., Woods, R. E., & Eddins, S. L. (2004). Digital image processing using MATLAB. *Prentice Hall, Upper Saddle River,* NJ.

Gonzalez, R., & Woods, R. (1992). *Digital image processing.* Addison Wesley.

Goode, A. *et al.* (2007). *Distributed Online Anomaly Detection in High-Content Screening.* CMU-CS-07-177, School of Computer Science, Carnegie Mellon University.

Graham, J. (1989). Resolution of composites in interactive karyotyping. In *Automation of Cytogenetics,* Berlin, Germany: Springer-Verlag, (pp. 191–203).

Granum, E., Gerdes, T., & Lundsteen, C. (1981). Simple weighted density distributions, WDD's for discrimination between G-banded chromosomes. *In Proc. Eur. Chrom. Anal. Workshop*, Edinburgh, U.K.

Gray, J., & Pinkel, D. (1992). Molecular cytogenetics in human cancer diagnosis. *Cancer, 69*, 1536–1542.

Gray-Weale, A. C., Graham, J. C., Burnett, J. R., et al. (1988). Carotid artery atheroma: comparison of preoperative B-mode ultrasound appearance with carotid endarterectomy specimen pathology. *Journal of Cardiovascular Surgery, 29*, 676-81.

Grigorescu S., Petkov N., & Kruizinga P. (2002). Comparison of Texture Features Based on Gabor Filters. *IEEE Transactions on Image Processing, 11*(10), 1160-1167

Grimson, W. E. L., Ettinger, G. J., White, S. J., Lozano-Perez, T., Wells, W. M., III., & Kikinis, R. (1996, April). An Automated Registration Methods for Frameless Stereotaxy, Image Guided Surgery, and Enhanced Reality Visulatization. *Medical Imaging, IEEE Transactions, 15*(2), 129-140.

Gronholdt, M. L., Nordestgaard, B. G., Schroeder, T. V., Vostrup, S., & Sillesen, H. (2001). Ultrasonic echolucent carotid plaques predict future strokes. *Circulation, 104*, 68-73.

Grossberg, M. D., & Nayar, S. K. (2004). Modelling the Space of Camera Response Functions. *IEEE Transactions on Pattern Analysis and Machine Intelligence, 26*(10).

GSI Lumonics (1999). *QuantArray Analysis Software*. Operator's Manual.

Gu, G. *et al.* (2006). *An Information-Theoretic Measure of Intrusion Detection Capability.* ASIACCS'06, March 21-24, Taipei, Taiwan, 90-101.

Gu, H., Zhang, Y., & Ji, Q. (2005). Task oriented facial behavior recognition with selective sensing. *Computer Vision and Image Understanding, 100*, 385-415.

Gudbjartsson, H., Maier, S. E., Mulkern, R. V., Morocz, I. A., Patz, S., & Jolesz, F. A. (1996). Line scan diffusion imaging. *Magnetic Resonance in Medicine, 36*, 509-519.

Guest, E., Berry, E., Baldock, R. A., Fidrich, M., & Smith, M. A. (2001). Robust point correspondence applied to two- and three-dimensional image registration. *IEEE Transactions in Pattern Analysis and Machine Intelligence, 23*(2), 165-179.

Guha, S., Rastogi, R., & Shim, K. (1999). ROCK: A robust clustering algorithm for categorical attributes. *Proc. of the 15th Int'l Conf. on Data Eng.*

Guo, G., & Dyer, C. R. (2005). Learning From Examples in the Small Sample Case: Face Expression Recognition. *IEEE Trans. Sys. Man and Cybernetics–PART B: Cybernetics, 35*(3), 477-488.

Guo, L., Lobenhofer, E. K., Wang, C., Shippy, R., Harris, S. C., Zhang, L., Mei, N.,Chen, T., Herman, D., Goodsaid, F. M., Hurban, P., Phillips, K. L., Xu, J., Deng, X., Sun, Y. A., Tong, W., Dragan, Y. P., & Shi, L. (2006). Rat Toxigonecomic Study Reveals Analytical Consistency Across Microarray Platforms. *Nat. Biotech., 24*, 1162-1169.

Gupta, N., & Gupta, N. (2007). A VLSI Architecture for Image Registration in Real Time. *IEEE Transactions on VLSI, 15*(9), 981-989.

Gupta, S., & Markey, M. K. (2005). Correspondence in texture features between two mammographic views. *Medical Physics, 32*(6), 1598-1606.

Gussenhoven, E. J., Essed, C. E., Lancée, C. T., Mastik, F., Frietman, P., van Egmond, F. C., et al. (1989). Arterial wall characteristics determined by intravascular ultrasound imaging: an in vitro study. *J Am Coll Cardiol, 14*(4), 947-52.

Haas C., Ermert H., Holt S., Grewe P., Machraoui A., & Barmeyer J. (2000). Segmentation of 3-D intravascular ultrasonic images based on a random field model. *Ultrasound in medicine & biology, 26*(2), 297–306.

Haeghen, V. Y., Naeyaert, J., Lemahieu, I., & Philips, W. (2000). An Imaging System with Calibrated Color Image Acquisition for Use in Dermatology. *IEEE Transactions on Medical Imaging, 19*(7).

Häfner, M., Brunauer, L., Payer, H., Resch, R., Wrba, F., Gangl, A., et al. (2007). Pit pattern classification of zoom-endoscopical colon images using evolved Fourier feature vectors *Proceedings of the 2007 IEEE Machine Learning for Signal Processing Workshop (MLSP'07)*, 99 - 104.

Häfner, M., Kendlbacher, C., Mann, W., Taferl, W., Wrba, F., Gangl, A., Vécsei, A., & Uhl, A. (2006). Pit pattern classification of zoom-endoscopic colon images using histogram techniques. *Proceedings of the 7th Nordic Signal Processing Symposium (NORSIG 2006)*, 58-61.

Häfner, M., Liedlgruber, M., Wrba, F., Gangl, A., Vécsei, A., & Uhl, A. (2006). Pit pattern classification of zoom-endoscopic colon images using wavelet texture features. *Proceedings of the International Conference on Advances in Medical Signal and Image Processing (MEDSIP 2006).*

Hagemann, A., Rohr, K., Stiehl, H. S., Spetzger, U, & Gilsbach, J. M. (1999). Biomechanical modeling of the human head for physically based, nonrigid image registration. *IEEE Transaction on Image Processing, 18,* 875–884.

Hajnal, J. V., Hill, D. L. G., & Hawkes, D. J. (2001). *Medical image registration.* CRC Press.

Hajnal, J. V., Saeed, N., Soar, E. J., Oatridge, A., Young, I. R., & Bydder, G. M. (1995). A registration and interpolation procedure for subvoxel matching of serially acquired MR images. *Journal of Computer Assisted Tomography, 19,* 289- 296.

Han, J. M. Kamber (2000). *Data Mining: Concepts and Techniques.* Morgan Kaufmann.

Hand, D. J. (1998). Intelligent data analysis: Issues and opportunities. *Intelligent Data Analysis, 2*(1), 67-79.

Hansen, L., Larsen, J., Nielsen, F. A., Strother, S., Rostrup, E., Savoy, R., et al. (1999). Generalizable patterns in neuroimaging: How many principal components? *NeuroImage, 9*, 534-544.

Hansen, M. H., & Yu, B. (2001). Model selection and the principle of minimum description length. *J. Am. Stat. Assoc., 96*(454), 746-774.

Haralick R.M., Shanmugam K., & Dinstein I. (1973). Texture Features for Image Classification. *IEEE Trans. Nov., SMC-3,* 610-621.

Haralick, R. M., & Shaphiro L. G. (1992), *Computer and Robot Vision.* vol. I., Boston, MA. Addison-Wesley.

Haralick, R. M., Shanmugan, K., & Dinstein, I. (1973). Textural features for image classification. *IEEE Transactions on Systems, Man and Cybernetics, 3*(6), 610-622.

Harrison, R. J. (n. d.). *Nucl. Med., 34,* 60.

Hasan, K. M., Parker, D. L., & Alexander, A. L. (2001). Comparison of gradient encoding schemes for diffusion-tensor MRI. *Journal of Magnetic Resonance Imaging, 13,* 769-780.

Haselgrove, J. C., & Moore, J. R. (1996). Correction for distortion of echo-planar images used to calculate the apparent diffusion coefficient. *Magnetic Resonance in Medicine, 36,* 960-964.

Hastie, T., Tibshirani, R., Eisen, M. B., Alizadeh, A., Levy, R., Staudt, L., Chan, W. C., Botstein, D., & Brown, P. (2002). 'Gene Shaving' as a Method for Identifying Distinct Sets of Genes with Similar Expression Patterns. *Genome Biology, 1,* research0003.1-0003.21.

Haykin, S. (1999). *Neural Networks: A Comprehensive Foundation*, NJ. Prentice-Hall.

Hayton, P. M., Brady, M., Tarassenko, L, & Moore, N. (1999). A non-rigid registration algorithm for dynamic breast MR images. *Artificial Intelligence 114,* 125-156

Hayton, P. M., Brady, M., Tarassenko, L., & Moore, N. (1997). Analysis of dynamic breast images using a model of contrast enhancement. *Medical Image Analysis, 1(3),* 207-224.

Heckbert, P., & Garland, M. (1997). Survey of Polygonal Surface Simplification Algorithms. *Siggraph 97 Course Notes, 25.* ACM Press.

Heckerman, D. E., Horvitz, E. J., & Nathwani, B. N. (1992). Toward normative expert systems. Part I: the pathfinder project. *Methods Inf Med, 31*(2), 90-105.

Hein, E., Albrecht, A., Melzer, D., Steinhöfer, K., Rogalla, P., Hamm, B., & Taoupitz, M. (2005). Computer-assisted diagnosis of focal liver lesions on CT images: Evaluation of the perceptron algorithm. *Academic Radiology. 12*(9), 1205-1210.

Helm, P. A., Tseng, H.-J., Younes, L., McVeigh, E. R., & Winslow, R. L. (2005). Ex vivo 3D diffusion tensor imaging and quantification of cardiac laminar structure. *Magnetic Resonance in Medicine, 54*, 850-859.

Herman, G. T., & Liu, H. K. (1977). Display of three dimensional information in computed tomography. *J Comput Assist Tomogr, 1*, 155–160.

Hernandez, T., & Kambhampati, S. (2004). Integration of biological sources: Current systems and challenges. *ACM SIGMOD, 33*(3), 51-60.

Hersh, W. (2006). Medical Image Retrieval Protocol. *ImageCLEFmed 2006*, available at http://www.clef-campaign.org/, last updated - 14 June 2006.

Herskovits, E. H., & Gerring, J. P. (2003). Application of a data-mining method based on Bayesian networks to lesion-deficit analysis. *NeuroImage, 19*(4), 1664-1673.

Hill, D. L. G, Hawkes, D. J., Harrison, N. A., & Ruff, C. F. (1993). A strategy for automated multimodality image registration incorporating anatomical knowledge and imager characteristics. In H. H. Barrett and A. F. Gmitro (Eds.) *Proc. 13th Int. Conf. Information Processing in Medical Imaging; Lecture Notes in Computer Science 687, June 1993* (pp. 182-196). New York: Springer-Verlag.

Hilsenbeck, S. G., Friedrichs, W. E., Schiff, R., O'Connell, P., Hansen, R. K., Osborne, C. K., & Fuqua, S. A. W. (1999). Statistical Analysis of Array Expression Data as Applied to the Problem of Tamoxifen Resistance. *J. Natl. Cancer Institute, 91*, 453-459.

Hirsch, J. G., Bock, M., Essig, M., & Schad, L. R. (1999). Comparison of diffusion anisotropy measurements in combination with the flair –technique. *Magnetic Resonance in Medicine, 17*, 705-716.

Hjelmas, E., & Low, B. K. (2001). Face detection: A survey. *Computer Vision and Image Understanding, 83*, 236-274.

Hodge, V. J., & Austin, J. (2004). A Survey of Outlier Detection Methodologies. *Artificial Intelligence Review, 22*, 85–126.

Hoffmann, R., Seidl, T., & Dugas, M. (2002). Profound effect of normalization on detection of differentially expressed genes in oligonucleotide microarray data analysis. *Genome Biology, 3*(7). research 0033.1-0033.11.

Holman, B. L., Zimmerman, R. L., Shapiro, J. R., Kaplan, M. L., Jones, A. G., & Hill, T. C. (1983). Biodistribution and dosimetry of *n*-isoproyl *p*-123I iodoamphetamine in the primate. *J. Nucl. Med., 24*, 922–31.

Holmes, J. H., & Peek, N. (2007). Intelligent data analysis in biomedicine. *J Biomedical Informatics, 40*(6), 605-608.

Horsch, K., Giger, M. L., Venta, L. A., & Vyborny, C. J. (2001). Automatic segmentation of breast lesions on ultrasound. *Medical Physics, 28*(8), 1652–1659.

Horsch, K., Giger, M. L., Vyborny, C. J., Lan, L., Mendelson, E. B., & Hendrick, R. E. (2006). Classification of breast lesions with multimodality computer aided diagnosis: Observer study results on an independent clinical data set. *Radiology, 240*(2), 357-368.

Horsch, K., Giger, M. L., Vyborny, C. J., & Venta, L. A. (2004). Performance of computer aided diagnosis (CAD) in the interpretation of lesions on breast sonography. *Academic Radiology, 11*(3), 272-280.

Horsfield, M. A., & Morgan, B. M. A. (2004). Algorithms for Calculation of Kinetic Parameters From T1-Weighted Dynamic Contrast-Enhanced Magnetic Resonance Imaging. *Journal of Magnetic Resonance Imaging, 20*, 723-729.

Horsfield, M., & Jones, D. (2002). Applications of diffusion-weighted and diffusion tensor MRI to white matter diseases – a review. *NMR in Biomedicine, 15*, 570-57.

Hsinchun, C., Fuller, S. S., Friedman, C., & Hersh, W. (Ed.). (2005). *Medical Informatics: Knowledge Management and Data Mining in Biomedicine.* (Integrated Series in Information Systems), Springer.

Hsu, C., & Lin, C. (2002). A Comparison of Methods for Multi-Class Support Vector Machines. *IEEE Transactions on Neural Networks, 13*(2), 415-425.

Hsu, C., Chang, C., & Lin, C. A Practical Guide to Support Vector Classification.

Hsu, C.-W., & Lin, C.-J. (2002). A comparison of methods for multiclass support vector machines. *IEEE Transactions on Neural Networks, 13*, 415-425.

Hsu, E. W., & Mori, S. (1995). Analytical expressions for the NMR apparent diffusion coefficients in an anisotropic system and a simplified method for determining fiber orientation. *Magnetic Resonance in Medicine, 34*, 194-200.

Hsu, W., & Bui, A. A. (2006). A framework for visually querying a probabilistic model of tumor image features. In D.W. Bates (Ed.), *AMIA Annu Symp Proc*, 354-358.

Hu, N., Downey, D. B., Fenster, A., & Ladak, H. M. (2003). Prostate boundary segmentation from 3D ultrasound images. *Medical Physics, 30*(7), 1648-1659.

Huang, C. H., Lanza, V., Rajasekaran, S., & Dubitzky, W. (2005). HealthGrid - Bridging life science and information technology. *Journal of Clinical Monitoring and Computing, 19*(4-5), 259-262.

Huang, X. *et al.* (2007). *System and Method for Whole Body Landmark Detection, Segmentation and Change Quantification in Digital Images.* Patent WO2007044508.

Huang, Y. L., & Chen, D. R. (2004). Watershed segmentation for breast tumor in 2-D sonography. *Ultrasound in Medicine & Biology, 30*(5), 625–632.

Huang, Y. L., Chen, J. H., & Shen, W .C. (2006). Diagnosis of hepatic tumors with texture analysis in non-enhanced computed tomography images. *Academic Radiology, 13*(6), 713-720.

Human Chromosome Study Group (1960). A proposed standard of nomenclature of human mitotic chromosomes. *Cereb. Palsy Bull.*

Huo, Z., Giger, M. L., & Vyborny, C. J. (2001). Computerized analysis of multiple-mammographic views: Potential usefulness of special view mammograms in computer-aided diagnosis. *IEEE Transactions on Medical Imaging, 20*(12), 1285-1292.

Hurlstone, D. P. (2002). High-Resolution Magnification Chromoendoscopy: Common Problems Encountered in "Pit Pattern" Interpretation and Correct Classification of Flat Colorectal Lesions. *American Journal of Gastroenterology, 97*, 1069-1070.

Hurlstone, D. P., Cross, S. S., Adam, I., Shorthouse, A. J., Brown, S., Sanders, D. S., & Lobo, A. J. (2004). Efficacy of High Magnification Chromoscopic Colonoscopy for the Diagnosis of Neoplasia in Flat and Depressed Lesions of the Colorectum: a Prospective Analysis. *Gut, 53*, 284-290.

Hutton, B. F., Braun, M., Thurfjell, L., & Lau, D. Y. H. (2002). Image registration: an essential tool for nuclear medicine. *European Journal of Nuclear Medicine and Molecular Imaging, 29*, 559–577.

ICRP. (1988). Radiation dose to patients from radiopharmaceuticals. *ICRP Publication, 53. Ann. ICRP 18*(1–4) (Oxford: Pergamon).

Ideker, T., Galitski, T., & Hood, L. (2001). A new approach to decoding life: systems biology. *Annu Rev Genomics Hum Genet, 2*, 343-372.

Ideker, T., Thorsson, V., Siehel, A. F., & Hood, L. E. (2000). Testing for Differentially Expressed Genes by Maximum Likelihood Analysis of Microarray Data. *J. Comput. Biol., 7*, 805-817.

Ikedo, Y. *et al.* (2007). Development of a fully automatic scheme for detection of masses in whole breast ultrasound images. *Medical Physics, 34*(11), 4378-4388.

Ilgner J., Palm C., Schutz A., Spitzer K., Westhofen M., & Lehmann T. (2003). Colour Texture Analysis for Quantitative Laryngoscopy. *Acta Otolaryngol, 123*, 730-734.

Insana, M. F., & Brown, D. G. (1993). *Acoustic scattering theory applied to soft biological tissues. In Ul-*

trasonic Scattering in biological tissues, Boca Raton, CRC Press.

International Commission on Radiological Protection (ICRP) 1975 report of the Task Group on Reference Man *ICRP Publication 23* (New York: Pergamon)

International Telecommunication Union (2002). ITU-R-BT.500-11 Methodology for the subjective assessment of the quality of television pictures. *Recommendation on Broadcasting Service*.

Irizarry, R. A., Hobbs, B., Collin, F., Beazer-Barclay, Y. D., Antonellis, K. J., Scherf, U., & Speed, T. P. (2003). Exploration, Normalization, and Summaries of High Density Oligonucleotide Array Probe Level Data. *Biostatistics, 4*, 249-264.

Islam, A., & Pearlman, W. A. (1999). An embedded and efficient low-complexity hierarchical image coder. *SPIE Visual Comm. and Image Processing*, (pp. 294).

Issa, B., Buckley, D. L., & Turnbull, L. W. (1999). Heterogeneity analysis of Gd-DTPA uptake: Improvement in breast lesion differentiation. *Journal of Computer Assisted Tomography, 23*(4), 615-621.

Iyatomi, H. *et al.* (2006). Quantitative assessment of tumor extraction from dermoscopy images and evaluation of computer-based extraction methods for an automatic melanoma diagnostic system. *Melanoma Research, 16*(2), 183-19.

Izrailev, F. M. (1990). Simple models of quantum chaos:spectrum and eigenfunctions. *Phys. Rep., 196*, 299-392.

J Magn Reson Imag (1999). *Special issue: Cardiovascular MRI, 10*(5).

Jackowski, M., Kao, C. Y., Qiu, M., Constable, R. T., & Staib, L. H. (2005). White matter tractography by anisotropic waveform evolution and diffusion tensor imaging. *Medical Image Analysis, 9*, 427-440.

Jackson, A. (2004). Analysis of Dynamic Contrast Enhanced MRI. *British Journal of Radiology, 77*(suppl 2), 5154-5166.

Jackson, A. (April, 2003). Quantitative characterization of tumor micro vasculature using dynamic contrast enhanced MRI. *Medica Mundi 47/1.*

Jackson, A., Buckley, D., & Parker, G. J. M. (2005). *Dynamic contrast-enhanced magnetic resonance imaging in oncology.* Springer-Verlag Berlin Heidelberg.

Jackson, A., O'Connor, J. P., Parker, G. J., & Jayson, G. C. (2007). Imaging tumor vascular heterogeneity and angiogenesis using dynamic contrast-enhanced magnetic resonance imaging, *Clinical Cancer Research, 13*(12), 3449-3459.

Jain, A. K., & Dubes, R. C. (1988). *Algorithms for Clustering Data*. Prentice Hall.

Jain, A. N., Tokuyasu, T. A., Snijders, A. M., Segraves, R., Albertson, D. G., & Pinkel, D. (2002). Fully automatic quantification of microarray image data. *Genome Research, 12*, 325–332.

Jan, S. (2004). GATE: a simulation toolkit for PET and SPECT. *Phys. Med. Biol., 49*(2004), 4543–4561.

Jerebko, A. K., Malley, J. D., Franaszek, M., & Summers, R. M. (2003). Multiple neural network classification scheme for detection of colonic polyps in CT colonography data sets. *Academic Radiology, 10*(2), 154-160.

Jesneck, J. L., Nolte, L. W., Baker, J. A., Floyd, C. E., & Lo, J. Y. (2006). Optimized approach to decision fusion of heterogeneous data for breast cancer diagnosis. *Medical Physics, 33*(8), 2945-2954.

Ji, L. (1989). Intelligent Splitting in the chromosome domain. *Pattern Recognition, 22*, 519-532.

Ji, L. (1994). Fully automatic chromosome segmentation. *Cytometry, 17*, 196-208.

Jiang, Y., Metz, C. E., & Nishikawa, R. M. (1996). A receiver operating characteristic partial area index for highly sensitive diagnostic tests. *Radiology, 201*(3), 745-750.

Jiang, Y., Nishikawa, R. M., Schmidt, R. A., Metz, C. E., Giger, M. L., & Doi, K. (1999). Improving breast cancer diagnosis with computer-aided diagnosis. *Academic Radiology, 6*(1), 22-33.

Joachims, T. (1999). Making large-Scale SVM Learning Practical. B. Schölkopf, C. Burges, & A. Smola (Eds.), *Advances in Kernel Methods - Support Vector Learning*. MIT Press.

Joakimsen, O., Bønaa, K. H., Mathiesen, E. B., et al. (2000). Prediction of Mortality by Ultrasound Screening of a General Population for Carotid Stenosis: The Tromsø Study. *Stroke*, *31*, 1871-6.

Johnson, H., & Christensen, G. (2002). Consistent landmark and intensity-based image registration. *IEEE Transactions in Medical Imaging, 21*, 450-461.

Johnson, J. M., Kennelly, M. M., Decesare, D., et al. (1985). Natural history of asymptomatic carotid plaque. *Archives of Surgery*, *120*, 1010-2.

Johnson, S. B. (1996). Generic data modeling for clinical repositories. *J Am Med Inform Assoc, 3*(5), 328-339.

Johnson, T. K., McClure, D., & McCourt, S. (1999). MABDOSE. I: characterization of a general purpose dose estimation code. *Med Phys.* 1999, *26*, 1389 –1395.

Johnson, T. K., McClure, D., & McCourt, S. (2000). MABDOSE. II: validation of a general purpose dose estimation code. *Med Phys., 26*, 1396 –1403.

Jolliffe, I. T. (2002). *Principal Component Analysis*. Springer.

Jones, M. W., & Chen, M. (1994). A new approach to the construction of surfaces from contour data. *Comput Graph Forum, 13*, 75–84.

Jones, D. K. (2004). The effect of gradient sampling schemes on measures derived from diffusion tensor MRI: a Monte Carlo study. *Magnetic Resonance in Medicine, 51,* 807-815.

Jones, D. K., Horsfield, M. A., & Simmons, A. (1999). Optimal strategies for measuring diffusion in anisotropic systems by magnetic resonance imaging. *Magnetic Resonance in Medicine, 42,* 515-525.

Jones, D. K., Symms, M. R., Cerignani, M., & Howard, R. J. (2005). The effect of filter size on VBM analyses of DT-MRI data. *NeuroImage, 26,* 546-554.

Jung, Y. H., Kim, J. S., Hur, B. S., & Kang, M. G. (2005). Design of Real-Time Image Enhancement Preprocessor for Cmos Image Sensor. *IEEE Transactions on Consumer Electronics, 46*(1).

Kadah, Y. M., Frag, A. A., Zurada, J. M., Badawi, A. M., & Youssef, A.B. M. (1996). Classification algorithms for quantitative tissue characterization of diffuse liver disease from ultrasound images. *IEEE Transactions on Medical Imaging, 15*(4), 466-478.

Kagawa, R., Moritake, K., Shima, T., et al. (1996). Validity of B-mode ultrasonographic findings in patients undergoing carotid endarterectomy in comparison with angiographic and clinicopathologic features. *Stroke*, *27*, 700-5.

Kahn, C. E., Roberts, L. M., Shaffer, K. A., & Haddawy, P. (1997). Construction of a Bayesian network for mammographic diagnosis of breast cancer. *Computers in Biology and Medicine, 27*(1), 19-29.

Kallergi, M. (2004). Computed-aided diagnosis of mammographic microcalcification clusters. *Medical Physics, 31*(2), 314-326.

Kanade, T., Cohn, J. F., & Tian, Y. (2000). Comprehensive database for facial expression analysis. *Proc. IEEE Int'l Conf. Face and Gesture Recognition,* (pp. 46-53).

Karahaliou, A., Boniatis, I., Skiadopoulos, S., Sakellaropoulos, P., Arikidis, N., Likaki, E., Panayiotakis, G., & Costaridou, L. (2008, in press). Breast cancer diagnosis: Analyzing texture of tissue surrounding microcalcifications. *IEEE Transactions on Information Technology in Biomedicine* (DOI: 10.1109/TITB.2008.920634).

Karahaliou, A., Skiadopoulos, S., Boniatis, I., Sakellaropoulos, P., Likaki, E., Panayiotakis, G., & Costaridou, L. (2007). Texture analysis of tissue surrounding microcalcifications on mammograms for breast cancer diagnosis. *The British Journal of Radiology, 80*(956), 648-656.

Karahaliou, A., Vassiou, K., Skiadopoulos, S., Kanavou, D., Yiakoumelos, A., & Costaridou, L. (2008, in press). Quantifying heterogeneity of lesion uptake in Dynamic Contrast Enhanced MRI for breast cancer diagnosis.

Nuclear Instruments and Methods in Physics Research Section A.

Karampinos, D. C., King, K. F., Sutton, B. P., & Georgiadis, J. G. (2007). *In vivo study of cross-sectional skeletal muscle fiber asymmetry with diffusion-weighted MRI.* Paper presented at the IEEE Engineering in Medicine and Biology Conference, Lyon, France.

Kardoulas, D. G., Katsamouris, A. N., Gallis, P. T. et al. (1996). Ultrasonographic and histologic characteristics of symptom-free and symptomatic carotid plaque. *Cardiovascular Surgery, 4,* 580-90.

Karkanis, S. A., Galousi, K., & Maroulis, D. (1999). Classification of Endoscopic Images Based on Texture Spectrum. ACAI99. *Workshop on Machine Learning in Medical Applications*, Chania, Greece, (pp. 63-69).

Karkanis, S. A., Iakovidis, D. K., Maroulis, D. E., Karras, A. D., & Tzivras, M. (2003). Computer-Aided Tumor Detection in Endoscopic Video using Color Wavelet features. *IEEE Transactions on Information Technology in Biomedicine, 7*(3), 141-152.

Karkanis, S., Iakovidis, D., Karras, D., & Maroulis, D. (2001). Detection of Lesions in Endoscopic Video using Textural Descriptors on Wavelet Domain supported by Artificial Neural Network Architectures. *Proceedings of the. International Conference on Image Processing (ICIP'01)*, 833-836.

Karkanis, S., Iakovidis, D., Maroulis, D., Theofanous, N., & Magoulas, G. (2000). Tumor Recognition in Endoscopic Video Images using Artificial Neural Network Architectures. *Proceedings of the 26th EUROMICRO Conference (EUROMICRO'00),* 423-429.

Karkanis, S., Magoulas, G., Grigoriadou, M., & Schurr, M. (1999). Detecting Abnormalities in Colonoscopic Images by Textural Description and Neural Networks. *Proceedings of the Workshop on Machine Learning in Medical Applications, Advance Course in Artificial Intelligence (ACAI'99)*, 59-62.

Karnan, M., & Thangavel, K. (2007). Automatic detection of the breast border and nipple position on digital mammograms using genetic algorithm for asymmetry approach to detection of microcalcifications. *Computer Methods and Programs in Biomedicine, 87*(1), 12-2.

Karvelis, P., Fotiadis, D., Syrrou, M., & Georgiou, I., (2005). Segmentation of chromosomes images based on a recursive watershed transform. *3rd European Medical & Biological Engineering Conference*, (EMBEC 2005), (pp. 497-502, 20-25).

Karvelis, P., Tzallas, A., Fotiadis, D., & Georgiou, I. (2007). A Multichannel Watershed-Based Segmentation Method for Multispectral Chromosome Classification. *IEEE Trans. Med. Imaging.*

Karypis, G., Han, E. H., & Kumar, V. (n.d.). CHAMELEON: A Hierarchical Clustering Algorithm Using Dynamic Modelling. *IEEE Computer: Special Issue and Data Analysis and Mining.*

Kass, M., Witkin, A., & Terzopoulos, D. (1987). Snakes: Active contours models. *Proc Int'l Conference Computer Vision*, (pp. 259-269).

Katehakis, D. G., Tsiknakis, M., & Orphanoudakis, S. (2002). *Towards an Integrated Electronic Health Record - Current Status and Challenges, Business Briefing: Global Healthcare 2002*, The Official Publication of the World Medical Association, January 2002.

Kato, S., Fu, K., Sano, Y., Fujii, T., Saito, Y., Matsuda, T., et al. (2006). Magnifying colonoscopy as a non-biopsy technique for differential diagnosis of non-neoplastic and neoplastic lesions. *World journal of gastroenterology : WJG*, 12(9), 1416-20.

Kaufman, L., & Rousseeuw, P. J. (1989). Finding Groups in Data - An Introduction to Cluster Analysis. *Wiley,* NY.

Kaufman, L., & Rousseeuw, P. J. (1990). *Finding Groups in Data: an Introduction to Cluster Analysis.* JohnWiley & Sons.

Kawasaki, M., Takatsu, H., Noda, T., Sano, K., Ito, Y., Hayakawa, K., et al. (2002). In vivo quantitative tissue characterization of human coronary arterial plaques by use of integrated backscatter intravascular ultrasound and comparison with angioscopic findings. *Circulation, 105*(21), 2487-92.

Kay, S. M. (1993). Fundamentals of Statistical Signal Processing, Volume I: Estimation Theory. N. J., USA: Prentice Hall.

Kelm, B. M. *et al.* (2007). Automated Estimation of Tumor Probability in Prostate Magnetic Resonance Spectroscopic Imaging: Pattern Recognition vs. Quantification. *Magnetic Resonance in Medicine*, *57*, 150–159.

Keppel, E. (1975). Approximating complex surfaces by triangulation of contour lines. *IBM J Res Dev 19*(1), 2–11.

Kerr, M. K., Martin, M., & Churchill, G. A. (2000). Analysis of Variance for Gene Expression Microarray Data. *J. Computational Biol. 7*, 819-837.

Keyserlingk, J. R., Ahlgren, P. D., Yu, E., Belliveau, N., & Yassa, M. (2007). Functional infrared imaging of the breast: Historical perspectives, current applications, and future considerations. In J. D. Bronzino & N. A. Diakides (Ed.), *Medical Infrared Imaging* (pp. 10.1 – 10.30).Boca Raton, FL: CRC Press.

Kier, C., Toth, D., Meyer-Wiethe, K., Schindler, A., Cangür, H., Seidel, G., & Aach, T. (February 2005). *Cerebral perfusion imaging with bolus harmonic imaging.*

Kim, S. Y., Lee, J. W., Sohn, I. S. (2006). Comparison of Various Statistical Methods for Identifying Differential Gene Expression in Replicated Microarray Data. *Statistical Methods in Medical Research, 15*, 3-20.

Kingsley, P. B., & Monahan, W. G. (2004). Selection of the optimum b factor for diffusion-weighted magnetic resonance imaging assessment of ischemic stroke. *Magnetic Resonance in Medicine, 51,* 996-1001.

Kinkel, K., Helbich, T. H., Esserman, L. J., Barclay, J., Schwerin, E. H., Sickles, E. A., & Hylton, N. M. (2000). Dynamic high-spatial-resolution MR imaging of suspicious breast lesions: Diagnostic criteria and interobserver variability. *AJR. American Journal of Roentgenology, 175*(1), 35-43.

Klachaturian, M. H., Wisco, J. J., & Tuch, D. S. (2007). Boosting the sampling frequency of *q*-ball imaging using multiple wavevector fusion. *Magnetic Resonance in Medicine, 57,* 289-296.

Klein, H. M., Gunther, R. W., Verlande, M., Schneider, W. D. Vorwerk, D., Kelch J., et al (1992). 3D-surface reconstruction of intravascular ultrasound images using personal computer hardware and a motorized catheter control. *Cardiovasc Intervent Radiol, 15*(2), 97-101.

Klein, M., (2001). Combining and relating ontologies: an analyis of problems and solutions. In: Gomez-Perez A et al., editors. *Workshop on ontologies and information sharing, IJCAI'01*, Seattle.

Klein, S. A. (1993) Image quality and image compression: a psychophysicist's viewpoint. *Digital and human vision*, (pp. 73–88).

Klein, S., Staring, M., & Pluim, J. P. (2007). Evaluation of optimization methods for nonrigid medical image registration using mutual information and B-splines. *IEEE Trans Image Process, 16(12),* 2879-2890.

Kline, J. A., Novobilski, A. J., Kabrhel, C., Richman, P. B., & Courtney, D. M. (2005). Derivation and validation of a Bayesian network to predict pretest probability of venous thromboembolism. *Annals of Emergency Medicine, 45*(3), 282-290.

Klingensmith, J. D., & Vince, D. G. (2002).B-spline methods for interactive segmentation and modeling of lumen and vessel surfaces in three-dimensional intravascular ultrasound. *Comput Med Imaging Graph, 26*(6), 429-38.

Klingensmith, J. D., Shekhar, R., & Vince, D. G. (2000). Evaluation of three dimensional segmentation algorithms for the identification of luminal and medial-adventitial borders in intravascular ultrasound images. *IEEE Transaction on Medical Imaging, 19*(10), 996–1011.

Klingensmith, J. D., Tuzcu, E. M., Nissen, S. E., & Vince, D. G. (2003). Validation of an automated system for luminal and medial-adventitial border detection in three-dimensional intravascular ultrasound. *The International Journal of Cardiovascular Imaging, 19*(1), 93–104.

Knoll, C., Alcaniz, M., Grau, V., Monserrat, C., & Juan, M.C. (1999). Outlining of the prostate using snakes with shape restrictions based on the wavelet transform. *Pattern Recognition, 32*, 1767-1781.

Kocur, C. M., Rogers, S. K., Myers, L. R., Burns, T., Kabrisky, M., Hoffmeister, J. W., Bauer, K. W., & Steppe, J. M. (1996). Using neural networks to select wavelet features for breast cancer diagnosis. *IEEE Engineering in Medicine and Biology, 15*(3), 95-102.

Kohonen, T. (1984). *Self-Organization and Associative Memory*. Berlin - Springer Verlag.

Kohonen, T. (1990). The self-organizing map. *Proceedings of the IEEE, 78*(9), 1464-1480.

Kolbert, K. S., Sgouros, G., Scott, A. M., Bronstein, J. E., Malane, R. A., Zhang, J., Kalaigian, H., McNamara, S., Schwartz, L., & Larson, S. M. (1997). Implementation and evaluation of patient-specific three-dimensional internal dosimetry. *J. Nucl. Med., 38*, 301–8.

Koning, G., Dijkstra, J., Von Birgelen, C., Tuinenburg, J. C., Brunette, J., Tardif, J. C., et al (2002). Advanced contour detection for three – dimensional intracoronary ultrasound: a validation in – vitro and in vivo. *Int J Cardiovasc Imag, 18*, 235-48.

Konofagou, E., & Hynynen, K. (2003). Localized Harmonic Motion Imaging: Theory, Simulations and Experiments. *Ultrasound Med. Biol., 29*, 1405-13.

Konofagou, E., Hannigan, T., & Ophir, J. (2000). Shear strain estimation and lesion mobility assessment in elastography. *Ultrasonics, 38*, 400-404.

Kontos, D., & Megalooikonomou, V. (2004). Fast and effective characterization of 3D Region of Interest in medical image data. Medical Imaging 2004: Image *Processing, edited by J. Michael Fitzpatrick, Milan Sonka, Proceedings of SPIE Vol. 5370* (SPIE, Bellingham, WA, 2004) (pp. 1324-1331)

Koral, K. F., Francis, I. R., & Kroll, S. (2002). Volume reduction versus radiation dose for tumors in previously untreated lymphoma patients who received iodine-131 tositumomab therapy. Conjugate views compared with a hybrid method. *Cancer, 94*, 1258–1263.

Kou, Z., Ji, L., & Zhang, X. (2002). Karyotyping of Comparative Genomic Hybridization Human Metaphases by Using Support Vector Machines. *Cytometry, 47*, 17-23.

Kovalski, G., Beyar, R., Shofti, R., & Azhari, H. (2000). Three-dimensional automatic quantitative analysis of intravascular ultrasound images. *Ultrasound in medicine & biology, 26*(4), 527–537.

Kramer, D., & Aghdasi, F. (1999). Texture analysis techniques for the classification of microcalcifications in digitized mammograms. In *Proc. 5th IEEE AFRICON Conf.* (pp. 395-400), Cape Town, Africa.

Krivacic, R. T. *et al.* (2004). A rare-cell detector for cancer. *Proc. of the National Academy of Sciences of the United States of America, Clinical Cancer Research, 101*(29), 10501 – 10504.

Krouskop, T. A., Dougherty, D. R., & Vinson, F. S. (1987). A pulsed Doppler ultrasonic system for making noninvasive measurements of the mechanical properties of soft tissue. *J. Rehabil. Res. Dev., 24*(2), 1-8.

Kruse, S. A., Smith, J. A., Lawrence, A. J., Dresner, M. A., Manduca, A., Greenleaf, J. F., & Ehman, R. L. (2000). Tissue characterization using magnetic resonance elastography: preliminary results. *Phys. Med. Biol., 45*, 1579-1590.

Kudo, S., Hirota, S., Nakajima, T., Hosobe, S., Kusaka, & H., Kobayashi, T. (1994). Colorectal tumours and pit pattern. *Journal of Clinical Pathology, 47*(10), 880-885.

Kudo, S., Tamura, S., Nakajima, T., Yamano, H., Kusaka, H., & Watanabe, H. (1996). Diagnosis of colorectal tumorous lesions by magnifying endoscopy. *Gastrointestinal endoscopy, 44*(1), 8-14.

Kuhl, C. K., Mielcareck, P., Klaschik, S., Leutner, C., Wardelmann, E., Gieseke, J. & Schild, H. H. (1999). Dynamic breast MR imaging: Are signal intensity time course data useful for differential diagnosis of enhancing lesions? *Radiology, 211*(1), 101-110.

Kuhn, K., Baker, S. C., Chudin, E., Lieu, M. H., Oeser, S., Bennett, H., et al. (2004). A novel, high-performance random array platform for quantitative gene expression profiling. *Genome Res, 14*(11), 2347-2356.

Kuncheva, L. (2004). *Combining Pattern Classifiers - Methods and Algorithms*. Wiley.

Kutcher, G. J., Burman, C., Brewster, L., Goitein, M., & Mohan, R. (1991). Histogram reduction method for calculating complication probabilities for 3-dimensional treatment planning evaluations. *Int. J. Radiat. Oncol. Biol. Phys., 21*, 137-46.

Kwong, K. K., McKinstry, R. C., Chien, D., Crawley, A. P., Pearlman, J. D., & Rosen, B. R. (1991). CSF-suppressed quantitative single-shot diffusion imaging. *Magnetic Resonance in Medicine, 21*, 157-163.

Kyriacou, E., Pattichis, M., Pattichis, C. S., Mavrommatis, A., Christodoulou, C. I., Kakkos,S., Nicolaides, A. (2007). Classification of Atherosclerotic Carotid Plaques Using Morphological Analysis on Ultrasound images. *Journal of Applied Intelligence*, Springer. ISSN: 0924-669X (Print) 1573-7497 (Online).

Kyriacou, E., Pavlopoulos, S., Koutsouris, D., Zoumpoulis, P., & Theotokas, I. (1997). Computer assisted characterization of liver tissue using image texture analysis techniques on B-scan images. In *19th Annual International Conference of the IEEE Engineering in Medicine and Biology Society. Vol. 2.* (pp. 806-809).

Ladak, H. M., Mao, F., Wang, Y., Downey, D. B., Steinman, D. A., & Fenster, A. (2000). Prostate boundary segmentation from 2D ultrasound images. *Medical Physics, 27*, 1777-1788.

Laliberte, F., Gagnon, L., & Sheng, Y. (2003). Registration and fusion of retinal images: an evaluation study. *IEEE Transactions in Medical Imaging, 22*(5). 404-418.

Langsfeld, M., Gray-Weale, A. C., & Lusby, R. J. (1989). The role of plaque morphology and diameter reduction in the development of new symptoms in asymptomatic carotid arteries. *Journal of Vascular Surgery, 9*, 548-57.

Lasko, T. A., Bhagwat, J. G., Zou, K. H., & Ohno-Machado, L. (2005). The use of receiver operating characteristic curves in biomedical informatics. *Journal of Biomedical Informatics 38*(5), 404-415.

Lavrac, N., Kononenko, I., Keravnou, E., Kukar, M., & Zupan, B. (1998). Intelligent data analysis for medical diagnosis: Using machine learning and temporal abstraction. *AI Communications, 11*(3), 191-218.

Laws, K. I. (1980) Rapid texture identification, In *SPIE Conference for Missile Guidance. Vol. 238.* (pp. 376-380).

Lazar, M., & Alexander, A. L. (2001). Error analysis of white matter tracking algorithms (streamlines and tensorlines) for DT-MRI. *Proceedings of International Society of Magnetic Resonance in Medicine*, (pp. 506), Glasgow, UK.

Lazar, M., & Alexander, A. L. (2003). An error analysis of white matter tractography methods: synthetic diffusion tensor field stimulations. *NeuroImage, 20*, 1140-1153.

Lazar, M., Weinstein, D. M., & Tsuruda, J. S. (2003). White matter tractography using diffusion tensor deflection. *Human Brain Mapping, 18*, 306-321.

Lazar, M., Weinstein, D., Hasan, K., & Alexander, A. L. (2000). Axon tractography with tensorilines. *Proceedings of International Society of Magnetic Resonance in Medicine*, (pp. 482), Denver, CO.

Le Bihan, D. (1991). Molecular diffusion nuclear magnetic resonance imaging. *Magnetic Resonance in Medicine, 7*, 1-30.

Le Bihan, D., Breton, E., & Lallemand, D. (1986). MR imaging of intravoxel incoherent motions: application to diffusion and perfusion in neurologic disorders. *Radiology, 161*, 401-407.

Le Callet, P., & Barba, D. (2001) Critère de qualité visuelle d'images couleur - application à l'évaluation réaliste de codeurs d'images. *Colloque GRETSI.*

Leahy, A. L., McCollum, P. T., Feeley, T. M., et al. (1988). Duplex ultrasonography and selection of patients for carotid endarterectomy: Plaque morphology or luminal narrowing? *Journal of Vascular Surgery, 8,* 558-62.

Lebrun, G., Charrier, C., Lezoray, O., & Cardot H. (2007). A fast and efficient segmentation scheme for cell microscopic image. *Cellular and Molecular Biology, Biomedical Signal and Image Processing, 53*(2), 51-61.

Lebrun, G., Charrier, C., Lezoray, O., & Cardot, H. (2008). Tabu search model selection for SVM. *International Journal of Neural Systems, 18*(1), 19-31.

Ledesma-Carbayo, M. J., Kybic, J., Desco, M., Santos, A., Sühling, M., Hunziker, P., & Unser, M. (2005). Spatio-temporal nonrigid registration for ultrasound cardiac motion estimation. *IEEE Transactions on Medical Imaging, 24*(9), 1113-1126.

Lee, C. C, Chen, S. H., & Chiang, Y. C. (2007). Classification of liver disease from CT images using a support vector machine. *Journal of Advanced Computational Intelligence and Intelligent Informatics, 11*(4), 396-402.

Lee, C. C., Chen, S. H., Tsai, H. M., Chung, P. C., & Chiang, Y. C. (2006). Discrimination of liver diseases from CT images based on Gabor filters. In *19th IEEE International Symposium on Computer-Based Medical Systems. Vol. 1.* (pp.203-206)

Lee, C. P., & Wang, T. G. (1993). Acoustic radiation pressure. *J. Acoust. Soc. Am., 94,* 1099-1109.

Lee, C.-H. *et al.* (2005). Segmenting Brain Tumors with Conditional Random Fields and Support Vector Machines. *Lecture Notes in Computer Science, 3765,* 469-478.

Lee, D., Baek, S., & Sung, K. (1997). Modified k-means Algorithm for Vector Quantizer Design. *IEEE Signal Processing Letters,* 4(1), 2-4.

Lee, J., Kim, N., Lee, H., Seo, J. B., Won, H. J., Shin, Y. M., Shin, Y. G., & Kim, S.H. (2007). Efficient liver segmentation using level-set method with optimal detection of the initial liver boundary from level-set speed images. *Computer Methods and Programs in Biomedicine, 88*(1), 26-38.

Lee, K. W., Wood, N. B., & Xu, X. Y. (2004). Ultrasound image-based computer model of a common carotid artery with a plaque. *Medical Engineering Physics, 26*(10), 823-840.

Lee, R. T., & Libby, P. (1997). The unstable atheroma. *Arteriosclerosis Thrombosis Vascular Biology, 17*(10), 1859-1867.

Lehmann, T. Goenner, C., & Spitzer K. (1999). Survey: Interpolation Methods in Medical Image Processing. *IEEE Transactions on Medical Imaging,18*(11), 1049-1075.

Lehmann, T. M. *et al.* (2005). Automatic categorization of medical images for content-based retrieval and data mining. *Computerized Medical Imaging and Graphics, 29,* 143–155.

Lehtinen, J. (1999). Distortion of a Wavelet Image Codec. *Acta Cyberntica, 14,* 342-356.

Leibovici, L., Fishman, M., Schonheyder, H. C., Riekehr, C., Kristensen, B., Shraga, I., et al. (2000). A causal probabilistic network for optimal treatment of bacterial infections. *IEEE Transactions on Knowledge and Data Engineering, 12*(4), 517-528.

Leichter, I., Fields, S., Nirel, R., Bamberger, P., Novak, B., Lederman, R., & Buchbinder, S. (2000). Improved mammographic interpretation of masses using computer-aided diagnosis. *European Radiology 10*(2), 377-383.

Leichter, I., Lederman, R., Buchbinder, S., Bamberger, P., Novak, B., & Fields, S. (2000). Optimizing parameters for computer-aided diagnosis of microcalcifications at mammography. *Academic Radiology, 7*(6), 406-412.

Leither, D. M., & Wolynes, P.G. (1997) Vibrational mixing and energy flow in polyatomics: quantitative prediction using local random matrix theory. *J. Phys. Chem. A, 101,* 541-548.

Lengyel, J., Greenberg, D. P., & Pop, R. (1995). Time–dependent three-dimensional intravascular ultrasound. In: Robert Cook, (Ed). *The SIGGRAPH 95 Conference on Comp Graphics,* (pp. 457-64).

Lerner, B. (1998). Toward a completely automatic neural-network-based human chromosome analysis. *IEEE Trans. Trans. Syst., Man, Cybern.*, pt. B, Cybern., *28*, 544–552.

Lerner, B., Guterman, H., & Dinstein, I. (1998). A Classification-driven Partially Occluded Object Segmentation (CPOOS) method with application to chromosome analysis. *IEEE Transactions on Signal Processing, 46*, 2841-2847.

Lerner, B., Guterman, H., Dinstein, I., & Romem, Y. (1995). Medial axis transform-based features and a neural network for human chromosome classification. *Pattern Recognition, 28*, 1673-1683.

Lerner, R. M., Parker, K. J., Holen, J., Gramiak, R., & Waag, R. C. (1988). Sono-elasticity: medical elasticity images derived from ultrasound signals in mechanically vibrated targets. In L.W. Kessler (Ed.), *Acoustical Imaging* (pp. 317-327). Plenum Press, New York.

Levner, I., & Zhang, H. (2007). Classification-Driven Watershed Segmentation. *IEEE Transactions on Image Processing, 16*(5), 1437-1445.

Lezoray, O., & Cardot, H. (2002). Cooperation of color pixel classification schemes and color watershed : a study for microscopical images. *IEEE transactions on Image Processing, 11*(7), 783-789.

Li, Q., Fraley, C., Bumgarner, R. E., Yeung, K. Y., & Raftery, A. E. (2005). Donuts, scratches and blanks: robust model-based segmentation of microarray images. *Bioinformatics, 21*(12), 2875-2882.

Li, S. Z., & Jain, A. K. (2005). *Handbook of face recognition*. New York, USA: Springer.

Li, S., & Li, W. (2000). Shape-adaptive discrete wavelet transform for arbitrary shaped visual object coding. *IEEE Trans. Circuits Syst. Video Technol., 10*, 725–743.

Liedlgruber, M., & Uhl, A. (2007). Statistical and structural wavelet packet features for Pit pattern classification in zoom-endoscopic colon images (P. Dondon, V. Mladenov, S. Impedovo, & S. Cepisca, Hrsg.). *Proceedings of the 7th WSEAS International Conference on Wavelet Analysis & Multirate Systems (WAMUS'07)*, 147-152.

Lien, J. J., Kanade, T., Cohn, J. F. & Li, C. C. (2000). Detection, tracking and classification of action units in facial expression. *Robotics and Autonomous Systems, 31*, 131-146.

Likar, B., & Pernus, F. (1999). Automatic extraction of corresponding points for the registration of medical images. *Medical Physics, 26*, 1678–1686.

Lin, C. Y., Sun, S. W., Hong, C. Y., & Chang, C. (2005). Unsupervised identification of white matter tracts in a mouse brain using a directional correlation-based region growing (DCRG) algorithm. *NeuroImage, 28*, 380-388.

Lin, C.-P., Wedeen, V. J., Chen, J.-H., Yao, C., & Tseng, W. I. (2003). Validation of diffusion spectrum magnetic resonance imaging with manganese-enhanced rat optic tracts and *ex vivo* phantoms. *Neuroimage, 19*, 482-495.

Lin, S. M., Du, P., Huber, W., & Kibbe, W.A. (2008). Model-based variance-stabilizing transformation for Illumina microarray data. *Nucleic Acids Res., 36*(2), e11. Epub 2008.

Linde, Y., Buzo, A., & Gray, R. M. (1980). An Algorithm for Vector Quantizer Design. *IEEE Transactions on Communications*, (pp. 702-710).

Linfoot, E. H. (1958). Quality Evaluation of Optical Systems. *Optica Acta, 5*(1-2), 1-13.

Lisboa, P. J. G. (2002). A review of evidence of health benefit from artificial neural networks in medical intervention. *Neural Networks, 15*(1), 11-39.

Liu, A., Williams, L., Lopatin, G., Yamauchi, D., Wong, J., & Raubitschek, A. (1999). A radionuclide therapy treatment planning and dose estimation system. *J. Nucl. Med., 40*, 1151–3.

Liu, A., Zhang, Y., Gehan, E., & Clarke, R. (2002). Block Principal Component Analysis with Application to Gene Microarray Data Classification. *Stat. Med. 21*, 3465-3474.

Liu, C., Xia, T., & Li, H. (2004). ROI and FOI algorithms for wavelet-based video compression. *5th Pacific Rim Conf. Multimedia*, Tokyo, (pp. 241).

Liu, W., & Wang, Z. (2006). Facial Expression Recognition Based on Fusion of Multiple Gabor Features. *Int'l Conf Pattern Recognition,* (pp. 536-539).

Liu, Z., Ha, J., Xiong, Z., Wu, Q., & Castleman, K. (2002). Cascaded Differential and Wavelet Compression of Chromosome Images. *IEEE Trans. on Biomedical Engineering, 49*, 323-283.

Liu, Z., Ha, J., Xiong, Z., Wu, Q., & Castleman, K. (2002). Lossy-to-lossless ROI coding of chromosome images using modified SPIHT and EBCOT. *IEEE International Symposium on Biomedical Imaging*, (pp.317).

Ljungberg M and Strand SE, Comput. Methods Prog. Biomed. 29 1989 257–72.

Lobregt, S., & Viergever, M. A. (1995). Discrete dynamic control model. *IEEE Trans Med Imag, 14*, 12-24.

Loeckx, D., Slagmolen, P., Maes, F., Vandermeulen, D., & Suetens, P. (2007). Nonrigid image registration using conditional mutual information. In *Proceedings of the International Conference on Information Processing in Medical Imaging (IPMI),* The Netherlands, July 2-6, 2007 (pp. 725-37).

Loevinger R, Budinger T and Watson E 1988 *MIRD Primer for Absorbed Dose Calculations* (New York: Society of Nuclear Medicine)

Lopes, A., & Brodlie, K.(2003). Improving the robustness and accuracy of the marching cubes algorithm for isosurfacing. *IEEE Transactions on Visualization and ComputerGraphics, 9*, 16–29.

Lorensen, W. E., & Cline, H. E. (1987). Marching cubes: A high resolution 3D surface construction algorithm. *In Proceedings of the 14th annual conference on Computer graphics and interactive techniques.* (pp. 163–169). ACM Press.

Lorensen, W., Cline, H., Nafis, C., Kikinis, R., Altobelli, D., & Gleason, L. (1993). Enhancing Reality in the Operating Room. *Proceedings of the 1993 IEEE Visualization Conference* (pp. 410-415).

Lori, N. F., Akbuda, E., Snyder, A. Z., Shimony, J. S., & Conturo, T. E. (1999). Diffusion tensor tracking of human neuronal fiber bundles: Simulation of effects of noise, voxel size and data interpolation. *Proceedings of International Society of Magnetic Resonance in Medicine*, (pp. 775), Denver, CO.

Lu, W., Olivera, G. H., Chen, Q., Chen M-L., & Ruchala, K. J. (2006). Automatic re-contouring in 4D radiotherapy. *Physics in Medicine and Biology, 51*, 1077–1099.

Lucas, P. J., van der Gaag, L. C., & Abu-Hanna, A. (2004). Bayesian networks in biomedicine and health-care. *Artif Intell Med, 30*(3), 201-214.

Lucht, R., Knopp, M. V., & Brix, G. (2000). Elastic Matching of Dynamic MR Mammographic Images. *Magnetic Resonance in Medicine, 43,* 9-16.

Lucht, R., Knopp, M. V., & Brix, G. (2001). Classification of signal-time curves from dynamic MR mammography by neural networks. *Magnetic Resonance Imaging, 19*(1), 51–57.

Luebke, D. (2001). A Developer's Survey of Polygonal Simplification Algorithms. *IEEE Computer Graphics & Applications,* (pp. 24-35).

Lukac, R., & Plataniotis, K. (2006). *Color Image Processing: Methods and Applications.* Boca Raton, FL: CRC Press / Taylor & Francis.

Luna-Acosta, G. A., Mndez-Bermdez, J. A., & Izrailev, F. M. (2001). Periodic chaotic billiards: Quantum-classical correspondence in energy space. *Phys. Rev. E, 64*, 036206+18.

Lundsteen, C., Gerdes, T., Maahr, J., & Philip, J., (1987) Clinical performance of a system for semiautomated chromosome analysis. *American Journal of Human Genetics, 41*, 493-502.

Lyons, M. J., Budynek, J., & Akamatsu, S. (1999). Automatic classification of single facial images. *IEEE Trans. Pattern Analysis and Machine Intelligence, 21*(12), 1357-1352.

Lyons, M., & Akamatsu, (1998). Coding Facial Expressions with Gabor Wavelets. *Int'l Conf Automatic Face and Gesture Recognition*, (pp. 200-205).

MacQueen, J. B. (1967). Some Methods for classification and Analysis of Multivariate Observations. *In 5-th Berkeley Symposium on Mathematical Statistics and Probability, 1*, 281-297. Berkeley:University of California Press.

Madabhushi, A., & Metaxas, D. N. (2003). Combining low-, high-level and empirical domain knowledge for automated segmentation of ultrasonic breast lesions. *IEEE Transaction on Medical Imaging, 22*(2), 155–169.

Maes, F., Collignon, A., Vandermeulen, D., Marchal, G., & Suetens, P. (1997). Multimodality image registration by maximization of mutual information. *IEEE Transaction on Medical Imaging, 16,* 187–198.

Maes, F., Vandermeulen, D., & Suetens, P. (1999). Comparative evaluation of multiresolution optimization strategies for multimodality image registration by maximization of mutual information. *Medical image analysis, 3,* 373-377.

Maes, F., Vandermeulen, D., & Suetens, P. (2003). Medical Image Registration Using Mutual Information. *Proceedings of the IEEE, 91(10),* 1699-1722.

Mainardi L. T., Passera K. M., Lucesoli A., Vergnaghi D., Trecate G., Setti E., Musumeci R., & Cerutti S. (2008). A non-rigid registration of MR breast images using complex-valued Wavelet Transform. *Journal of Digital Imaging, 21(1),* 27-36.

Mainardi, L. T., Passera, K. M., Lucesoli, A., Potepan, P., Setti, E., & Musumeci, R. (2006). A method for dynamic subtraction mr imaging of the liver. *BMC Medical Imaging, 6,* 5.

Maintz, A. J. B., & Viergever, M. A. (1998). An overview of medical image registration methods. *Med. Image Anal., 2,* 1–37.

Maintz, J. B. A., & Viergever, M. A. (1998). A survey of medical image registration. *Medical Image Analysis, 2*(1), 1-36.

Maintz, J. B. A., van den Elsen, P. A., & Viergever, M. A. (1995). Comparison of feature-based matching of CT and MR brain images. In N. Ayache, (Eds.) *Proc. 1st Int. Conf. Computer Vision, Virtual Reality and Robotics in Medicine; Lecture Notes in Computer Science 905*, Nice, France, April 1995, (pp. 219-228) New York, Springer-Verlag

Makela, T., Clarysse, P., Sipila, O., Pauna, N., Pham, Q. C., Katila, T., & Magnin, I. E. (2002). A review of cardiac image registration methods. *IEEE Transactions on Medical Imaging, 21,* 1011–1021.

Malvern, L. E. (1969). *Introduction to the Mechanics of a Continuous Medium.* Englewood Cliffs, NJ: Prentice-Hall.

Mandelbrot, B. B. (1983). *Fractal geometry of nature.* NY. W. H. Freeman and Co.

Manduca, A., Dutt, V., Borup, D. T., Muthupillai, R., Ehman, R. L., & Greenleaf, J. F. (1998). *Reconstruction of Elasticity and Attenuation Maps in Shear Wave Imaging: An Inverse Approach, Medical Image Computing and Computer-Assisted Interventation — MICCAI'98, 1496,* Lecture Notes in Computer Science, Springer Berlin / Heidelberg, (pp. 606-613).

Manduca, A., Oliphant, T. E., Dresner, M. A., Mahowald, J. L., Kruse, S. A., Amromin, E., Felmlee, J. P., Greenleaf, J. F., & Ehman, R. L. (2001). Magnetic resonance elastography: non-invasive mapping of tissue elasticity. *Medical Image Analysis, 5*(4), 237-254.

Manjunath, B. S., & Ma, W. Y. (1996). Texture features for browsing and retrieval of image data. *IEEE Trans. Pattern Analysis and Machine Intelligence, 18*(8), 837-842.

Mann, H. B., & Whitney, D. R. (1947). On a test of whether one of two random variables is stochastically larger than the other. *Annals of Mathematical Statistics, 18*, 50-60.

Maragos, P. (1989). Pattern spectrum and multiscale shape representation. *IEEE Transactions on Pattern Analysis and Machine Intelligence, 11*, 701-715.

Marcus, A. (1998). Metaphor design for user interfaces. *Conference on Human Factors in Computing Systems*, 129-130.

Markou, M., & Singh, S. (2003). Novelty Detection: A Review, Part 1: Statistical Approaches. *Signal Processing, 83*, 2499–2521.

Markou, M., & Singh, S. (2003). Novelty Detection: A Review, Part 2: Neural network-based approaches. *Signal Processing, 83*, 2481–2497.

Maroulis, D., Iakovidis, D., Karkanis, S., & Karras, D. (2003). CoLD: a versatile detection system for colorectal lesions in endoscopy video-frames. *Computer methods and programs in biomedicine*, 70(2), 151-66.

Marret, H., Sauget, S., Giraudeau, B., Brewer, M., Ranger-Moore, J., Body, G., & Tranquart, F. (2004). Contrast-Enhanced Sonography helps in discrimination of benign from malignant adnexal masses. *J Ultrasound Med.*

Martín, L., Bonsma, E., Anguita, A., Vrijnsen, J., García-Remesal, M., Crespo, J., Tsiknakis, M., & Maojo, V. (2007). Data Access and Management in ACGT: Tools to Solve Syntactic and Semantic Heterogeneities Between Clinical and Image Databases. In: *Advances in Conceptual Modeling – Foundations and Applications*, (pp. 24-33).

Martin-Sanchez, F., et al (2004). Synergy between medical informatics and bioinformatics: facilitating genomic medicine for future health care. *Journal of Biomedical Informatics*, *37*(1), 30-42.

Mascalchi, M., Tessa, C., Moretti, M., Della Nave, R., Boddi, V., Martini, S., Inzitari, D., & Villari, N. (2002). Whole brain apparent diffusion coefficient histogram: a new tool for evaluation of leukoaraiosis. *Journal of Magnetic Resonance Imaging, 15,* 144-148.

Masutani, Y., Aoki, S., Abe, O., Hayashi, N., & Otomo, K. (2003). MR diffusion tensor imaging: recent advance and new techniques for diffusion tensor visualization. *European Journal of Radiology, 46,* 53-56.

Masutani, Y., Uozumi, K., Akahane, M., & Ohtoo, K. (2006). Liver CT image processing: A short introduction of the technical elements. *European Journal of Radiology, 58*(2), 246-251.

Matsopoulos, G. K., Asvestas, P. A., Mouravliansky, N. A., & Delibasis, K. K. (2004). Multimodal registration of retinal images using self organizing maps. *IEEE Transactions in Medical Imaging, 23*, 1557-1563.

Mattiello, L., Basser, P. J., & Bihan, D. L. (1994). Analytical expression for the b matrix in NMR diffusion imaging and Spectroscopy. *Journal of Magnetic Resonance, 108,* 131-141.

Mattiello, L., Basser, P. J., & Bihan, D. L. (1997). The b-matrix in diffusion tensor echo-planar imaging. *Magnetic Resonance in Medicine, 37,* 292-300.

Mavrommatis, A. (2006). *Morphology of Carotid US Images*, MSc thesis, Univ. of Cyprus, Nicosia, Cyprus.

Maynard, S. E., Min, J. Y., Merchan, J., Lim, K. H., Li, J., Mondal, S., et al.(2003). Excess placental soluble fms-like tyrosine kinase 1 (sFlt1) may contribute to endothelial dysfunction, hypertension, and proteinuria in preeclampsia. *J Clin Invest, 111*, 649-58.

McVeigh, E. R. (1996). MRI of myocardial function: motion tracking techniques. *Magnetic Resonance Imaging, 14*(2), 137-150.

McClelland, J. R., Blackall, J. M., Tarte, S., Chandler, A. C., Hughes, S., Ahmad, S., Landau, D. B., &Hawkes, D. J. (2006). A continuous 4D motion model from multiple respiratory cycles for use in lung radiotherapy. *Medical Physics, 33*, 3348–3358.

McCormack, M.J., Kenney, A.R., Bryant C.W., Covington C.D., Dickinson, R.L., Coggins R.E. et al. (2007). Patent No. WO/2007/030696. Geneva: World Intellectual Property Organization.

McGee, S. (2002). Simplifying likelihood ratios. *Journal of general internal medicine: Official journal of the Society for Research and Education in Primary Care Internal Medicine*, *17*(8), 646-9.

McInerney, T., & Terzopoulos, D. (1996). Deformable models in medical image analysis: a survey. *Medical Image Analysis*, *1*(2), 91-108.

McIsaac, A. I., Thomas, J. D., & Topol, E. J. (1993). Toward the quiescent coronary plaque. *Journal of the American College of Cardiology, 22*(4), 1228-1241.

McKeown, M. J. (2000). Detection of consistently task-related activations in fMRI data with hybrid independent component analysis. *Neuroimage, 11*, 24-35.

McMurtry, L. W., Donaghy, M. J., Vlassoff, A., & Douch, P. G. C. (2000). Distinguishing morphological features of the third larval stage of ovine Trichostrongylus. *Veterinary Parasitology, 90*(1-2), 73-81.

Meairs, S., & Hennerici, M. (1999). Four-dimensional ultrasonographic characterization of plaque surface motion in patients with symptomatic and asymptomatic carotid artery stenosis. *Stroke, 30*(9), 1807-1813.

Mehta, M. L. (1991). Random matrices. Boston: *Academic Press.*

Meihle, A. (1973). *Surgery of the facial nerve.* Philadelphia, USA: Saunders.

Meijering, E. H. W., Niessen, W. J., & Viergever, M. A. (1999). Retrospective motion correction in digital subtraction angiography: a review. *IEEE Transactions on Medical Imaging, 18,* 2–21.

Meinel, L. A., & Reinhardt, J. M (2006). Breast MRI computer-aided diagnosis systems. In: J. S. Suri, R. M. Rangayyan (Eds.). *Recent Advances in Breast Imaging, Mammography, and Computer-Aided Diagnosis of Breast Cancer* (pp. 791-832). Bellingham, Washington, USA, SPIE Press.

Meinel, L. A., Stolpen, A. H., Berbaum, K. S., Fajardo, L. L., & Reinhardt, J. M. (2007). Breast MRI lesion classification: Improved performance of human readers with a backpropagation neural network computer-aided diagnosis (CAD) system. *Journal of Magnetic Resonance Imaging, 25*(1), 89-95.

Melhem, E. R., Mori, S., Mukundan, G., Kraut, M. A., Pomper, M. G., & van Zijjl, P. C. M. (2002). Diffusion Tensor MR Imaging of the Brain and White Matter Tractography. *American Journal of Radiology, 178,* 3-16.

Menegaz, G., & Grewe L. (2002). 3D/2D object-based coding of head MRI data. *2002 International Conference on Image Processing,* (1), 181-184.

Menze, B. H. *et al.* (2006). *Optimal Classification of Long Echo Time In Vivo Magnetic Resonance Spectra in the Detection of Recurrent Brain Tumors.* Multidimensional Image Processing, IWR, University of Heidelberg.

Merla, A. (2007). Computational physiology in a thermal image setting. In: *Proceedings of S.Co.2007, Fifth Conference on Complex Models and Computational Intensive Methods for Estimation and Prediction,* Book of Short Papers, ISBN 978-88-6129-114-0, (pp. 338-343).

Merla, A., & Romani, G. L. (2006). Functional Infrared Imaging in Clinical Applications. In J. D. Bronzino & N. A. Diakides, (Ed.), *Medical Imaging Devices and Systems, The Biomedical Engineering Handbook* (pp. 32.1 – 32.13).Boca Raton, FL: CRC Press.

Merla, A., & Romani, G. L. (2006). Functional infrared imaging in medicine: a quantitative diagnostic approach. In *Proceedings of the 2006 IEEE Engineering Medicine Biology Society, 1,* 224-7.

Merla, A., & Romani, G. L. (2007). Biomedical applications of functional infrared imaging. In J. D. Bronzino & N. A. Diakides (Ed.), *Medical Infrared Imaging* (pp. 15.1 – 15.20). Boca Raton, FL: CRC Press.

Merla, A., & Romani, G. L. (2007). Thermal signatures of emotional arousal: a functional infrared imaging study. In *Proceedings of the 2007 IEEE Engineering Medicine Biology Society,* (pp. 247-9).

Merla, A., Di Donato, L., & Romani, G. L. (2001). Assistance to surgery by means of infrared functional imaging: preliminary results. In *Proceedings of the 2001 IEEE Engineering Medicine Biology Society,* Proceedings CD track 1264.

Merla, A., Di Donato, L., Di Luzio, S., & Romani, G. L. (2002). Quantifying the Relevance and Stage of Disease with the Tau image Technique. *IEEE Engineering in Medicine and Biology Magazine, 21*(6), 86 – 91.

Merla, A., Di Donato, L., Rossini, P. M., & Romani, G. L. (2004). Emotion detection through Functional Infrared

Imaging: preliminary results. *Biomedizinische Technick, 48*(2), 284-286.

Merla, A., Di Donato, L., Salsano, F., & Romani, G. L. (2002). Raynaud's Phenomenon: infrared functional imaging applied to diagnosis and drugs effects. *International Journal of Immunopathology and Pharmacology, 15*(1), 41-52.

Merla, A., Di Romualdo, S., Di Donato, L., Proietti, M., Salsano, F., & Romani, G. L. (2007). Combined thermal and laser Doppler imaging in the assessment of cutaneous tissue perfusion. In: *Proceedings of the 2007 IEEE Engineering Medicine Biology Society,* (pp. 2630-3).

Merla, A., Ledda, A., Di Donato, L., & Romani, G. L. (2002). Use of infrared functional imaging to detect impaired thermoregulatory control in men with asymptomatic varicocele. *Fertility and Sterility, 78*(1), 199-200.

Merla, A., Ledda, A., Di Donato, L., & Romani, G. L. (2004). Assessment of the effects of the varicocelectomy on the thermoregulatory control of the scrotum. *Fertility and Sterility, 81*(2), 471-2.

Messmer, P. *et al.* (2006). A CT Database for Research, Development and Education: Concept and Potential. *Journal of Digital Imaging, 0*(0), 1-6, Online publication 07 August 2006.

Mettlin, C. (1995). American society national cancer detection project. *Cancer, 75,* 1790-1794.

Metzler, V., Seidel, G., Wiesmann, M., Meyer-Wiethe, K., & Aach, T. (2004). *Perfusion Harmonic Imaging of the Human Brain.*

Meurie, C., Lebrun, G., Lezoray, O., & Elmoataz, A. (2003). A supervised segmentation scheme for cancerology color images. *IEEE ISSPIT* (pp. 664-667).

Meurie, C., Lezoray, O., Charrier, C., & Elmoataz, A. (2005). Combination of multiple pixel classifiers for microscopic image segmentation. *International Journal of Robotics and Automation, 20*(2), 63-69.

Meyer, F. (2001). An Overview of Morphological Segmentation. *IJPRAI, 15*(7), 1089-1118.

Meyer, J., Phillips, M. H., Cho, P. S., Kalet, I., & Doctor, J. N. (2004). Application of influence diagrams to prostate intensity-modulated radiation therapy plan selection. *Physics in Medicine and Biology, 49*(9), 1637-1653.

Michie, D., Spiegelhalter, D., & Taylor, C. (1994). *Machine learning, neural and statistical classification.*

Mieusset, R., Bujan, L., Plantavid, M., Mansat, A., Grandjean, H., & Pontonnier, F. (1991) Scrotal hyperthermia: frequency in an infertile population and associated alterations in testicular function. *Advanced Experimental Medicine and Biology, 286,* 203-9.

Minami, G., Xiong, Z., Wang, A., & Mehrotra, S. (2001). 3-D wavelet coding of video with arbitrary regions of support. *IEEE Trans. Circuits Syst. Video Technol., 11,* 1063–1068.

Minati, L., & Weglarz, W. P. (2007). Physical foundations, models and methods of diffusion magnetic resonance imaging of the brain: a review. *Concepts in Magnetic Resonance A, 30,* 278-307.

Minhas, A. S., & Reddy, M. R. (2005). Neural network-based approach for AD in the lungs region by electrical impedance tomography. *Physiol. Meas., 26,* 489–502

Minka, T. (1999). Automatic choice of dimensionality for PCA. *MIT, Technical Report, 514.*

Mintz, G. S., Nissen, S. E., Anderson, W. D., Bailey, S. R., Elber, R., Fitzgerald, P. J., et al (2001). American college of cardiology clinical expert consensus document on standards for acquisition, measurement and reporting of intravascular ultrasound studies: a report of the American College of Cardiology task force on clinical expert consensus documents (committee to develop a clinical expert consensus on standards for acquisition, measurement and reporting of intravascular ultrasound studies [IVUS]). *J Am Coll of Cardiol, 37,* 1478– 1492.

Mir, A. H., Hanmandlu M., & Tandon S. N. (1995). Texture analysis of CT images. *IEEE Engineering in Medicine and Biology Magazine, 14*(6), 781-786.

Miyaji, S., Hamada, T., & Matsumoto, S. (2000). Development of a Digital Compressed Picture Quality Assessment

System Considering Human Visual Perception. *Systems and Computers in Japan*, *5*, 97–109.

Mock, U., Georg, D., Bogner, J., Auberger, T., & Potter, R. (2004). Treatment planning comparison of conventional, 3D conformal, and intensity-modulated photon (IMRT) and proton therapy for paranasal sinuscarcinoma. *Int J Radiat Oncol Biol Phys*, *58*(1), 147–154. [3D reduces dose delivered].

Mokhtari-Dizajl, M., Montazeri, M., & Saberi, H. (2006). Differentiation of mild and severe stenosis with motion estimation in ultrasound images. *Ultrasound in Medicine and Biology*, *32*(10), 1493-1498.

Moller, M., Nilsson, H., Caspersson, T., & Lomakka, G. (1970). Identification of human chromosome regions by aid of computerized pattern analysis. *Exp. Cell. Res.*, *70*, 475–478.

Montgomery, D. W. G. *et al.* (2007). Fully automated segmentation of oncological PET volumes using a combined multiscale and statistical model. *Medical Physics*, *34*(2), 722-736.

Monti, S. (1999). *Learning hybrid Bayesian networks from data.* (Ph.D. Dissertation, University of Pittsburgh, 1999).

Monti, S., & Carenini, G. (2000). Dealing with the expert inconsistency in probability elicitation. *IEEE Transactions on Knowledge and Data Engineering*, *12*(4), 499-508.

Moosmann, M., Eichele, T., Nordby, H., Hugdahl, K., & Calhoun, V. D. (2008). Joint independent component analysis for simultaneous EEG-fMRI: Principle and simulation. *International Journal of Psychophysiology*, *67*(3), 212-221.

Moradi, M., Setarehdan, S., & Ghaffari, S. (2003). Automatic Locating the Centromere on Human Chromosome Pictures. *16th IEEE Symposium on Computer-Based Medical Systems (CBMS'03)*, (pp. 56-61).

Moran, G., Stokes, C., Thewes, S., Hube, B., Coleman, D. C., & Sullivan, D. (2004). Comparative genomics using Candida albicans DNA microarrays reveals absence and divergence of virulence-associated genes in Candida dubliniensis. *Microbiology*, *150*, 3363-3382.

Mori, S., & van Zijil, P. C. M. (2002). Fiber tracking: principles and strategies – a technical review. *NMR in Biomedicine*, *15*, 468-480.

Mori, S., Crain, B. J., & van Zijl, P. C. (1998). 3D brain fiber reconstruction from diffusion MRI. *Proceedings of International Conference on Functional Mapping of the Human Brain*, Montreal.

Mori, S., Fredericksen, K., van Zijil, P. C. M., Stieltjes, B., Kraut, A. K., Solaiyappan, M., & Pomper, M. D. (2002). Brain white matter anatomy of tumor patients using diffusion tensor imaging. *Annals of Neurology*, *51*, 377-380.

Mori, S., Grain, B. J., Chacki, V. P., & van Zijl, P. C. (1999). Three-dimensional tracking of axonal projections in the brain by magnetic resonance imaging. *Annals of Neurology*, *45*, 26-269.

Mori, S., Kaufmann, W. E., Davatzikos, C., Stieltjes, B., Amodei, L., Fredericksen, K., Pearlson, G. D., Malhem, E. R., Solaiyappan, M., Raymond, G. V., Moser, H. W., & van Zijil, P. C. M. (2002). Imaging cortical association tracts in human brain. *Magnetic Resonance Imaging*, *47*, 215-223.

Moseley, M. E., Cohen, Y., & Kucharcyzk, J. (1990). Diffusion-weighted MR imaging of anisotropic water diffusion in cat central nervous system. *Radiology*, *176*, 439-445.

Moseley, M. E., Cohen, Y., & Mintorovitch, J. (1990). Early detection of regional cerebral ischemic injury in cats: evaluation of diffusion and T2-weighted MRI and spectroscopy *Magnetic Resonance in Medicine*, *14*, 330-346.

Mougiakakou, S. G., Valavanis I. K., Nikita A., & Nikita K. (2007). Differential diagnosis of CT focal liver lesions using texture features, feature selection and ensemble driven classifiers. *Artificial Intelligence in Medicine*, *41*(1), 25-37.

Mougiakakou, S. G., Valavanis, I. K., Mouravliansky, N. A., Nikita, A., & Nikita K. S. (in press). DIAGNOSIS: A telematics enabled system for medical image archiving, management and diagnosis assistance. *IEEE Transactions on Instrumentation and Measurements*.

Müller, A., Neitmann, A., Merkle, N., Wohrle, J., Hombach, V., & Kestler, H. A. (2005). Contour detection of short axis slice MR images for contraction irregularity assessment. *Computers in Cardiology, 32*, 21-24.

Müller, H. *et al.* (2005). Benefits of Content-based Visual Data Access in Radiology. *RadioGraphics, 25*, 849-858.

Murphy, J. R. (2004) Statistical errors in immunologic research. *Journal of Allergy and Clinical Immunology, 114*(6), 1259-1263.

Murphy, K. P. (2002). *Dynamic Bayesian Networks: Representation, Inference and Learning.* (Ph.D. Dissertation, University of California, Berkeley, 2002).

Muthupillai, R., Lomas, D. J., Rossman, P. J., Greenleaf, J. F., Manduca, A., & Ehman, R. L. (1995). Magnetic resonance elastography by direct visualization of propagating acoustic strain waves. *Science, 269*, 1854-57.

Nadkarni, P. M., Marenco, L., Chen, R., Skoufos, E., Shepherd, G., & Miller, P. (1999). Organization of heterogeneous scientific data using the EAV/CR representation. *J Am Med Inform Assoc, 6*(6), 478-493.

Naegele-Jackson, S., Holleczek, P., Rabenstein, T., Maiss, J., & Sackmann, M. (2002). Influence of compression and network impairments on the picture quality of video transmissions in tele-medicine. *In Proceedings of the 35th Annual Hawaii International Conference on System Sciences,* (pp. 2060–2068).

Nagarajan, R. (2003). Intensity-Based Segmentation of Microarray Images. *IEEE Trans. On Medical Imaging, 22*(7), 882–889.

Nair, A., Kuban, B. D., Obuchowski, N., Vince, D. G. (2001). Assessing spectral algorithms to predict atherosclerotic plaque composition with normalized and raw intravascular ultrasound data. *Ultrasound Med Biol, 27*(10), 1319-31.

Nanayakkara, N. D., Samarabandu, J., & Fenster, A. (2006). Prostate segmentation by feature enhancement using domain knowledge and adaptive region based operations", *Physics in Medicine and Biology, 51*, 1831–1848

Napoli, J., Stutsman, S., Chu, J. C. H., Gong, X., Rivard, M. J., Cardarelli, G., Ryan, T. P., & Favalora, G. E. (2008). Radiation therapy planning using a volumetric 3-D display: PerspectaRAD. *Proceedings of SPIE-IS&T Electronic Imaging, SPIE, 6803.*

Nash, J. M., Carter, J. N., & Nixon, M. S. (1997). Dynamic feature extraction via the velocity Hough transform. *Pattern Recognition Letters, 18*, 1035-1047.

Nasrabadi, N. M., & King, R. A. (1998). Image coding using vector quantization: a review. *IEEE Trans.Com., 36*, 957-971.

Nealen, A., Muller, M., Keiser, R., Boxerman, E., & Carlson, M. (2005). Physically based deformable models in computer graphics. In *Eurographics 2005, State of the Art Report* 2005.

Nelder, J. A., & Mead, R. (1965). A Simplex Method for Function Minimization. *Computer Journal, 7*, 308-313.

Nelson WR, Hirayama H, and Rogers DW, "The EGS4 code system," SLAC Report No. 265 (SLAC, Stanford, CA, 1985).

Nelson, S. J., Day, M. R., Buffone, P. J., Wald, L. L., Budinger, T. F., Hawkins, R., Dillon, W. P., Huhn, S., Prados, M.D., Chang, S., & Vigneron, D. B.(1997). Alignment of volume MR images and high resolution [18F]fluorodeoxyglucose PET images for the evaluation of patients with brain tumors. *Journal of Computer Assisted Tomography, 21(2),* 183-91.

Nelson, T. R., Downey, D. B., Pretorius, D. H., & Fenster, A. (1999). *Three-dimensional Ultrasound.* Philadelphia, PA: Lippincot, Williams & Wilkins.

Neofytou, M. S., Pattichis, C. S., Pattichis, M. S., Tanos, V., Kyriacou, E. C., & Koutsouris, D. (2007). A Standardised Protocol for Texture Feature Analysis of

Endoscopic Images in Gynaecological Cancer. *BioMedical Engineering OnLine, 6*(44). http://www.biomedical-engineering-online.com/content/6/1/44.

Neofytou, M. S., Pattichis, C. S., Pattichis, M. S., Tanos, V., Kyriacou, E., & Koutsouris, D. (2005). The Effect of Color Correction of Endoscopy Images for Quantitative Analysis in Endometrium. *27th Annual International conference of the IEEE Engineering in Medicine and Biology Society*, 1-4 September, Shanghai, China, (pp. 3336- 3339).

Neofytou, M. S., Pattichis, C. S., Pattichis, M. S., Tanos, V., Kyriacou, E., & Koutsouris, D. (2004). Multiscale Texture Feature Variability Analysis in Endoscopy Imaging Under Different Viewing Positions. *CD-ROM Proceedings of the II EFOMP Mediterranean Conference on Medical Physics*, 28-30 April, Limassol, Cyprus.

Neofytou, M. S., Pattichis, C. S., Pattichis, M. S., Tanos, V., Kyriacou, E., Pavlopoulos, S., & Koutsouris, D. (2004). Texture Analysis of the Endometrium During Hysteroscopy: Preliminary Results. *26th Annual International conference of the IEEE Engineering in Medicine and Biology Society,, 2*, 1483-1486. 1-5 September, San Francisco, California, USA.

Neofytou, M. S., Pattichis, C. S., Pattichis, M. S., Tanos, V., Kyriacou, E., & Koutsouris, D. (2006). Texture-Based Classification of Hysteroscopy Images of the Endometrium. *28th Annual International conference of the IEEE Engineering in Medicine and Biology Society*, 30-3 September, New York, USA, (pp. 3005-3008).

Nevo, S. T., van Stralen, M., Vossepoel, A. M., Reiber, J. H. C., de Jong, N., van der Oteen, A. F. W., & Bosch, J. G. (2007). Automated tracking of the mitral valve annulus motion in apical echocardiographic images using multidimensional dynamic programming. *Ultrasound in Medicine and Biology, 33*(9), 1389-1399.

Newton, J. (2002). *Analysis of Microarray Gene Expression Data Using Machine Learning Techniques*. Technical Report, University of Alberta, Canada.

Ng, R., & Han, J. (1994). Efficient and effective clustering method for spatial data mining. *In Proc. of the 20th VLDB Conference*, (pp.144–155), Santiago, Chile.

Nguyen, D. V., Wang, N., & Carrol, R. J. (2004). Evaluation of Missing Value Estimation for Microarray Data. *Journal of Data Science, 2*, 347-370.

Nguyen, T. D., Kim, S. H., & Kim, N. C. (2005). An Automatic Body ROI Determination for 3D Visualization of a Fetal Ultrasound Volume. R. Khosla et al. (Eds.): *KES 2005, LNAI 3682,* (pp. 145–153).

Nicolaides, A., Sabetai, M., Kakkos, S.M., Dhanjil, S., Tegos, T., Stevens, J. M., Thomas, D. J., Francis, S., Griffin, M., Geroulakos, G., Ioannidou, E., & Kyriacou, E. (2003). The Asymptomatic, Carotid, Stenosis and Risk of Stroke (ACSRS) study. *International Angiology, 22(3),* 263-272.

Nightingale, K., McAleavey, S., & Trahey, G. (2003). Shear-wave generation using acoustic radiation force: In vivo and ex vivo results. *Ultrasound Med. Biol., 29,* 1715-1723.

Nightingale, K., Soo, M. S., Nightingale, R., & Trahey, G. (2002). Acoustic radiation force impulse imaging (ARFI): In vivo demonstration of clinical feasibility. *Ultrasound Med. Biol., 28*(2), 227-235.

Nikiforidis, G. C., & Sakellaropoulos, G. C. (1998). Expert system support using Bayesian belief networks in the prognosis of head-injured patients of the ICU. *Med Inform (Lond), 23*(1), 1-18.

Nissen, S. E., Di Mario, C., & Tuzcu, E. M. (1998). Intravascular Ultrasound Angioscopy, Doppler and Pressure Measurements. In E. J. Topol (Ed.), *Comprehensive Cardiovascular Medicine* (pp. 2471-2501). Lippincott-Raven Publishers, Philadelphia.

Noble, D. (2002). Modeling the Heart from Genes to Cells to the Whole Organ. Science, *295*(5560), 1678-1682.

Noble, J. A., & Boukerroui, D. (2006). Ultrasound Image Segmentation: A Survey. *IEEE Transactions on Medical Imaging, 25*, 987-1010.

Nowakowski, A. (2007). Quantitative active dynamic thermal IR-imaging and thermal topography in medical diagnostics. In J. D. Bronzino, & N. A. Diakides (Ed.), *Medical Infrared Imaging* (pp. 7.1 – 7.29).Boca Raton, FL: CRC Press.

Nowell, P., & Hungerford, D. (1960). A minute chromosome in human chronic granulocytic leukemia. *Science, 132*, 1197–1200.

Nucifora, P. G. P., Verma, R., Lee, S., & Melherm, E. R. (2007). Diffusion-Tensor MR Imaging and Tractography: Exploring Brain Microstructure and Connectivity. *Radiology, 245,* 367-384.

Nuis, A. (1997). Health protection of individuals against the dangers of ionising radiation in relation to medical exposure: Council directive 97/43 EURATOM 30-6-1997

Nyborg, W. L. (1998). Acoustic streaming. In M.F. Hamilton & D.T. Blackstock (Eds.), *Nonlinear Acoustics* (pp. 207-231). New York: Academic Press.

Nyul, L. G., & Uduppa, J. K. (1999). On standardizing the MR image intensity scale. *Magnetic Resonance in Medicine, 42,* 1072-1081.

O'Donnell, T. F. Jr., Erdoes, L., Mackey, W. C., et al. (1985). Correlation of B-mode ultrasound imaging and arteriography with pathologic findings at carotid endarterectomy. *Archives of Surgery, 120*, 443-9.

Ogunyemi, O. (2006). Methods for reasoning from geometry about anatomic structures injured by penetrating trauma. *J Biomedical Informatics, 39*(4), 389-400.

Okada, T., Miki, Y., Fushimi, Y., Hanakawa, T., Kanagaki, M., Yamamoto, A., Urayama, S., Fukyama, H., Hiraoka, M., & Togashi, K. (2006). Diffusion-Tensor Fiber Tractography: Intaindividual Comparison of 3.0-T and 1.5-T MR imaging. *Radiology, 238,* 668-678.

Olivès, J.-L. (1998). *Optimisation globale d'un système imageur à l'aide de critères de qualité visuelle.* PhD thesis de l'Ecole Nationale Supérieure de l'Aéronautique et de l'Espace ENSAE.

Olszewski, M. E., Wahle, A., Mitchell, S. C., & Sonka, M. (2004). Segmentation of intravascular ultrasound images: A machine learning approach mimicking human vision. *In International Congress Series, 1268*, 1045–1049.

Ophir, J., Alam, S. K., Garra, B., Kallel, F., Konofagou, E. E., Krouskop, T., & Varghese, T. (1999). Elastography: ultrasonic estimation and imaging of the elastic properties of tissues. *Proceedings of the Institution of Mechanical Engineers, 213*(3), 203-233.

Ophir, J., Cespedes, I., Ponnekanti, H., Yazdi, Y., & Li, X. (1991). Elastography: a quantitative method for imaging the elasticity of biological tissues. *Ultrasonic Imaging, 13*, 111-134.

Ophir, J., Kallel, F., Varghese, T., Konofagou, E., Alama, S. K., Krouskop, T., Garra, B., & Righetti, R. (2001). Imagerie acoustique et optique des milieux biologiques - Optical and acoustical imaging of biological media: Elastography. *Comptes Rendus de l Académie des Sciences – Series IV - Physics, 2*(8), 1193–1212.

Osman MM, Cohade C, Nakamoto Y, Wahl RL, Respiratory motion artifacts on PET emission images obtained using CT attenuation correction on PET-CT, Eur J Nucl Med Mol Imaging (2003) 30:603–606.

Ozarslan, E., & Mareci, T. H. (2003). Generalized diffusion tensor imaging and analytical relationships between diffusion tensor imaging and high angular resolution diffusion imaging. *Magnetic Resonance in Medicine, 50,* 955-965.

Padhani, A. R., & Husband, J.E. (2001). Dynamic contrast-enhanced MRI studies in oncology with an emphasis on quantification, validation and human studies. *Clinical Radiology, 56,* 607–620.

Pagani, E., Bammer, R., Horsfield, M. A., Rovaris, M., Gass, A., Ciccarelli, O., & Filippi, M. (2007). Diffusion MR Imaging in Multiple Sclerosis: Technical Aspects and Challenges. *American Journal of Neuroradiology, 28,* 411-420.

Pan, W. (2002). A Comparative Review of Statistical Methods for Discovering Differentially Expressed Genes in Replicated Microarray Experiments. *Bioinformatics, 18*, 546-554.

Panagiotou, S. (2006). *Classification of Plaques Using SVM Class.* MSc thesis, Univ. of Cyprus, Nicosia Cyprus.

Panagopoulos, Th., Papaodysseus, C., Exarhos, M., Triantafillou, C., Roussopoulos, G., & Roussopoulos,

P. (2004). Prehistoric Wall-Paintings Reconstruction Using Image Pattern Analysis And Curve Fitting. *IEEE Systems Man and Cybernetics, 1*, 108-113.

Pantic, M., & Rothkrantz, L. (2000). Automatic analysis of facial expressions: The state of the art. *IEEE Trans. Pattern Analysis and Machine Intelligence, 22*(12), 1424-1445.

Pantic, M., & Rothkrantz, L. (2000). Expert system for automatic analysis of facial expressions. *Image and Vision Computing, 18*(11), 881-905.

Pantic, M., Valstar, M. F., Rademaker, R., & Maat, L. (2005). Web-based database for facial expression analysis. *Proc. IEEE Int'l Conf. Multimedia and Expo,* (pp. 317-321).

Papadakis, N. G., Martin, K. M., Mustafa, M. H., Wilkinson, I. D., Griffiths, P. D., Huang, C. L. H., & Woodruff, P. W. R. (2002). Study of the effect of CSF suppression on white matter diffusion anisotropy mapping of healthy human brain. *Magnetic Resonance in Medicine, 48,* 394-398.

Papadopoulos, A., Fotiadis, D. I., & Likas, A. (2005). Characterization of clustered microcalcifications in digitized mammograms using neural networks and support vector machines. *Artificial Intelligence in Medicine, 34*(12), 141-150.

Papaodysseus, C., Exarhos, M., Panagopoulos, Th., Triantafillou, C., Roussopoulos, G., Pantazi, Af., Loumos, V., Fragoulis, D., & Doumas, C. (2005). Identification of Geometrical Shapes in Paintings and its Application to Demonstrate the Foundations of Geometry in 1650 BC. *IEEE Transactions on Image Processing, 14*(7).

Paquerault, S., Yarusso, L. M., Papaioannou, J., Jiang, Y., & Nishikawa, R. M. (2004). Radial gradient-based segmentation of mammographic microcalcifications: Observer evaluation and effect on CAD performance. *Medical Physics, 31*(9), 2648-2657.

Pardo, X. M., Radeva, P., & Cabello, D. (2003). Discriminant snakes for 3-D reconstruction of anatomical organs. *Medical Image Analysis*, 7(3), 293–310.

Park, J. M., Franken, E. A. Jr., Garg, M., Fajardo, L. L., & Niklason, L. T. (2007). Breast tomosynthesis: Present considerations and future applications. *Radiographics, 27* (Suppl 1), S231-240.

Parker, G. J. (2000). Tracing fiber tracts using fast marching. *Proceedings of International Society of Magnetic Resonance*, (pp. 85), Denver, CO.

Parker, G. J., Haroon, H. A., & Wheeler-Kingshott, C. A. (2003). A framework for a streamline-based probabilistic index of connectivity (PICo) using a structural interpretation of MRI diffusion measurements. *Journal of Magnetic Resonance Imaging, 18,* 242-254.

Parker, G. J., Stephan, K. E., & Barker, G. J. (2002). Initial demonstration of in vivo tracing of axonal projections with the human brain using diffusion tensor imaging and fast marching tractography. *NeuroImage, 15,* 797-809.

Parker, K. J., Taylor, L. S., & Gracewski, S. (2005). A unified view of imaging the elastic properties of tissue. *J. Acoust. Soc. Am., 117*, 2705-2712.

Parmigiani, G., Garett, E. S., Irizarry, R. A., & Zeger, S. L. (2003). *The Analysis of Gene Expression Data: Methods and Software*. Springer.

Patel, A. C, & Markey, M. K. (2005) Comparison of three-class classification performance metrics: A case study in breast cancer CAD. In M. P. Eckstein, Y. Jiang Y (Ed.), *SPIE Medical Imaging 2005: Image Perception, Observer Performance, and Technology Assessment. Vol.* 5749. (pp. 581-589).

Pathak, S. D., Chalana, V., Haynor, D. R., & Kim, Y. (2000). Edge-guided boundary delineation in prostate ultrasound images. *IEEE Transactions on Medical Imaging, 19*, 1211-1219.

Patlak, C., Blasberg, R., & Fenstermacher, J. (1983). Grafical evaluation of blood flow-to-brain Barrier transfer constant form multiple time uptake data. *J.Cereb. Blood Flow Metab, 3,* 1-7.

Patriarche, J., & Erickson, B. (2004). A Review of the Automated Detection of Change in Serial Imaging Studies of the Brain. *Journal of Digital Imaging, 17(3),*158-174.

Pattichis, C. S., Pattichis, M. S., & Micheli-Tzanakou, E. (2001). Medical Imaging Fusion Applications: An Overview. In *Proc. of the 35th Asilomar Conference on Signals, Systems, and Computers,* Pacific Grove, California (USA), November 2001 (pp. 1263-1267), IEEE Signal Processing Society Staf.

Pauwels S, Barone R, Walrand S, . Practical dosimetry of peptide receptor radionuclide therapy with 90Y-labeled somatostatin analogs. J Nucl Med. 2005;46(suppl 1):92S–98S.

Pavlidis, I. (2003). Continuous physiological monitoring. In: *Proceedings of the 25th Annual International Conference of the IEEE Engineering in Medicine and Biology Society, 2,* 1084–1087.

Pavlidis, I., Dowdall, J., Sun, N., Puri, C., Fei, J., & Garbey, M. (2007): Interacting with human physiology. *Computer Vision Image Understanding,* doi:10.1016/j.cviu.2006.11.018

Pavlidis, I., & Cooper, M. (2001). The face of fear. *The Lancet, 357,* 1757.

Pavlidis, I., Eberhardt, N. L., & Levine, J. A. (2002). Human behaviour: Seeing through the face of deception. *Nature, 415,* 35.

Pavlidis, I., Levine, J., & Baukol, P. (2001). Thermal image analysis for anxiety detection. In: *Proceedings of the 2001 IEEE International Conference on Image Processing, 2,* 315–318.

Pearl, J. (1988). *Probabilistic Reasoning in Intelligent Systems: Networks of Plausible Inference.* San Francisco, CA: Morgan Kaufmann.

Pelizzari, C. A. (1998). Image Processing in Stereotactic Planning: Volume Visualization and Image Registration. *Medical Dosimetry, 23*(3), 137–145.

Penedo, M., Pearlman, W. A., Tahoces, P. G., Souto, M., & Vidal, J. J. (2003). Region-based wavelet coding methods for digital mammography. *IEEE Transactions on Medical Imaging, 22,* 1288 – 1296.

Peng, H. L., & Arfanakis, K. (2007). Diffusion tensor encoding schemes optimized for white matter fibers with selected orientations. *Magnetic Resonance Imaging, 25,* 147-153.

Peng, Y. *et al.* (2006). Knowledge-discovery incorporated evolutionary search for microcalcification detection in breast cancer diagnosis. *Artificial Intelligence in Medicine, 37*(1), 43-53.

Penney, G. P., Schnabel, J. A., Rueckert, D., Viergever, M. A., & Niessen, W. J. (2004). Registration-Based Interpolation. *IEEE Transactions on Medical Imaging, 23*(7), 922-926.

Perez, A., Dennis, R. J., Gil, J. F. A., Rondon, M. A., & Lopez, A. (2002). Use of the mean, hot deck and multiple imputation techniques to predict outcome in intensive care unit patients in Colombia. *Statistics in Medicine, 21,* 3885-3896.

Perona, P., & Malik. J. (1990). Scale space and edge detection using anisotropic diffusion. *IEEE Transactions on Pattern Analysis and Machine Intelligence, 12*(7), 629-639.

Petland, A., Moghaddam, B., & Starner, T. (1994). View-based and modular eigenspaces for face recognition. *Proc IEEE Conf. Computer Vision and Pattern Recognition,* (pp. 84-91).

Petrou, M., & Sevilla, G. P. (2006). *Image Processing, Dealing with Texture.* John Wiley and Sons.

Pham, D. L., Xu, C., & Prince, J. L. (2000). Current methods in medical image segmentation. *Annual Review of Biomedical Engineering, 2*(1), 315–337.

Phillips, R., Ward, R., & Beavis, A. (2005). Immersive visualization training of radiotherapy treatment. In *Medicine Meets Virtual Reality Conference (MMVR 13)* (pp. 390–396) (Long-Beach, California), IOS Press.

Pierpaoli, C. (2002). Inferring structural and architectural features of brain tissue from DT-MRI measurements. *CNS Spectrums , 7,* 10-515.

Pierpaoli, C., Jezzard, P., Basser, P. J., Barnett, A., & Di, C. G. (1996). Diffusion tensor MR imaging of the human brain. *Radiology, 201,* 637-648.

Pipe, J. G., & Zwart, N. (2006). Turboprop: improved PROPELLER imaging. *Magnetic Resonance in Medicine, 55,* 380-385.

Pipe, J. G., Farthing, V. G., & Forbes, K. P. (2002). Multishot diffusion-weighted FSE using PROPELLER MRI. *Magnetic Resonance in Medicine, 47,* 42-52.

Piper, J., & Granum, E. (1989). On fully automatic feature measurement for banded chromosome classification. *Cytometry, 10,* 242-255.

Pisano, E. D, Gatsonis, C., Hendrick, E., Yaffe, M., Baum, J. K., Acharyya, S., Conant, E. F., Fajardo, L. L., Bassett, L., D'Orsi, C., Jong, R., & Rebner, M. (2005). Diagnostic performance of digital versus film mammography for breast-cancer screening. *The New England Journal of Medicine, 353*(17), 1773-1783.

Pitiot, A., Thompson, P. & Toga, A. (2002). Adaptive elastic segmentation of brain MRI via shape model guided evolutionary programming. *IEEE Transactions in Medical Imaging, 21,* 910–923.

Pizer, S., Fritsch, D., Yushkevich, P., Johnson, V., & Chaney, E. (1996). Segmentation, registration, and measurement of shape variation via image object shape. *IEEE Transactions in Medical Imaging, 18,* 851–865.

Plataniotis, K. N., & Venetsanopoulos, A. N. (2000). *Color Image Processing and Applications.* Springer Verlag. Berlin.

Platt, J. (1998). Sequential minimal optimization: A fast algorithm for training support vector machines. In *Advances in Kernel Methods - Support Vector Learning,* (pp. 185-208).

Platt, J. (1999). Probabilistic outputs for support vector machines and comparisons to regularized likelihood methods. In *Advances in Large Margin Classifiers,* (pp. 61-74).

Plerou, V., Gopikrishnan, P., Rosenow, B., Amaral, L. A. N., Guhr, T., & Stanley, H. E. (2002). Random matrix approach to cross correlations in financial data. *Phys. Rev. E, 65,* 066126+18 .

Plissiti, M. E., Fotiadis, D. I., Michalis, L. K., Bozios, G. E. (2004). An automated method for lumen and media-adventitia border detection in a sequence of IVUS frames. *IEEE Trans Inf Technol Biomed, 8*(2), 131-41.

Pluim, J. P. W., Maintz, J. B. A., & Viergever, M. A. (2003). Mutual-Information-Based Registration of Medical Images: A Survey. *IEEE Transactions on Medical Imaging, 22*(8), 986-1004.

Pokrajac, D. *et al.*, (2005). Applying spatial distribution analysis techniques to classification of 3D medical images. *Artificial Intelligence in Medicine, 33,* 261—28.

Pollack, J. R., Perou, C. M., Alizadeh, A. A., Eisen, M. B., Pergamenschikov, A., Williams, C. F., Jeffrey, S. S., Botstein, D., & Brown, P. O. (1999). Genome-wide analysis of DNA copy-number changes using cDNA microarrays. *Nat Genet, 23,* 41-46.

Pommert, A., & Höhne, K.H. (2002). Evaluation of Image Quality in Medical Volume Visualization: The State of Art. *Lecture Notes in Computer Science, 2489,* 598–605.

Ponnekanti, H., Ophir, J., Huang, Y., & Cespedes, I. (1995). Fundamental mechanical limitations on the visualization of elasticity contrast in elastography. *Ultrasound Med. Biol., 21,* 533-543.

Popescu, M., Gader, P., Keller, J., Klein, C., Stanley, J., & Caldwell, C. (1999). Automatic karyotyping of metaphase cells with overlapping chromosomes. *Computers in Biology and Medicine, 29,* 61-82.

Potamias, G., & Moustakis, V. (2001). Knowledge Discovery from Distributed Clinical Data Sources: The Era for Internet-Based Epidemiology. In *Procs 23rd Annual International Conference of the IEEE Engineering in Medicine and Biology Society,* Istanbul, Turkey, (pp. 25-28).

Prastawa, M. *et al.* (2004). A brain tumor segmentation framework based on outlier detection. *Medical Image Analysis, 26*(8), 275–283.

Pratikakis, I. *et al.*, (2005). Three-Dimensional Multiscale watershed segmentation of MR images, *in Medical*

Image Analysis Methods, Editor. Lena Costaridou, CRS - Taylor & Francis, 271—314.

Press, W. H., Teukolsky, S. A., Vetterling, W. T., & Flannery, B. P. (1992). *Numerical recipes in C: the art of scientific computing.*

Qi, H., Kuruganti, P. T., & Snyder, W. E. (2007). Detecting beast cancer from thermal infrared images by asymmetry analysis. In J. D.Bronzino & N. A. Diakides (Ed.), *Medical Infrared Imaging* (pp. 11.1 – 11.14).Boca Raton, FL: CRC Press.

Quackenbush, J. (2002). Microarray Data Normalization and Transformation. *Nat. Genetics, 32,* 496-501.

Radeva, P., Suri, J. S., & Laxminarayan, S. (2003). *Angiography and plaque imaging: Advanced segmentation techniques.* Boca Raton, FL: CRC Press.

Radke, R. J. *et al.* (2005). Image Change Detection Algorithms: A Systematic Survey. *IEEE Transactions on Image Processing, 14*(3), 294-307.

Raguin, L. G., Hernando, D., Karampinos, D. C., Ciobanu, L., Sutton, B. P., Liang, Z.-P., et al. (2006). *Quantitative analysis of q-space MRI data: theoretical and experimental validation.* Paper presented at the International Society of Magnetic Resonance in Medicine (ISMRM), 14th Scientific Meeting, Seattle, WA, USA.

Rahnenführer, J., & Bozinov, V. (2004). Hybrid clustering for microarray image analysis combining intensity and shape features. *BMC Bioinformatics, 5,* 47.

Rajpoot, K., & Rajpoot, N. (2004). Wavelets and support vector machines for texture classification. *Multitopic Conference, 2004. Proceedings of INMIC 2004. 8th International,* 328-333.

Rajpoot, N. (2003). Local Discriminant Wavelet Packet Basis for Texture Classification. *Proceedings of the International Society for Optical Engineering SPIE Wavelets: Applications in Signal and Image Processing X,* 774-783.

Ramakrishnan, N., Antoniotti, M., & Mishra, B. (2005). Reconstructing Formal Temporal Models of Cellular Events using the GO Process Ontology. *Bio-Ontologies SIG Meeting, ISMB 2005,* Detroit, U.S.A..

Rasheed, Q., Dhawale, P. J., Anderson, J., & Hodgson, J. M. (1995). Intracoronary ultrasound-defined plaque composition: computer-aided plaque characterization and correlation with histologic samples obtained during directional coronary atherectomy. *Am Heart J, 129*(4), 631-7.

Raychaudhuri, S., Stuart, J. M., & Altman, R. B. (2000). Principal Component Analysis to Summarize Microarray Experiments: *Application to Sporulation Time Series, Pac. Symp. Biocomput., 5,* 452-463.

Rayleigh, L. (1902). On the pressure of vibrations. *Phil. Mag., 3,* 338-346.

Reilly, L. M., Lusby, R. J., Hughes, L., et al. (1983). Carotid plaque histology using real-time ultrasonography. Clinical and therapeutic implications. *American Journal of Surgery, 146,* 188-93.

Reumann, K., & Witkam, A. P. M. (1974). Optimizing Curve Segmentation in Computer Graphics. *International Computing Symposium. Amsterdam, North Holland,* (pp. 467- 472).

Richard, W. D., & Keen, C. G. (1996). Automated texture-based segmentation of ultrasound images of the prostate. *Computerized Medical Imaging and Graphics, 20*(3), 131-140.

Ried, T., Liyanage, M., Manoir, S., Heselmeyer, K., Auer, G., Macville, M., & Schröck, E., (1997). Tumor cytogenetics revisited: comparative genomic hybridization and spectral karyotyping. *J. Mol. Med., 75,* 801-814.

Rieseberg, S., Merboldt, K. D., Kuntzel, M., & Frahm, J. (2005). Diffusion tensor imaging using partial Fourier STEAM MRI with projection onto convex subsets reconstruction. *Magnetic Resonance in Medicine, 54,* 486-490.

Rietzel, E., Chen, G. T., Choi, N. C., & Willet, C. G. (2005). Four-dimensional image-based treatment planning: Target volume segmentation and dose calculation in the presence of respiratory motion. *International*

Journal of Radiation Oncology Biology and Physics, 61, 1535–1550.

Rivest, J.-F., Beucher, S., & Delhomme, J. P. (1992). Marker-controlled segmentation: an application to electrical borehole imaging. *Journal of Electronic Imaging, 1*(2), 136-142.

Rizzo, G., Castiglioni, I., Arienti, R., Cattaneo, G. M., Landoni, C., Artioli, D., Gilardi, M. C., Messa, C., Reni, M., Ceresoli, G. L., & Fazio, F. (2005). Automatic registration of PET and CT studies for clinical use in thoracic and abdominal conformal radiotherapy. *Quarterly Journal of Nuclear Medicine and Molecular Imaging, 49(3)*, 267-279.

Robb, R. A. (1999). Virtual endoscopy: development and evaluation using the Visible Human Datasets, *Computerized Medical Imaging and Graphics*, (24), 133–151.

Robb, R. A., & Hanson, D. P. (2006). Biomedical Image Visualization Research Using the Visible Human Datasets. *Clinical Anatomy, 19*, 240–253.

Robb, R. A., Greenleaf, J. F., Ritman, E. L., Johnson, S. A., Sjostrand, J. D., Herman, G. T., & Wood, E. H. (1974). Three-dimensional visualization of the intact thorax and contents: a technique for cross-sectional reconstruction from multiplanar x-ray views. *Comput Biomed Res, 7*, 395–419.

Robinson, D., & Milanfar, P. (2004). Fundamental Performance Limits in Image Registration. *IEEE Transactions on Image Processing, 13*(9), 1185-1199.

Roelandt, J. R., di Mario, C., Pandian, N. G., Wenguang, L., Keane, D., Slager, C. J., et al. (1994). Three-dimensional reconstruction of intracoronary ultrasound images. Rationale, approaches, problems, and directions. *Circulation, 90*(2), 1044–55.

Roerdink, J. B. T. M., & Meijster, A. (2000). The watershed transform: definitions, algorithms and parallelization strategies. *Fundamenta Informaticae, 41*(1-2), 187-228.

Roganski, A. (2002). Infrared Detectors: an overview. *Infrared Physics and Technology, 43*(5), 187- 210.

Rohde, G. K., Barnet, A. S., Basser, P. J., Marenco, S., & Pierpaoli, C. (2004). Comprehensive approach for correction of motion and distortion in diffusion-weighted MRI. *Magnetic Resonance in Medicine, 51*, 103-114.

Rohde, G. K., Barnett, A. S., Basser, P. J., & Pierpaoli, C. (2005). Estimating intensity variance due to noise in registered images: applications to diffusion tensor MRI. *NeuroImage, 26*, 673-684.

Rohlfing, T., & Maurer, C. R. Jr (2003). Volume–Preserving Nonrigid Registration of MR Breast Images Using Free-Form Deformation With an Incompressibility Constraint. *IEEE Transactions on Medical Imaging, 22(6)*, 730 – 741.

Román-Roldán R., Gómez-Lopera J. F., Atae-Allah C., Martínez-Aroza J., & & Luque-Escamilla, P. L. (2001). A measure of quality for evaluating methods of segmentation and edge detection. *Pattern Recognition, 34*, 969-980.

Rosenblatt, F. (1958). The Perceptron: A Probabilistic Model for Information Storage and Organization in the Brain. *Psychological Review, 65*(6), 386-408.

Rosenfield, K., Losordo, D. W., Ramaswamy, K., Pastore, J. O., Langevin, R. E., Razvi, S., et al. (1991). Three dimensional reconstruction of human coronary and peripheral arteries from images recorded during two-dimensional intravascular ultrasound examination. *Circulation, 84*(5), 1938-56.

Roses, A. D. (2000). Pharmacogenomics and the practice of medicine. *Nature*; *405*, 857-65.

Rousseeuw, P. J. *et al.* (2006). Robustness and Outlier Detection in Chemometrics. *Critical Reviews in Analytical Chemistry, 36*, 221–242.

Rowley, H., Baluja, S., & Kanade, T. (1998). Neural network-based face detection. *IEEE Trans. Pattern Analysis and Machine Intelligence, 20*(1), 23-38.

Rubin, D. L., Shah, N. H., & Noy, N. F. (2008). Biomedical ontologies: a functional perspective. *Brief Bioinform, 9*(1), 75-90.

Rueckert D., Sonoda, L. I., Hayes, C., Hill, D. L. G., Leach, M. O., & Hawkes, D. J. (1999). Nonrigid registration using free-form deformation: application to breast MR images. *IEEE Transactions on Medical Imaging, 18(8),* 712-721

Rueckert D., Sonoda, L. I., Hayes, C., Hill, D. L. G., Leach, M. O., & Hawkes, D. J. (1999). Nonrigid registration using free-form deformation: application to breast MR images. *IEEE Transactions on Medical Imaging, 18(8),* 712-721

Russ, J. C. (1992). *The image processing handbook*. FL. Boca Raton CRC.

Russo, V., Setola, R., Del Vescovo, R., Grasso, R. F., & Zobel, B. B. (2007). DyCoH: an innovative tool to Dynamic Contrast Enhancement analysis. *29th Annual International Conference of the IEEE Engineering in Medicine and Biology Society.*

Ruta D., & Gabrys B. (2000). An overview of classifier fusion methods. *Computing and Information Systems*, 7, 1-10.

Sabetai, M. M., Tegos, T. J., Nicolaides, A. N. et. al. (2000). Reproducibility of computer-quantified carotid plaque echogenicity. Can we overcome the subjectivity?. *Stroke*, *39(9),* 2189-2196.

Sahgal, A., Larson, D. A., & Chang, E. L. (2008). Stereotactic body radiosurgery for spinal metastases: a critical review. *International Journal of Radiation Oncology, Biology, Physics., 71*(3), 652-65.

Sahiner, B., Chan, H. P., Roubidoux, M. A., Helvie, M. A., Hadjiiski, L. M., Ramachandran, A., Paramagul, C., LeCarpentier, G. L., Nees, A., & Blane, C. (2004). Computerized characterization of breast masses on threedimensional ultrasound volumes. *Medical Physics, 31*(4), 744–754.

Sahiner, B., Chan, H-P, Roubidoux, M. A., Hadjiiski, L. M., Helvie, M. A., Paramagul, C., Bailey, J., Nees, A. V., & Blane, C. (2007). Malignant and benign breast masses on 3D US volumetric images: Effect of computer-aided diagnosis on radiologist accuracy. *Radiology, 242*(3), 716-724.

Said, A., & Pearlman, W. A. (1996). A new, fast and efficient image codec based on set partitioning in hierarchical trees. *IEEE Trans. Circuits Syst. Video Technol., 6*, 243–250.

Saito, N. (1997). Classification of Geophysical Acoustic Waveforms and Extraction of Geological Information Using Time-Frequency Atoms. *1996 Proceedings of the Computing Section of the American Statistical Association*, 322-327.

Saito, N., & Coifman, R. R. (1995). Local Discriminant Bases and their Applications. *J. Mathematical Imaging and Vision*, *5*(4), 337-358.

Salonen, R. M., Nyyssonen, K., Kaikkonen, J., et al. (2003). Six-year effect of combined vitamin C and E supplementation on atherosclerotic progression: the Antioxidant Supplementation in Atherosclerosis Prevention (ASAP) Study. *Circulation, 107*, 947-53.

Samant, S. S., Xia, J., Muyan-Özçelik, P., & Owens, J. D. (2008). High performance computing for deformable image registration: Towards a new paradigm in adaptive radiotherapy. *Medical. Physics., 35*(8), 3546-3553.

Sampat, M., Bovik, A., Aggarwal, J., & Castleman, K. (2002). Pixel-by-Pixel classification of MFISH images. In *Proc. of the 24th IEEE EMBS Ann. Intern. Conf.*, (pp. 999-1000).

Sampat, M., Bovik, A., Aggarwal, J., & Castleman, K. (2005). Supervised parametric and non-parametric classification of chromosome images. *Pattern Recognit., 38*, 1209-1223.

Sampat, P. M., Markey, M. K., & Bovik, A. C. (2005). Computer-aided detection and diagnosis in mammography. In: A. C. Bovik (Ed.), *Handbook of Image and Video Processing 2nd ed.* (pp. 1195-1217). San Diego, Elsevier Academic Press.

Sandrin, L., Cassereau, D., & Fink, M. (2004). The role of the coupling term in transient elastography. *J. Acoust. Soc. Am., 115*, 73-83.

Sandrin, L., Catheline, S., Hennequin, X., & Fink, M. (1999). Time-resolved 2-D pulsed elastography. *Ultrasonic Imaging, 21*, 259-272.

Sanz-Requena, R., Moratal, D., García-Sánchez, D. R., Bodí, V., Rieta, J. J., Sanchis, J. M. (2007). Automatic segmentation and 3D reconstruction of intravascular ultrasound images for a fast preliminar evaluation of vessel pathologies. *Comput Med Imaging Graph, 31*(2), 71-80.

Saracoglu, K., Brown, J., Kearney, L., Uhrig, S., Azofeifa, J., Fauth, C., Speicher, M., & Eils, R. (2001). New concepts to improve resolution and sensitivity of molecular cytogenetic diagnostics by multicolor fluorescence in situ hybridization. *Cytometry, 44*, 7-15.

Sariyanni, C. P. A., Asvestas P., Matsopoulos, G. K., Nikita, K. S., Nikita, A.S., & Kelekis, D. (2001). A Fractal Analysis of CT Liver Images for the Discrimination of Hepatic Lesions: A Comparative Study. In *23rd Annual EMBS International Conference. Vol. 2.* pp.1557-1560.

Sarvazyan, A. P., Rudenko, O. V., Scott, D., Swanson, J., Fowlkes, B., & Emelianov, S. Y. (1998). Shear wave elasticity imaging: a new ultrasonic technology of medical diagnostics. *Ultrasound Med. Biol., 24*(9), 1419-1435.

Scarcanski, J., Gavião, W., Cunha, S., & João, F. (2005). Diagnostic Hysteroscopy Video Summarization and Browsing. *27th Annual International conference of the IEEE engineering in Medicine and Biology Society*, Shanghai, China, (pp. 5680-5683).

Scharpf, R. B., Iacobuzio-Donahue, C. A., Sneddon, J. B., & Parmigiani, G. (2007). When should one subtract background fluorescence in 2-color microarrays? *Biostatistics, 8*(4), 695-707.

Schelkens, P., Munteanu, A., Barbarien, J., Galca, M., Giro-Nieto, X., & Cornelis J., (2003). Wavelet Coding of Volumetric Medical Datasets, *IEEE Transactions On Medical Imaging, 22*(3), 441-458.

Schena, M. (2003). *Microarray analysis.* New Jersey: John Wiley & Sons.

Schena, M., Shalon, D., Davis, R. W., & Brown, P. O. (1995). Quantitative motoring of gene expression patterns with a complementary DNA Microarray. *Science, 270*, 467-470.

Schiemann, T., Tiede, U., & Höhne, K. H. (1997). Segmentation of the visible human for high-quality volume-based visualization. *Medical Image Analysis, 1*(4), 263-70.

Schmidt, C., Fagerberg, B., Wikstrand, J., et al. (2003). On behalf of the RIS study group. Multiple risk factor intervention reduces cardiovascular risk in hypertensive patients with echolucent plaques in the carotid artery. *Journal of Internal Medicine, 253*, 430-8.

Schmitt, M., Teodorescu, H. N., Jain, A., Jain, S., & Jain, L. (2002). *Computational intelligence processing in medical diagnosis.* NY. Physica-Verlag.

Schnabel, J. A., Rueckert, D., Quist, M., Blackall, J. M., Castellano Smith, A. D., Hartkens, T., Penney, G. P., Hall, W. A., Liu, H., Truwit, C. L., Gerritsen, F. A., Hill, D. L. G., & Hawkes, D. J. (2001). A Generic Framework for Non-Rigid Registration Based on Non-Uniform Multi-Level Free-Form Deformations. In *Proceedings of Medical Image Computing and Computer-Assisted Intervention (MICCAI)*, Utrecht, The Netherlands, 14-17 October 2001 (pp. 573-581).

Schnall, M. D., & Ikeda, D. (1999). Lesion diagnosis working group report. *Journal of Magnetic Resonance Imaging, 10*(6), 982–990.

Schnall, M. D., Rosten, S., Englander, S., Orel, S. G., & Nunes, L. W. (2001). A combined architectural and kinetic interpretation model for breast MR images. *Academic Radiology, 8*(7), 591-597.

Schneiderman, H., & Kanade, T. (2000). A statistical model for 3d object detection applied to faces and cars. *Proc. IEEE Int'l Conf. Computer Vision and Pattern Recognition*, (pp. 746-751).

Schroeder, W., Martin, K., & Lorensen, W. (1998). *The Visualization Toolkit: An Object-Oriented Approach to 3D Graphics.* Prentice Hall.

Schuurbiers, J. C., Von Birgelen, C., Wentzel, J. J., Bom, N., Serruys, P. W., De Feyter, P. J., et al (2000). On the IVUS plaque volume error in coronary arteries when neglecting curvature. *Ultrasound Me Biol, 26*(9), 1403-11.

Schwartzkopf, W., Bovik, A., & Evans, B. (2005). Maximum-likelihood techniques for joint segmentation-classification of multispectral chromosome images. *IEEE Trans. Med. Imag., 24*, 1593-1610.

Schwarz, G. (1978). Estimating the dimension of a model. *Annals of Statistics, 6*(2), 461-464.

Šeba, P. (2003). Random matrix analysis of human EEG data. *Phys. Rev. Lett., 91*(19), 198104+4.

Sebastiani, P., Ramoni, M. F., Nolan, V., Baldwin, C. T., & Steinberg, M. H. (2005). Genetic dissection and prognostic modeling of overt stroke in sickle cell anemia. *Nature Genetics, 37*, 435-440.

Seemann, G., Hoeper, Ch., Doessel, O., Holden, A. V., & Zhang, H. (2006). Heterogeneous three-dimensional anatomical and electrophysiological model of human atria. *Phil. Trans. R. Soc., A 364*, 1465–1481.

Ségonne, F. (2005). *Segmentation of Medical Images under Topological Constraints*. PhD Thesis. Department of Electrical Engineering and Computer Science. Massachusetts Institute of Technology.

Sellberg, M. S., & Vanderploeg, M. J. (1994). Virtual human: A computer graphics model for biomechanical simulations and computer-aided instruction. *Proceedings of the 16th Annual International Conference of the IEEE Engineering in Medicine and Biology Society, Engineering Advances: New Opportunities for Biomedical Engineers, IEEE*, New York, NY, (pp. 329–330).

Seltzer, S. E., Getty, D. J., Pickett, R. M., Swets, J. A., Sica, G., Brown, J., Saini, S., Mattrey, R.F., Harmon, B., Francis, I. R., Chezmar, J., Schnall, M. O., Siegelman, E. S., Ballerini, R., & Bhat, S. (2002). Multimodality diagnosis of liver tumors: Feature analysis with CT, Liver-specific and Contrast-enhanced MR, and a computer model. *Academic Radiology, 9*(3), 256-259.

Selvi, S. T. *et al.* (2005). *Breast Cancer Detection Using MMRF*. Proceedings of the International Conference on Information and Automation, December 15-18, Colombo, Sri Lanka, 127-132.

Serocka, P., (2007). Visualization of High-Dimensional Biomedical Image Data In: *Advances in Multimedia Information Processing*. Springer.

Serra, J. (1982). *Image Analysis and Mathematical Morphology*. London, England: Academic Press.

Serra, J. (1988). *Image Analysis and Mathematical Morphology: Theoretical Advances*. London: Academic Press.

Sgouros G, Barest G, Thekkumthala J. Treatment planning for internal radionuclide therapy: three-dimensional dosimetry for nonuniformly distributed radionuclides. *J Nucl Med.* 1990; 31:1884 –1891.

Sgouros G, Chiu S, Pentlow KS. Three-dimensional dosimetry for radioimmunotherapy treatment planning. *J Nucl Med.* 1993;34:1595–1601.

Sgouros G, Kolbert KS, Sheikh A. (2004). Patient-specific dosimetry for 131I thyroid cancer therapy using 124I PET and 3-dimensional-internal dosimetry (3D-ID) software. *J Nucl Med.* 45:1366 –1372.

Sgouros G, Squeri S, Ballangrud AM. (2003) Patient-specific, 3-dimensional dosimetry in non-Hodgkin's lymphoma patients treated with 131I-anti-B1 antibody: assessment of tumor dose-response. *J Nucl Med.* 44:260 –268.

Sgouros G. (2005). Dosimetry of internal emitters. *J Nucl Med.* Jan;46 Suppl 1:18S-27S.

Shapiro, J. M. (1999). Embedded image coding using zerotrees of wavelet coefficients. *IEEE Trans. Signal Processing, 31*(12), 3445-3462.

Shapiro, S. S., & Wilk, M. B. (1965). An Analysis of Variance Test for Normality (complete samples). *Biometrika, 52, 3, & 4*, 591-611.

Shastri, D., Merla, A., Tsiamyrtzis, P., & Pavlidis, I. (2007). Imaging facial signs of neuro-physiological responses. In *Proceedings of the 10th International Conference on Medical Image Computing and Computer-Assisted Intervention-MICCAI*, Brisbane, Australia, October 29 – November 2.

Shekhar, R., Cothren, R. M., Vince, D. G., Chandra, S., Thomas, J. D., & Cornhill, J. F. (1999). Three-dimensional segmentation of luminal and adventitial borders in serial intravascular ultrasound images. *Computerized Medical Imaging and Graphics, 23*, 299–309.

Shen, D., Zhan, Y., & Davatzikos, C. (2003). Segmentation of Prostate Boundaries From Ultrasound Images Using Statistical Shape Model. *IEEE Transactions on Medical Imaging, 22*(4), 539-551.

Shen, D., Herskovits, E. H., & Davatzikos, C. (2001). An adaptive-focus statistical shape model for segmentation and shape modeling of 3D brain structures. *IEEE Transactions on Medical Imaging, 20*, 257-270.

Shen, L., & Bai, L. (2006). A review on Gabor wavelets for face recognition. *Pattern Analsysis and Applications, 9*, 273-292.

Sheraizin, S., & Sheraizin, V. (2005). Endoscopy Imaging Intelligent Contrast Improvement. *27th Annual International conference of the IEEE engineering in Medicine and Biology Society*, 1-4 September, Shanghai, China, (pp. 6551-6554).

Shi, et al. (2006). CT Colonography: Influence of 3D Viewing & polyp Candidate Features on Interpretation with Computer-Aided Detection. Radiology, 239,768-776.

Shim, V. B., Pitto, R. P., Streicher, R. M., Hunter, P. J., & Anderson, I. A. (2007). The use of sparse CT datasets for auto-generating accurate FE models of the femur and pelvis. *Journal of Biomechanics, 40*, 26–35.

Shimizu, A., Kawamura, T., & Kobatake, H. (2005). Proposal of computer-aided detection system for three dimensional CT images of liver cancer. *International Congress Series, 1281*, 1157-1162.

Shinkareva, S. V. *et al.* (2006). Classification of functional brain images with a spatio-temporal dissimilarity map. *NeuroImage, 33*, 63–71.

Shwe, M. A., Middleton, B., Heckerman, D. E., Henrion, M., Horvitz, E. J., Lehmann, H. P., et al. (1991). Probabilistic diagnosis using a reformulation of the INTERNIST-1/QMR knowledge base. I. The probabilistic model and inference algorithms. *Methods Inf Med, 30*(4), 241-255.

Shyu, C. R., Brodley, C. E., Kak, A. C., Kosaka, A., Aisen, A. M., & Broderick, L. S. (1999). ASSERT: A physician-in-the-loop content-based retrieval system for HRCT image databases. *Computer Vision and Image Understanding, 75*(1), 111-132.

Siddiqui, K. I., Hero, A., & Siddiqui, M. (2002). Mathematical Morphology applied to Spot Segmentation and Quantification of Gene Microarray Images. *In. Asilomar Conference on Signals and Systems.*

Siegel, JA, Stabin, MG, Brill, AB. The importance of patientspecific radiation dose calculations for the administration of radionuclides in therapy. *Cell Mol Biol (Noisy-Le-Grand)* 2002; 48(5):451-9.

Siegel, J.A., Thomas, S.R., Stubbs, J.B., Stabin, M.G., Hays, M.T., Koral, K.F., Robertson, J.S., Howell, R.W., Wessels, B.W., Fisher, D.R., Weber, D.A., Brill, A.B.: MIRD pamphlet no. 16: Techniques for quantitative radiopharmaceutical biodistribution data acquisition and analysis for use in human radiation dose estimates. *J Nucl Med* 40 (1999) 37S–61S

Sierra, R., Bajka, M., & Szekely, G. (2003). Evaluation of Different Pathology Generation Strategies for Surgical Training Simulators. *Computer Assisted Radiology and Surgery: Proceedings of the 17th International Congress and Exhibition* (pp. 376-381).

Sinha, S., Sinha, U., & Edgerton, V. R. (2006). In vivo diffusion tensor imaging of the human calf muscle. *Journal of Magnetic Resonance Imaging, 24*, 182-190.

Skare, S., & Andersson, J. L. (2001). On the effects of gating in diffusion imaging of the brain using single shot EPI. *Magnetic Resonance in Medicine, 19*, 1125-1128.

Skare, S., Hedehus, M., Moseley, M. E., & Li, T. Q. (2000). Condition number as a measure of noise performance of diffusion tensor data acquisition schemes with MRI. *Journal of Magnetic Resonance, 147*, 340-352.

Sklansky, J., & Ballard, D. (1973). Tumor Detection in Radiographs. *Computers and Biomedical Research, 6*(4), 299-321.

Sklansky, J., Tao, E. Y., Bazargan, M., Ornes, Ch. J., Murchison, R. C., & Teklehaimanot, S. (2000). Computer-aided, case-based diagnosis of mammographic regions of interest containing microcalcifications. *Academic Radiology, 7*(6), 395-405.

Skorpil, M., Engstroem, M., & Nordell, A. (2007). Diffusion-direction-dependent imaging: a novel MRI approach for peripheral nerve imaging. *Magnetic Resonance Imaging, 25*, 406-411.

Skorpil, M., Karlsson, M., & Nordell, A. (2004). Peripheral nerve diffusion tensor imaging. *Magnetic Resonance Imaging, 22*, 743-745.

Slager, C. J., Wentzel, J. J., Schuurbiers, J. C. H., Oomen, J. A. F., Kloet, J., Krams, R., et al. (2000). True 3-Dimensional reconstruction of coronary arteries in patients by fusion of angiography and IVUS (ANGUS) and its quantitative validation. *Circulation, 102*, 511-16.

Sluimer, I. et al. (2006). Computer Analysis of Computed Tomography Scans of the Lung: A Survey. *IEEE Trans. on Medical Imaging, 25*(4), 385-405.

Snyder WS, Fisher HL, Ford MR, Warner GG. Estimates of absorbed fractions for monoenergetic photon sources uniformly distributed in various organs of a heterogeneous phantom. *J Nucl Med.* 1969;10(suppl):7S–52S.

Snyder WS, Ford MR, Warner GG. *Estimates of Specific Absorbed Fractions for Photon Sources Uniformly Distributed in Various Organs of a Heterogeneous Phantom.* MIRD Pamplet No. 5, rev. New York, NY: Society of Nuclear Medicine; 1978.

Soille, P. (1999). *Morphological image analysis: principles and applications.* Berlin, Heidelberg: Springer Verlag.

Soille, P. (2004). *Morphological Image Analysis: Principles and Applications*, Springer-Verlag, Berlin and New York, corrected 2nd printing of the 2nd edition.

Soltanian-Zadeh, H., Rafiee-Rad, F., & Pourabdollah-Nejad, S. D. (2004). Comparison of multiwavelet, wavelet, Haralick, and shape features for microcalcification classification in mammograms. *Pattern Recognition, 37*(10), 1973-1986.

Sonka, M., Zhang, X. M., Siebes, M., Bissing, M. S., DeJong, S. C., Collins, S. M., & McKay C. R. (1995). Segmentation of intravascular ultrasound images: A knowledge-based approach. *IEEE Transaction on Medical Imaging, 14*(4), 719–732.

Sorensen, A. G., Wu, O., Copen, W. A., Davis, T. L., Gonzalez, R. G., & Koroshetz, W. J. (1999). Human acute cerebral ischemia: Detection of changes in water diffusion anisotropy by using MR imaging. *Radiology, 212,* 785-792.

Sotiriou, C., & Piccart, M. J. (2007). Taking gene-expression profiling to the clinic: when will molecular signatures become relevant to patient care. *Nature Reviews*; *7*, 545-53.

Specht, D. F. (1990). Probabilistic Neural Networks. *INNS Neural Networks 3*(1), 109-118.

Speed, T. (2003). *Statistical Analysis of Gene Expression Microarray Data.* Chapman & Hall/CRC.

Speicher, M., Ballard, S., & Ward, D. (1996). Karyotyping human chromosomes by combinatorial Multi-Fluor FISH. *Nat. Gen., 12*, 341-344.

Spinosa, E. J., & de Carvalho, A. (2005). Support vector machines for novel class detection in Bioinformatics. *Genet. Mol. Res., 4*(3), 608-615.

Spirka, T. A., & Damaser, M. S. (2007). Modeling physiology of the urinary tract. *Journal of Endourology, 21*(3), 294-299.

Spitzer, V. M., & Whitlock, D. G. (1998). The visible human data set: the anatomical platform for human simulation. *Anat. Rec. (New Anat.,) 253*, 49–57.

Spitzer, V., Spitzer, G., Lee, C., Reinig, K., Granas, L., Graus, K., & Smyth, P. (2004). VH Dissector: A platform for curriculum development and presentation for the anatomical arts and sciences. In *Medicine Meets Vitual*

Reality 12 (Newport Beach, California), IOS Press, (pp. 127–129).

Srikanchana, R., Thomasson, D., Choyke, P., & Dwyer, A. (2004). A Comparison of Pharmacokinetic Models of Dynamic Contrast Enhanced MRI. *17th IEEE Symposium on Computer-Based Medical System.*

Stabin M 1996 MIRDOSE—the personal computer software for use in internal dose assessment in nuclear medicine *J. Nucl. Med.* 37 538–46

Stabin M G 1994 A model of the prostate gland for use in internal dosimetry *J. Nucl. Med.* 35 516–20

Stabin M G, Konijnenberg M, Knapp F F Jr and Spencer R H 2000 Monte Carlo modeling of radiation dose distributions in intravascular radiation therapy *Med. Phys.* 27 1086–92

Stabin MG and Konijnenberg M 2000 Re-evaluation of absorbed fractions for photons and electrons in small spheres *J. Nucl. Med.* 41 149–60

Stabin MG, Flux GD, Internal dosimetry as a tool for radiation protection of the patient in nuclear medicine, Biomed Imaging Interv J 2007; 3(2):e28.

Stabin MG. 1996 MIRDOSE: personal computer software for internal dose assessment in nuclear medicine. *J Nucl Med.*; 37:538 –546.

Stanley, R., Keller, J., Gader, P., & Caldwell, C. (1998). Data-driven homologue matching for chromosome identification. *IEEE Trans. Med. Imag., 17,* 451–462.

Steele, A. (2002). *Medical Informatics Around the World: An International Perspective Focusing on Training Issues.*, Universal Publishers, ISBN: 1581126344.

Steens, S. C., Admiraal-Behloul, F., Schaap, J. A., Hoogenraad, F. G. C, Wheeler-Kingshott, C. A. M., le Cessie, S., Tofts, P. S., & van Buchem, M. A. (2004). Reproducibility of brain ADC histograms. *European Radiology, 14,* 425-430.

Steinwart, I. (2004). Sparseness of support vector machines-some asymptotically sharp bounds. *Proceedings of NIPS* (pp. 169-184).

Stejskal, E. O., & Tanner, T. E. (1965). Spin diffusion measurements: spin echoes in the presence of a time-dependent field gradient. *Journal of Chemical Physics, 42,* 288-292.

Sterpetti, A. V., Schultz, R. D., Feldhaus, R. J., et al. (1988). Ultrasonographic features of carotid plaque and the risk of subsequent neurologic deficits. *Surgery, 104,* 652-60.

Stieltjes, B., Kaufmann, W. E., van Zijil, P. C. M., Fredericksen, K., Pearlson, G. D., & Mori, S. (2001). Diffusion tensor imaging and axonal tracking in the human brainstem, *NeuroImage, 14,* 723-735.

Stoitsis, J., Golemati, S., & Nikita K. S. (2006). A modular software system to assist interpretation of medical images - Application to vascular ultrasound images. *IEEE Transactions on Instrumentation and Measurement, 55*(6), 1944-1952.

Stoitsis, J., Valavanis, I., Mougiakakou, S. G., Golemati, S., Nikita, A., & Nikita, K. S. (2006). Computer aided diagnosis based on medical image processing and artificial intelligence methods. *Nuclear Instruments & Methods in Physics Research A, 569*(2), 591-595.

Storey, J. D., & Tibshirani, R. (2003). Statistical significance for genomewide studies. *Proc. Nat. Acad. Sci., 100,* 9440-9445.

Stoutjesdijk, M. J., Fuetterer, J. F., Boetes C., van Dieand, L. E., Jager, G., & Barentsz, J. O. (2005). Variability in the description of morphologic and contrast enhancement characteristics of breast lesions on magnetic resonance imaging. *Investigative Radiology, 40*(6), 355–362.

Strzelecki, M. *et al.* (2006). Classification and segmentation of intracardiac masses in cardiac tumor echocardiograms. *Computerized Medical Imaging and Graphics, 30,* 95–107.

Studholme, C., Hill, D. L. G., & Hawkes, D. J. (1999). An overlap invariant entropy measure of 3-D medical image alignment. *Pattern Recognition, 32,* 71–86.

Subramanian, A., Tamayo, P., Mootha, V. K., Mukherjee, S., Ebert, B. L., Gillette, M. A., Paulovich, A., Pomeroy,

S. L., Golub, T. R., Lander, E. S., & Mesirov, J. P. (2005). Gene Set Enrichment Analysis: A Knowledge-Based Approach for Interpreting Genome-Wide Expression Profiles. *Proc. Nat. Acad. Sci. 102*, 15545-15550.

Subramanian, K. R., Brockway, J. P., & Carruthers, W. B. (2004). Interactive detection and visualization of breast lesions from dynamic contrast enhanced MRI volumes. *Computerized Medical Imaging and Graphics, 28*(8), 435-444.

Sudipto G., Rajeev, R., & Kyuseok, S. (1998). CURE: An efficient clustering algorithm for large databases. *In Proc. of 1998 ACM-SIGMOD Int. Conf. on Management of Data.*

Sugimoto, T., Ueha, S., & Itoh, K. (1990). Tissue hardness measurement using the radiation force of focused ultrasound. *Proc. IEEE Ultrason. Symp.*, (pp. 1377-1380).

Sühling, M., Jansen, C., Arigovindan, M., Buser, P., Marsch, P., Unser, M., & Hunziker, P. (2004). Multiscale motion mapping – A novel computer vision technique for quantitative, objective echocardiographic motion measurement independent of Doppler – First clinical description and validation. *Circulation, 110*(19), 3093-3099.

Sujana, H., Swarnamani, S., & Suresh, S. (1996). Application of artificial neural networks for the classification of liver lesions by image texture parameters. *Ultrasound in Medicine and Biology, 22*(9), 1177-1181.

Sujansky W. (2001). Heterogeneous database integration in biomedicine. *J Biomed Inform, 34*(4), 285–98.

Summers, P., Staempfli, P., Jaermann, T., Kwiecinski, S., & Kollias, S. (2006). A preliminary study of the effects of trigger timing on diffusion tensor imaging of the human spinal cord. *American Journal of Neuroradiology, 27*, 1952-1961.

Sumner, T., Evans, J., & Buckland, A. (1971). A new technique for distinguishing between human chromosomes. *Nature New Biol., 232*, 31-32.

Sun, N., Garbey, M., Merla, A., & Pavlidis, I. (2005). Imaging the cardiovascular pulse. In: *Proceedings of the IEEE Computer Society Conference on Computer Vision and Pattern Recognition, 1*, 416-421.

Sun, Y. N., Horng, M. H., Lin, X. Z., & Wang, J. Y. (1996). Ultrasound image analysis for liver diagnosis: A noninvasive alternative to determine liver disease. *IEEE Engineering in Medicine and Biology Magazine*, 93-101.

Sundar, H., Shen, D., Biros, G., Xu, C., & Davatzikos, C. (2007). Robust computation of mutual information using spatially adaptive meshes. In *Proceedings of Medical Image Computing and Computer-Assisted Intervention (MICCAI)*, Brisbane, Australia, October 29 - November 2, 2007 (pp. 950-958).

Sundersingh, B. J. (2000). *Qualitative Evaluation of Data Compression in Real-Time Ultrasound Imaging.* PhD Thesis University of Tennessee, Memphis.

Sung, K. K., & Pogio, T. (1998). Example-based learning for view-based human face detection. *IEEE Trans. Pattern Analysis and Machine Intelligence, 20*(1), 39-51.

Sunko, F. M., Ordaas, S., Butakoff, C., Cruz, S., & Frangi, A. F. (2007). Active shape models with invariant optima features: Application to facial analysis. *IEEE Trans. Pattern Analysis and Machine Intelligence, 29*(7), 1105-1117.

Suri, J. S., Chandrasekhar, R., Lanconelli, N., Campanini, R., Roffilli, M., Chang, R.-F., Guo, Y., Sivaramakrishna, R. et al (2006). The current status and likely future of breast imaging CAD. In: J. S. Suri, R. M. Rangayyan (Eds.). *Recent Advances in Breast Imaging, Mammography, and Computer-Aided Diagnosis of Breast Cancer* (pp. 901-961). Bellingham, Washington, USA, SPIE Press.

Sweeney, W., Musavi, M., & Guigi, J. (1994). Classification of chromosomes using a probabilistic neural network. *Cytometry, 16*, 17–24.

Taboada, A., & Sahli, H. (2008). Experimental System for Image Anomaly Detection Based on Features and Distances. *Ingeniería Electrónica, Automática y Comunicaciones, 29*(2).

Taira, R. K., Bui, A. A. T., Kangarloo, H. K. R., Taira, A., Bui, H., & Kangarloo, E. (2002). Identification of Patient Name References within Medical Documents Using Semantic Selectional Restrictions. *Proc AMIA Fall Symposium*, (pp. 757-761).

Takagi, A., Hibi, K., Zhang, X., Teo, T. J., Bonneau, H. N., Yock, P. G., & Fitzgerald P. J. (2000). Automated contour detection for highfrequency intravascular ultrasound imaging: A technique with blood noise reduction for edge enhancement. *Ultrasound in medicine & biology*, *26*, 1033–1041.

Takano, M., Inami, S., Jang, I. K., Yamamoto, M., Murakami, D., Seimiya, K., et al (2007). Evaluation by optical coherence tomography of neointimal coverage of sirolimus-eluting stent three months after implantation. *Am J Cardiol, 99*(8), 1033-8.

Taktak, A. G., Fisher, A. C., & Damato, B. (2004). Modelling survival after treatment of intraocular melanoma using artificial neural networks and Bayes theorem. *Phys. Med. Biol., 49*, 87–98.

Tarca, A. L., Romero, R., & Draghici, S. (2006). Analysis of microarray experiments of gene expression profiling. *Am J Obstet Gynecol, 195*(2), 373-388.

Tasdoken, S., & Cuhadar, A. (2003). ROI Coding with Integer Wavelet Transforms and Unbalanced Spatial Orientation Trees. *25th Annual International Conference of the IEEE-EMBS.*

Taubman, D. (2000). High performance scalable image compression with EBCOT, *IEEE Trans. Image Processing, 9*, 1158–1170.

Tay, S., Blanche, P.-A., Voorakaranam, R. A., Tunc, V., Lin, W., Rokutanda, S., Gu, T., Flores, D., Wang, P., Li, G., St Hilaire, P., Thomas, J., Norwood, R. A., Yamamoto, M., & Peyghambarian, N. (2008). An updatable holographic three-dimensional display. *Nature Letters, 451*, 694-698.

Tegos, T. J., Sametai, M. M., Nicolaides, A. N. et al. (2000). Comparability of the ultrasonic tissue characteristics of carotid plaques. *Journal of Ultrasound Medicine, 19*, 399-407.

Teschner, M., Kimmerle, S., Heidelberger, B., Zachmann, G., Raghupathi, L., Fuhrmann, A., Cani, P. M., Faure, F., Magenat-Thalmann, N., Strasser, W., & Volino, P. (2005). Collision detection for deformable objects. *Computer Graphics Forum, 24*(1), 61–81.

The ACMI Corporation [www.acmicorp.com]

The company Richard WOLF GmbH [http://www.richard-wolf.com/default.aspx]

The Edmund Optics company [www.edmundoptics.com]

The MathWorks company for software [www.mathworks.com]

The Pinnacle Systems company [www.pinnaclesys.com]

Theiler, J., Eubank, S., Longtin, A., Galdrikian, B., & Farmer, J. D. (1992). Testing for nonlinearity in time series: The method of surrogate data. *Physica D, 58*, 77-94.

Theodoropoulos, G., Loumos, V., Anagnostopoulos, C., Kayafas, E., & Martinez-Gonzales, B. (2000). A digital image analysis and neural network based system for identification of third-stage parasitic strongyle larvae from domestic animals. *Computer Methods and Programs in Biomedicine, 62*(2), 69-76.

Thiele, D. L., Kimme-Smith, C., Johnson, T. D., McCombs, M., & Bassett, L. W. (1996). Using tissue texture surrounding calcification clusters to predict benign vs malignant outcomes. *Medical Physics, 23*(4), 549-555.

Thiran, P., Hainaut, J. L., & Houben, G. J. (2005). Database Wrappers Development: Towards Automatic Generation. In: *Proc of the Ninth European Conference on Software Maintenance and Reengineering* (CSMR'05), 207-216.

Thirion, J. P. (1998). Image matching as a diffusion process: an analogy with maxwell's demons. *Med Image Analysis, 2*, 243–260.

Thirion, J. P., & Calmon, G. (1999). Deformation analysis to detect and quantify active lesions in three-dimensional medical image sequences. *IEEE Transactions on Medical Imaging, 18,* 429- 441.

Thompson, M., McInnes, R. & Willard, H. (1992). *Genetics in Medicine* 5th Edition, WB Saunders Company, Philadelphia.

Thompson, P. M., Woods, R. P., Mega, M. S., & Toga, A. W. (2000). Mathematical/computational challenges in creating deformable and probabilistic atlases of the human brain. *Human Brain Mapping, 9*, 81–92.

Tian, Y., Kanede, T., & Cohn J.F. (2001). Recognizing action units for facial expression analysis. *IEEE Trans. Pattern Analysis and Machine Intelligence, 23*(2), 97-115.

Timp, S., Varela, C., & Karssemeijer, N. (2007). Temporal change analysis for characterization of mass lesions in mammography. *IEEE Transactions on Medical Imaging, 26*(7), 945-953.

Tjoa, P. M., & Krishnan, M. S. (2003). Feature Extraction for the Analysis of Colon Status from the Endoscopic Images. *BioMedical Engineering OnLine.* [http://www.biomedical-engineering-online.com/content/2/1/9].

Tofts, P. S., & Kermode, A. G., (1991). Measurement of Blood-Brain Barrier Permeability and Leakage Space using Dynamic MR Imaging. Fundamental concepts. *Magnetic Resonance in Medicine, 17*, 357-367.

Tofts, P. S., Brix, G., Buckley, D. L., Evelhoch, J. L., Henderson, E., Knopp, M. V, Larsson, H. B. W., Lee, T-Y., Mayer, A. A., Parker, G. J. M., Port, R. E., Taylor, J., & Wiesskoff, R. M. (1999). Estimating Kinetic Parameters From Dynamic Contrast Enhanced T1-Weighted MRI of a Diffusable Tracer: Standardized Quantities and Symbols. *Journal of Magnetic Resonance Imaging, 10*, 223-232.

Toga, A. W., & Thompson, P. M. (2001). The role of image registration in brain mapping. *Image Vision Comput, 19,* 3–24.

Tomasi, C., & Manduchi, R. (1998). Bilateral filtering for gray and color images. In *6th IEEE International Conference on Computer Vision.* (pp. 839-846).

Torkkola, K., Gardner, R. M., Kaysser-Kranich, T., & Ma, C. (2001). Self-Organizing Maps in Mining Gene Expression Data. *Information Sciences, 139*, 79-96.

Torr, G. R. (1984). The acoustic radiation force. *Am. J. Phys., 52*, 402-408.

Tourassi, G. D. (2005). Current status of computerized decision support systems in mammography. *Studies in Fuzziness and Soft Computing: Intelligent Paradigms for Healthcare Enterprises 184,* (pp. 173–208). Springer-Verlag Berlin Heidelberg.

Tournier, J. D., Calamante, F., Gadian, D. G., & Connelly, A. (2004). Direct estimation of the fiber orientation density distribution function from diffusion-weighted MRI data using spherical deconvolution. *Neuroimage, 23*, 1176-1185.

Tropea, B. I., Schwarzacher, S. P., Chang, A., Asvar, C., Huie, P., Sibley, R. K., & Zarins, C. K. (2000). Reduction of aortic wall motion inhibits hypertension-mediated experimental atherosclerosis. *Arteriosclerosis Thrombosis Vascular Biology, 20*(9), 2127-2133.

Troyanskaya, O., Cantor, M., Sherlock, G., Brown, P., Hastie, T., Tibshirani, R., Botstein, D., & Altman, R. B., (2001). Missing Value Estimation Methods for DNA Microarrays. *Bioinformatics 17*, 520-525.

Tseng, G. C., Oh, M. K., Rohlin, L., Liao, J. C., & Wong, W. H. (2001). Issues in cDNA Microarray Analysis: Quality Filtering, Channel Normalization, Models of Variations and Assessment of Gene Effects. *Nucleic Acids Research, 29*, 2549-2557.

Tsougos I, Mavroidis P Rajala J, Theodorou K, Jarvenpaa R, Pitkanen MA, Holli K, Ojala AT, Lind BK, Hyodynmaa S, Kappas C. 2005 Evaluation of dose-response models and parameters predicting radiation induced pneumonitis using clinical data from breast cancer radiotherapy *Phys. Med. Biol.* 50 3535-54

Tsujii, O., Freedman, M. T., & Mun, S. K. (1999). Classification of microcalcifications in digital mammograms using trend-oriented radial basis function neural network. *Pattern Recognition, 32*(5), 891-903.

Tuch, D. S. (2004). q-ball imaging. *Magnetic Resonance in Medicine, 52*, 1358-1372.

Tuch, D. S., Reese, T. G., Wiegell, M. R., Makris, N., Belliveau, J. W., & Wedeen, V. J. (2002). High angular resolution diffusion imaging reveals intravoxel white matter fiber tractography. *Magnetic Resonance in Medicine, 48*, 577-582.

Tuch, D. S., Wiegell, M. R., Reese, T. G., Belliveau, J. W., & Wedeen, V. (2001). Measuring cortico-cortical connectivity matrices with diffusion spectrum imaging. *Proceedings of International Society of Magnetic Resonance in Medicine*, (pp. 502), Glasgow, UK.

Tung, S., Wu C-S, & Su, M. (2001). Magnifying Colonoscopy in Differentiating Neoplastic From Nonneoplastic Colorectal Lesions. *American Journal of Gastroenterology, 96*, 2628-2632.

Turaga, D. S., Chen, Y. & Caviedes, J. (2004). No reference PSNR estimation for compressed pictures. *Signal Processing Image Communication, 19*, 173-184.

Turner, R., Le Bihan, D. J., & Chesnick, A. S. (1991). Echo-planar imaging of diffusion and perfusion. *Magnetic Resonance in Medicine, 19*, 247-253.

Tusher, V. G., Tibshirani, R., & Chum, G. (2001). Significance Analysis of Microarrays Applied to the Ionizing Radiation Response. *Proc. Nat. Acad. Sci., 98*, 5116-5121.

Twellmann, T., Lichte, O., & Nattkemper, T. W. (2005). An adaptive tissue characterisation network for model-free visualisation of dynamic contrast-enhanced magnetic resonance data. *IEEE Transactions on Medical Imaging, 24*(10), 1256-1266.

Tzouio-Mazoyer, N., Landeau, B., Papathanasiou, D., Crivello, F., Etard, O., Delcroix, N., Mazoyer, B., & Joliot, M. (2002). Automated anatomical labeling of activations in SPM using a macroscopic anatomical parcellation of the MNI MRI single-subject brain. *NeuroImage, 15*, 273-289.

Tzouvelekis, A., Harokopos, V., Paparountas, T., Oikonomou, N., Chatziioannou, A., Vilaras, G., Tsiambas, E., Karameris, A., Bouros, D., & Aidinis, V. (2007). Comparative expression lprofiling in pulmonary fibrosis suggests a role of hypoxia-inducible factor-1α in disease pathogenesis. *American Journal of Respiratory and Critical Care Medicine, 176*(11), 1108-1119.

Ueno, I., & Pearlman, W. (2003). Region of Interest coding in volumetric images with shape-adaptive wavelet transform. *SPIE/IS&T Electronic Imaging 2003.*

Uenohara, M., & Kanade, T. (1995). Vision-Based Object Registration for Real-Time Image Overlay. In N. Ayache (Ed.), *Computer Vision, Virtual Reality and Robotics in Medicine: CVRMed '95* (pp. 14-22). Berlin: Springer-Verlag.

Valavanis, I. K, Mougiakakou, S. G., Nikita, A., & Nikita, K. S. (2007). Evaluation of texture features in hepatic tissue tissue discrimination. In *29th IEEE Conference in Engineering in Medicine and Biology.* (pp. 3741-3744).

van den Elsen, P. A., Maintz, J. B. A., Pol, E-J. D., & Viergever M. A. (1995). Automatic registration of CT and MR brain images using correlation of geometrical features. *IEEE Transactions on Medical Imaging, 14(2)*, 384 - 396.

van den Elsen, P. A., Pol E-J. D., Sumanaweera, T. S., Hemler, P. F., Napel S., & Adler, J. (1994). Grey value correlation techniques used for automatic matching of CT and MR brain and spine images. In R. A. Robb, (Ed.), *Proc. of SPIE, Visualization in Biomedical Computing, September 1994, 2359* (pp. 227–237)

van den Elsen, P. A., Pol E-J. D., Sumanaweera, T. S., Hemler, P. F., Napel S., & Adler, J. (1994). Grey value correlation techniques used for automatic matching of CT and MR brain and spine images. In R. A. Robb, (Ed.), *Proc. of SPIE, Visualization in Biomedical Computing, September 1994, 2359* (pp. 227–237)

Van der Geest, R. J., & Reiber, J. H. C. (1999). Quantification in cardiac MRI. *Journal of Magnetic Resonance Imaging, 10*(5), 602-608.

Van der Geest, R. J., Buller, V. G., Jansen, E., Lamb, H. J., Baur, L. H., van der Wall, E. E., de Roos, A., & Reiber, J. H. C. (1997). Comparison between manual and semiautomated analysis of left ventricular volume parameters from short-axis MR images. *Journal of Computer Assisted Tomography, 21*(5), 756-765.

Van Ginneken, B., Frangi, A. F., Staal, J. J., Ter Har Romeny, B. M., & Viergever, M. A. (2002). Active shape model segmentation with optimal features. *IEEE Trans. Medical Imaging, 21*(8), 924-933.

Van Stralen, M., Leung, K. Y. E., Voormolen, M. M., de Jong, N., van der Steen, A. F. W., Reiber, J. H. C., & Bosch, J. G. (2008). Time continuous detection of the left ventricular long axis and the mitral valve plane in 3-D echocardiography. *Ultrasound in Medicine and Biology, 34*(2), 196-207.

VanBemmel, J. H., & Musen, M. A. (Ed.) (1997). *Handbook of Medical Informatics*. Stanford University, Stanford, Springer.

Vanderheydt, L., Oosterlinck, A., Daele, J., & Berghe, H., (1980). Design of graph-representation and a fuzzy-classifier for human chromosomes. *Pattern Recognit., 12*, 201–210.

Vapnik, V.N. (1998). *Statistical Learning Theory*. Wiley.

Veldkamp, W. J. H., & Karssemeijer, N. (1998). Accurate segmentation and contrast measurement of microcalcifications in mammograms: A phantom study. *Medical Physics, 25*(7), 1102-1110.

Veldkamp, W. J. H., Karssemeijer, N., Otten, J. D. M., & Hendriks, J. H. C. L. (2000). Automated classification of clustered microcalcifications into malignant and benign types. *Medical Physics, 27*(11), 2600-2608.

Veldman, T., Vignon, C., Schröck, E., Rowley, J., & Ried, T. (1997). Hidden chromosome abnormalities in haematological malignancies detected by multicolor spectral karyotyping. *Nat. Genet., 15*, 406-410.

Vincent, L. (1993). Morphological grayscale reconstruction in image analysis: Applications and efficient algorithms. *IEEE Trans. Image Processing, 2*, 176-201.

Vincent, L., & Soille, P. (1991). Watershed in Digital Spaces: An Efficient Algorithm Based on Immersion Simulations. *IEEE Transactions on Pattern Analysis and Machine Intelligence, 13*, 583-598.

Viola, P. (1995). *Alignment by maximization of mutual information* (Tech. Rep. No. 1548). Massachusetts Institute of Technology.

Viola, P., & Jones, M. (2001). Rosubt real-time object detection. *Int'l Workshop on Statistical and Computational theories of Vision - Modeling, Learning, Computing and Sampling.*

Viola, P., & Jones, M. (2004). Robust real-time face detection. *J. Computer Vision, 57*(2), 137-154.

Vomweg, T. W., Buscema, M., Kauczor, H. U., Teifke, A., Intraligi, M., Terzi, S., Heussel, C. P., Achenbach, T., Rieker, O., Mayer, D., & Thelen, M. (2003). Improved artificial neural networks in prediction of malignancy of lesions in contrast-enhanced MR-mammography. *Medical Physics, 30*(9), 2350-2359.

Von Birgelen, C., van der Lugt, A., Nicosia, A., Mintz, G. S., Gussenhoven, E. J., de very, E., et al (1996). Computerized assessment of coronary lumen and atherosclerotic plaque dimensions in three-dimensional intravascular ultrasound correlated with histomorphometry. *Am J Cardiol, 78*(11), 1202-9.

Vossepoel, A. (1987). *Analysis of Image Segmentation for Automated Chromosome Identification,* Ph.D. dissertation, Univ. Leiden, Leiden, The Netherlands.

Voultsidou, M., Dodel, S., & Herrmann, J. M. (2005). Neural networks approach to clustering of activity in fMRI data. *IEEE Trans. Med. Imaging, 12*(8), 987-996.

Vovk, U. *et al.* (2007). A Review of Methods for Correction of Intensity Inhomogeneity in MRI. *IEEE Transactions on Medical Imaging, 26*(3), 405-421.

Wachowiak, M. P., & Peters, T. M. (2006). High-Performance Medical Image Registration Using New Optimization Techniques. *IEEE Transactions on Information Technology in Biomedicine, 10*(2), 344-353.

Wahle, A., Olszewski, M. E., & Sonka, M. (2004). Interactive virtual endoscopy in coronary arteries based on multimodality fusion. *IEEE Trans Med Imag, 23*(11), 1391-403.

Wahle, A., Prause, G. P. M., DeJong, S. C., & Sonka, M. (1999). Geometrically correct 3-D reconstruction of intravascular ultrasound images by fusion with biplane angiography – methods and validation. *IEEE Trans Med Imag, 18*(8), 686-98.

Wang, X., Ghosh, S., & Guo, S. W. (2001). Quantitative quality control in microarray image processing and data acquisition. *Nucleic Acids Research, 29*(15), e75.

Wang, X.Y., & Feng, D. D. (2005). Biomedical image registration for diagnostic decision making and treatment monitoring. In F. Dong, G. Ghinea and S. Y. Chen (Ed.), *User Centered Design for Medical Visualization* Premier Reference Source.

Wang, Y., & Castleman, K. (2005). Normalization of multicolor fluorescence in situ hybridization (M-FISH) images for improving color karyotyping. *Cytometry, 64*, 101-109.

Wang, Y., Cardinal, H. N., Downey, D. B., & Fenster, A. (2003). Semiautomatic three-dimensional segmentation of the prostate using two dimensional ultrasound images. *Medical physics, 30*(5), 887-897.

Washington, C. W., & Miga, M. I. (2004). Modality Independent Elastography (MIE): A New Approach to Elasticity Imaging. *IEEE Transactions on Medical Imaging, 23*(9), 1117-1128.

Watson CC, Casey ME, Bendriem B, Carney JP, Townsend DW, Eberl S, Meikle S, DiFilippo FP, Optimizing Injected Dose in Clinical PET by Accurately Modeling the Counting-Rate Response Functions Specific to Individual Patient Scans, J Nucl Med 2005; 46:1825–1834.

Watson E W and Stabin M G 1984 BASIC alternative software package for internal dose calculations Computer Applications in Health Physics: Proc. 17th Midyear Topical Symposium of the Health Physics Society (Pasco, WA, 5–9 February 1984) pp 7.79–7.86

Weatherburn, G. C., Ridout, D., Strickalnd, N. H., Robins, P., Glastonbury, C. M., Curati, W., Harvey, C., & Shadbolt, C. (2003). A comparison of conventional film, CR hard copy and PACS soft copy images of the chest: Analyses of ROC curves and inter-observer agreement. *European Journal of Radiology, 47*, 206-214.

Webb, A. (2003). *Introduction to Biomedical Imaging*. IEEE Press Series in Biomedical Engineering.

Wedeen, V. J., Hagmann, P., Tseng, W. I., Reese, T. G., & Weisskoff, R. M. (2005). Mapping complex tissue architecture with diffusion spectrum magnetic resonance imaging. *Magnetic Resonance in Medicine, 54*, 1194-1206.

Wedeen, V. J., Reese, T. G., Tuch, D. S., Weigel, M. R., Dou, J.-G., Weisskoff, R. M., et al. (2000). *Mapping fiber orientation spectra in cerebral white matter with Fourier-transform MRI*. Paper presented at the International Society for Magnetic Resonance in Medicine (ISMRM), Denver, CO.

Wei, L. *et al.* (2005). Relevance vector machine for automatic detection of clustered microcalcifications. *IEEE Transactions on Medical Imaging, 24*(10), 1278-1285.

Weinstein, D., Kindlmann, G., & Lundberg, E.C. (1999). Tensorline: advection diffusion based propagation through diffusion tensor fields. *Proceedings IEEE Visualization*, (pp. 249-253), San Francisco, CA.

Wenska, J. S., Dryer, C. R., & Rosenfeld, A. (1976). A Comparative Study of Texture Measures for Terrain Classification. *IEEE Trans. Syst., Man, Cyber., SMC-6*, 269-285.

Wenzl, R., Lehner, R., Vry, U., Pateisky, N., Sevelda, P., & Husslein, P. (1994). Three-Dimensional Video-endoscopy: Clinical use in Gynaecological Laparoscopy. *Lancet, 344*, 1621–1622.

Werring, D. J., Toosy, A. T., Clark, C. A., Parker, G. J., Barker, G. J., Miller, D. H., & Thompson, A. J. (2000). Diffusion tensor imaging can detect and quantify corticospinal tract degeneration after stroke. *Journal of Neurology, Neurosurgery, and Psychiatry, 69*, 269-272.

Westerbring-van der Putten, E. P., Goossens, R. H. M., Jakimowicz, J. J., & Dankelman, J. (2008). Haptics in minimally invasive surgery – a review. *Minimally Invasive Therapy, 17*(1), 3–16.

Westervelt, P. J. (1951). The theory of steady forces caused by sound waves. *J. Acoust. Soc. Am., 23*, 312-315.

Westin, C. F., Maier, S. E., Mamata, H., Nabavi, A., Jolesz, F. A., & Kikinis, R. (2002). Processing and visualization for diffusion tensor MRI. *Medical Image Analysis, 6,* 93-108.

Weszka, J. S., Dryer, C. R., & Rosenfeld A. (1976). A comparative study of texture measures for terrain classification. *IEEE Transactions on Systems, Man and Cybernetics, 6*, 269-285.

Widder, B., Paulat, K., Hachspacher, J., et al. (1990). Morphological characterization of carotid artery stenoses by ultrasound duplex scanning. *Ultrasound in Medicine and Biology, 16*, 349-54.

Wiecek, B., Strzelecki, M., Jakubowska, T., & Wysocki, M. (2007). Advanced thermal image processing. In J. D. Bronzino, & N. A. Diakides, (Ed.), *Medical Infrared Imaging* (pp. 12.1 – 12.13).Boca Raton, FL: CRC Press.

Wiener, J. I., Schilling, K. J., Adami, C., & Obuchowski, N. A. (2005). Assessment of suspected breast cancer by MRI: A prospective clinical trial using a combined kinetic and morphologic analysis. *AJR. American Journal of Roentgenology, 184*(3), 878-886.

Wigner, E. P. (1967). Random matrices in physics. *SIAM Rev., 9*, 1-23.

Wilhjelm, J. E., Gronholdt, L. M., et al. (1998). Quantitative Analysis of Ultrasound B-Mode Images of Carotid Atherosclerotic Plaque: Correlation with Visual Classification and Histological Examination. *IEEE Transactions on Medical Imaging, 17*(6), 910-922.

Williams, M. B, Yaffe, M. J, Maidment, A. D, Martin, M. C, Seibert, J. A, & Pisano, E. D. (2006). Image quality in digital mammography: Image acquisition. *Journal of the American College of Radiology, 3*(8), 589-608.

Wilson, L. S., Robinson, D. E., & Dadd, M. J. (2000). Elastography- the movement begins. *Phys. Med. Biol., 45*, 1409-1421.

Woods, B. J., Clymer, B. D., Kurc, T., Heverhagen, J. T., Stevens, R., Orsdemir, A., Bulan, O., & Knopp, M. V. (2007). Malignant-lesion segmentation using 4D co-occurrence texture analysis applied to dynamic contrast-enhanced magnetic resonance breast image data. *Journal of Magnetic Resonance Imaging, 25*(3), 495-501.

Woods, R. P., Mazziotta, J. C., & Cherry, S. R. (1993). MRI-PET registration with automated algorithm, *Journal of Computer Assisted Tomography, 17(4),* 536–546.

World Health Organization website, www.who.int/ncd/cvd.

Wu, C. M, Chen, Y. C., & Hsieh, K. S. (1992). Texture features for classification of ultrasonic liver images. *IEEE Transactions on Medical Imaging, 11*(2), 141-151.

Wu, H., & Yan, H. (2003). Microarray Image Processing Based on Clustering and Morphological Analysis. *In First Asia Pacific Bioinformatics Conference*, (pp. 111-118).

Wu, Q., & Markey, M. K (2006). Computer-aided diagnosis of breast cancer in MR imaging. In: J. S. Suri, R. M. Rangayyan (Eds.). *Recent Advances in Breast Imaging, Mammography, and Computer-Aided Diagnosis of Breast Cancer* (pp. 791-832). Bellingham, Washington, USA, SPIE Press.

Wu, Y., Ianakiev. K., & Govindaraju, V. (2002). Improved k-nearest neighbor classification, *Pattern Recognition, 35*(10), 2311-2318.

Wu, Y.-C., & Alexander, A. L. (2007). Hybrid diffusion imaging. *Neuroimage, 36*, 617-629.

Wu, Z., Irizarry, R., Gentleman, R. C., Murillo, F. M., & Spencer, F. (2004). A Model Based Background Adjustment for Oligonucleotide Expression Arrays. *Collection of Biostatistics Research Archive, 1.*

Wyatt, J. C., & Wright, P. (1998). Design should help use of patients' data. *Lancet, 352*(9137), 1375-1378.

Xiao, G. F., Brady, M., Noble, J. A., & Zhang, Y. Y. (2002). Segmentation of ultrasound B-mode images with intensity inhomogeneity correction. *IEEE Transaction on Medical Imaging, 21*(1), 48–57.

Xiaoxue, Y. *et al.* (2004). *Abnormality detection in retinal images*. Technical Report MIT-3845, MIT, Massachusetts Institute of Technology.

Xie, X. (2006). *Defect Detection in Random Colour Textures*. PhD Thesis. Faculty of Engineering. Department of Computer Science. University of Bristol.

Xing, D., Papadakis, N. G., Huang, C. L., Lee, V.M., Carpenter, T. A., & Hall, L. D. (1997). Optimised diffusion-weighting for measurement of apparent diffusion coefficient (ADC) in human brain. *Magnetic Resonance Imaging, 15,* 771-784.

Xiong, Z., Wu, X., & Yun, D. Y. (1998). Progressive coding of medical volumetric data using three-dimensional integer wavelet packet transform. *IEEE Multimedia Signal Processing*, (pp. 553-558).

Xu XG, Chao T Cand Bozkurt A 2000 VIP-man: an image-based whole-body adult male model constructed from colour photographs of the visible human project for multi-particle Monte Carlo calculations *Health Phys.* 78 476–86

Xu, R. *et al.*, (2006). Target Detection with Improved Image Texture Feature Coding Method and Support Vector Machine. *International Journal of Intelligent Technology*, *1*(1), 47-56, ISSN 1305-6417.

Xue, R., van Zijil, P. C. M., Vrain, B. J., Solaiyappan, M., & Mori, S. (1999). In vivo three-dimensional reconstruction of rat brain axonal projections by diffusion tensor imaging. *Magnetic Resonance in Medicine, 42,* 1123-1127.

Yamakoshi, Y., Sato, J., & Sato, T. (2000). Ultrasonic imaging of internal vibration of soft tissue under forced vibration. *IEEE Trans. Ultrason., Ferroelect. Freq. Contr.*, *37*, 45-53.

Yang S.-B. (2005). Smooth side-match weighted vector quantizer with variable block size for image coding. *IEEE Proceedings Vision and Image and Signal Processing, 152*, 763-770.

Yang, M. H., Kriegman, D. J., & Ahuja, N. (2002). Detecting faces in images: a survey. *IEEE Trans. on Pattern Analysis and Machine Intelligence,* 24(1), 34-58.

Yang, Y. H., Buckley, M. J., & Speed, T. P. (2001). Analysis of cDNA microarray images. *Brief Bioinform, 2*(4), 341-349.

Yang, Y. H., Dudoit, S., Luu, P., Lin, D. M., Peng, V., Ngai, J., & Speed, T. P. (2002). Normalization for cDNA Microarray Data: A Robust Composite Method Addressing Single and Multiple Slide Systematic Variation. *Nucleic Acids Research, 30*(15).

Ye, Z., Zhan, Y., & Song, S. (2004). Facial expression features extraction based on Gabor wavelet transformation. *IEEE Int'l Conf Systems, Man and Cybernetics*, (pp. 2215-2219).

Yetik, I. S., & Nehorai, A. (2006). Performance Bounds on Image Registration. *IEEE Transactions on Signal Processing, 54*(5), 1737-1749.

Yeung, K. W., & Ruzzo, W. L. (2001). Principal Component Analysis for Clustering Gene Expression Data. *Bioinformatics, 9,* 763-774.

Yin, L., Wei, X., Sun, Y., Wang, J., & Rosato, M. (2006). A 3D facial expression database for facial behavior research. *Proc. IEEE Int'l Conf. Face and Gesture Recognition*, (pp. 211-216).

Yokoi, H., & Fujino, M. A. (2006). Activities for Endoscopy Information Systems Standardization in Japan. *28th Annual International conference of the IEEE engineering in Medicine and Biology Society*, New York, USA, (pp. 5667-5670).

Yu, C. M., Sanderson, J., E., Marwick, T. H., & Oh, J. K. (2007). Tissue Doppler imaging – A new prognosticator for cardiovascular diseases. *Journal of the American College of Cardiology*, *49*(9), 1903-1914.

Yu, J., Smith, V.A., Wang, P.P., Hartemink, A.J., & Jarvis, E.D. (2004). Advances to Bayesian network inference for generating causal networks from observational biological data. *Bioinformatics, 20*(18), 3594-3603.

Yu, J.S., Kim, Y. H., & Rofsky, N. (2005). Dynamic subtraction magnetic resonance imaging of cirrhotic liver: assessment of high signal intensity lesions on nonenhanced T1-weighted images. *Journal of Computer Assisted Tomography, 29(1),* 51-58.

Zacharaki, E. I., Matsopoulos, G. K., Asvestas, P. A., Gröndahl, K., & Gröndahl, H. G. (2004). A digital subtraction radiography scheme based on automatic multiresolution registration. *Dentomaxillofacial Radiology, 33*, 1-14.

Zagrodsky, V., Walimbe, V., Castro-Pareja, C. R., Qin, J. X., Song, J. M., & Shekhar, R. (2005). Registration-assisted segmentation of real-time 3-D echocardiographic data using deformable models. *IEEE Transactions on Medical Imaging, 24*(9), 1089-1099.

Zaidi H, Labbe C and Morel C, Parallel Comput. 24 (1998) 1523–36.

Zemp, R. J., Tavakkoli, J., & Cobbold, R. S. C. (2003). Modeling of nonlinear ultrasound propagation in tissue from array transducers. *J. Acoust. Soc. Am., 113*, 139-152.

Zhan, W., & Yang, Y. (2006). How accuately can the diffusion profiles indicate multiple fiber orientations? A study on general fiber crossings in diffusion MRI. *Journal of Magnetic Resonance, 183*, 193-202.

Zhan, W., Gu, H., Silbersweig, D. A., Stern, E., & Yang, Y. (2003). Circular spectrum mapping for intravoxel fiber structures based on high angular resolution apparent diffusion coefficients. *Magnetic Resonance in Medicine, 49*, 1077-1088.

Zhan, W., Stein, E. A., & Yang, Y. (2004). Mapping the orientation of intravoxel crossing fibers based on the phase information of diffusion circular spectrum. *Neuroimage, 23*, 1358-1369.

Zhan, W., Stein, E. A., & Yang, Y. (2006). A rotation-invariant spherical harmonic decomposition method for mapping intravoxel multiple fiber structures. *Neuroimage, 29*, 1212-1223.

Zhang, S., & Laidlaw, D. (2001). Elucidating neural structure in diffusion tensor MRI volumes using streamtubes and streamsurfaces. *Proceedings of International Society of Magnetic Resonance in Imaging*, (pp. 505), Glasgow, UK.

Zhang, X., Fujita, H., Kanematsu, M., Zhou, X., Hara. T., Kato, H., Yokoyama, R., Hoshi, H. (2005). Improving the classification of cirrhotic liver by texture features. In *27th IEEE Conference of Engineering in Medicine and Biology.* (pp. 867-870).

Zhang, X., McKay, C. R., & Sonka, M. (1998). Tissue characterization in intravascular ultrasound images. *IEEE Trans Med Imag, 17*(6), 889-99.

Zhang, Z., Lyons, M., Schuster, M., & Akamatsu, S. (1998). Comparison Between Geometry-Based and Gabor-Wavelet-Based Facial Expression Recognition Using Multi-Layer Perceptron. *Int'l Conf Automatic Face and Gesture Recognition*, (pp. 454-459).

Zhong, J., & Ning, R. (2005). Image Denoising based on wavelets and multifractals for singularity detection. *IEEE Transactions on Image Processing, 14*, 1435-1447.

Zimmerman, S., Johnston, D., Arrighi, F., & Rupp, M. E. (1986). Automated homologue matching of human G-banded chromosomes. *Comput. Biol. Med., 16*, 223–233.

Zitova, B., & Flusser, J. (2003). Image registration methods: a survey. *Image and Vision Computing, 21*, 977–1000.

Zou, Q., Chu, W. W., Morioka, C., Leazer, G. H., & Kangarloo, H. (2003). IndexFinder: A method of extracting key concepts from clinical texts for indexing. In M. Musen (Ed.), *AMIA Annu Symp Proc*, 763-767.

About the Contributors

Dimitris Arabadjis received his Diploma in Electrical and Computer Engineering from the National Technical University of Athens in 2006. He has been a PhD. student in the School of Electrical and Computer Engineering of NTUA since 2006. His research interests and recent work are on the following subjects: applications of information theory to archaeology, automatic reassembling of fragmented objects, image processing, pattern recognition, finite precision error, numerical solutions of differential equations, etc. He has two publications in international Journals on these subjects.

Nikolaos Arikidis was born in Athens, Greece, in 1974. He received BSc (1997) in Medical Instrumentation Technology from the Technological Educational Institute of Athens, Greece, and M.Sc. (1999) in Biomedical Engineering Instrumentation from the University of Dundee, UK. He is Biomedical Engineer in "Sotiria" Hospital, Athens, Greece, and PhD. candidate in the Department of Medical Physics, University of Patras, Greece. His research interests include medical image segmentation and wavelet analysis.

Konstantinos Arfanakis is Associate Professor of Biomedical Engineering at the Illinois Institute of Technology, USA. His research interests include the development of magnetic resonance imaging (MRI) data acquisition, image reconstruction, data analysis, and visualization techniques, and the application of these methods for the diagnosis and monitoring of neurological disease. His recent research contributions can be grouped into the following categories: a) functional MRI, b) diffusion tensor imaging (DTI) and structural connectivity of the brain, c) lesion detection, d) neuronal structural integrity in seizure disorders, e) microstructural correlates of psychiatric disorders, f) early diagnosis of Alzheimer's disease.

Charalambos N. Bougias was born in Ioannina, Greece, in 1973. He received the Diploma Degree from the Department of Radiology Technologist, Athens, Greece, in 1998. He is currently working at the department of Nuclear Medicine, University Hospital of Ioannina. His research interests include fMRI, protocol optimization of the diffusion tensor imaging and advanced neuro imaging with MRI.

Christos V. Bourantas was born in Levadia, Greece in 1974. He graduated from the Medical School, University of Ioannina, Greece in 1999 and awarded his PhD. degree in Cardiology in 2005 from Medical School, University of Ioannina, Greece. Currently he is working as specialist registrar in Cardiology at "Laikon" General Hospital, Athens. He is also a Horonary Lecturer in Academic Cardiology, Hull University, Kingston-upon-Hull, United Kingdom. His research interests focus on cardiac imaging, image processing and 3-D reconstruction methodologies.

Dr. Alex Bui received his PhD in Computer Science in 2000 and is now an Associate Professor of Radiological Sciences at UCLA. He is the Director of the UCLA-National Library Medicine (NLM) training program in medical informatics. Dr. Bui's research interests focus on distributed information architectures for biomedical research and clinical environments, probabilistic data modeling, and visualization of medical information.

Christophe Charrier, received his PhD from the university of Saint-Etienne in 1998 in the field of Computer Engineering and Image Processing. From 1998 to 2001, he was a postdoctoral researcher at the LRTS, Laval University, Quebec City, with Pr. Gilles Y. Delisle. In 2001, he joined the Communication Networks and Services department of technology of the Université de Caen Basse Normandie as an associate professor. His research concerns color image compression, human vision, color image quality, data fusion and data classification.

Dr Aristotelis A. Chatziioannou received a Diploma in Electrical & Computer Engineering and a PhD. in Metabolic Engineering and Medical Informatics from the National Technical University of Athens (NTUA) Greece. Since September of 2005 he is with the Institute of Biological Research & Biotechnology in the National Hellenic Research Foundation. His published work includes various peer reviewed journal papers a book chapter and more than (30) international conference proceedings. His scientific activities include metabolic engineering, genomics, biological ontologies, bioinformatics, computational biology, biomedical image processing. Dr. Chatziioannou is a member of the Technical Chamber of Greece, the Hellenic Computer Society, the Hellenic Society of Artificial Intelligence, the Hellenic Society of Biochemistry & Molecular Biology and a founding member of the Hellenic Society of Computational Biology and Bioinformatics. He is reviewer in various scientific journals

Christodoulos I. Christodoulou received his diploma in Electrical Engineering with specialization in Telecommunications at the Technical University RWTH Aachen, Germany in 1987 and the PhD. degree in Electronics Engineering from the Queen Mary University of London, in 2000. He carries out his research work in cooperation with the department of Computer Science of the University of Cyprus and with the Cyprus Institute of Neurology and Genetics. His research interests include Intelligent Information Systems, Artificial Neural Networks, Signal and Image Processing, Pattern Recognition, Biosignal Analysis, and Computer Applications in Medicine and Meteorology. His research work in the above areas has been published in a number of refereed journal papers, book chapters and conference papers.

Richard S.C. Cobbold received the BSc degree in physics from Imperial College, University of London in 1956, and obtained the M.Sc. and PhD. degrees from the University of Saskatchewan, Canada in 1961 and 1965 respectively. Since 1966 he has been with the Institute of Biomedical Engineering where he was Director from 1974 through to 1983. He is currently Professor Emeritus in the Institute and in the Department of Electrical and Computer Engineering. His research interests center around the fundamental aspects of ultrasound, Doppler ultrasound and its application for vascular assessment. He is the author of two books, a number of research papers and several book chapters. A third book, *Foundations of Biomedical Ultrasound*, was published by Oxford University Press in 2006. He was elected a Fellow of the Royal Society of Canada in 1976 and was appointed Canada-UK Rutherford lecturer in 1995.

Lena Costaridou received BSc (1979) in Physics from the University of Patras, Greece, M.Sc. (1982) in Medical Engineering from the Department of Electrical Engineering and Applied Sciences of the George Washington University, USA, and PhD. (1997) in Medical Physics from the University of Patras, Greece. She is an Assistant Professor at the Department of Medical Physics, School of Medicine, University of Patras, Greece. Her research interests include medical image processing and analysis with emphasis on tissue quantification and characterization in the frame of Computer Assisted Diagnosis systems and quality of medical imaging systems. She is author/co-author of 60 articles in international refereed journals and over 70 international conference papers, and reviewer for several international journals. She is the editor of the book "Medical Image Analysis Methods" (CRC Press, 2005).

Alberto Taboada Crispi, Electronic Engineer (Universidad Central de Las Villas (UCLV), Santa Clara, Cuba, 1985), Master of Sciences (Electronics, UCLV, 1997), PhD (Electrical Engineering and Computer Science, University of New Brunswick, Canada, 2002). From 1985 to 1988, he worked as an Engineer at the University Hospital "Arnaldo Milián Castro", Santa Clara, Cuba. Then, he joined the Electrical Engineering Faculty at UCLV as Professor and Researcher. Now, he is with the Center for Studies in Electronics and Information Technologies at UCLV. His research interests are in Instrumentation, Digital Signal and Image Processing, Pattern Recognition, and Biomedical Applications.

Robert J. Dawe holds a BS degree in biomedical engineering from the Illinois Institute of Technology, USA and is now pursuing a PhD degree in the same field. His research interests include diffusion tensor imaging and postmortem MRI of the human brain. He is a recipient of the ARCS Foundation scholarship for college scientists.

Cecile Delgorge-Rosenberger graduated from Ecole Nouvelle d'Ingénieurs en Communication (ENIC), Lille, France, in 1999, with an Engineering Degree in New Information and Communication Technologies. In 2001, she received the Master Degree in Signals and Images in Biology and Medicine, from University of Angers, France. In dec. 2005, she obtained the PhD. in Industrial Sciences and Technologies in the Laboratory of Vision and Robotics from University of Orleans, France. Her PhD. work is a contribution to the European project, named OTELO (mObile Tele-Echography using an ultra-Light rObot). Her research work is in acquisition, compression, transmission and evaluation techniques for ultrasound images.

I. Dimou received an MSc in informatics from the Technical University of Crete since 2002 and a Bachelor's in telecommunications and electronics engineering since 1998. In 2005 he worked as a research assistant at the Katholieke Univeriseit Leuven, Belgium in research related to the development of intelligent diagnostic tools for cancer. He is currently a PhD candidate at the Technical University of Crete, where he has also worked as a teaching assistant. He has actively participated in various research projects in his field. His research interests are mainly focused on practical and theoretic aspects of biomedical informatics applications with the use of intelligent tools including probabilistic methods, support vector machines and classifier fusion.

Charalampos Doukas has received a diploma in Information and Communication Systems Engineering from the University of the Aegean and is currently a PhD Student at the same department. His research activities are focused on medical image processing, telemedicine and applications of artificial intelligence on medical informatics. He is an author/co-author of 8 journal papers and book chapters and more than 15 international conference papers. He is a member of IEEE - Societies: Engineering in Medicine and Biology, Computer, Communications, ACM, the Technical Chamber of Greece, and the Greek Computer Society and the Hellenic Organization of Biomedical Engineering. Charalampos Doukas is currently working as a research associate at the University of the Aegean and Athens Information Technology.

Hubert Elie is doctor in pathology and head of the pathological histology and cytology department, Centre Hospitalier du Cotentin, Cherbourg, France.

Abderrahim Elmoataz is a full-time professor of computer Science at the Computer Science Department of the Université de Caen Basse-Normandie, France. His research concerns graph-based and discrete variational methods for image and data processing.

Alfred Gangl is professor of Gastroenterology and Hepatology at the Department of Gastroenterology and Hepatology of the Medical University of Vienna (since 1982) which he heads. After he graduated as Doctor universae medicinae in 1966 at the University of Vienna, he worked in different Austrian hospitals. Apart from that he spent two years as a Research Fellow at the Medical Center of the University of California. He is a member of several associations and societies in the field of gastroenterology and hepatology. His research interests and scientific activities include all aspects of diagnosis and treatment of gastrointestinal and liver diseases.

John G. Georgiadis is the Kritzer Professor of Mechanical Science and Engineering at the University of Illinois at Urbana-Champaign, USA. He has expertise in the area of quantitative visualization of flow and mass transport in biological and engineered systems, and the use of in vivo Magnetic Resonance Imaging (MRI) to improve medical diagnostics and to quantify energy utilization in the human body. He is currently directing research projects focusing on MRI studies in brain and skeletal muscle. He received his Diploma in Mechanical Engineering (1984) from the National Technical University of Athens, Greece, and his MS (1985) and PhD (1987) degrees in Mechanical Engineering from UCLA.

Panagiotis Georgoulias is a Lecturer of Nuclear Medicine in the Medical School of the University of Thessaly. He received his Medical Degree in 1991 from the University of Athens and his PhD in 1999 from the University of Crete. His main research interests are focused on the field of Nuclear Medical Imaging, and Nuclear Cardiology.

Nikolaos Giannakeas was born in Athens, Greece in 1980. He graduated from the Physics Department of the University of Ioannina, Greece in 2003. He is currently working towards the PhD degree in the Medical School of the University of Ioannina. His research interests include microarray image and data analysis, biomedical engineering and bioinformatics.

Alexia Giannoula was born in 1979 in Greece. She received the BSc degree in computer science from the Aristotle University of Thessaloniki, Greece, in 2001. From 2001 to 2002, she worked as a research assistant at the Artificial Intelligence & Information Analysis laboratory of the Aristotle University of Thessaloniki. In 2004, she obtained the M.A.Sc. degree in electrical and computer engineering (communications) from the University of Toronto, Canada, and in 2008, the PhD. degree in electrical and computer engineering from the Institute of Biomaterials & Biomedical Engineering, University of Toronto, Canada. Her research interests include the acoustic radiation force of ultrasound for elasticity imaging, the principles of shear-wave propagation and also, signal processing, multimedia coding and biometrics.

Spyretta Golemati received the Diploma in Mechanical Engineering from the National Technical University of Athens, Greece, in 1994 and the M.Sc. and PhD. degrees in Bioengineering from Imperial College of Science, Technology and Medicine, University of London, UK, in 1995 and 2000, respectively. She is currently a Lecturer in Biomedical Engineering at the National Kapodistrian University of Athens, Greece. Her research interests include medical imaging, image and signal processing, and cardiovascular and respiratory mechanics. She has co-authored more than 60 papers in international refereed journals, book chapters in books and conference proceedings. She is a member of the Institute of Electrical and Electronic Engineers and the Technical Chamber of Greece.

Michael Häfner was born on December 9 1968 in Vienna, Austria. He studied Medicine in Vienna and Perugia, Italy and graduated on January 23 1995. He started collaborating at the Department of Gastroenterology and Hepatology of the Medical University of Vienna in 1994, where he also was trained in Internal Medicine. He is specialist in Gastroenterology and Hepatology with his main focus on interventional endoscopy. Michael Haefner is currently secretary of the Austrian Society of Gastroenterology and Hepatology and organiser of several courses on interventional endoscopy, including an annual postgraduate course on endoscopy in Vienna. He acts as tutor at various national and international hands-on training courses. Recently he spent half a year in Malaysia to start up an endoscopy unit in Kuala Lumpur.

J. Michael Herrmann received a Diploma in Mathematics and PhD. In Computer Science from Leipzig University, Germany, in 1993. He has been a Postdoctoral Researcher at Leipzig University, at NORDITA, Copenhagen, at the Laboratory for Information Representation at RIKEN in Japan, and at the Max Planck Institute for Fluid Dynamics in Göttingen. After having held an assistant professorship at the Physics Department of Göttingen University, he is now a lecturer for robotics at the school of Informatics of Edinburgh University, Scotland. His research interests include dynamical systems and the computational neuroscience of behavior.

William Hsu is a doctoral student in the Medical Imaging Informatics group at UCLA. He received his BS in Biomedical Engineering in 2004 at Johns Hopkins University. His research interests include information visualization, knowledge representation, and human computer interaction. His dissertation work is related to exploring novel visualizations and methods for interaction that assist physicians and patients with understanding the diverse data captured in medical records.

Stavros Kakkos holds a Medical Degree (1990, University of Patras, Greece), a Doctorate in Medicine (1995, University of Patras) and a license to practice General Surgery (1997, Greece). In 1999 he received a Master's degree in Vascular Technology and Medicine and in 2004 a PhD in Vascular Surgery both by the University of London, UK. During 2004-2008 he continued clinical training in

Vascular Surgery (UK & USA). He is currently an Assistant Professor at the Dept of Vascular Surgery, University of Patras, Greece. Dr Kakkos has received numerous awards and distinctions for his clinical and research activities.

Kangarloo is a Professor of Pediatrics, Radiology, and Bioengineering at UCLA. Dr. Kangarloo is an experienced medical informatics researcher and is the principal investigator of several National Institutes of Health-funded grants in the areas of imaging informatics. He leads a multi-disciplinary team of computer scientists, engineers, physicists, and clinical researchers and is a co-Director of the UCLA Biomedical Informatics Center.

Anna Karahaliou was born in Patras, Greece, in 1977. She received BSc (2001) in Physics from University of Patras, Greece, and M.Sc. (2003) in Medical Physics from the University of Patras, Greece. She is currently PhD. candidate in the Department of Medical Physics, University of Patras, Greece. Her research interests include medical image processing and analysis and pattern recognition.

Petros Karvelis was born in Mesolongi, Greece in 1978. He graduated from the Computer Science Department, School of Natural Sciences, of the University of Ioannina, Greece in 2001. His thesis was on Computational Geometry – "Tetrahedralization algorithms of convex polyhedron". He received a M.Sc. thesis in the area of Computer Science in the Department of Computer Science, School of Natural Sciences, University of Ioannina in 2004. The title of the M.Sc. thesis was – Segmentation of human chromosome images. Today he is PhD candidate of the Department of Computer Science, School of Natural Sciences, University of Ioannina and his PhD thesis concerns the – Processing and Analysis of human chromosome images for the detection of chromosome abnormalities.

Dimitrios C. Karampinos received a Diploma degree in Mechanical Engineering (2003) from the National Technical University of Athens, Greece and is now pursuing a PhD. degree in Mechanical Science and Engineering at the University of Illinois at Urbana-Champaign, USA. His research work has been focused on the development of acquisition and model-based analysis techniques in diffusion, perfusion, elastography and flow quantification MRI of the human brain and skeletal muscle.

Thomas Kilindris received his Electrical Engineering Diploma in 1991 from the Aristotelian University of Thessaloniki. He is occupied at the Laboratory of Medical Phyhsics and Informatics at the Medical School of the University of Thessaly, Hellas. His research interests include biomedical image and signal processing, parallel processing methods for dose calculation and design and optimization of treatment planning systems for stereotactic radiotherapy. He is the co-author of "*PARALLEL EIKONA: a parallel digital image processing package*" (John Wiley & Sons, Inc., 1993).

Veliou S. Konstantia was born in Ioannina,Greece, in 1973.She received the Diploma Degree from the Department of medicine , Boulgary, in 1997.She is radiologist and currently working at the department of MR imaging ,Magnitiki Tomografia of Epirous.Her research interests include fMRI, and neuro imaging with MR.

Anastasios Koutlas was born in Ioannina, Greece in 1981. He graduated with BSc Honours in Computing Science, from University of Manchester Institute of Science and Technology (UMIST) in 2003.

He is currently working for a PhD. in Medical Physics Department, in the Medical School of University of Ioannina. His research interests include facial expression recognition and machine learning.

Efthyvoulos Kyriacou is an Associate Professor with the Department of Computer Science and Engineering of Frederick University Cyprus. His research interests focus on Telematics, image processing, neural networks and their applications in medicine. He has published several journal and conference papers in the above fields. He is an associate editor of IEEE transaction on Information Technology in Biomedicine, while he is an active reviewer of many other scientific journals. He is a member of IEEE EMB and Computer Societies, the Hellenic society of Biomedical Engineering and the Cyprus Society of Medical Physics and Biomedical Engineering.

Gilles Lebrun received his PhD from the university of Caen Basse-Normandie in 2006 the field of computer science. He is actually assistant professor of computer science in the Services and Network Communication of the université de Caen Basse-Normandie. His research concerns machine learning paradigm and their application to image processing problems.

Michel Lecluse is cytological technician in the pathological histology and cytology department, Centre Hospitalier du Cotentin, Cherbourg, France.

Michael Liedlgruber received his Master's degree in Computer Sciences from the University of Salzburg (Austria) in May 2006. His Master's thesis has already been devoted to pit pattern classification using wavelets. Currently he is working on his PhD thesis at the Department of Computer Sciences (University of Salzburg) in the same field of research. His main research interests include image processing and pattern recognition.

Olivier Lezoray received the M.S and Doctoral degrees, both in Computer Science, from Université de Caen Basse-Normandie, France, respectively in 1996 and 2000. From 1999 to 2000, he was assistant professor with the Computer Science Department of the Université de Caen Basse-Normandie. Since 2000, he has been an associate professor with the Cherbourg Institute of Technology in the Communications, Networks and Services Department. His research concerns color image segmentation and filtering (graph-based variational and morphological methods) and machine learning techniques for image mining (neural networks and support vector machines).

Christos P. Loizou: Received the BSc degree in electrical engineering, the M.Sc. degree in computer science and telecommunications from the University of Kaiserslautern, Kaiserslautern, Germany, and the PhD. degree from the Department of Computer Science, Kingston University, U.K. He is currently an Assistant Professor in the Department of Computer Science, Intercollege, Limassol, Cyprus, since 2000. He has been involved in numerous projects funded by the Cyprus Institute Promotion and Foundation. He has published 1 book, 6 chapters in books, 6 refereed journal articles, and 24 conference proceeding papers. His current research interests include medical imaging, signal and image processing, pattern recognition, biosignal analysis and computer applications in medicine. He is a Senior Member of the IEEE.

George Loudos is an Assistant Professor in the Department of Medical Instruments Technolody, Technological Educational Institute of Athens. He received the Diploma in electrical engineering and the PhD. degree from the National Technical University of Athens (NTUA), Greece, in1998 and his PhD in Biomedical Engineering in 2003. His research interests are focused on the field of Nuclear Medical Imaging, including dedicated systems for small animal imaging and scintimammography, SPECT and PET, Monte Carlo simulations of PET/SPECT systems. In addition he is working in the field of Telemedicine and more specifically Telecardiology.

Panagiota Loumou was born in Athens, Greece in 1985. She is a graduate student at the National Technical University of Athens, Department of Electrical & Computer Engineering. She is a member of the Multimedia Laboratory of the same department and has participated in several European Programs as a Project Team Member. Her research interests involve biomedical engineering, image processing, web development and social networks.

D. Lowe is Professor of Information Engineering at Aston University and a leading innovator in the research and development of applications for neural networks, forecasting and pattern recognition. While at the Royal Signals and Radar Establishment in Malvern, UK, Professor Lowe specialized in automatic speech recognition and generic pattern processing. In 1993, he joined Aston University as a founding Professor in the Neural Computing Research Group. Professor Lowe is a past Chairman of the IEE International Conference on Artificial Neural Networks, and remains active on various committees of international neural network, biomedical and financial conferences. He is also a member of several strategic government advisory committees on technology development.

Luca Mainardi is Assistant Professor at the Department of Bioengineering of the Politecnico di Milano. His teaching activities concern Biomedical Signal Processing and Bioelectricity and Biolectromagnetism. His research concerns biomedical signal and image processing and biomedical system modelling. He is the responsible of the Biomedical Signal Processing Laboratory at the Department of Bioengineering and he is Member of the Scientific Board of the Laboratory of Advanced Radiological Analysis (LARA) at the National Cancer Institute of Milano. He is author of more than 50 peer reviewed international papers. Member of the Board of Gruppo Nazionale di Bioingegneria in the years 2004-2007.

Ilias G. Maglogiannis received a Diploma in Electrical & Computer Engineering and a PhD. in Biomedical Engineering and Medical Informatics from the National Technical University of Athens (NTUA) Greece in 1996 and 2000 respectively, with scholarship from the Greek Government. From 1996 until 2000 he worked as a Researcher in the Biomedical Engineering Laboratory in NTUA and he has been engaged to several European and National Projects. Since February of 2001 he is with the Dept of Information and Communication Systems Engineering in University of the Aegean. His published scientific work includes three (3) books (Springer, IOS press and Morgan Claypool Publishers) and five (5) lecture notes (in Greek) on Biomedical Engineering and Multimedia topics, forty one (41) journal papers and more than seventy (70) international conference papers. He is an Associate Editor for the IEEE Transactions on Information Technology in Biomedicine Journal and editorial board member of the Journal on Information Technology in Healthcare. He has served as guest editor in IEEE EMB

Magazine (special issue on Signal and Distributed Data Processing for Networked eHealth Applications), Oncology Reports (special issue on Computational analysis and decision support systems in oncology), Simulation: Transactions of the Society for Modelling and Simulation International (special issue on Performance Modelling and Simulation in Healthcare Information Systems), Applied Intelligence (special issue on Artificial Intelligence Application and Innovations) and Section Editor in Handbook of Computational Intelligence in Medical Systems. He has served in program and organizing committees in national and international conferences (26) and he is a reviewer for several scientific journals (15). His scientific activities include medical bioinformatics, medical image processing and telemedicine. Dr. Maglogiannis is a member of IEEE - Societies: Engineering in Medicine and Biology, Computer, Communications, SPIE - International Society for Optical Engineering, ACM, the Technical Chamber of Greece, the Greek Computer Society and the Hellenic Organization of Biomedical Engineering. Dr. Maglogiannis is also a national representative for Greece in the IFIP technical committee TC 12 (Artificial Intelligence - Knowledge-Oriented Development of Applications) and member of the Working Group on Leading-edge Applications of the eMobility technology platform.

George K. Matsopoulos received the Diploma in Electrical Engineering in 1989 from the National Technical University of Athens (NTUA), Athens, Greece. He received the M.Sc. degree in 1989 and the PhD. degree in Bioengineering in 1993 from the University of Strathclyde, Glasgow, U.K. He is currently an Assistant Professor at the School of Electrical and Computer Engineering at the National Technical University of Athens. His research interests include nonlinear image processing applied to medical applications, biomedical signal processing, 2-D and 3-D registration of medical images, computer vision applications, classification and experts systems and Web-based medical systems for telemedicine application and remote image processing. Dr. Matsopoulos is a member of the IEEE, the Technical Chamber of Greece and the Hellenic Society of Biomedical Engineering.

Cyril Meurie received his PhD from the Université de Caen Basse-Normandie, France in 2005 in the field of computer science. From 2004 to 2006, he was assistant professor at the computer Science Department of the Université de Caen Basse-Normandie. He is actually a two-year postdoctoral researcher at the INRETS (French National Institute for Transport and Safety Research), Lille, France. His research concerns color image segmentation (variational and morphological method) with application in vidéo-surveillance (critical event detection, people tracking, passengers counting...) in transport environment.

Arcangelo Merla holds a PhD in advanced biomedical technologies and bioimaging from the University of Chieti (Italy) and a MS (laurea) in physics from the University of Bologna (Italy). His expertise is in the area of biomedical imaging and modelling, with special reference to thermal and infrared imaging. He is the Director of the functional Infrared Imaging Lab at the ITAB – Institute of Advanced Biomedical Technologies at the Foundation University G. D'Annunzio of Chieti-Pescara, and Professor of Applied Physics at the School of Medicine of the University of Chieti-Pescara, Italy.

Lampros K. Michalis was born in 1960 in Arta, Greece. He graduated with distinction from the Medical School, University of Athens, Greece in 1984. In 1989 he was awarded with Distinction for his MD Thesis from the Athens Medical School, Greece. Since 1995, he has been in the Medical School, University of Ioannina, Greece, where he is currently a Professor of Cardiology. He is in charge of the

Coronary Care Unit and the Catheter Laboratory of the University Hospital of Medical School, Ioannina, Greece. His research interests focus on vibrational angioplasty using guide-wires, bioengineering and interventional cardiology.

Maykel Orozco Monteagudo was graduated with high honors in Computer Sciences from Universidad Central de Las Villas (UCLV), Santa Clara, Cuba, in 2002. He is a Master of Sciences (Computer Sciences, UCLV, 2006) and he is currently starting his PhD studies. From 2002 to 2005, he worked as professor of Department of Mathematics at UCLV. Then, he joined the Center for Studies in Electronics and Information Technologies at UCLV to work as professor and researcher. His interests are in Programming, Artificial Intelligence, and Digital Signal Processing.

Stavroula G. Mougiakakou received the diploma and the PhD degree from the National Technical University of Athens (NTUA), Greece, in 1997 and 2003, respectively. From 2003 to 2005, she was with the Greek Ministry of Public Order as Special Consultant in IT projects. Since 2005 she is working as a Researcher at the Institute of Communication and Computer Systems, NTUA. Her research interests include intelligent medical decision support systems, physiological control systems, "artificial pancreas", medical informatics, bioinformatics, and eHealth. She has co-authored 18 papers in refereed international journals and book chapters, more than 40 papers in international conference proceedings and held one patent. She has been involved as technical project manager in several European and National funded R&D projects in the area of biomedical engineering. Dr. Mougiakakou is a member of the Institute of Electrical and Electronics Engineers, and the Technical Chamber of Greece.

Panagiotis Moulos holds a Diploma in Applied Mathematics and Physics, from the National Technical University of Athens (NTUA) and a Master of Science Degree in Bioinformatics from the Free University of Brussels (ULB). His scientific activities include system biology, bioinformatics with emphasis in microarray analysis, genomics, computational biology. Mr. Moulos is a member the Hellenic Society of Biochemistry & Molecular Biology.

Katerina K. Naka was born in Ioannina, Greece, in 1971. She graduated with distinction from the Medical School, University of Ioannina, Ioannina, Greece in 1994. She received the PhD. degree from the University of Wales College of Medicine, Cardiff, Wales, United Kingdom in 2003. She has completed her training in Cardiology and is currently a Lecturer in Cardiology, in the Medical School, University of Ioannina, Ioannina, Greece. Her research interests focus on vascular endothelial function, large arterial mechanics, heart failure and bioengineering.

Anrew Nicolaides is Professor Emeritus at Imperial College. He was the Professor of Vascular Surgery at Imperial College School of Medicine and Consultant Vascular Surgeon at St Mary's Hospital Medical School from 1983–2000 and Medical Director of the Cyprus Institute of Neurology and Genetics from 2001-2004. His research group is known internationally in several areas, which include noninvasive vascular screening and diagnostic investigation, early detection and prevention of cardiovascular and venous disease. His research is now directed towards the genetic risk factors and biomarkers for cardiovascular disease (arterial and venous), identification of individuals at risk and the development of effective methods of prevention, especially stroke.

Alexandra Nikita received the M.D. degree from the University of Athens, Athens, Greece, in 1993. From 1994 since 1998, she was resident at the 2nd Department of Radiology, University of Athens, Greece. In 1998, she successfully passed the Greek radiological exams and obtained the title of radiologist. Since May 2000, she works at the University as scientific collaborator at the 2nd Department of Radiology, University of Athens. She has co-authored 15 papers in refereed international journals and 50 papers in international conference proceedings. She is a member of the Athens Medical Association, the Hellenic Radiological Society, the Cardiovascular Interventional Radiological Society of Europe (CIRSE) and the Radiological Society of North America (RSNA).

Konstantina S. Nikita received the Diploma degree in electrical engineering and the PhD. degree from National Technical University of Athens (NTUA), Greece, in 1986 and 1990, respectively, and the M.D. degree from the Medical School, University of Athens, in 1993. Since 1990, she has been working as a Researcher with the Institute of Communication and Computer Systems, NTUA. In 1996, she joined the Department of Electrical and Computer Engineering, NTUA, where she is currently a Professor. Her current research interests include medical imaging, biomedical signal and image processing and analysis, biomedical informatics, health telematics, simulation of physiological systems, computational bioelectromagnetics, biological effects, and medical applications of electromagnetic waves. She has authored or coauthored 90 papers in refereed international journals and chapters in books, and more than 150 papers in international conference proceedings. She was the coauthor of one book in Greek and the coeditor of one book in English published by Springer. She holds two Greek patents. She has been the Technical Manager with several European and National Research and Development Projects in the field of biomedical engineering. Dr. Nikita is a member of the Technical Chamber of Greece, the Athens Medical Association, and the Hellenic Society of Biomedical Engineering. She was the recipient of the 2003 Bodossakis Foundation Academic Prize for exceptional achievements in "Theory and Applications of Information Technology in Medicine."

Marios S. Neofytou received his diploma degree in Electrical & Computer Engineering from the National Technical University of Athens (NTUA) in 2000 and his PhD. degree in Biomedical Engineering from the department of Electrical & Computer Engineering of the National Technical University of Athens, Greece, in 2007. From 2000 to 2003 he was a research graduate student at the Institute of Communication and Computer Systems – NTUA, working in the area of Biomedical Engineering in several EU funded research projects (EMERGENCY-112, MEDISIGNAL etc) concerning telemedicine, medical imaging and medical informatics. From 2003-2007, he is the Administrator of the Medical Informatics Laboratory of the Computer Science Department of the University of Cyprus. He is working in research projects (IPPOKRATHS, CATIA, InteMEDnet etc.) dealing with e-learning, medical imaging and image processing. He has published several journals and conference papers in the fields of telemedicine, medical imaging and medical informatics. Dr. Neofytou is a member of IEEE EMB Society, IEEE Computer Society and the Hellenic society of Biomedical Engineering.

Denis Hernández Pacheco: was graduated as Telecommunications and Electronics Engineer from Universidad Central de Las Villas (UCLV), Santa Clara, Cuba, in 2006. Since then, he has been with the Center for Studies in Electronics and Information Technologies at UCLV, working as professor and researcher. His interests are in Programming, and Digital Signal and Image Processing.

Mihalis Panagopoulos was born in Athens, Greece. He received his Diploma in Electrical and Computer Engineering from the National Technical University of Athens in 2002. He received his PhD. degree in Computer Engineering from NTUA in 2008. His main research interests involve: Image processing, pattern recognition, curve fitting, finite precision error, biomedical engineering and application of pattern recognition methods and statistics to archeology. He has eight publications in international journals on these subjects.

George Panayiotakis was born in Chania, Greece, in 1956. He received BSc (1979) in Physics and PhD. (1986) in Medical Physics from the University of Patras, Greece. He is professor in the Department of Medical Physics, School of Medicine, University of Patras, Greece and head of the Medical Radiation Physics Unit at the University Hospital of Patras. He is a member of the Steering Committee of the Interdepartmental Program of Postgraduate Studies in Medical Physics, as well as of the Steering Committee of the Interdepartmental Program of Postgraduate Studies in Electronics and Information Processing, both offered by the University of Patras. He is a consultant to the National Food and Drug Administration, Greece. He is a member of the overseas advisor committee of the British Journal of Radiology and reviewer for several international journals. He has published over 160 papers in international peer-reviewed journals and over 200 papers in international conferences. His research interests focus on medical radiation physics, medical imaging, medical image detectors, simulation of medical imaging systems using Monte Carlo techniques, and include medical image processing and analysis.

Constantin Papaodysseus received his Diploma in Electrical and Computer Engineering from National Technical University of Athens (NTUA) and his M.Sc. degree from Manchester University, U.K. He received his PhD. degree in Computer Engineering from NTUA. From 1996 he was an Ass. Professor at NTUA, Dpt. of Electrical and Computer Engineering. From 2001 he is an associate Professor at the same department. His research interests include music and speech processing and automatic recognition, image processing, applied mathematics, quantization error analysis, adaptive algorithms, biomedical engineering, etc. He has more than forty-five publications in international Journals and many publications in international conferences on these subjects.

Katia Passera took her Master degree in Biomedical Engineering on April 2004 at the Department of Biomedical Engineering, Politecnico di Milano (Italy) with a thesis awarded by the Bioengineering National Group. She took the European PhD degree in Bioengineering on June 2008 defending a thesis on image registration and segmentation. She is collaborating with the Department of Imaging Diagnosis and Radiotherapy, National Cancer Institute of Milan. The research topic concerns the registration and elaboration of biomedical images, in particular Dynamic Contrast-Enhanced Magnetic Resonance Imaging in applications orientated to improve the diagnosis and treatment of tumors.

Constantinos Pattichis is a Professor in the Computer Science department of the University of Cyprus. His current research interests include ehealth, medical imaging, biosignal analysis, and intelligent systems. He has been involved in numerous projects related to health telematics funded by EU, the National Research Foundation of Cyprus, the INTERREG and other bodies, with a total funding managed close to 5 million Euros. He has published 47 refereed journal and 110 conference papers, and 18 chapters in books in these areas. He served as Chairperson of the Cyprus Association of Medical Physics and Biomedical Engineering(96-98), and the IEEE Cyprus Section(98-00). He is a Senior Member of IEEE.

Marios S. Pattichis is an Associate Professor with the Department of Electrical and Computer Engineering and an Associate Professor with the Department of Radiology at the University of New Mexico (UNM), Albuquerque, New Mexico. His research interests are in the areas of medical image and video processing, digital image and video models, radar image processing, SIMD, and reconfigurable computer architecture applications. He is an associate editor for Pattern Recognition. At UNM, he received the 2004 ECE distinguished teaching award and the 2006 School of Engineering Harrison Faculty Recognition Award. He is a Senior Member of IEEE.

Christophe Rosenberger is Full Professor at ENSICAEN, France. He obtained his PhD. degree from the University of Rennes I in 1999. He works at the GREYC Laboratory in the Image Research Unit. His research interests include evaluation of image processing algorithms and biometric systems. He also works on biometric authentication algorithm for e-transactions .

Panayiotis Roussopoulos was born in Athens, Greece, in 1971. He received his Diploma in Physics from the university of Patras in 2002. He has been a PhD. student in the School of Electrical and Computer Engineering of NTUA since 2002. His research interests and recent work are on the following subjects: applications of information theory to archaeology, image processing, pattern recognition, finite precision error, numerical solutions of differential equations in physics, etc. He has nine publications in international Journals on these subjects.

Alexander Falcón Ruiz: was graduated with high honors as Telecommunications and Electronics Engineer from Universidad Central de Las Villas (UCLV), Santa Clara, Cuba, in 2003. From 2003 to 2005, he worked as professor of Department of Digital Systems at the University of Informatics Sciences, Havana, Cuba. Since then, he works as professor and researcher in the Center for Studies in Electronics and Information Technologies at UCLV. His interests are in Instrumentation, Programming, and Digital Signal Processing.

Valentina Russo received her Laurea degree in Computer Scince from University of Roma Tre (Italy) in the 2006. From 2004 she worked on the development of innovative tools to support the Dynamic Contrast Enhancement analysis cooperating with the Complex System and Security Lab of the University CAMPU Bio-Medico. Actually she is PhD Student in System Engineering at University "La Sapienza" of Rome. Her research interests include development of biomedical systems and automatic image analysis and processing. She is the co-author of 4 scientific papers.

Farhang Sahba received the BSc degree in electronics engineering from the Isfahan University of Technology, Isfahan, in 1992, the MS degree in telecommunications from the Toosi University of Technology, Tehran, in 1995, and the PhD. degree in systems design engineering from the University of Waterloo, Canada, in 2007. He has worked in the area of medical image analysis for several years. His main research interests include Medical Imaging, Machine Intelligence, Pattern Recognition and Computer Vision.

Hichem Sahli: received the PhD degree in computer sciences from the Ecole Nationale Sup. De Physique Strasbourg - France in 1991. From 1991-1996, he was attaché de recherche at the Ecole des Mines de Paris. He held visiting professor appointments from 1997 to 1998 at the Vrije Universiteit

Brussel (VUB). Since 1999 he is professor at the Dept. of Electronics and Informatics (ETRO) of the VUB, and group-coordinator at the Interuniversitair Micro-Elektronica Centrum vzw (IMEC). Within ETRO, he coordinates the research team in computer vision, with research fields in inverse problems in computer vision, image and motion analysis, and subsurface imaging.

Roberto Setola received his Laurea degree in Electronic Engineering (1992) and his PhD in Electronic Engineering and Computer Science (1996) from the University of Naples. From 1999 to 2004, he worked at the Italian Prime Minister's Office. At present, he is an Assistant Professor of Automatic Control at University CAMPUS Bio-Medico of Roma and lead of the Complex System and Security Lab. His research interests include modelling and control, control of complex systems, surgery robotics, and biomedical systems. He is the author of more than 100 scientific papers.

Spyros Skiadopoulos was born in Piraeus, Greece, in 1972. He received BSc (1995) in Physics from the Aristotle University of Thessaloniki, Greece, and M.Sc. (1997) and PhD. (2003) in Medical Physics from the University of Patras, Greece. He is Medical Radiation Physicist at "Olympion" Hospital of Patras and postdoctoral fellow in the Department of Medical Physics, University of Patras, Greece. His research interests include medical image processing and analysis and medical image quality evaluation methods.

John S. Stoitsis received the Diploma of Electrical and Computer Engineering from the Aristotle University of Thessaloniki in 2002, and the M.Sc. and PhD. degree in Biomedical Engineering from the University of Patras in 2004 and 2007, respectively. His research interests include biomedical image and signal processing, medical informatics, computer aided diagnosis and neuroscience. He has authored or co-authored seven papers in international journals and chapters in books, and more than ten papers in international conferences. He is a member of the Institute of Electrical and Electronics Engineers and the Technical Chamber of Greece.

Vasilios Tanos received his diploma degree in Medical School of Cyrillus and Methodius University, Skopje, Yugoslavia in 1986, and his PhD degree in The Hebrew University of Jerusalem (Department of Biochemistry), Human Sciences in 2003. He is a Visiting Professor in Obstetrics and Gynaecology in the Department of Obstetrics and Gynaecology, in the Ioannina University, the Faculty of Medicine and a Visiting Professor in Obstetrics and Gynaecology, in the Department of Obstetrics and Gynaecology, the Faculty of Medicine, in the Hebrew University of Jerusalem. He has worked in several European and local funded project such as IPPOKRATHS, CATIA, TeleGYN etc. He has several publications in international journals and conferences. He is working in the ARETAEION Hospital, Nicosia where he is the director of the gynaecology clinic.

Ricky Taira received a PhD in biomedical physics in 1988 from UCLA and is currently a Professor of Radiological Sciences. His past research interests have included development of picture archive and communication systems (PACS), medical knowledge bases (the KMeD project), and currently, natural language processing of medical corpora and formal ontological representations of disease entities.

Evanthia E. Tripoliti was born in Chios, Greece, in 1978. She received the Diploma Degree from the Department of Computer Science, University of Ioannina, Greece, in 2001 and the MS Degree in the area of Technology and Applications in the Department of Computer Science, University of Ioannina,

Greece, in 2003. She is currently working toward the Ph. D Degree at the Department of Computer Science, University of Ioannina. Since 1999, she has been with the Unit of Medical Technology and Intelligent Information Systems, Department of Computer Science University of Ioannina, Greece and her research interests include digital processing of medical images (MRI, fMRI, DTI).

Kiki Theodorou received her Bachelor degree in Physics in 1994, a Masters degree in Medical Physics in 1996 and her PhD in Medical Physics in 1999. She is an Assistant Professor in the Medical School at the University of Thessaly, in Medical Physics and Medical Informatics. Her main research interests are focused on Medical Imaging, Medical Image Processing, High Field Magnetic Resonance Imaging, Stereotactic Radiotherapy and Monte Carlo Simulations in Radiation Dosimetry.

George Theodoropoulos is an Associate Professor at the Agricultural University of Athens, Department of Anatomy & Physiology of Domestic Animals. He received his Diploma of Veterinary Medicine from the Aristotle University of Thessaloniki (1979) and his M.Sc. degree in Veterinary Pathology (Veterinary Parasitology) from the Iowa State University (1984). He received his PhD. degree in Comparative Pathology, from the University of California, Davis (1988). His research interests include host-parasite interactions, epidemiology of parasites, multimedia computer systems in Veterinary Medicine, etc. He has more than forty-five publications in international Journals and many publications in international conferences on these subjects.

Dimitrios G. Tsalikakis was born in Thessaloniki, Greece, in 1977. He is a researcher at the Unit of Medical Technology and Intelligent Information Systems and external lecturer at the University of Western Macedonia, Greece. He received the Diploma degree in Mathematics from the University of Ioannina, Greece in 2001 and the PhD degree in computation electrophysiology from the University of Ioannina, Greece in 2006. His research interests include cardiac modeling, monophasic action potential analysis, automated systems analysis, virtual instrumentation, computational electrophysiology, spatial extended cardiac models, phase resetting techniques and scientific computing. He has published several papers in refereed journals and international conferences.

Manolis Tsiknakis received the B.Eng. degree in electronic engineering, in 1983, the M.Sc. degree in microprocessor engineering, in 1985, and the PhD. degree in control systems engineering from the University of Bradford, Bradford, U.K., in 1989. Since 1992, he has been with the Institute of Computer Science, Foundation for Research and Technology–Hellas, Heraklion, Greece, where he is currently a Principal Researcher in many collaborative R&D projects, the Head of the Center of eHealth Technologies, and the technical coordinator of the development of HYGEIAnet, the regional health information network of Crete. He is the initiator and Co-Chair of the ERCIM Biomedical Informatics Working Group. His current research interests include biomedical informatics, component-based software engineering, biomedical information integration, ambient intelligence in eHealth and mHealth service platforms, and IT adoption related issues.

Ioannis Tsougos received his Bachelor degree in Physics in 1998, a Masters degree in Medical Physics in 2001 and his PhD in Medical Physics and Radiation Biology in 2005. His current position is a lecturer with tenure in the Medical School at the University of Thessaly, in Medical Physics and

Radiobiology. His main research interests are focused on in vivo Radiation Dosimetry and Radiation Biology, Nuclear Imaging and High Field Magnetic Resonance Imaging.

Andreas Uhl is an associate professor at the Department of Computer Sciences (University of Salzburg) where he heads the Multimedia Processing and Security Lab. His research interests include image and video processing and compression, wavelets, media security, medical imaging, biometrics, and number-theoretical numerics.

Andreas Vécsei graduated (Dr. med. univ.) at the University of Vienna. His post-graduate training in Austria and Kerala (India) made him receive his license to practice general pediatrics (Facharzt für Kinder- und Jugendheilkunde). After having been instructed in pediatric gastroenterology according to the syllabus of GPGE (Gesellschaft für pädiatrische Gastroenterologie und Ernährung; an association of German-speaking pediatric gastroenterologists) at the Medical University of Vienna and Munich, he received his certificate in 2006. Since 2006 he is in charge of the Endoscopy Unit of the St. Anna Children's Hospital, Vienna. His current research interests include Helicobacter pylori infection, celiac disease and computer-assisted evaluation of endoscopic images including the assessment of villous atrophy on endoscopic examination of the small intestine.

Ioannis K. Valavanis was born in Athens, Greece, in 1980. He received his diploma in Electrical and Computer Engineering in 2003 from the National Technical University of Athens (NTUA), Greece and his Master degree in 2006 from University of Athens, Greece. He is currently a PhD student at the laboratory of Biomedical Simulations and Medical Imaging (BIOSIM) at NTUA. His research interests include medical image processing, bioinformatics, artificial intelligence methods and their application in biological and medical data. He has co-authored more than ten papers in international journals or conferences. Mr. Valavanis is a member of the Technical Chamber of Greece.

Marotesa Voultsidou received a Diploma in Physics from the University of Crete at Heraklion, Greece, 1997. In 1999 she receive her Master degree also in Physics. In 2006 she received her PhD form the Department of Physics at the University of Crete. Her research interests include dynamical systems, graph theory and neural modeling.

Friedrich Wrba is professor of Pathology at the Department of Clinical Pathology of the University of Vienna. After training as a general practitioner in various Austrian hospitals he started his special training in clinical Pathology, which he finished successfully at the Department of Clinical Pathology at the University of Vienna in the year 1987. In 1990-1992 he spent 2.5 years as a Visiting Research Fellow at the Imperial Cancer Research Fund Laboratories in London, England, (Walter Bodmer's laboratory). Since 1991 he is lecturer and Professor of Pathology, and staff member of the department. His areas of special interest are gastroenterology, hepatology, and molecular pathology.

M. Zervakis holds a PhD degree from the University of Toronto, Department of Electrical Engineering, since 1990. He joined the Technical University of Crete on January 1995, where he is currently full professor at the department of Electronic and Computer Engineering. Prof. Zervakis is the director of the Digital Image and Signal Processing Laboratory (DISPLAY) and is involved in research on modern aspects of signal processing, including estimation and constrained optimization, multi-channel and multi-band signal processing, wavelet analysis for data/image processing and compression, biomedical imaging applications, neural networks and fuzzy logic in automation applications.

Index

D

E

F

G

H

I

K

L

M

N

O

P

Q

R

S

T

U

V

W

X